MW01393348

MYASTHENIA GRAVIS AND RELATED DISORDERS

BIOCHEMICAL BASIS FOR DISEASE OF THE NEUROMUSCULAR JUNCTION

ANNALS OF THE NEW YORK ACADEMY OF SCIENCES
Volume 998

MYASTHENIA GRAVIS AND RELATED DISORDERS

BIOCHEMICAL BASIS FOR DISEASE OF THE NEUROMUSCULAR JUNCTION

Edited by Mark A. Agius, David P. Richman, Robert H. Fairclough, and Ricardo A. Maselli

The New York Academy of Sciences
New York, New York
2003

Copyright © 2003 by the New York Academy of Sciences. All rights reserved. Under the provisions of the United States Copyright Act of 1976, individual readers of the Annals *are permitted to make fair use of the material in them for teaching or research. Permission is granted to quote from the* Annals *provided that the customary acknowledgment is made of the source. Material in the* Annals *may be republished only by permission of the Academy. Address inquiries to the Permissions Department (editorial@nyas.org) at the New York Academy of Sciences.*

Copying fees: *For each copy of an article made beyond the free copying permitted under Section 107 or 108 of the 1976 Copyright Act, a fee should be paid through the Copyright Clearance Center, Inc., 222 Rosewood Drive, Danvers, MA 01923 (www.copyright.com).*

♾ *The paper used in this publication meets the minimum requirements of the American National Standard for Information Sciences—Permanence of Paper for Printed Library Materials, ANSI Z39.48-1984.*

Library of Congress Cataloging-in-Publication Data

International Conference on Myasthenia Gravis and Related Disorders
(10th: 2002: Key Biscayne, Fla.).
Myasthenia gravis and related disorders: biochemical basis for disease of the neuromuscular junction / edited by Mark A. Agius ... [*et al.*].
p.; cm. — (Annals of the New York Academy of Sciences; v. 998)
Includes bibliographical references and index.
ISBN 1-57331-396-3 (cloth: alk. paper) — ISBN 1-57331-397-1 (paper: alk. paper)
1. Myasthenia gravis—Pathophysiology—Congresses. 2. Myoneural junction—Congresses. 3. Neuromuscular diseases—Pathophysiology—Congresses.
[DNLM: 1. Myasthenia Gravis—Congresses. 2. Autoimmune Diseases—immunology—Congresses. 3. Myasthenic Syndromes, Congenital—Congresses. 4. Neuromuscular Junction—physiopathology—Congresses. 5. Receptors, Cholinergic—immunology—Congresses. 6. Thymoma—physiopathology—Congresses.
WE 555 I614m 2003] I. Agius, Mark A. II. Title. III. Series.
Q11.N5 vol. 998
[RC935.M8]
500 s—dc21
[616.7/4

2003013764

GYAT / PCP

Printed in the United States of America
ISBN 1-57331-396-3 (cloth)
ISBN 1-57331-397-1 (paper)
ISSN 0077-8923

ANNALS OF THE NEW YORK ACADEMY OF SCIENCES

Volume 998
September 2003

MYASTHENIA GRAVIS AND RELATED DISORDERS

BIOCHEMICAL BASIS FOR DISEASE OF THE NEUROMUSCULAR JUNCTION

Editors
MARK A. AGIUS, DAVID P. RICHMAN, ROBERT H. FAIRCLOUGH, AND RICARDO A. MASELLI

This volume is the result of the **Tenth International Conference on Myasthenia Gravis and Related Disorders**, presented by the New York Academy of Sciences and the Myasthenia Gravis Foundation of America, Inc., and held May 29 to June 1, 2002, in Key Biscayne, Florida.

CONTENTS

Part IV. Autoimmunity: General Concepts

Part V. Immunology of Autoimmune Disorders Involving the Neuron and Presynaptic Nerve Terminal

Part VI. Immunology of Postsynaptic Autoimmune Disorders: The Thymus

Part VII. Immunology of Postsynaptic Autoimmune Disorders: T Cells and Immunoregulation

Part VIII. Immunology of Postsynaptic Autoimmune Disorders: Antigenic Targets and Human Disease

Part IX. Immunology of Postsynaptic Autoimmune Disorders: Antigenic Targets and Experimental Myasthenia

Part X. Epidemiology and Measurements in Myasthenia Gravis

Part XI. Current Diagnosis and Treatment: Pre- and Postsynaptic Immune Syndromes

Part XII. Future Therapies in Myasthenia

Financial assistance was received from:

Cosponsor

- MYASTHENIA GRAVIS FOUNDATION OF AMERICA, INC.

Corporate Supporters

- ALPHA THERAPEUTIC CORPORATION
- CRESCENT HEALTHCARE, INC.
- ICN PHARMACEUTICALS, INC.
- LOUIS STOKES VETERANS AFFAIRS MEDICAL CENTER, CLEVELAND, OHIO
- ZLB BIOPLASMA, INC.

MGFA Chapter Support

- CAROLINAS CHAPTER OF MGFA
- CONNECTICUT “HOPE” CHAPTER OF MGFA
- GREAT LAKES CHAPTER OF MGFA
- MARYLAND/DC/DELAWARE CHAPTER OF MGFA
- MASSACHUSETTS/NEW HAMPSHIRE CHAPTER OF MGFA
- MGNET
- MYASTHENIA GRAVIS ASSOCIATION OF ILLINOIS
- MYASTHENIA GRAVIS FOUNDATION OF CALIFORNIA
- WEST CENTRAL FLORIDA CHAPTER OF MGFA

Individual Supporters

- DEBORA K. BOELZ
- PETER CARBERRY
- BARRY AND SHERRY GOLD
- WILLIAM AND MARCIA LORIMER
- ROBERT PASCUZZI
- JOSEPH TISHLER
- TINA VASSAR
- GERALDINE WEINRIB

Additional Supporters

- NATIONAL INSTITUTE OF NEUROLOGICAL DISORDERS AND STROKE, NATIONAL INSTITUTES OF HEALTH
- UNIVERSITY OF CALIFORNIA, DAVIS

Continuing Medical Education Sponsorship

- MINNESOTA MEDICAL ASSOCIATION

The New York Academy of Sciences believes it has a responsibility to provide an open forum for discussion of scientific questions. The positions taken by the participants in the reported conferences are their own and not necessarily those of the Academy. The Academy has no intent to influence legislation by providing such forums.

Introduction

MARK A. AGIUS

Department of Neurology, University of California at Davis, Davis, California 95616, USA

The Tenth International Myasthenia Gravis Conference more than any other prior conference in this series documents that a large number of molecules located both presynaptically as well as postsynaptically at the neuromuscular junction are potential targets of biochemical dysfunction resulting in clinical disease. These molecules may be targets of genetic-, toxic-, or immune-mediated dysfunction. The same molecules that may be rendered dysfunctional as a consequence of genetic mutations may also be candidate targets for toxic- or immune-mediated disorders. These conditions may demonstrate phenotypic and genotypic overlap. In this context, the various forms of myasthenia gravis represent a diverse subgroup of disorders of the neuromuscular junction that demonstrate both weakness as well as fatigability, that is, increased weakness with increased effort.

Presynaptic molecules involved in synapse function include calcium channels, the machinery of neurotransmitter packaging and release, and synaptic vesicle recycling. Thus, a genetic abnormality of calcium channels is a representative example of how a disordered presynaptic molecule may result in congenital myasthenia. The nicotinic acetylcholine receptors and molecules of their clustering mechanisms along with synapse-specific genes are in turn representative postsynaptic molecules whose dysfunction may result in disease. The three-dimensional structure of acetylcholine binding protein, a homologue protein to the extrasynaptic portion of the acetylcholine receptor, has recently been solved crystallographically. The structure/function analysis of the nicotinic acetylcholine receptor at the neuromuscular junction has resulted in a proposed activation model of the acetylcholine receptor and regulation of its assembly. Representative examples of disorders of synaptic and postsynaptic molecules resulting in clinical disease include subunits of the acetylcholine receptors, acetylcholinesterase, and rapsyn, a component of the acetylcholine receptor clustering mechanism.

Potential immune targets at the neuromuscular junction include calcium channels, potassium channels, neuronal and muscle nicotinic acetylcholine receptors, as well as the muscle-specific kinase and other molecules of the acetylcholine receptor clustering mechanism. Thymoma associated with myasthenia gravis and other neurological disorders represents one of the commonest paraneoplastic syndromes. Well differentiated thymic epithelial cell tumors may lead to abnormal positive selection of autoreactive thymocytes. In contrast, myasthenia gravis in patients with thymic germinal

Address for correspondence: Mark A. Agius, Department of Neurology, University of California at Davis, 1515 Newton Court, Room 510, Davis, CA 95616-8603. Voice: 530-754-5020; fax: 530-754-5036.

maagius@ucdavis.edu

Ann. N.Y. Acad. Sci. 998: xiii–xiv (2003). © 2003 New York Academy of Sciences.
doi: 10.1196/annals.1254.001

centers may possibly arise consequent to antigenic presentation in structurally abnormal thymic medulla.

There are a number of apparently distinct peripheral immune regulatory mechanisms, including those subserved by cytokines as well as by direct cell-cell interaction, including CD 25+ subsets and cells of the innate immune system, such as NK cells. Our understanding of the role of T cells and T cell subgroups, of B cells and antibody specificities, and of components of the innate immune system, including macrophages and complement, is enhanced by the experimental models of immune myasthenia. T cell and B cell epitope spread is documented in experimental immune myasthenia and may be relevant in the progression of ocular myasthenia to generalized disease.

Epidemiological studies document a progressive increase in the apparent prevalence of immune myasthenia over the past few decades. Immune myasthenia commonly presents over the age of 50 years. Present classifications of immune myasthenia based on age of onset, thymic pathology, pure ocular involvement, and presence or absence of acetylcholine receptor antibodies are limited because of subgroup heterogeneity. A revised and simplified classification of immune myasthenia is based on serum antibody pattern and presumed mechanism of disease. Patients with type 1 immune myasthenia have relatively high acetylcholine receptor antibodies. Those with type 2 disease have relatively low acetylcholine receptor antibodies along with titin antibodies. Patients with type 3 immune myasthenia have muscle-specific kinase antibodies only. Type 4 disease represents immune myasthenia wherein the targets are as yet undefined. This group is likely to be heterogeneous.

The natural history of immune myasthenia appears to involve recurring waves of inflammation that result in target molecule(s) damage. Epitope spread along with the loss of membrane and membrane folds and associated integral and peripheral membrane proteins contribute to pathogenicity and may contribute to chronic immune stimulation. A strategy of treatment based on induction of a remission and maintenance of the remission obtained is effective in immune myasthenia in ways similar to other autoimmune disorders. Also, it is likely that early intervention with immune suppression may contribute to limiting epitope spread and consequent long-term disease severity.

Safer and specific therapies in myasthenia gravis are still required because of the potential for serious side effects associated with present broad immunosuppressive therapies. In this context, studies such as those testing mycophenolate mofetil in a multicentered, double-blinded, placebo-controlled fashion have benefited from the establishment of a quantitative measurement of muscle function endorsed by the Myasthenia Gravis Foundation of America. Future therapies targeting antigen-specific autoreactive T and B cells and antibodies in immune myasthenia are likely to be developed and employed in concert with strategies directed at subsets of immune cells with specific phenotypes and regulatory or effector function.

Neurophysiology of the Neuromuscular Junction: Overview

ROBERT L. RUFF

Neurology Service and Rehabilitation and SCI&D Care Line,
Louis Stokes Cleveland VA Medical Center, and
Department of Neurology, Case Western Reserve University, Cleveland, Ohio, USA

ABSTRACT: This manuscript reviews the physiology of neuromuscular transmission with emphasis on four features: (1) the structure of the neuromuscular junction, (2) release of vesicles of acetylcholine from the nerve terminal, (3) the roles of postsynaptic Na^+ channels and acetylcholine receptors in converting the chemical signal from the nerve terminal into a propagated action potential on the muscle fiber, and (4) the safety factor for neuromuscular transmission. It also introduces new information about how the neuromuscular junction maintains physiological integrity during muscle fiber stretch and contraction.

KEYWORDS: neuromuscular junction; neuromuscular transmission; sodium channels; acetylcholine esterase; transmitter release; quantal transmitter release; safety factor; contractility; skeletal muscle

INTRODUCTION

The five aims of this manuscript are (1) to describe the structure of the neuromuscular junction, (2) to review the factors that trigger release of vesicles of acetylcholine from the nerve terminal, (3) to describe the two ion channels on the postsynaptic membrane, sodium (Na^+) channels and acetylcholine receptors, that are critical for converting the chemical signal from the nerve terminal into a propagated action potential on the muscle fiber, (4) to define the safety factor for neuromuscular transmission and to indicate the features of the neuromuscular junction that contribute to the safety factor, and (5) finally to describe new information about how the neuromuscular junction maintains physiological integrity during muscle contraction.

KEY FEATURES OF MOTOR NERVES

Skeletal muscle fibers are innervated by large motor neurons in the anterior horn (anterior horn cells) of the spinal cord.[1] Anterior horn cells give rise to single large myelinated axons. Action potentials travel along motor axons by saltatory conduction, with action potentials jumping from node of Ranvier to node of Ranvier, with little

Address for correspondence: Robert L. Ruff, Neurology Service 127(W), Cleveland VAMC, 10701 East Boulevard, Cleveland, OH 44106. Voice/fax: 216-421-3040.
robert.ruff@med.va.gov

Ann. N.Y. Acad. Sci. 998: 1–10 (2003). © 2003 New York Academy of Sciences.
doi: 10.1196/annals.1254.002

current leaving in the axon in the internodal region. Two structural features of myelinated axons optimize saltatory conduction: (1) The internodal regions of the axons are covered by insulating layers of myelin, which reduces the current loss in the internodal region by increasing the transmembrane resistance and decreasing the capacitative coupling between the axon and the extracellular space.[2,3] (2) The nodes of Ranvier have high concentrations of Na^+ channels, which produce the depolarizing current of the action potential. Vertebrate nodes of Ranvier contain about 2000 channels/μm^2.[4] The high density of Na^+ channels reduces the threshold for generating an action potential.[4,5] In addition, nodes of Ranvier have few potassium (K^+) channels,[5] which minimizes inhibition of the action potential and enables the action potential to propagate along the axon at rates > 50 m/s.[2]

DISTAL MOTOR NERVE PROPERTIES

Within the target muscle, the end of each motor axon branches into 20 to 100 thinner terminal fibers. Each terminal motor nerve fiber ends in a single nerve terminal that innervates a single muscle fiber. The muscle fibers innervated by all of the terminal branches of a single motor axon are called a motor unit. The terminal motor nerve branches are ≤100 μm long and are unmyelinated.[3] The unmyelinated terminal motor nerve branches contain delayed rectifier and inward rectifier potassium (K^+) channels as well as Na^+ channels.[5,6] Therefore, the amplitude and duration of the action potential in the terminal nerve fibers are controlled by K^+ channels as well as by Na^+ channels. The nerve terminal has few Na^+ channels; hence, the action potential passively propagates within the nerve terminal (see FIG. 1). The lack of nerve terminal Na^+ channel and the presence of K^+ channels prevent action potentials from reflecting out of the nerve terminal and reverberating among the distal nerve branches. In neuromyotonia, also called Isaacs' syndrome, a single action potential propagating down a motor nerve produces repeated action potentials in the nerve terminals.[7] Neuromyotonia can result from autoantibodies that disrupt nerve terminal delayed rectifier K^+ channels.[7,8] Neuromyotonia demonstrates that the nerve terminal K^+ channels regulate nerve terminal excitability.[9]

ACETYLCHOLINE IS THE TRANSMITTER AT THE NEUROMUSCULAR JUNCTION

Acetylcholine (ACh) is stored in vesicles in the nerve terminal (see FIG. 1).[3,10] ACh-containing vesicles are aligned near release sites, called active zones, in the nerve terminal, where the vesicles will fuse with the presynaptic nerve terminal membrane.[3] Release sites are positioned over the clefts between the tops of the secondary synaptic folds of the postsynaptic muscle membrane.[3,11,12] Transmitter release requires Ca^{2+} entry into the nerve terminal. The Ca^{2+} channels responsible for ACh release are P/Q-type.[13] N-type calcium channels are probably also present on mammalian motor nerve terminals.[14–17] The Ca^{2+} channels that trigger ACh release are distributed as 2 parallel double rows with approximately 5 channels per row, a spacing of about 20 nm between rows, and a spacing of about 60 nm between the double rows of channels at the active zone.[18,19] High concentration of Ca^{2+}

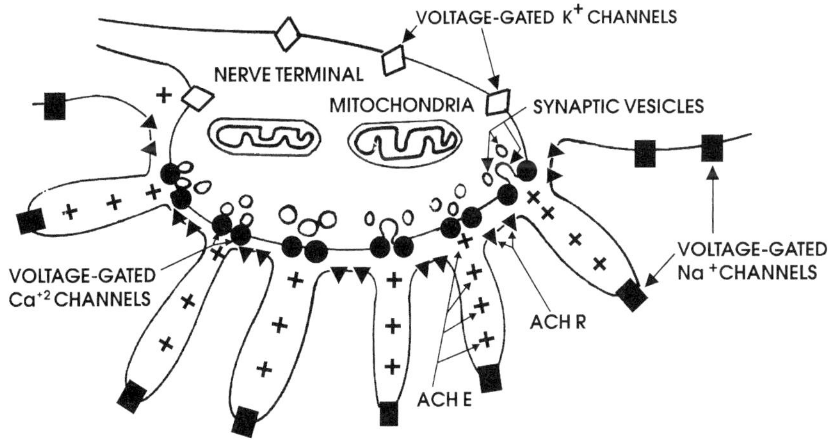

FIGURE 1. This is a cartoon depiction of the neuromuscular junction. The nerve terminal is located above the secondary synaptic folds of the postsynaptic muscle membrane. The nerve terminal contains mitochondria, which produce the energy needed to synthesize ACh and package the ACh into synaptic vesicles. Synaptic vesicles can fuse with the nerve terminal membrane after an action potential enters the nerve terminal. The nerve terminal contains voltage-gated K^+ channels (◇) and Ca^{2+} channels (●). Active zones, where Ca^{2+} channels are concentrated and synaptic vesicles fuse with the presynaptic membrane, are precisely aligned above troughs between secondary synaptic folds of the postsynaptic membrane. Within the synaptic cleft, the extracellular matrix contains AChE (+) that is bound to the basal lamina of the postsynaptic membrane. The secondary synaptic folds contain a high density of AChR (▼) on the tops of the secondary folds close to the nerve terminal membrane and a high density of Na^+ channels at the bottom of the troughs of the secondary synaptic folds (■).

channels at the active zones enables the Ca^{2+} concentration to locally rise to 100 to 1000 μM quickly in the regions of the nerve terminal where vesicle fusion occurs.[11,12] A usual nerve terminal action potential does not fully activate the Ca^{2+} channels because the duration of the action potential is ≤1 ms and the nerve terminal Ca^{2+} channels are activated with a time constant of ≥1.3 ms.[15] Increasing the duration of the nerve terminal action potential by blocking delayed rectifier potassium channels with tetraethylammonium (TEA) or 3,4-diaminopyridine (3,4-DAP) will increase calcium entry and increase ACh release.[15,20,21] In Lambert-Eaton Myasthenic Syndrome (LEMS), antibodies directed against nerve terminal Ca^{2+} channels reduce the number of Ca^{2+} channels.[22–29] Neuromuscular transmission is impaired due to a paucity of vesicles released from the nerve terminal in response to an action potential. Treatment with 3,4-DAP improves neuromuscular transmission in LEMS by increasing the time that Ca^{2+} channels are stimulated, resulting in increased Ca^{2+} entry that partially compensates for the deficiency of Ca^{2+} channels.[30,31]

The fusion of synaptic vesicles and the presynaptic nerve terminal membrane may be opposed by electrostatic forces due to the similar polarity of surfaces of the nerve terminal and vesicle membranes. Ca^{2+}, by binding to the membrane surfaces, may neutralize the negative surface charges.[32] Calcium may also open calcium-activated cationic channels, and the entry of cations may also reduce the negative surface charges on the vesicle and nerve terminal membranes.[33] Calcium also triggers conformation changes in large molecules that allow synaptic vesicles to detach from the cytoskeleton and that actively trigger membrane fusion.[34] Calcium entry may trigger alteration of several key nerve terminal proteins including synaptotagmin,[35,36] synexin, and members of the family of synapse-associated proteins (SNAP).[37]

Synaptic vesicle fusion is a complex process that involves multiple proteins. The process of synaptic vesicle fusing with the nerve terminal membrane to release ACh and the process of recycling of nerve terminal membrane to reform synaptic vesicles are described elsewhere in this volume.[38,39]

THE ROLE OF THE SYNAPTIC CLEFT

The space between the nerve terminal and the postsynaptic membrane, the synaptic cleft, is about 50 nm (see FIG. 1).[3] ACh diffuses across the synaptic cleft to activate ACh receptors (AChRs). Each synaptic vesicle releases about 10,000 ACh molecules into the synaptic cleft.[40] ATP is also released from synaptic vesicles, and the released ATP may modulate transmitter release of postsynaptic transmitter sensitivity.[41] An action potential in the nerve terminal stimulates between 50 to 300 synaptic vesicles to fuse (i.e., the normal quantal content is between 50 to 300).[42] Diffusion of ACh across the synaptic cleft is very rapid due to the small distance to be traversed and the high diffusion constant for ACh.[43] Acetylcholine esterase (ChE) in the basal lamina of the postsynaptic membrane and the synaptic cleft accelerates the disappearance of ACh from the synaptic cleft, as does diffusion of ACh out of the cleft.[44] Inactivation of ChE prolongs the duration of action of ACh on the postsynaptic membrane and slows the decay of the ACh-induced endplate current.[45,46] The concentration of ChE is approximately 3000 molecules/μm^2 of postsynaptic membrane,[44] which is about 5- to 8-fold lower than the concentration of AChRs.[47] The concentration of ChE in the secondary synaptic folds is very high. Most of the ACh entering a synaptic cleft is hydrolyzed. Consequently, the secondary synaptic folds act like sinks that terminate the action of ACh and prevent AChRs from being activated more than once in response to released ACh.[48,49]

The extracellular matrix in the neuromuscular junction is a complex collection of proteins that regulate the synthesis of postsynaptic proteins as well as regulate the concentration of ACh. The endplate basement membrane is enriched with collagen IV (α2, α4, and α5 chains) and contains several forms of laminin, laminin-4, laminin-9, and laminin-11, which bind to α-dystrophoglycan in the endplate membrane. Laminin-4 also binds to integrin. The laminin family of proteins form a complex network in the synaptic space that anchors other extracellular matrix proteins including agrin, perlecan, and entactin. The collagen-tailed form of ChE in the synapse binds to perlecan, which in turn binds to α-dystrophoglycan. In addition to binding laminin and perlecan, α-dystrophoglycan also binds agrin, integrin, and the MASC (myotube-associated specificity component)/MuSK (muscle-specific kinase) complex. Agrin, MASC, and MuSK are associated with the formation and maintenance of AChR clustering.[34,50,51] Rapsyn is the molecule that specifically links AChRs.[52]

The high synthesis of AChR component subunits at the neuromuscular junction is due in part to ARIA (AChR-inducing activity), a molecule that is released by the nerve terminal.[53] ARIA activates ErbB receptor tyrosine kinases in the postsynaptic membrane. The ErbB receptors regulate the expression of AChR subunits by the subsynaptic nuclei. AChBP (acetylcholine binding protein) is a recently described globular protein secreted by the specific subset of oligodendroglia and Schwann cells that are located around nerve terminals.[54] Production of AChBP is regulated by synaptic activity and by binding ACh. AChBP may reduce the effective concentration of ACh in the synaptic cleft.

POSTSYNAPTIC MEMBRANE SPECIALIZATION

The postsynaptic membrane area is increased by folding into secondary synaptic clefts or folds (see FIG. 1). The AChRs are concentrated at the tops of the secondary synaptic folds and firmly anchored to the dystrophin-related protein complex through rapsyn.[52,55] Rapsyn is important in clustering AChRs at the endplate during synaptogenesis, and rapsyn-deficient transgenic mice do not cluster AChRs, utrophin, and other dystrophin-related complex proteins.[55–58] Clusters of AChRs are connected to the cytoskeleton via associations with the dystrophoglycan and sarcoglycan protein complexes.[34,50] The dystroglycan and sarcoglycan complexes connect to utrophin, which in turn connects to cytoskeleton by binding to actin. Utrophin and dystrobrevin also connect to $\alpha 1$ syntrophin and $\alpha 2$ syntrophin, which in turn associate with NOS (nitric oxide synthetase).[59,60] NOS produces the free radical gas nitric oxide (NO) that participates in cell signaling. The presence of NOS at the neuromuscular junction suggests that NO could diffuse from its site of synthesis to affect target proteins in the nerve and muscle. The interactions between ACh and the AChRs that produce a depolarizing generator potential that depolarizes the endplate region sufficiently to trigger action potentials are reviewed elsewhere in this volume.[61–63]

The concentration of AChRs at the endplate is ~15,000–20,000 receptors/μm^2.[47] Away from the endplate, the concentration of AChRs is about 1000-fold lower with a slight increase in AChR density at the tendon ends of the muscle fibers.[64] The relatively high concentration of AChRs at the endplate results in part because the muscle fiber nuclei near the endplate preferentially produce the mRNA that encodes for AChR subunits.[56,58] AChRs continually turnover, with old receptors internalized and degraded. The removed receptors are replaced with new receptors. The AChRs are not recycled. Early in development, the half-life of AChRs is short, about 13–24 hours.[65] At a mature endplate, the half-life of AChRs is about 8–11 days. Cross-linking of receptors by antibodies dramatically shortens AChR half-life by accelerating internalization of the receptors.[66,67] The details of AChR structure are covered elsewhere in this volume.[68]

Na^+ channels are concentrated in the depths of the secondary synaptic clefts.[55,69–74] Both the Na^+ channels and AChRs are rigidly located in the endplate membrane.[55–58,69–74] Na^+ channels are locked in the membrane by their associations with ankyrin, the sarcoglycan complex, the dystroglycan complex, dystrobrevins, and dystrophin/utrophin.

The increased density of Na^+ channels raises the safety factor for neuromuscular transmission.[71–77] In addition, a high concentration of Na^+ channels may be needed at the endplate because two action potentials must be generated, one traveling toward each tendon end of the muscle fiber. The density of Na^+ channels varies with fiber type.[72–74] Fast twitch fibers have about 500–550 Na^+ channels/μm^2 on the endplate membrane and slow twitch fibers have about 100–150 Na^+ channels/μm^2. In acquired autoimmune myasthenia gravis, antibodies directed at AChRs attack the endplate membrane.[78] The antibodies fix complement, resulting in loss of endplate membrane. Na^+ channels as well as AChRs are lost from the endplate in myasthenia gravis, and the loss of endplate Na^+ channels reduces the safety factor for neuromuscular transmission.[77]

THE QUANTAL NATURE OF NEUROMUSCULAR TRANSMISSION

The size of the depolarization of the endplate membrane produced by a single motor nerve action potential (endplate potential) is determined by the product of the number of vesicles (or quanta) of ACh released (quantal content) and size of the endplate depolarization to a single vesicle (quantal size), with an adjustment for the AChR reversal potential.[2] Diseases that interfere with ACh release such as LEMS alter the quantal content. Conditions that reduce the sensitivity of the postsynaptic membrane to ACh such as myasthenia gravis reduce quantal size.

THE SAFETY FACTOR FOR NEUROMUSCULAR TRANSMISSION

The safety factor (SF) for neuromuscular transmission can be defined as

$$SF = EPP/(E_{AP} - RP)$$

where EPP is the endplate potential amplitude, RP is the resting membrane potential, and E_{AP} is the threshold potential for initiating an action potential.[79] The safety factor for neuromuscular transmission of fast twitch mammalian skeletal muscle fibers is large compared with slow twitch fibers for several reasons.[80] The structure and transmitter release properties of axons innervating fast and slow twitch fibers are different. The quantal contents of rodent fast twitch fibers are higher than slow twitch fibers.[80,81] The postsynaptic sensitivities of fast twitch fibers are also greater than slow twitch fibers. Endplates on fast twitch fibers depolarize more in response to quantitative iontophoresis of ACh.[82] Fast twitch endplates have a higher concentration of Na^+ channels compared to slow twitch endplates.[71–74,76,77] The increased Na^+ current on fast twitch fibers may be needed because fast twitch fibers require larger depolarizations to initiate contraction compared with slow twitch fibers.[83] The differences in synaptic transmission for fast and slow twitch fibers may compensate for the different functional properties of fast and slow twitch motor units. Slow twitch motor units in mammals are tonically active at slow rates, whereas fast twitch motor units are phasically active at high rates.[84] Under these conditions, transmitter depletion and other factors may not appreciably compromise neuromuscular transmission for slow twitch fibers, while fast twitch fibers may suffer from reduction in the endplate potential amplitude during activity.[80,85–87] The effective safety factor for slow twitch motor units from rat soleus muscle at a steady state firing rate of 10 Hz is about 1.8.[80] The safety factor for neuromuscular transmission for fibers from the fast twitch rat extensor digitorum longus muscle stimulated at 40 Hz drops from 3.7 for the first stimulation to 2.0 after 200 stimuli.[80]

HOW THE NEUROMUSCULAR JUNCTION RESPONDS TO CHANGES IN MUSCLE LENGTH

Given the complex molecular composition of the nerve terminal, the extracellular matrix, and the endplate membrane and the precise alignment of the active zones on the nerve terminal with the clefts between the endplate synaptic folds, how does the neuromuscular junction accommodate to muscle fiber stretching and contracting? Surprisingly, the high efficiency of neuromuscular transmission is maintained during muscle stretch and contraction. The safety factor for neuromuscular transmission does not change for muscles at different lengths from 80% to 125% of the resting length. The constancy of neuromuscular transmission is accomplished by the neuromuscular junction remaining rigid so that the endplate membrane did not deform when the muscle fiber changed length.[88] The change in muscle fiber length was accomplished by folding and unfolding of the extrajunctional membrane while the endplate region remained rigid. The extreme stiffness of the endplate membrane adds mechanical and electrical stability to the neuromuscular junction, which enables the active zones on the nerve terminal to remain precisely aligned with the clefts of the synaptic folds and enables the safety factor for neuromuscular transmission to remain constant during muscle activity.

ACKNOWLEDGMENTS

Robert L. Ruff was supported by the Offices of Medical Research and Rehabilitation Research and Development of the Research and Development Service of The Department of Veterans Affairs. Suzanne S. Powell assisted in compiling and editing this manuscript.

REFERENCES

1. Burke, R.E. 2001. The structure and function of motor units. *In* Disorders of Voluntary Muscle, pp. 3–25. Cambridge Univ. Press. Cambridge.
2. Ruff, R.L. 1986. Ionic channels: II. Voltage- and agonist-gated and agonist-modified channel properties and structure. Muscle Nerve **9:** 767–786.
3. Salpeter, M.M. 1987. The Vertebrate Neuromuscular Junction. Alan R. Liss. New York.
4. Ruff, R.L. 1986. Ionic channels: I. The biophysical basis for ion passage and channel gating. Muscle Nerve **9:** 675–699.
5. Black, J.A., J.D. Kocsis & S.G. Waxman. 1990. Ion channel organization of the myelinated fiber. Trends Neurosci. **13:** 48–54.
6. Reid, G. *et al.* 1999. Human axons contain at least five types of voltage-dependent potassium channel. J. Physiol. **518:** 681–696.
7. Shillito, P. *et al.* 1995. Acquired neuromyotonia: evidence for autoantibodies directed against K^+ channels of peripheral nerves. Ann. Neurol. **38:** 714–722.

8. NEWSOM-DAVIS, J. *et al.* 2003. Autoimmune disorders of neuronal potassium channels. This volume.
9. NAGADO, T. *et al.* 1999. Potassium current suppression in patients with peripheral nerve hyperexcitability. Brain **122:** 2057–2066.
10. KATZ, B. 1966. Nerve Muscle and Synapse. McGraw–Hill. New York.
11. AUGUSTINE, G.J., E.M. ADLER & M.P. CHARLTON. 1991. The calcium signal for transmitter secretion from presynaptic nerve terminals. Ann. N.Y. Acad. Sci. **635:** 365–381.
12. SMITH, S.J. & G.J. AUGUSTINE. 1988. Calcium ions, active zones, and synaptic transmitter release. Trends Neurosci. **10:** 458–464.
13. PROTTI, D.A. *et al.* 1993. Mammalian neuromuscular transmission blocked by funnel web toxin. Ann. N.Y. Acad. Sci. **681:** 405–407.
14. CATTERALL, W.A. *et al.* 1993. Molecular properties of calcium channels in skeletal muscle and neurons. Ann. N.Y. Acad. Sci. **681:** 342–355.
15. STANLEY, E.F. 1993. Presynaptic calcium channels and the transmitter release mechanism. Ann. N.Y. Acad. Sci. **681:** 368–372.
16. WRAY, D. & V. PORTER. 1993. Calcium channel types at the neuromuscular junction. Ann. N.Y. Acad. Sci. **681:** 356–367.
17. NUDLER, S. *et al.* 2003. Ca^{2+} channels and synaptic transmission at the adult, neonatal, and P/Q-type deficient neuromuscular junction. This volume.
18. ENGEL, A.G. 1991. Review of evidence for loss of motor nerve terminal calcium channels in Lambert-Eaton myasthenic syndrome. Ann. N.Y. Acad. Sci. **635:** 246–258.
19. PUMPLIN, D.W., T.S. REESE & R. LLINAS. 1981. Are the presynaptic membrane particles calcium channels? Proc. Natl. Acad. Sci. USA **78:** 7210–7213.
20. LINDGREN, C.A. & J.W. MOORE. 1991. Calcium current in motor nerve endings of the lizard. Ann. N.Y. Acad. Sci. **635:** 58–69.
21. STANLEY, E.F. & C. COX. 1991. Calcium channels in the presynaptic nerve terminal of the chick ciliary ganglion giant synapse. Ann. N.Y. Acad. Sci. **635:** 70–79.
22. LEYS, K. *et al.* 1991. Calcium channel autoantibodies in the Lambert-Eaton myasthenic syndrome. Ann. Neurol. **29:** 307–414.
23. LAMBERT, E.H., L.M. EATON & E.D. ROOKE. 1956. Defect of neuromuscular transmission associated with malignant neoplasm. Am. J. Physiol. **187:** 612–613.
24. MOTOMURA, M. *et al.* 1995. An improved diagnostic assay for Lambert-Eaton myasthenic syndrome. J. Neurol. Neurosurg. Psychiatr. **58:** 85–87.
25. NAGEL, A. *et al.* 1988. Lambert-Eaton syndrome IgG depletes presynaptic membrane active zone particles by antigenic modulation. Ann. Neurol. **24:** 552–558.
26. LANG, B. *et al.* 1993. Autoantibody specificities in Lambert-Eaton myasthenic syndrome. Ann. N.Y. Acad. Sci. **681:** 382–391.
27. VIGLIONE, M.P., J.K.W. BLANDINO & Y.I. KIM. 1993. Effects of Lambert-Eaton syndrome serum and IgG on calcium and sodium currents in small-cell lung cancer cells. Ann. N.Y. Acad. Sci. **681:** 418–421.
28. ROSENFELD, M.R. *et al.* 1993. Sera from patients with Lambert-Eaton myasthenic syndrome recognize the β-subunit of Ca^{2+} channel complexes. Ann. N.Y. Acad. Sci. **681:** 408–411.
29. MASELLI, R.A. 2003. Effect of inherited abnormalities of calcium regulation on human neuromuscular transmission. This volume.
30. MCEVOY, K.M. *et al.* 1989. 3,4-Diaminopyridine in the treatment of Lambert-Eaton myasthenic syndrome. N. Engl. J. Med. **321:** 1567–1571.
31. SANDERS, D.B. 2003. Lambert-Eaton myasthenic syndrome: diagnosis and treatment. This volume.
32. NILES, W.D. & F.S. COHEN. 1991. Video-microscopy studies of vesicle-planar membrane adhesion and fusion. Ann. N.Y. Acad. Sci. **635:** 273–306.
33. EHRENSTEIN, G. *et al.* 1991. Evidence of a model of exocytosis that involves calcium-activated channels. Ann. N.Y. Acad. Sci. **635:** 297–306.
34. VINCENT, A. 2001. The neuromuscular junction and neuromuscular transmission. *In* Disorders of Voluntary Muscle, pp. 142–167. Cambridge Univ. Press. Cambridge.
35. PERIN, M.S. *et al.* 1990. Phospholipid binding by a synaptic vesicle protein homologous to the regulatory region of protein kinase C. Nature **345:** 260–263.

36. PERIN, M.S. *et al.* 1991. Domain structure of synaptotagmin (p65). J. Biol. Chem. **266:** 623–629.
37. ZIMMERBERG, J., M. CURRAN & F.S. COHEN. 1991. A lipid/protein complex hypothesis for exocytotic fusion pore formation. Ann. N.Y. Acad. Sci. **681:** 307–317.
38. CREMONA, O. *et al.* 2003. Protein ubiquitylation and synaptic function. This volume.
39. JAHN, R. 2002. Presynaptic vesicle docking and fusion. This conference.
40. MILEDI, R., P.C. MOLENAAR & R.L. POLAK. 1983. Electrophysiological and chemical determination of acetylcholine release at the frog neuromuscular junction. J. Physiol. (Lond.) **334:** 245–254.
41. ETCHEBERRIGARAY, R. *et al.* 1991. Endoplasmic reticulum as a source of Ca^{2+} in neurotransmitter secretion. Ann. N.Y. Acad. Sci. **635:** 90–99.
42. KATZ, B. & R. MILEDI. 1979. Estimates of quantal content during chemical potentiation of transmitter release. Proc. R. Soc. Lond. **205:** 369–378.
43. LAND, B.R. *et al.* 1984. Diffusion and binding constants for acetylcholine derived from the falling phase of miniature endplate currents. Proc. Natl. Acad. Sci. USA **81:** 1594–1598.
44. MCMAHAN, U.J., J.R. SANES & L.M. MARSHALL. 1978. Cholinesterase is associated with the basal lamina at the neuromuscular junction. Nature **271:** 172–174.
45. KATZ, B. & R. MILEDI. 1973. The binding of acetylcholine to receptors and its removal from the synaptic cleft. J. Physiol. (Lond.) **231:** 549–574.
46. SINGH, G. 2002. Postsynaptic toxins of the neuromuscular junction: organophosphates. This conference.
47. LAND, B.R., E.E. SALPETER & M.M. SALPETER. 1981. Kinetic parameters for acetylcholine interaction in intact neuromuscular junction. Proc. Natl. Acad. Sci. USA **78:** 7200–7204.
48. COLQUHOUN, D. & B. SAKMANN. 1985. Fast events in single-channel currents activated by acetylcholine and its analogues at the frog muscle end-plate. J. Physiol. (Lond.) **369:** 501–557.
49. ENGEL, A.G. *et al.* 2003. Congenital myasthenic syndromes: multiple molecular targets at the neuromuscular junction. This volume.
50. HOLLAND, P.C. & S. CARBONETTO. 2001. The extracellular matrix of skeletal muscle. *In* Disorders of Voluntary Muscle, pp. 103–121. Cambridge Univ. Press. Cambridge.
51. GAUTAM, M., P.G. NOAKES & L. MOSCOSO. 1996. Defective neuromuscular synaptogenesis in agrin-deficient mutant mice. Cell **85:** 525–535.
52. GAUTAM, M., P.G. NOAKES & J. MUDD. 1995. Failure of postsynaptic specialization at neuromuscular junctions of rapsyn-deficient mice. Nature **377:** 232–236.
53. WANAMAKER, C.P. *et al.* 2003. Regulation of nicotinic acetylcholine receptor assembly. This volume.
54. SMIT, A.B. *et al.* 2001. A glia-derived acetylcholine-binding protein that modulates synaptic transmission. Nature **411:** 261–267.
55. FLUCHER, B.E. & M.P. DANIELS. 1989. Distribution of Na^+ channels and ankyrin in neuromuscular junctions is complementary to that of acetylcholine receptors and the 43 kD protein. Neuron **3:** 163–175.
56. SANES, J.R. *et al.* 1991. Selective expression of an acetylcholine receptor–lacZ transgene in synaptic nuclei of adult muscle fibers. Development **113:** 1181–1191.
57. MARTINOU, J.C. *et al.* 1991. Acetylcholine receptor–inducing activity stimulates expression of the epsilon-subunit gene of the muscle acetylcholine receptor. Proc. Natl. Acad. Sci. USA **88:** 7669–7673.
58. MERLIE, J.P. & J.R. SANES. 1985. Concentration of acetylcholine receptor mRNA in synaptic regions of adult muscle fibers. Nature **317:** 66–68.
59. BRENMAN, J.E. *et al.* 1996. Interaction of nitric oxide synthase with the postsynaptic protein PSD-95 and α1-synthophin mediated by PDZ domains. Cell **84:** 757–767.
60. KUSNER, L.L. & H.J. KAMINSKI. 1996. Nitric oxide synthase is concentrated at the skeletal muscle endplate. Brain Res. **730:** 238–242.
61. SMIT, A.B. *et al.* 2003. Structure and function of AChBP, homologue of the ligand-binding domain of the nicotinic acetylcholine receptor. This volume.
62. FAIRCLOUGH, R.H. *et al.* 2003. Agonist-induced transitions of the acetylcholine receptor. This volume.

63. SINE, S.M. *et al.* 2003. Mechanistic diversity underlying fast channel congenital myasthenic syndromes. This volume.
64. KUFFLER, S.W. & D. YOSHIKAMI. 1975. The distribution of acetylcholine sensitivity at the post-synaptic membrane of vertebrate skeletal twitch muscles: iontophoretic mapping in the micron range. J. Physiol. (Lond.) **244:** 703–730.
65. SALPETER, M.M. & R.H. LORING. 1985. Nicotinic acetylcholine receptors in vertebrate muscle: properties, distribution, and neural control. Prog. Neurobiol. **25:** 297–325.
66. KAO, I. & D. DRACHMAN. 1977. Myasthenic immunoglobulin accelerates acetylcholine receptor degradation. Science **196:** 526–528.
67. MERLIE, J.P., S. HEINEMANN & J.M. LINDSTROM. 1979. Acetylcholine receptor degradation in adult rat diaphragms in organ culture and the effect of anti-acetylcholine receptor antibodies. J. Biol. Chem. **254:** 6320–6327.
68. LINDSTROM, J. 2003. Nicotinic acetylcholine receptors of muscles and nerves: comparison of their structures, functional roles, and vulnerability to pathology. This volume.
69. HAIMOVICH, B. *et al.* 1987. Localization of sodium channel subtypes in rat skeletal muscle using channel-specific monoclonal antibodies. J. Neurosci. **7:** 2957–2966.
70. ROBERTS, W.M. 1987. Sodium channels near end-plates and nuclei of snake skeletal muscle. J. Physiol. (Lond.) **388:** 213–232.
71. RUFF, R.L. 1992. Na current density at and away from end plates on rat fast- and slow-twitch skeletal muscle fibers. Am. J. Physiol. **262**(Cell Physiol. 31)**:** C229–C234.
72. RUFF, R.L. & D. WHITTLESEY. 1992. Na^+ current densities and voltage dependence in human intercostal muscle fibres. J. Physiol. (Lond.) **458:** 85–97.
73. RUFF, R.L. & D. WHITTLESEY. 1993. Na^+ currents near and away from endplates on human fast and slow twitch muscle fibers. Muscle Nerve **16:** 922–929.
74. RUFF, R.L. & D. WHITTLESEY. 1993. Comparison of Na^+ currents from type IIa and IIb human intercostal muscle fibers. Am. J. Physiol. **265**(Cell Physiol. 34)**:** C171–C177.
75. CALDWELL, J.H., D.T. CAMPBELL & K.G. BEAM. 1986. Sodium channel distribution in vertebrate skeletal muscle. J. Gen. Physiol. **87:** 907–932.
76. MILTON, R.L., M.T. LUPA & J.H. CALDWELL. 1992. Fast and slow twitch skeletal muscle fibres differ in their distributions of Na channels near the endplate. Neurosci. Lett. **135:** 41–44.
77. RUFF, R.L. & V.A. LENNON. 1998. Endplate voltage-gated sodium channels are lost in clinical and experimental myasthenia gravis. Ann. Neurol. **43:** 370–379.
78. VINCENT, A. *et al.* 2003. Antibodies in myasthenia gravis and related disorders. This volume.
79. BANKER, B.Q., S.S. KELLY & N. ROBBINS. 1983. Neuromuscular transmission and correlative morphology in young and old mice. J. Physiol. (Lond.) **339:** 355–375.
80. GERTLER, R.A. & N. ROBBINS. 1978. Differences in neuromuscular transmission in red and white muscles. Brain Res. **142:** 255–284.
81. TONGE, D.A. 1974. Chronic effects of botulinum toxin on neuromuscular transmission and sensitivity to acetylcholine in slow and fast skeletal muscle of the mouse. J. Physiol. (Lond.) **241:** 127–139.
82. STERZ, R., M. PAGALA & K. PEPER. 1983. Postjunctional characteristics of the endplates in mammalian fast and slow muscles. Pflüg. Arch. **398:** 48–54.
83. LASZEWSKI, B. & R.L. RUFF. 1985. The effects of glucocorticoid treatment on excitation-contraction coupling. Am. J. Physiol. **248**(Endocrinol. Metab. 11)**:** E363–E369.
84. HENNIG, R. & T. LØMO. 1985. Firing patterns of motor units in normal rats. Nature **314:** 164–166.
85. KELLY, S.S. & N. ROBBINS. 1986. Sustained transmitter output by increased transmitter turnover in limb muscles of old mice. J. Neurosci. **6:** 2900–2907.
86. LEV-TOV, A. 1987. Junctional transmission in fast- and slow-twitch mammalian muscle units. J. Neurophysiol. **57:** 660–671.
87. LEV-TOV, A. & R. FISHMAN. 1986. The modulation of transmitter release in motor nerve endings varies with the type of muscle fiber innervated. Brain Res. **363:** 379–382.
88. RUFF, R.L. 1996. Effects of length changes on Na^+ current amplitude and excitability near and far from the end-plate. Muscle Nerve **19:** 1084–1092.

Ca^{2+} Channels and Synaptic Transmission at the Adult, Neonatal, and P/Q-Type Deficient Neuromuscular Junction

SILVANA NUDLER,[a] JOAQUIN PIRIZ,[a] FRANCISCO J. URBANO,[a,b] MARCELO D. ROSATO-SIRI,[a,c] ERIKA S. PIEDRAS RENTERIA,[d,e] AND OSVALDO D. UCHITEL[a,f]

[a]*Laboratorio de Fisiología y Biología Molecular, Departamento de Fisiología, Biología Molecular y Celular, Facultad de Ciencias Exactas y Naturales, Universidad de Buenos Aires, IFIBYNE-CONICET, Buenos Aires, Argentina*

[d]*Department of Molecular and Cellular Physiology, Stanford University, Stanford, California, USA*

ABSTRACT: Different types of voltage-activated Ca^{2+} channels have been established based on their molecular structure and pharmacological and biophysical properties. One of them, the P/Q-type, is the main channel involved in nerve-evoked neurotransmitter release at neuromuscular junctions and the immunological target in Eaton-Lambert Syndrome. At adult neuromuscular junctions, L- and N-type Ca^{2+} channels become involved in transmitter release only under certain experimental or pathological conditions. In contrast, at neonatal rat neuromuscular junctions, nerve-evoked synaptic transmission depends jointly on both N- and P/Q-type channels. Synaptic transmission at neuromuscular junctions of the ataxic P/Q-type Ca^{2+} channel knockout mice is also dependent on two different types of channels, N- and R-type. At both neonatal and P/Q knockout junctions, the K^+-evoked increase in miniature endplate potential frequency was not affected by N-type channel blockers, but strongly reduced by both P/Q- and R-type channel blockers. These differences could be accounted for by a differential location of the channels at the release site, being either P/Q- or R-type Ca^{2+} channels located closer to the release site than N-type Ca^{2+} channels. Thus, Ca^{2+} channels may be recruited to mediate neurotransmitter release where P/Q-type channels seem to be the most suited type of Ca^{2+} channel to mediate exocytosis at neuromuscular junctions.

KEYWORDS: calcium channels; neuromuscular junction; transmitter release; miniature endplate potentials; calcium dependence

[b]Present address: Department of Physiology and Neuroscience, NYU School of Medicine, 550 First Avenue, New York, NY 10016.

[c]Present address: Biophysics Sector, S.I.S.S.A./I.S.A.S., Via Beirut 2–4, 34014 Trieste, Italy.

[e]Present address: Department of Physiology, Loyola University Chicago, Maywood, IL 60153.

[f]Address for correspondence: Osvaldo D. Uchitel, Departamento de Fisiología, Biología Molecular y Celular, Facultad de Ciencias Exactas y Naturales, Universidad de Buenos Aires, Ciudad Universitaria, Pabellón II piso 2, Buenos Aires 1428, Argentina. Voice: +54 11 4576 3368; fax: +54 11 4576 3321.

odu@fbmc.fcen.uba.ar

Ann. N.Y. Acad. Sci. 998: 11–17 (2003). © 2003 New York Academy of Sciences.
doi: 10.1196/annals.1254.003

Voltage-dependent calcium channels (VDCCs) are transmembrane proteins that open in response to membrane depolarization and allow Ca^{2+} ions to enter the cell from extracellular space. They play a key role in neuronal signaling as mediators of Ca^{2+} entry during the process of neurotransmitter release.[1,2] Ca^{2+} influx through VDCCs is considered to increase intracellular Ca^{2+} concentration in a bell-shape microdomain close to the channel mouth.[3] This means that intracellular Ca^{2+} constitutes a complex signal, which can be modulated by factors that alter Ca^{2+} buffering and/or diffusion, with a large effect on Ca^{2+}-triggered cellular events like synaptic neurotransmitter release.[4]

Neuronal VDCCs have been subdivided according to their electrophysiological and pharmacological properties into (i) low voltage-activated or T-type channels and (ii) high-voltage activated channels, a class that includes the L-, N-, P/Q-, and R-types. The high-voltage activated types have mainly been characterized by their different sensitivity to pharmacological modulators and inhibitory toxins.[5]

VDCCs consist of an α_1 subunit that forms the core of the channel, in addition to β, α_2–δ, and possibly γ subunits that modulate the functional properties of the α_1 subunit. Molecular cloning has identified 10 different genes ($Ca_v1.1$ to $Ca_v3.3$) encoding α_1 subunit genes (called α_{1A}, α_{1B}, ..., α_{1S}), which are the main subunits of many of the previously characterized native Ca^{2+} channel subtypes. Four different genes encoding β subunits (i.e., β_1–β_4), 3 genes encoding the α_2–δ complex, and 5 genes encoding neuronal γ subunits have also been identified.[6]

CALCIUM CHANNELOPATHIES

Mutations in Ca^{2+} channel genes lead to channel dysfunction and altered channel properties. These disturbances may cause abnormally increased or decreased Ca^{2+} entry that could have profound influence on various Ca^{2+} signaling pathways, including neurotransmitter release.[7–9] Although different Ca^{2+} channel subunits have been implicated in several CNS diseases, mutations of the $Ca_v2.1$ gene that encodes the α_{1A} subunit of the P/Q channel are perhaps the best known.[9] Indeed, mutations in the $Ca_v2.1$ gene have been found to be responsible for the human episodic neurological disorders, familial hemiplegic migraine (FHM), episodic ataxia type 2, and spinocerebellar ataxia type 6.[10–12] Likewise, natural $Ca_v2.1$ mutations have been reported for the tottering (tg) and leaner (tg^{la}) mice, of which the homozygous rodents exhibit symptoms of ataxia and epilepsy.[13,14] Furthermore, P/Q knockout mice generated by elimination of $Ca_v2.1$ display a neurological deficit characterized by progressive ataxia and dystonia until they are finally unable to walk, followed by death (~P20).[15]

CALCIUM CHANNELS AND NERVE-EVOKED RELEASE AT THE ADULT NEUROMUSCULAR JUNCTION

Different types of VDCCs can support neurotransmitter release at many synapses.[16,17] At mature rat, mouse, and human neuromuscular junctions, neurotransmitter release is blocked completely by the P/Q-type channel blocker, ω-agatoxin IVA, indicating that neurotransmitter release is mediated almost exclusively by this type of channel.[18–21] The reduction in neurotransmitter release observed in Lambert-Eaton Myasthenic Syndrome (LEMS) patients and in passive transfer animal models of the disease resulted from an autoimmune reaction against the P/Q-type voltage-gated Ca^{2+} channels located in the presynaptic motor nerve terminal.[22]

Expression of L-type VDCCs at presynaptic motor nerve terminals has been revealed by specific antibodies to the α_{1D} subunit (Pagani *et al.*, personal communication) and by the inhibitory effect of nitrendipine on perineurial calcium currents at adult mice neuromuscular junctions.[23] However, L-type channels were only coupled to neurotransmitter release after neuromuscular junctions were treated with okadaic acid,[24] with immunoglobulin from either LEMS[25] or amyotrophic lateral sclerosis patients,[26] during reinnervation,[27] and during functional recovery from botulinum toxin type-A poisoning.[28]

CALCIUM CHANNELS AND NERVE-EVOKED RELEASE AT THE NEONATAL AND P/Q DEFICIENT NEUROMUSCULAR JUNCTION

Unlike at mature mammalian neuromuscular junctions, at neonatal rat neuromuscular junctions both the P/Q Ca^{2+} channel blocker ω-agatoxin IVA and the N-type channel blocker ω-conotoxin GVIA were capable of inhibiting neurotransmitter release, with ω-agatoxin IVA being more effective. Therefore, during the first week after birth, neurotransmitter release was jointly dependent on P/Q- and N-type channels, with different degrees of efficiency.[29,30]

Further insight into the relation between Ca^{2+} channels and neurotransmitter release is gained by studying synaptic transmission at neuromuscular junctions from a P/Q-type channel deficient mouse.[14] Electrophysiological studies at the neuromuscular junction have shown that basic features of transmission are retained and mediated by both N- and R-type channels. However, synaptic transmission features reduced quantal content and increased variance in synaptic transmission delay, with little or no paired-pulse facilitation.[31,32]

CALCIUM CHANNELS AND K^+-EVOKED NEUROTRANSMITTER RELEASE

Spontaneous release of acetylcholine in mammalian neuromuscular junctions depends on the intracellular free Ca^{2+} concentration of the nerve terminal, which in turn depends on the external Ca^{2+} concentration linked to ion influx through VDCCs. Thus, activation of Ca^{2+} channels by K^+ depolarization results in a several-fold increase in miniature endplate potential (MEPP) frequency. At adult neuromuscular junctions, the increase can be prevented by blocking the P/Q-type channels with ω-agatoxin IVA.[19] At neonatal neuromuscular junctions, where transmitter release is jointly mediated by N- and P/Q-type channels, ω-agatoxin IVA strongly reduces the frequency of MEPPs, while the N-type channel blocker ω-conotoxin GVIA as well as the L-type channel blocker nitrendipine were completely ineffective (FIG. 1, left). Similarly, at the KO neuromuscular junction where transmitter release is jointly mediated by N- and R-type channels, the R-type channel blocker SNX-482[33] strongly reduces the frequency of MEPPs induced by K^+ depolarization.

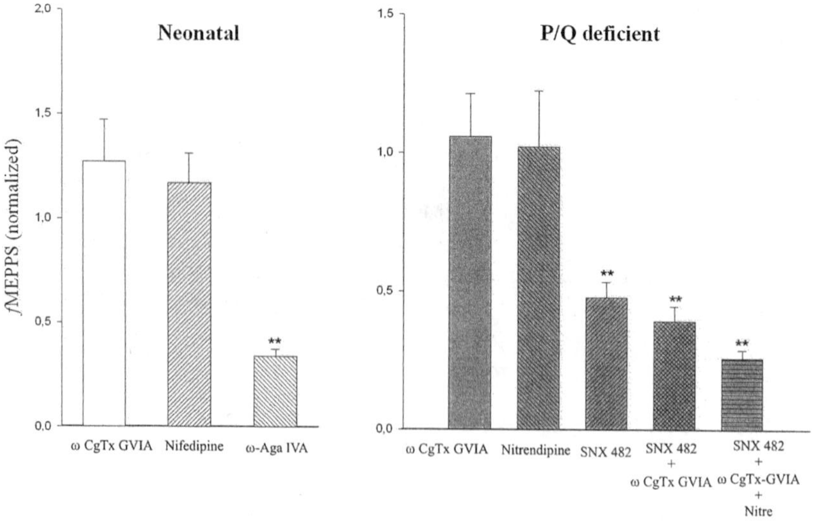

FIGURE 1. Effect of calcium channel blockers on K^+-evoked release of neurotransmitter at neuromuscular junctions of neonatal rats and P/Q-type channel deficient mice. The bar diagram illustrates the blockade exerted by ω-conotoxin GVIA (1 μM), nitrendipine (5 μM), nifedipine (10 μM), ω-agatoxin IVA (100 nM), and SNX-482 (1 μM) on the K^+-evoked increase in MEPP frequency. Each bar represents the mean ± SEM of at least 10 fibers per muscle of at least 2 muscles; $^{**}p < 0.001$.

In contrast, N- or L-type channel blockers applied alone do not affect K^+-evoked MEPP frequency, although a small, but significant, inhibitory effect was observed when applied together with the SNX-482 (FIG. 1, right).

LOCALIZATION OF Ca^{2+} CHANNELS AT THE RELEASE SITE

The lack of sensitivity of K^+-evoked MEPP frequency to N-type channel blockers and the lower Ca^{2+} dependence of N-type-mediated synaptic transmission at neonatal neuromuscular junctions suggest that N-type channels might be located further away from the Ca^{2+} sensor as compared with P/Q- or R-type channels present at the same release site. One prediction resulting from this hypothesis is that Ca^{2+} entering via N-type Ca^{2+} channels will diffuse along a greater distance before reaching the Ca^{2+} sensor, which increases the likelihood of Ca^{2+} being bound by a Ca^{2+} buffer, particularly by a fast chelator like BAPTA.[34] Indeed, when nerve transmission was only mediated by P/Q-type channels (e.g., in adult animal junctions), intracellular BAPTA did not affect neurotransmitter release.[23] On the other hand, at both early stages of development and P/Q knockout, the N-type blocker effect was strongly reduced at BAPTA-loaded junctions, without affecting the effect of P/Q- or R-type blockers.[30,31] Thus, reduction of quantal output by occluding Ca^{2+} influx through N-

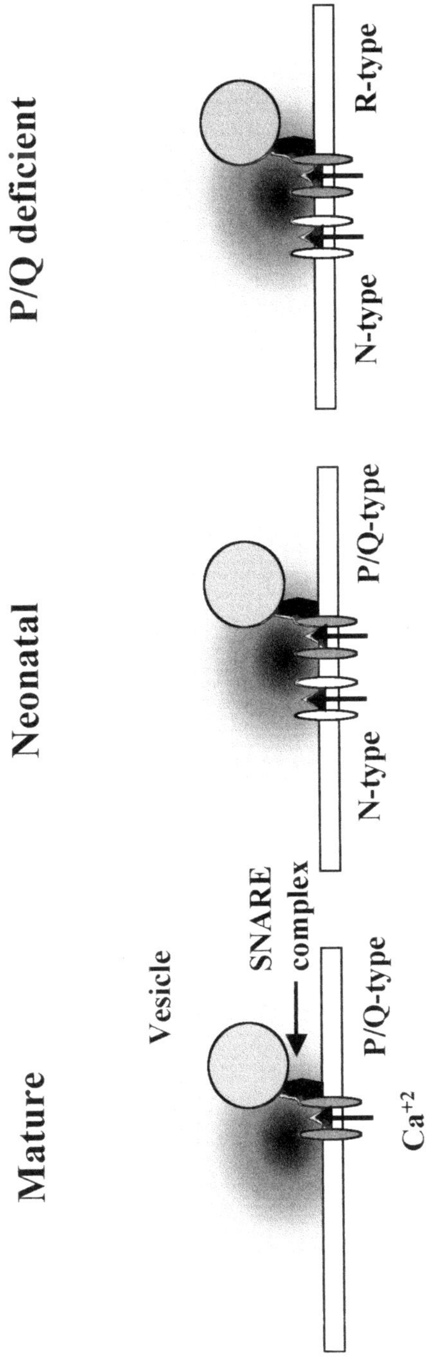

FIGURE 2. Hypothetical distribution of VDCCs at mammalian motor nerve terminals. A schematic view of the localization of calcium channels in motor nerve terminals. At mature rat motor nerve terminals, only P/Q-type VDCCs mediate neurotransmitter release. At neonatal rat neuromuscular junctions, P/Q- and N-type VDCCs mediate neurotransmitter release at the same active site. In this model, the synprint regions of P/Q- and N-type VDCCs "compete" to attach the SNARE complex. During development, P/Q-type VDCCs would show more affinity than N-type VDCCs, with displacement of the latter far from the release machinery. This specific spatial distribution of calcium channels might explain the different efficacies observed in neurotransmitter release coupling.[30] At neuromuscular junctions from a P/Q-type channel deficient mouse, R-type and N-type mediate neurotransmitter release at the same active site. R-type VDCCs are located closer to the calcium sensor than N-type VDCCs. Intracellular calcium concentration is represented by gray color intensity.

type channels supports the hypothesis of different locations of Ca^{2+} channels at the release site, with the N-type being located further away (FIG. 2).

CONCLUSIONS

Thus, the general conclusion is that different Ca^{2+} channels have an intrinsic capability of mediating neurotransmitter release. However, it is P/Q-type channels that appear to be most favorably suited to interact with the release machinery as a result of a close association with release sites in comparison with other types of Ca^{2+} channels. These different interactions may result in alterations in the efficiency, timing, and plasticity of synaptic transmission underlying neurological syndromes like paraneoplastic Lambert-Eaton Myasthenic Syndrome and the congenital episodic ataxias and migraines.

ACKNOWLEDGMENTS

This work was supported by NIH Grant No. R03TW01312-02, Ministerio de Salud, Beca Carrillo Oñativia (Argentina), ANCyT 6220, the Muscular Dystrophy Association, and UBACYT grants (to Osvaldo D. Uchitel). Francisco J. Urbano was a UNESCO/IUPAB fellow.

REFERENCES

1. KATZ, B. 1969. The Release of Neural Transmitter Substances. Liverpool University Press. Liverpool.
2. LLINAS, R., I.Z. STEINBERG & K. WALTON. 1976. Presynaptic calcium currents and their relation to synaptic transmission: voltage clamp study in squid giant synapse and theoretical model for the calcium gate. Proc. Natl. Acad. Sci. USA **73:** 2913–2922.
3. LLINAS, R. & H. MORENO. 1998. Local Ca^{2+} signaling in neurons. Cell Calcium **24:** 359–366.
4. CATTERALL, W.A. 2000. Structure and regulation of voltage-gated Ca^{2+} channels. Annu. Rev. Cell Dev. Biol. **16:** 521–555.
5. UCHITEL, O.D. 1997. Toxins affecting calcium channels in neurons. Toxicon **35:** 1161–1191.
6. ERTEL, E.A. *et al.* 2000. Nomenclature of voltage-gated calcium channels. Neuron **25:** 533–535.
7. HANS, M. *et al.* 1999. Functional consequences of mutations in the human alpha1A calcium channel subunit linked to familial hemiplegic migraine. J. Neurosci. **19:** 1610–1619.
8. KRAUS, R.L. *et al.* 1998. Familial hemiplegic migraine mutations change alpha1A Ca^{2+} channel kinetics. J. Biol. Chem. **273:** 5586–5590.
9. TORU, S. *et al.* 2000. Spinocerebellar ataxia type 6 mutation alters P-type calcium channel function. J. Biol. Chem. **275:** 10893–10898.
10. JEN, J. 1999. Calcium channelopathies in the central nervous system. Curr. Opin. Neurobiol. **9:** 274–280.
11. OPHOFF, R.A. *et al.* 1998. P/Q-type Ca^{2+} channel defects in migraine, ataxia, and epilepsy. Trends Pharmacol. Sci. **19:** 121–127.
12. ZHUCHENKO, O. *et al.* 1997. Autosomal dominant cerebellar ataxia (SCA6) associated with small polyglutamine expansions in the alpha1A-voltage-dependent calcium channel. Nat. Genet. **15:** 62–69.

13. FLETCHER, C.F. *et al.* 1996. Absence epilepsy in tottering mutant mice is associated with calcium channel defects. Cell **87:** 607–617.
14. DOYLE, J. *et al.* 1997. Mutations in the Cacnl1a4 calcium channel gene are associated with seizures, cerebellar degeneration, and ataxia in tottering and leaner mutant mice. Mamm. Genome **8:** 113–120.
15. JUN, K. *et al.* 1999. Ablation of P/Q-type Ca(2+) channel currents, altered synaptic transmission, and progressive ataxia in mice lacking the alpha(1A)-subunit. Proc. Natl. Acad. Sci. USA **96:** 15245–15250.
16. REUTER, H. 1996. Diversity and function of presynaptic calcium channels in the brain. Curr. Opin. Neurobiol. **6:** 331–337.
17. CATTERALL, W.A. 1998. Structure and function of neuronal Ca^{2+} channels and their role in neurotransmitter release. Cell Calcium **24:** 307–323.
18. UCHITEL, O.D. *et al.* 1992. P-type voltage-dependent calcium channel mediates presynaptic calcium influx and transmitter release in mammalian synapses. Proc. Natl. Acad. Sci. USA **89:** 3330–3333.
19. PROTTI, D.A. & O.D. UCHITEL. 1993. Transmitter release and presynaptic Ca^{2+} currents blocked by the spider toxin omega-Aga-IVA. Neuroreport **5:** 333–336.
20. PROTTI, D.A. *et al.* 1996. Calcium channel blockers and transmitter release at the normal human neuromuscular junction. Neurology **46:** 1391–1396.
21. KATZ, E. *et al.* 1997. Effects of Ca^{2+} channel blocker neurotoxins on transmitter release and presynaptic currents at the mouse neuromuscular junction. Br. J. Pharmacol. **121:** 1531–1540.
22. VINCENT, A., D. BEESON & B. LANG. 2000. Molecular targets for autoimmune and genetic disorders of neuromuscular transmission. Eur. J. Biochem. **267:** 6717–6728.
23. URBANO, F.J. & O.D. UCHITEL. 1999. L-type calcium channels unmasked by cell-permeant Ca^{2+} buffer at mouse motor nerve terminals. Pflüg. Arch. **437:** 523–528.
24. URBANO, F.J., R.S. DEPETRIS & O.D. UCHITEL. 2001. Coupling of L-type calcium channels to neurotransmitter release at mouse motor nerve terminals. Pflüg. Arch. **441:** 824–831.
25. XU, Y.F., S.J. HEWETT & W.D. ATCHISON. 1998. Passive transfer of Lambert-Eaton myasthenic syndrome induces dihydropyridine sensitivity of ICa in mouse motor nerve terminals. J. Neurophysiol. **80:** 1056–1069.
26. FRATANTONI, S.A. *et al.* 2000. Amyotrophic lateral sclerosis IgG-treated neuromuscular junctions develop sensitivity to L-type calcium channel blocker. Muscle Nerve **23:** 543–550.
27. KATZ, E. *et al.* 1996. Calcium channels involved in synaptic transmission at the mature and regenerating mouse neuromuscular junction. J. Physiol. **497**(part 3)**:** 687–697.
28. SANTAFE, M.M. *et al.* 2000. Multiple types of calcium channels mediate transmitter release during functional recovery of botulinum toxin type A–poisoned mouse motor nerve terminals. Neuroscience **95:** 227–234.
29. ROSATO-SIRI, M.D. & O.D. UCHITEL. 1999. Calcium channels coupled to neurotransmitter release at neonatal rat neuromuscular junctions. J. Physiol. **514**(part 2)**:** 533–540.
30. ROSATO-SIRI, M.D. *et al.* 2002. Differential Ca^{2+}-dependence of transmitter release mediated by P/Q- and N-type calcium channels at neonatal rat neuromuscular junctions. Eur. J. Neurosci. **15:** 1874–1880.
31. URBANO, F.J. *et al.* 2001. Short term facilitation and Ca^{2+} dependence of transmitter release are altered at the neuromuscular junction of P/Q Ca^{2+} channel knock out mice. Biophys. J. **80:** 234a.
32. DEPETRIS, R.S. *et al.* 2001. Loss of temporal precision of neurotransmitter release at neuromuscular junctions of mice lacking P/Q-type Ca^{2+} channels. Soc. Neurosci.
33. NEWCOMB, R. *et al.* 1998. Selective peptide antagonist of the class E calcium channel from the venom of the tarantula *Hysterocrates gigas*. Biochemistry **37:** 15353–15362.
34. ADLER, E.M. *et al.* 1991. Alien intracellular calcium chelators attenuate neurotransmitter release at the squid giant synapse. J. Neurosci. **11:** 1496–1507.

Effect of Inherited Abnormalities of Calcium Regulation on Human Neuromuscular Transmission

RICARDO A. MASELLI, WENDY BOOKS, AND VANESSA DUNNE

Department of Neurology, University of California, Davis, Davis, California 95616, USA

ABSTRACT: Synaptotagmins are abundant synaptic proteins that represent the best candidate for the calcium sensor at the nerve terminal. The pore-forming, voltage-sensing transmembrane alpha-1 subunit of the P/Q voltage-gated calcium channel (or $Ca_v2.1$) encoded by the CACNA1A gene is another major component of the process of action potential–evoked exocytosis at the adult mammalian neuromuscular junction. Defects of these proteins, in nonhuman species, result in severe disruption of rapid synaptic transmission. This paper investigates the molecular bases of inherited presynaptic deficits of neuromuscular transmission in humans. Patients with congenital presynaptic failure, including two patients with episodic ataxia type 2 (EA-2) due to CACNA1A mutations, were studied with muscle biopsy, microelectrode studies, electron microscopy, DNA amplification, and sequencing. All patients, including EA-2 patients, showed selective failure of the action potential–dependent release without reduction of the spontaneous release of neurotransmitter. In addition, patients with EA-2 showed partial blockade of neuromuscular transmission with the N-type blocker ω-conotoxin not seen in controls. The EM showed a varied degree of increased complexity of postsynaptic folds. Mutational analysis in candidate genes, including human synaptotagmin II, syntaxin 1A, synaptobrevin I, SNAP 25, CACNA1A, CACNB2, and Rab3A, was unrevealing. Although no mutations in candidate genes were found in patients with inborn presynaptic failure, functional and structural similarities between this group and patients with EA-2 due to CACNA1A mutations suggest a common pathogenic mechanism.

KEYWORDS: synaptotagmins; inherited presynaptic deficits; acetylcholine; CACNA1A mutations; presynaptic congenital myasthenic syndromes; calcium

INTRODUCTION

Presynaptic disorders of neuromuscular transmission represent a complex group of diseases, resulting from impaired release of acetylcholine (ACh) from the motor nerve terminal. Various autoimmune, toxic, and hereditary mechanisms have been

Address for correspondence: Ricardo A. Maselli, M.D., Department of Neurology, University of California, Davis, 1515 Newton Court, Room 510, Davis, CA 95616. Voice: 530-754-5011; fax: 530-754-5036.

ramaselli@ucdavis.edu

Ann. N.Y. Acad. Sci. 998: 18–28 (2003). © 2003 New York Academy of Sciences.
doi: 10.1196/annals.1254.004

implicated in the pathogenesis of presynaptic disorders. Hereditary mechanisms are responsible for a small group of these conditions, which are referred to as presynaptic congenital myasthenic syndromes (CMSs).

The presynaptic CMSs, so far described, can be divided into three major types. One type results from an impaired mechanism of resynthesis of ACh due to defects in the choline acetyltransferase gene (CHAT).[1–3] Another type is characterized by reduced quantal release and paucity of synaptic vesicles at the nerve terminal.[4] The last type comprises a more heterogeneous group of disorders that resemble the Lambert-Eaton myasthenic syndrome (LEMS).[5,6] Although the genetic defects underlying the last two types are unknown, a reasonable prediction would be that they involve genes encoding proteins that participate in the process of calcium-dependent exocytosis, including the alpha-1A subunit (or $Ca_V2.1$) of the P/Q-type calcium channel gene (CACNA1A).

To date, only pathogenic mutations in CACNA1A have been described in humans, although not in association with presynaptic CMS, but as the cause of three dominantly inherited disorders: familial hemiplegic migraine (FHM), episodic ataxia type 2 (EA-2), and spinocerebellar ataxia type 6 (SCA-6).[7,8] These diseases comprise a wide range of symptoms, including complicated migraine, ataxia, nystagmus, dysarthria, diplopia, muscle fatigue, seizures, coma, and a progressive cerebellar syndrome.[9–11]

The fundamental role that the P/Q-type calcium channel plays at the human adult neuromuscular junction has prompted researchers to examine neuromuscular transmission in patients with CACNA1A mutations by way of single-fiber electromyography (SFEMG) or microelectrode studies.[12,13] Not only have these studies confirmed the underlying failure of neuromuscular transmission, but they have also demonstrated a remarkable remodeling of calcium channel types at the nerve terminal in two patients with EA-2, which may provide some clues about the underlying mechanism of these disorders.[13,14]

This communication reports on the results of a mutational analysis performed in a group of patients with presynaptic deficit of quantal release not associated with paucity of synaptic vesicles at the nerve terminal (FIG. 1). It also describes findings of the ultrastructure and the *in vitro* physiology of the neuromuscular junctions in these patients and in two patients with EA-2.

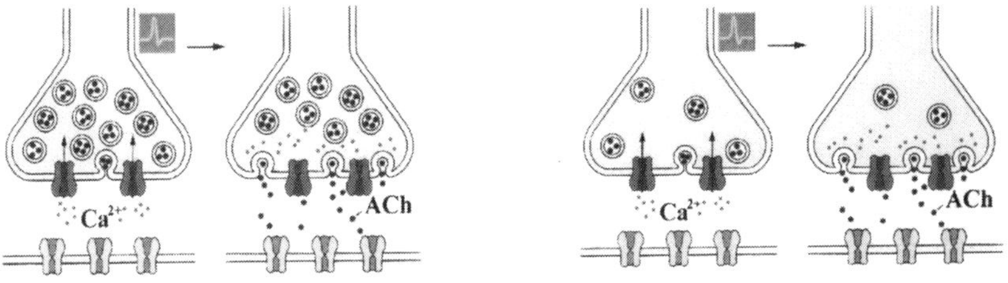

FIGURE 1. Schematic view of conditions characterized by reduced quantal release in association with normal (*left*) or reduced number (*right*) of synaptic vesicles at the nerve terminal.

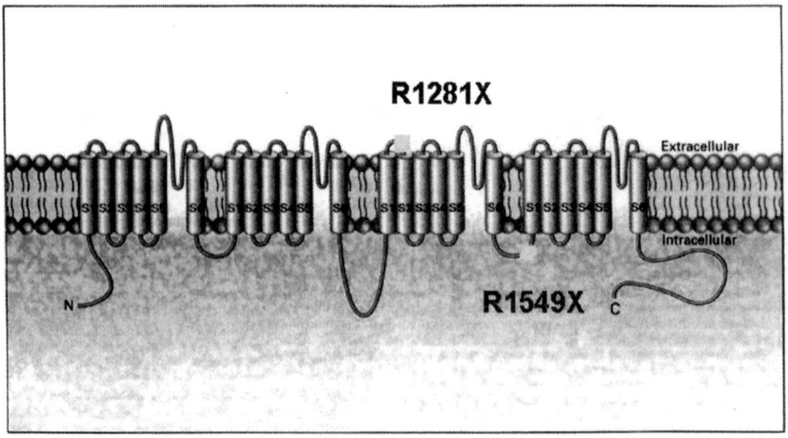

FIGURE 2. Position of heterozygous nonsense mutations of the two EA-2 patients in the α1A subunit of the calcium channel ($Ca_V2.1$) encoded by CACNA1A. (Modified from refs. 10 and 15.)

METHODS

Patients

Three of the patients who are currently 13, 15, and 19 years old have previously been described.[6] All three had muscle fatigue since early life without family history of neuromuscular problems. In addition, two of the patients had a history of incoordination, and on examination one patient had prominent horizontal nystagmus with a left cerebellar syndrome. The patients with EA-2 have previously been described in detail.[15,16] Both patients had a history of recurrent episodes of vertigo, gait instability, and episodic generalized weakness. The examination showed horizontal nystagmus in both patients. Each patient carries one heterozygous nonsense mutation in CACNA1A. The positions of the mutations were R1281X (patient 1) and R1549X (patient 2) (FIG. 2).

Muscle Biopsy

All patients had an anconeus muscle biopsy performed on the nondominant side. All muscle specimens were studied with routine histochemistry, *in vitro* microelectrode studies, and electron microscopy of the neuromuscular junction.

In Vitro *Microelectrode Studies*

Recording of miniature endplate potentials (MEPPs) and EPPs was performed as previously described.[17]

Electron Microscopy

Muscle bundles from the anconeus muscle were fixed in Karnovsky's solution and further dissected into bundles of about 40 fibers each. The bundles were divided into two parts following the longitudinal course of the fibers. One of the halves was reacted with Karnovsky-Roots solution to localize endplates. Regions of the unstained half matching the cholinesterase-reactive area of the stained half were embedded in EPON for electron microscopy.

Morphometric Analysis of the Neuromuscular Junction

Printouts of electron microscopy photographs were scanned, and the morphometric analysis was performed with the NIH image processing analysis program, as previously described.[6]

Mutational Analysis

All coding and flanking intron regions of candidate genes were amplified using polymerase chain reaction (PCR) and genomic DNA as a template, as previously described.[6] The genomic sequences of candidate presynaptic genes were obtained from GenBank. Also sequenced were all the coding and flanking intron regions of CHAT, the collagenic tail of the endplate acetylcholinesterase (COLQ), the four adult AChR subunit genes, and the promoter region of the ε-subunit gene. The N88K mutation in the rapsyn gene (RAPSN) was investigated by restriction analysis, as previously described.[18] Sequencing of PCR products was performed automatically using fluorescently labeled dideoxy chain terminators and an Applied Biosystems model 373 A DNA sequencer (Applied Biosystems, Foster City, CA).

RESULTS

Physiologic Findings

Reduction of Action Potential–Dependent Release without Decrease of Spontaneous Release of Neurotransmitter

The amplitudes and quantal content of nerve-evoked EPPs were reduced in all the patients, and the frequency distributions of EPP amplitudes in the patients were often arranged following Poisson's prediction, indicating very low probability of quantal release. Failures of stimulation pulses to elicit EPPs were common in the muscle biopsies of the patients, but not in control muscles. The mean quantal content of EPPs evoked by nerve stimulation at 1 Hz was 4.47 ± 1.2 in the three patients with presynaptic CMS, 6.05 ± 0.5 in the two patients with EA-2, and 12.60 ± 0.80 in controls ($p < 0.001$). In the muscle biopsies of the patients, nerve stimulation at fast rates failed to depress the EPP amplitudes. In contrast, in control muscles, nerve stimulation at 20 Hz resulted in transient depression of EPP amplitudes, probably as a result of depletion of synaptic vesicles at the nerve terminal. The lack of depression of EPP amplitudes during nerve stimulation at fast rates also suggested that the probability of quantal release in the patients was very low. The ratio obtained from dividing the quantal content of EPPs elicited by 20-Hz stimulation by that of EPPs resulting from 1-Hz stimulation (EPP 20/1 Hz) was 1.02 ± 0.06 (n = 20) in the patients with presynaptic CMS, 1.05 ± 0.08 (n = 11) in the EA-2 patients, and 0.73 ± 0.09 (n = 11) in controls ($p < 0.001$).

MEPP amplitudes were normal in the three patients with CMS. The mean MEPP amplitude in the CMS patients was 0.93 ± 0.13 and comparable to that of controls: 0.83 ± 0.04 mV. The mean MEPP amplitude of 0.79 ± 0.04 mV (n = 8) was normal in one patient with EA-2 (patient 2), while it was reduced to 0.68 ± 0.04 mV (n = 7) in the other patient with EA-2 (patient 1). MEPP frequencies expressed as MEPPs per minute were normal in two patients with presynaptic CMS [5.20 ± 0.9 (n = 9) and 3.3 ± 0.6 (n = 12)] and in patient 2 with EA-2 [3.6 ± 1.3 (n = 8)], in comparison with 4.06 ± 0.5 (n = 51) in controls, while it was increased to 12.2 ± 2.6 (n = 6) in one patient with CMS and to 8.75 ± 2.6 (n = 8) in patient 1 with EA-2.

Novel Sensitivity to N-Type Calcium Channel Blockade in EA-2 Patients

Exposure of EA-2 muscles to the L-type calcium channel blocker nifedipine (10 μM) resulted in no change of the basal EPP quantal content. The N-type blocker ω-conotoxin (ω-CgTx) (5 μM) resulted in a reduction of the EPP quantal content of 80% in EA-2 patient 2 and 58% in EA-2 patient 1, while control muscles showed no significant change. The P-type calcium channel blocker ω-agatoxin-IVA (ω-Aga-IVA) resulted in a reduction of the EPP quantal content of 95% in EA-2 patient 2, 88% in EA-2 patient 1, and 97% in control material.

Ultrastructural Findings

Normal or Mildly Overdeveloped Postsynaptic Folds

All the studied endplates showed a well-developed postsynaptic membrane folding pattern in all the patients. The endplate index (ratio of the length of postsynaptic membrane to presynaptic membrane) was within the normal range in all the patients, except in patient 2 with EA-2 in whom it was moderately increased.

Normal Size of Nerve Terminals

The presynaptic CMS patients showed axon termini of normal size. In the EA-2 patients, at the majority of the neuromuscular junctions, the size of the nerve terminal was also normal; however, at a few junctions, small nerve terminals apposed to normally developed postsynaptic membranes were seen, especially in patient 2.

Normal or Increased Number of Synaptic Vesicles

The size and distribution of synaptic vesicles were normal in two patients with presynaptic CMS, while the density of synaptic vesicles was moderately increased in one patient with presynaptic CMS and in the two patients with EA-2, in comparison with controls.

Other Findings in the Nerve Terminals

Agglutination of synaptic vesicles inside double membrane sacs was present in variable degrees in the three patients with presynaptic CMS.[6] In one patient, this finding was associated with prominent invagination of axolemmal membranes and increased number of coated pits, suggestive of increased exocytosis. The interpretation of accelerated exocytosis was also supported by the finding of increased MEPP frequency in the same patient. Membranous debris and lamellar whorls in the nerve terminal were also found in EA-2 patient 2. However, on serial sections, this membranous material appeared to be derived from the Schwann cell and not from the nerve terminal itself.

Mutational Analysis

Selection of Candidate Genes

The mutational analysis was primarily focused on genes encoding proteins that participate in the regulation of the action potential–evoked rise of intracellular calcium at the nerve terminal. The two most important proteins are the calcium acceptor synaptotagmin and the pore-forming alpha-1A (or $Ca_v2.1$) subunit of the neuronal P/Q voltage-gated calcium channel. The second line of candidate genes were those encoding proteins participating in the fusion of synaptic vesicles, including syntaxin, SNAP 25, and synaptobrevin, the GTP-binding protein Rab3, and the regulatory β-2 subunit of the voltage-gated calcium channel, recognized by LEMS antibodies.[19]

Synaptotagmins

Synaptotagmins I and II are abundant synaptic vesicle proteins that represent the best candidate for the Ca^{2+} sensor.[20,21] All synaptotagmins are characterized by a variable N-terminal, a transmembrane region, and two cytoplasmic C2 domains (C2A and C2B) followed by a short conserved C-terminus.[22,23] The C2A region binds phospholipids and syntaxin as a function of Ca^{2+} (FIG. 3).

The synaptotagmin isoform investigated in our patients by mutational analysis was synaptotagmin II, which was the isoform shown by previous studies expressed at the adult mammalian neuromuscular junction.[24,25] Using a mouse IgG monoclonal antibody directed against the RNQE sequence in the variable N-terminal domain of synaptotagmin II[26] (a generous gift from M. Takahashi), we confirmed the expression of synaptotagmin II at the human neuromuscular junction. Amplification and sequencing of the promoter and the eight coding regions of synaptotagmin II in the three presynaptic CMS revealed no abnormalities; specifically, no substitutions of the four aspartate residues (Asp 272, 278, 230, and 232) that coordinate Ca^{2+} molecules were seen.

Syntaxin 1A

The entire gene comprising 10 exons was analyzed. One silent polymorphism T→C at position 459 was detected with an allelic frequency of T 53.2% and C 46.8%. No pathogenic mutations were observed.

Synaptobrevins

The isoform expressed at the neuromuscular junction of adult mammals is synaptobrevin I.[27] Mutational analysis of the six coding regions of synaptobrevin I revealed one silent polymorphism A→C at position 356 with an allelic frequency of A 78% and C 22%. No pathogenic mutations were detected.

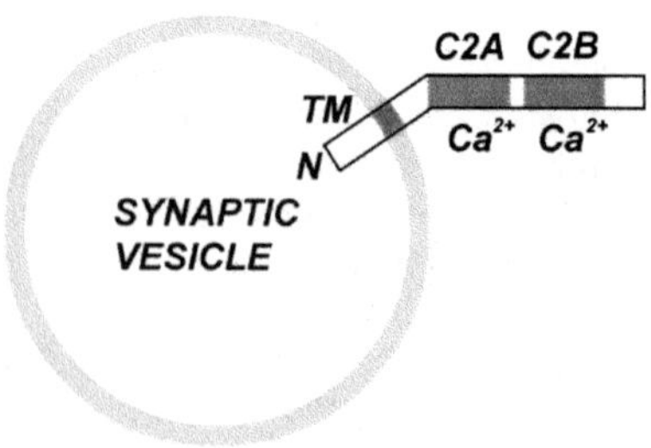


```
                                                                                          *
SytIV (Rat)       LPAMDEQSMTSDPYIKMTILPEKKHKVKTRVLRKTLDPVFDETFTFYGVPYPHIQELSLHFTVLSFDRFSRDDVIG
SytXI (Rat)     D LPVMDGQTQGSDPYIKMTILPDKRHRVKTRVLRKTLDPVFDETFTFYGIPYSQLQDLVLHFLVLSFDRFSRDDVIG
Syt V (Human)   D LAALDL-GGSSDPYVRVYLLXDKRRRYETKVHRQTLNPHFGETFAFK-VPYVELGGRVLVMAVYDFDRFSRNDAIG
SytII (Human)   D LPALDM-GGTSDPYVKVFLLPDKKKKYETKVHRKTLNPAFNETFTFK-VPYQELGGKTLVMAIYDFDRFFKHDIIG
SytII (Mouse)   D LPALDM-GGTSDPYVKVFLLPDKKKKYETKVHRKTLNPAFNETFTFK-VPYQELAGKTLVMAIYDFDRFSKHDIIG
SytII (Rat)     D LPALDM-GGTSDPYVKVFLLPDKKKKYETKVHRKTLNPAFNETFTFK-VPYQELGGKTLVMAIYDFDRFSKHDIIG
```

FIGURE 3. Synaptotagmins. **(Top)** Drawing of synaptotagmin showing the N-terminus (N), the transmembrane (TM), and the C2A and C2B domains. **(Bottom)** Alignment of the amino acid sequences of the Ca^{2+}-binding motif from the C2A region of several synaptotagmins showing high homology. Specifically, the four aspartate residues (Asp 272, 278, 230, and 232) that coordinate Ca^{2+} molecules are conserved in human synaptotagmins II and V. In contrast, in synaptotagmins IV and XI, which exhibit no Ca^{2+}-dependent phospholipid binding, aspartate is substituted by serine (*). (Modified from ref. 23.)

SNAP 25

Analysis of six exons with flanking intron regions showed no abnormalities.

Rab3A

Analysis of the five coding regions of Rab3A revealed no mutations or polymorphisms.

CACNB2

Amplification and sequencing of the 13 coding regions of CACNB2 showed a silent polymorphism C→T at position 1123. The allelic frequency was C 73.5% and T 26.5%. No pathogenic mutations were observed.

CACNA1A

Mutational analysis of CACNA1A, which involved the amplification and sequencing of the 47 coding regions of the gene, revealed several previously described polymorphisms,[6] but no pathogenic mutations.

DISCUSSION

We have presented here five patients with varied degrees of presynaptic defect due to selective impairment of the action potential–dependent release without reduction of spontaneous release of neurotransmitter. This type of neuromuscular transmission failure resembles that underlying LEMS, a classical presynaptic disorder resulting from a deficient quantal release of neurotransmitter. Two of the patients, who had fluctuating weakness, transient ataxia, and interictal nystagmus, were carriers of heterozygous nonsense mutations in the CACNA1A. Another patient with a long-standing history of muscle weakness and fatigue also had intermittent ataxia and prominent nystagmus.

The selection of synaptotagmin as one of the main targets of the mutational analysis in the patients with presynaptic CMS was based on the essential role that this protein plays in both synaptic vesicle exocytosis and endocytosis via its C2 domains. The devastating effect of mutations in the synaptotagmin gene has been directly demonstrated in mammals. Homozygous mice for a synaptotagmin I gene mutation die within 48 h after birth. Studies of hippocampal neurons cultured from these mice showed severe impairment of the action potential–dependent release, but normal spontaneous release.[28] Conceivably, a mutation resulting in a single amino acid change, such as the evolutionary substitution of aspartate by serine in the C2A domain of synaptotagmins IV and XI, may inactivate the calcium-binding properties of the protein that are essential for the action potential–triggered release of neurotransmitter.

The C2B domain of synaptotagmin plays a fundamental role in the process of vesicle retrieval through clathrin-mediated endocytosis.[29] In *Caenorhabditis elegans*, synaptotagmin is encoded by the gene *snt-1*.[30] Mutant nematodes with deficient *snt-1* show a striking reduction of synaptic vesicles in the nerve terminals.[31,32] Thus, the analysis of the synaptotagmin gene may also be relevant for the characterization of the genetic abnormality underlying presynaptic CMS with paucity of synaptic vesicles.

We have encountered no mutations in the synaptotagmin gene; however, we have only examined the gene encoding synaptotagmin II in a small number of patients. Examination of genes encoding other synaptotagmin isoforms in a large number of patients may be necessary to conclude whether congenital defects of synaptotagmin may be responsible for human pathology.

The other main focus of the mutational analysis was the genes encoding the voltage-gated calcium channel itself. This investigation was prompted by the clear similarities that we found between the findings of the *in vitro* studies in our patients and those encountered in LEMS, a disease resulting from an autoimmune attack of the presynaptic voltage-gated calcium channel. Furthermore, there was also a strong resemblance between the patients with presynaptic failure and the two patients with EA-2 due to heterozygous nonsense mutations in CACNA1A, the gene encoding the alpha-1 subunit of the P/Q-type calcium channel. However, in spite of these similarities, our preliminary study showed that there were no pathogenic mutations in CACNA1A or CACNB2.

A possible explanation for the absence of abnormalities in genes encoding fundamental proteins of the presynaptic apparatus in presynaptic CMS is that the majority of these proteins have several isoforms. Thus, a deficit in a given protein can be compensated by an alternative isoform encoded by a different gene. Indeed, in the patients with moderate presynaptic deficit due to heterozygous CACNA1A mutations, we found a striking rearrangement of presynaptic voltage-gated calcium channel types with a strong participation of N-type calcium channels in the action potential–evoked release of ACh not seen in controls. This compensatory effort may be insufficient to restore normal neuromuscular transmission because the N-type calcium channel is less efficient than the P-type to trigger neurotransmitter release.[33–35] Further, an upregulated expression of the N-type channel, which has different activation voltage than the P-type channel, may alter the calcium homeostasis at the nerve terminal, including the level of basal calcium, miniature potential frequencies, and the recycling of synaptic vesicles, at both the peripheral and central synapses. Lack of alternative isoforms of the presynaptic enzyme choline acetyltransferase may be, in part, the reason for the CMS due to abnormal ACh resynthesis, one of the first recognized forms of CMS.[1]

The mutational analysis in patients with presynaptic CMS was completed with the screening of genes encoding the vesicle protein synaptobrevin I or VAMP I (vesicle-associated membrane protein I), the plasma membrane proteins syntaxin 1A and SNAP 25, and the low molecular weight G protein Rab3, which hydrolyzes GTP. Botulinum toxins target synaptobrevin, syntaxin, and SNAP 25 and result in botulism, another classical presynaptic disorder of neuromuscular transmission.[36,37] Furthermore, *Drosophila* strains lacking either neural synaptobrevin or syntaxin[38,39] and the Rab3 knockout mice[40] showed complete blockade of synaptic transmission. No pathogenic mutations were found in any of these genes in our patients, but again we have analyzed only one isoform in a small group of patients. Therefore, we cannot conclusively rule out that genetic defects of these proteins may result in rare forms of CMS or other congenital neurologic disorders.

In summary, we have analyzed the function and structure of the neuromuscular junction in a small group of patients with congenital presynaptic failure of neuromuscular transmission and found similarities with that of patients with EA-2 due to known mutations in CACNA1A. The striking functional upregulation of non-P-type calcium channels that we found at the nerve terminals of EA-2 patients suggests that complex compensatory mechanisms may take place in response to genetic defects involving fundamental proteins of the presynaptic apparatus.

ACKNOWLEDGMENTS

This work was supported by the Muscular Dystrophy Association and the Myasthenia Gravis Foundation of California.

REFERENCES

1. Ohno, K., A. Tsujino, J.M. Brengman *et al.* 2001. Choline acetyltransferase mutations cause myasthenic syndrome associated with episodic apnea in humans. Proc. Natl. Acad. Sci. USA **98:** 2017–2022.
2. Byring, R.F., H. Pihko, A. Tsujino *et al.* 2002. Congenital myasthenic syndrome associated with episodic apnea and sudden infant death. Neuromuscul. Disord. **12:** 548–553.
3. Maselli, R.A., D. Chen, D. Mo *et al.* 2003. Choline acetyltransferase mutations in myasthenic syndrome due to deficient acetylcholine resynthesis. Muscle Nerve **27:** 180–187.
4. Walls, T.J., A.G. Engel, A.S. Nagel *et al.* 1993. Congenital myasthenic syndrome associated with paucity of synaptic vesicles and reduced quantal content. Ann. N.Y. Acad. Sci. **681:** 461–468.

5. ENGEL, A.G., K. OHNO & S.M SINE. 1999. Congenital myasthenic syndromes. *In* Myasthenia Gravis and Myasthenic Disorders, pp. 251–297. Oxford Univ. Press. London/New York.
6. MASELLI, R.A., B.S. KONG, C.M. BOWE *et al.* 2001. Presynaptic congenital myasthenic syndrome due to quantal release deficiency. Neurology **57:** 279–289.
7. OPHOFF, R.A., G.M. TERWINDT, M.N. VERGOUWE *et al.* 1996. Familial hemiplegic migraine and episodic ataxia type-2 are caused by mutations in the Ca^{2+} channel gene CACNL1A4. Cell **87:** 543–552.
8. ZHUCHENKO, O., J. BAILEY, P. BONNEN *et al.* 1997. Autosomal dominant cerebellar ataxia (SCA6) associated with small polyglutamine expansions in the alpha 1A–voltage-dependent calcium channel. Nat. Genet. **15:** 62–69.
9. JOUVENCEAU, A., L.H. EUNSON, A. SPAUSCHUS *et al.* 2001. Human epilepsy associated with dysfunction of the brain P/Q-type calcium channel. Lancet **358:** 801–807.
10. DUCROS, A., C. DENIER, A. JOUTEL *et al.* 2001. The clinical spectrum of familial hemiplegic migraine associated with mutations in a neuronal calcium channel. N. Engl. J. Med. **345:** 17–24.
11. WADA, T., N. KOBAYASHI, Y. TAKAHASHI *et al.* 2002. Wide clinical variability in a family with a CACNA1A T666m mutation: hemiplegic migraine, coma, and progressive ataxia. Pediatr. Neurol. **26:** 47–50.
12. JEN, J., J. WAN, M. GRAVES *et al.* 2001. Loss-of-function EA2 mutations are associated with impaired neuromuscular transmission. Neurology **57:** 1843–1848.
13. MASELLI, R., J. JEN, M. GRAVES *et al.* 2001. Patients with CACNA1A mutations and associated myasthenic weakness have presynaptic failure of neuromuscular transmission [abstract]. Neurology **56**(suppl. 3): A60.
14. MASELLI, R.A., J. WAN, B.S. DUNNE *et al.* 2003. Presynaptic failure of neuromuscular transmission and synaptic remodeling in EA-2. Submitted.
15. YUE, Q., J.C. JEN, M.M. THWE *et al.* 1998. *De novo* mutation in CACNA1A caused acetazolamide-responsive episodic ataxia. Am. J. Med. Genet. **77:** 298–301.
16. JEN, J., Q. YUE, S.F. NELSON *et al.* 1999. A novel nonsense mutation in CACNA1A causes episodic ataxia and hemiplegia. Neurology **53:** 34–37.
17. MASELLI, R.A., R.L. WOLLMAN, C. LEUNG *et al.* 1993. Neuromuscular transmission in amyotrophic lateral sclerosis. Muscle Nerve **16:** 1193–1203.
18. DUNNE, V.P. & R.A. MASELLI. 2003. Identification of pathogenic mutations in the rapsyn human gene. J. Hum. Genet. **48:** 204–207.
19. ROSENFELD, M.R., E. WONG, J. DALMAU *et al.* 1993. Cloning and characterization of a Lambert-Eaton myasthenic syndrome antigen. Ann. Neurol. **33:** 113–120.
20. KELLY, R.B. 1995. Neural transmission: synaptotagmin is just a calcium sensor. Curr. Biol. **5:** 257–259.
21. CHARVIN, N., C. L'EVEQUE, D. WALKER *et al.* 1997. Direct interaction of the calcium sensor protein synaptotagmin I with a cytoplasmic domain of the alpha 1A subunit of the P/Q-type calcium channel. EMBO J. **16:** 4591–4596.
22. SUTTON, R.B., B.A. DAVLETOV, A.M. BERGHUIS *et al.* 1995. Structure of the first C2 domain of synaptotagmin I: a novel Ca^{2+}/phospholipid-binding fold. Cell **80:** 929–938.
23. VON POSER, C., K. ICHTCHENKO, X. SHAO *et al.* 1997. The evolutionary pressure to inactivate: a subclass of synaptotagmins with an amino acid substitution that abolishes Ca^{2+} binding. J. Biol. Chem. **272:** 14314–14319.
24. ANGAUT-PETIT, D., P. JUZANS, J. MOLGO *et al.* 1995. Mouse motor nerve terminal immunoreactivity to synaptotagmin II during sustained quantal transmitter release. Brain Res. **681:** 213–217.
25. ANGAUT-PETIT, D., J. MOLGO, L. FAILLE *et al.* 1998. Incorporation of synaptotagmin II to the axolemma of botulinum type-A poisoned mouse motor endings during enhanced quantal acetylcholine release. Brain Res. **797:** 357–360.
26. NISHIKI, T., Y. TOKUYAMA, Y. KAMATA *et al.* 1996. The high-affinity binding of *Clostridium botulinum* type B neurotoxin to synaptotagmin II associated with gangliosides GT1b/GD1a. FEBS Lett. **378:** 253–257.
27. LI, J.Y., L. EDELMANN, R. JAHN & A. DAHLSTROM. 1996. Axonal transport and distribution of synaptobrevin I and II in the rat peripheral nervous system. J. Neurosci. **16:** 137–147.

28. GEPPERT, M., Y. GODA, R.E. HAMMER *et al.* 1994. Synaptotagmin I: a major Ca^{2+} sensor for transmitter release at a central synapse. Cell **79:** 717–727.
29. DE CAMILI, P. & K. TAKEI. 1996. Molecular mechanisms in synaptic vesicle endocytosis and recycling. Neuron **16:** 481–486.
30. BROSE, N., K. HOFMANN, Y. HATA & T.C. SÜDHOF. 1995. Mammalian homologs of *Caenorhabditis elegans* unc-13 gene define novel family of C2-domain proteins. J. Biol. Chem. **270:** 25273–25280.
31. JORGENSEN, E.M., E. HARTWIEG, K. SCHUSKE *et al.* 1995. Defective recycling of synaptic vesicles in synaptotagmin mutants of *Caenorhabditis elegans*. Nature **378:** 196–199.
32. NONET, M.L., O. SAIFEE, H. ZHAO *et al.* 1998. Synaptic transmission deficits in *Caenorhabditis elegans* synaptobrevin mutants. J. Neurosci. **18:** 70–80.
33. MINTZ, I.M., B.L. SABATINI & W.G. REGEHR. 1995. Calcium control of transmitter release at a cerebellar synapse. Neuron **15:** 675–688.
34. WU, L.G., R.E. WESTBROEK, J.G. BORST *et al.* 1999. Calcium channel types with distinct presynaptic localization couple differentially to transmitter release in single calyx-type synapses. J. Neurosci. **19:** 726–736.
35. URBANO, F.J., E.S. PIEDRAS-RENTERIA, K. JUN *et al.* 2003. Altered properties of quantal neurotransmitter release at endplates of mice lacking P/Q-type Ca^{2+} channels. Proc. Natl. Acad. Sci. USA **100:** 3491–3496.
36. TONELLO, F., S. MORANTE, O. ROSSETTO *et al.* 1996. Tetanus and botulism neurotoxins: a novel group of zinc-endopeptidases. Adv. Exp. Med. Biol. **389:** 251–260.
37. LALLI, G., J. HERREROS, S.L. OSBORNE *et al.* 1999. Functional characterisation of tetanus and botulinum neurotoxins binding domains. J. Cell Sci. **112:** 2715–2724.
38. SCHULZE, K.L., K. BROADIE, M.S. PERIN & H.J. BELLEN. 1995. Genetic and electrophysiological studies of *Drosophila* syntaxin-1A demonstrate its role in nonneuronal secretion and neurotransmission. Cell **80:** 311–320.
39. DEITCHER, D.L., A. UEDA, B.A. STEWART *et al.* 1998. Distinct requirements for evoked and spontaneous release of neurotransmitter are revealed by mutations in the *Drosophila* gene neuronal-synaptobrevin. J. Neurosci. **18:** 2028–2039.
40. TANAKA, M., J. MIYOSHI, H. ISHIZAKI *et al.* 2001. Role of Rab3 GDP/GTP exchange protein in synaptic vesicle trafficking at the mouse neuromuscular junction. Mol. Biol. Cell **12:** 1421–1430.

Transmitter Release Deficits at the Neuromuscular Synapse of Mice with Mutations in the $Ca_V2.1$ (α_{1A}) Subunit of the P/Q-Type Ca^{2+} Channel

J. J. PLOMP,[a,b] A. M. VAN DEN MAAGDENBERG,[c] M. D. FERRARI,[a] R. R. FRANTS,[c] AND P. C. MOLENAAR[b]

Departments of [a]Neurology, [b]Neurophysiology, and [c]Human and Clinical Genetics, Leiden University Medical Center, Leiden, the Netherlands

KEYWORDS: **P/Q-type Ca^{2+} channel; neuromuscular junction (NMJ); mutation**

INTRODUCTION

P/Q-type Ca^{2+} channels are expressed at many central synapses and also at the peripheral neuromuscular junction (NMJ). One important function of the channels is to mediate neurotransmitter release by allowing Ca^{2+} influx at presynaptic active zones. Mutations of channel subunits have been shown in inherited forms of migraine, ataxia, and epilepsy in humans and in a number of mouse mutants (for review, see ref. 1). It is likely that mutations will induce synaptic disturbances in the brain that will contribute to disease symptoms. Furthermore, neuromuscular transmission might be compromised due to NMJ malfunction. Indeed, impaired neuromuscular transmission was recently shown in patients with episodic ataxia type-2,[2] with mutations in CACNA1A, the gene that codes for the $Ca_V2.1$ pore-forming subunit of P/Q-type channels. We have earlier described synaptic defects at diaphragm NMJs of *Tottering* mice (missense mutation P601L in *Cacna1a*)[3] and have now studied two further natural mouse $Ca_V2.1$ mutants, that is, *Leaner* (splice mutation yielding truncated C-terminus) and *Rolling Nagoya* (R1262G missense mutation).

METHODS

Homozygous *Leaner* and *Rolling Nagoya* mice were obtained from breeding with heterozygous animals. In diaphragms *in vitro*, intracellular recordings were made with standard microelectrode equipment of the miniature endplate potential (MEPP, the spontaneous uniquantal ACh release event) and the endplate potential (EPP, the

Address for correspondence: Dr. J. J. Plomp, Ph.D., Department of Neurophysiology, Leiden University Medical Center, Wassenaarseweg 62, P. O. Box 9604, 2300 RC Leiden, the Netherlands. Voice: +31 71 527 6208; fax: +31 71 527 6782.
j.j.plomp@lumc.nl

Ann. N.Y. Acad. Sci. 998: 29–32 (2003). © 2003 New York Academy of Sciences.
doi: 10.1196/annals.1254.005

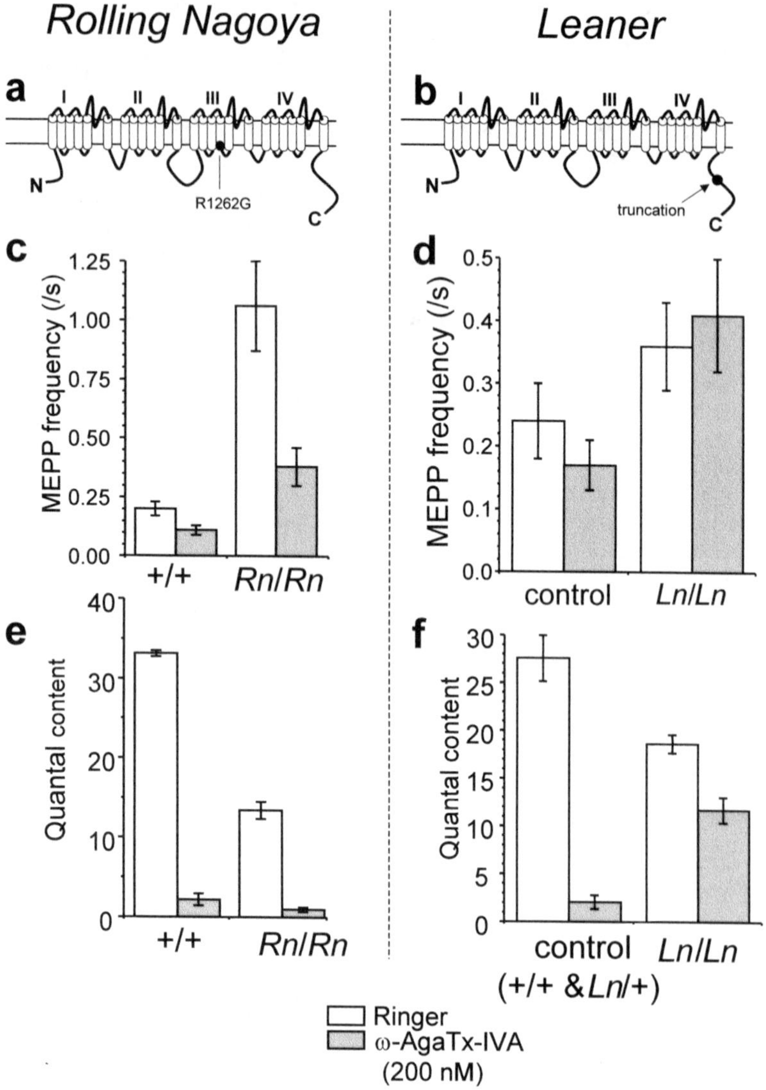

FIGURE 1. Summary of the results of the *in vitro* electrophysiological analysis of transmitter release at the NMJ of *Rolling Nagoya* (*left*) and *Leaner* mice (*right*). Shown are the sites of mutations in the $Ca_V2.1$ protein **(a, b)** and the resulting effects on spontaneous ACh release (MEPP frequency) **(c, d)** and evoked release (quantal content) at 0.3 Hz nerve stimulation **(e, f)**. Means ± SEM of 4–6 muscles (10–15 NMJs per muscle).

depolarization due to ACh release evoked by the nerve action potential resulting from stimulation of the phrenic nerve). We used μ-conotoxin GIIIB to block muscle Na^+ channels. At least 25 MEPPs and EPPs were recorded from each NMJ. Quantal content, that is, the number of ACh quanta released per nerve impulse, was calculated from EPP and MEPP amplitudes.

RESULTS

We found decreases in quantal content at 0.3 Hz stimulation (about 30%, $p < 0.01$, in *Leaner*, and about 60%, $p < 0.001$, in *Rolling Nagoya*; FIG. 1). At *Rolling Nagoya* and wild-type NMJs, evoked ACh release was reduced by >90% by 200 nmol of the P-type channel blocker, ω-agatoxin-IVA. However, at *Leaner* NMJs, the reduction was only 35%. N-type channel blocker, ω-conotoxin-GVIA, did not reduce quantal content at *Leaner* NMJs. Spontaneous ACh release (MEPP frequency) was increased by about 400% at *Rolling Nagoya* NMJs.

CONCLUSIONS

The increase in spontaneous ACh release at *Rolling Nagoya* NMJs, also observed by us previously at *Tottering* NMJs,[3] suggests increased Ca^{2+} influx under resting conditions via the mutated channels. It is clear that *Leaner* and *Rolling Nagoya* mutations in *Cacna1a* lead to reduction of nerve action potential–evoked ACh release at the NMJ. At *Leaner* motor nerve terminals, there might be compensatory expression of non-P/Q–non-N-type Ca^{2+} channels in view of the reduced sensitivity to ω-agatoxin-IVA and the lack of effect of ω-conotoxin-VIA. Chronic reduction of evoked ACh release per se is not the trigger for such a compensatory mechanism since *Rolling Nagoya* NMJs had a normal sensitivity for ω-agatoxin-IVA. The cytoplasmic C-terminus of $Ca_v2.1$ is known to be highly interactive with other functional and structural presynaptic proteins.[4] Disturbance of such interactions at *Leaner* NMJs due to the truncation of the C-terminus might trigger the compensatory phenomenon.

ACKNOWLEDGMENTS

This work was supported by the Prinses Beatrix Fonds [Grant No. MAR01-0105], the Hersenstichting Nederland [Grant No. 9F01(2).24], and the KNAW Van Leersumfonds.

REFERENCES

1. PLOMP, J.J., A.M. VAN DEN MAAGDENBERG, P.C. MOLENAAR *et al.* 2001. Mutant P/Q-type calcium channel electrophysiology and migraine. Curr. Opin. Invest. Drugs **2:** 1250–1260.
2. JEN, J., J. WAN, M. GRAVES *et al.* 2001. Loss-of-function EA2 mutations are associated with impaired neuromuscular transmission. Neurology **57:** 1843–1848.

3. PLOMP, J.J., M.N. VERGOUWE, A.M. VAN DEN MAAGDENBERG *et al.* 2000. Abnormal transmitter release at neuromuscular junctions of mice carrying the tottering alpha(1A) Ca(2+) channel mutation. Brain **123:** 463–471.
4. MAXIMOV, A., T.C. SUDHOF & I. BEZPROZVANNY. 1999. Association of neuronal calcium channels with modular adaptor proteins. J. Biol. Chem. **274:** 24453–24456.

Protein Ubiquitylation and Synaptic Function

OTTAVIO CREMONA,[a] CHIARA COLLESI,[a] AND ELISABETTA RAITERI[a,b]

[a]*Università Vita–Salute San Raffaele, San Raffaele Scientific Institute, 20132 Milano, Italy*

[b]*Università del Piemonte Orientale "A. Avogadro", 28100 Novara, Italy*

ABSTRACT: **Conjugation of ubiquitin to proteins is a well-established signal to regulate an ever expanding range of cellular processes. Here, we discuss recent findings that deeply link ubiquitin signaling to synaptic activity.**

KEYWORDS: **ubiquitin; synapse; neurotransmitter release; synaptic vesicle recycling**

INTRODUCTION

Posttranslational modification is a common means of regulating protein activity, localization, and stability. Rapid, reversible, and localized modifications carried out by pairs of complementary enzymes are quite versatile and can be sensitive to regulation themselves. Protein phosphorylation is the most investigated of such kinds of covalent modifications: it can cycle a protein through active and inactive states by means of the reciprocal action of protein kinases and phosphatases. Recently, an extraordinary wealth of data has brought attention to another very common post-translational modification—the covalent addition and removal of the protein ubiquitin. As for protein phosphorylation, ubiquitylation seems to be involved in virtually every aspect of eukaryotic biology and, not surprisingly, in some important human pathologies, including neurodegenerative diseases such as Parkinson's disease,[1] spinocerebellar ataxia type,[1,2] and gracile axonal dystrophy.[3]

In this short review, we will focus on recent developments in the ubiquitin field concerning synaptic physiology, while referring the reader to excellent reviews for other and more general aspects of the field.[4–12]

THE UBIQUITIN PATHWAY: POLYUBIQUITYLATION VERSUS MONOUBIQUITYLATION

In contrast to the addition of small molecules such as phosphates, ubiquitylation tags the substrate with one or multiple copies of a 76-amino-acid protein, ubiquitin, which is one of the most highly conserved proteins in eukaryotes. Its C-terminal

Address for correspondence: Ottavio Cremona, Università Vita–Salute San Raffaele, San Raffaele Scientific Institute, Via Olgettina 58, 20132 Milano, Italy. Voice: +39-02-2643-4748; fax: +39-02-2643-4844.
ottavio.cremona@hsr.it

Ann. N.Y. Acad. Sci. 998: 33–40 (2003). © 2003 New York Academy of Sciences.
doi: 10.1196/annals.1254.006

glycine forms a covalent isopeptide bond to the ε-amino group of lysine residues in substrate proteins (reviewed in refs. 4 and 6). Ubiquitin itself, via one of at least four of its seven lysine residues (K11, K29, K48, and K63), can serve as an acceptor to form a polyubiquitin chain containing from two to four ubiquitins.[7] A hierarchical set of three enzymes is required for ubiquitin modification: ubiquitin-activating (E1), ubiquitin-conjugating or ubiquitin-carrier (E2), and ubiquitin-protein ligase (E3) enzymes. While E1 is the product of a single gene in a given genome, there are tens of E2 genes in mammals and many more of E3 genes, which are classified in two families.[7] HECT (homologous to E6-AP carboxyl terminus) domain E3s form thiol-ester intermediates with ubiquitin during the ligation process, while RING FINGER (so-called for the structure of their metal-coordinating sites) E3s mediate the direct transfer of ubiquitin from E2 to substrates.

The wide variety of E3s provides specificity in determining which substrate proteins will be modified at particular times and locations. Productive ubiquitylation requires the successful interaction of the E3s with at least two other moieties, the E2 and the ubiquitylation signal in the targeting protein. This gives several opportunities to regulate the conjugation reaction by protein-protein interactions. Phosphorylation of the substrate is a particularly common mechanism (see, e.g., ref. 13) and, in some cases, the ability of E3s to recognize a phosphorylated signal depends on the presence of phosphoamino acid binding motifs in the E3 subunits (like the WW domains of the HECT-E3 Nedd4).[14] Phosphorylation of E3s is another way of regulating ubiquitin conjugation, which is particularly evident in the cell cycle, where proteolysis is tightly coupled to the activity of cyclin-dependent kinases.[15]

For many years, the best-known cellular role for ubiquitin conjugation has been the targeting of proteins for degradation to the 26S proteasome, a cytoplasmic proteolysis multisubunit complex that degrades soluble proteins tagged with a chain of at least four K48-linked ubiquitins (polyubiquitylation). However, more than 20 years ago, it was found that histones might carry single ubiquitin molecules.[16] Since then, it has become increasingly evident that several proteins that look polyubiquitylated by conventional biochemical analysis were in fact monoubiquitylated at multiple sites and that, in response to this posttranslational modification, their fate was not related to proteasome destruction. In fact, conjugation of a single ubiquitin moiety (or short ubiquitin chains mainly through K63-linked ubiquitin[7]) was found to serve as an active signal for a variety of key cellular functions, including protein traffic along the endocytic route, membrane traffic from several intracellular stations, budding of retrovirus from the plasma membrane, transcription regulation, and intracellular signaling (reviewed in ref. 8).

At least three distinct protein domains have been described to bind ubiquitin. The UBA (ubiquitin-associated) and CUE (from the first protein in which it was identified, the yeast Cue1p) motifs are moderately conserved 40-amino-acid sequences that are found in proteins related to very disparate functions, including ubiquitylation itself (only UBA motifs), membrane trafficking, and intracellular signaling.[17–19] Recently, the structure of the CUE domain complexed with monoubiquitin has been solved by NMR[20] and X-ray crystallography,[21] thus providing the first insights into the molecular determinants for ubiquitin recognition and, possibly, monoubiquitylation. The third ubiquitin-binding motif—the UIM (ubiquitin-interacting motif)—is a short sequence of approximately 15 amino acids that is well conserved among different proteins, including ubiquitylating and deubiquitylating enzymes and in accessory factors of the endocytic machinery.[22] Interestingly, the UIMs of these latter proteins do not only bind monoubiquitin, but are also required for intramolecular monoubiquitylation.[23–25]

As for other posttranslational modifications like protein phosphorylation, another important level of control of this pathway is the action of reverting enzymes, that is, the deubiquitinating enzymes (DUBs) that selectively remove ubiquitin from substrates. DUBs are thiol proteases encoded by tens of genes in mammals (reviewed in refs. 7, 26, and 27). The family of ubiquitin-specific processing enzymes (UBPs) is responsible for shortening multiubiquitin chains from proteins by sequentially removing the terminal ubiquityl group.

UBIQUITYLATION AND SYNAPTIC ACTIVITY

About 10 years ago, staining of synaptic membranes[28] and immunoblot analysis of various neuronal fractions from rat brain with anti-ubiquitin antibodies[29] showed that synapses are sites of intense ubiquitylation. More recently, this issue has been revisited in rat hippocampal neurons where the 1D profile of ubiquitinated proteins in postsynaptic densities has been analyzed under various stimulation conditions.[30] Upon tetrodotoxin synaptic block, ubiquitin conjugates decrease about 50%; on the contrary, increasing excitatory synaptic activity by the $GABA_A$ antagonist bicuculline results in a twofold increase of ubiquitylated substrates. The accelerated or reduced ubiquitylation in response to different levels of synaptic stimulation correlates with dramatic changes in protein turnover. Strikingly, inhibition of the proteasome system by a variety of drugs mimics the effect of neuronal inactivity on postsynaptic protein turnover, even in conditions of intense stimulation. Taken together, these data strongly suggest that ubiquitin participates as a key modulator of synaptic function in response to neuronal activity.

UBIQUITIN AT THE PRESYNAPSE

At the beginning of the 1990s, the *fat facets* gene (*faf*) was found to be essential for eye development in *Drosophila.*[31] The *faf* encodes for a DUB expressed throughout the developing nervous system. More recently, *faf* was identified in another genetic screen to uncover proteins whose neuronal overexpression alters synaptic growth at the *Drosophila* neuromuscular junction.[32] Although loss-of-function *faf* mutants do not have any evident neurological defect, overexpression of *faf* induces severe presynaptic overgrowth and defects in neurotransmitter release, including a marked reduction in the number of vesicles released by nerve terminal stimulation. Transgenic expression in *Drosophila* of the yeast DUB, UBP2, has a similar phenotype, thus giving a direct proof that perturbation of the ubiquitin pathway markedly affects presynaptic development and function. Another important piece of evidence in favor of this hypothesis was the isolation of mutants for another enzyme of the ubiquitin pathway, *highwire* (*hiw*), during a genetic screen to identify interactors of *faf* (more specifically, genes that enhance the *faf* overexpression phenotype).[32,33] Mutants of *hiw* and of its orthologue in nematodes, RPM-1, show the same synaptic overgrowth defects as *faf* overexpression mutants.[33,34] Not surprisingly, *hiw* is a RING

FINGER–type E3,[33] that is, an enzyme endowed with the opposite function of *faf* in the ubiquitin pathway.

Very recently, the genetic analysis of the *ataxia* mice showed that mutation in another DUB, USP14 (ubiquitin-specific protease 14), is responsible for defects in neurotransmitter release, as evidenced by severe alterations in short-term plasticity of central synapses.[35] Interestingly, USP14 can only process short ubiquitin chains—possibly single-conjugated ubiquitins—but not polyubiquitin.[36]

Taken together, these data give compelling genetic evidence that ubiquitylation is a key event for synaptic function. However, the search for ubiquitylated substrates, the next obvious step, is just beginning. In a genetic screen designed to identify *faf* substrates, a homologue of mammalian epsin, *liquid facet* (*lqf*), was detected.[37,38] Independently, an exhaustive homology search in data banks for UIM-containing proteins led to the identification of epsin and its major interactor in brain, Eps15, as ubiquitin-binding proteins.[22] Furthermore, epsin and Eps15 were found to be monoubiquitylated at multiple sites.[23–25] These proteins are accessory factors of clathrin-mediated endocytosis,[39,40] expressed in many tissues, but highly concentrated in brain.[40] At nerve terminals, they are thought to participate in the clathrin-dependent recycling of synaptic vesicle membrane components, a process necessary to maintain synaptic stability under prolonged nerve terminal stimulation (reviewed in refs. 41–43). Epsins and Eps15s are adaptors that bring together structural components of the clathrin coat (clathrin itself and the clathrin adaptor AP-2) and other endocytic factors, both proteins and lipids.[44–46] The precise function of epsin and Eps15 ubiquitylation is currently unknown. However, several scenarios can be envisaged:

- *(i)* UIMs might cooperate with other protein-protein interaction domains (i.e., the EH domains of Eps15 and the corresponding NPF motifs of epsin; the AP-2 and clathrin-binding motifs of both epsin and Eps15), and protein-lipid domains [i.e., the PI(4,5)P2-binding ENTH domain of epsin] to assemble the endocytic machinery;
- *(ii)* activation of UIMs by ubiquitin binding might modulate the affinities of other interaction domains in the adaptor proteins (i.e., the two UIMs of epsin are immediately adjacent to the phosphoinositide-binding ENTH domain);
- *(iii)* UIMs may assist E2 and E3 in the transfer of ubiquitin to substrates, increasing the efficiency and/or specificity of the reaction; and
- *(iv)* UIMs may protect monoubiquitylated substrates from polyubiquitylation and therefore degradation.

Turnover of synaptic vesicles seems to be a possible target of ubiquitylation, but is there any role for ubiquitin in the exocytosis of the neurotransmitter? At least, the integral membrane protein of the synaptic vesicle synaptophysin and the presynaptic membrane SNARE syntaxin are ubiquitylated.[47] For both proteins, specific E3 ubiquitin ligases that promote their degradation have been identified.[48,49] Interestingly, the same E3 that controls synaptophysin ubiquitylation, Siah-1, is also responsible for the ubiquitin tagging of Numb,[50] an endocytic protein that interacts with Eps15 EH domains.[51] Siahs are mammalian orthologues of the *Drosophila seven in absentia* gene, which controls eye development, similarly to *faf*.[52] These data might suggest that ubiquitylation can act as a common regulatory mechanism of exo/endocytic events at the presynapse.

UBIQUITIN AT THE POSTSYNAPSE

As reported above, postsynaptic densities are sites of intense ubiquitylation.[30,47] The targets of this activity are just starting to be unraveled. Regulation of the abundance of neurotransmitter receptors at the postsynaptic membrane is a potential mechanism for controlling synaptic strength, and this process is likely to depend on the exo/endocytosis of the receptors. Ubiquitylation is an attractive candidate for the retrieval of neurotransmitter receptors because it is a sufficient signal for endocytosis for a variety of other transmembrane receptors.[53,54] In *Xenopus* oocytes, α1 glycine receptors are polyubiquitylated in the plasma membrane upon agonistic stimulation.[55] Then, they are rapidly and efficiently retrieved and degraded along the endocytic route. Trafficking of AMPA receptors has been implicated in a variety of fundamental events of synaptic plasticity, including long-term potentiation[56] and long-term depression.[57] GLR-1, an AMPA receptor of nematodes, is ubiquitylated *in vivo*.[58] Mutations in this protein that prevent ubiquitin conjugation result in increased accumulation of GLR-1 at postsynaptic sites and in defects in locomotion consistent with increased synaptic strength. By contrast, overexpression of ubiquitin reduces the GLR-1 amount at the synapse. This effect is counteracted by inactivation of a clathrin adaptor, unc-11, an orthologue of mammalian AP180. Taken together, these data strongly support the idea that regulation of receptor trafficking at the postsynapse depends on a network of clathrin and ubiquitin interactions.

Besides neurotransmitter receptors, Ehlers[30] identified a number of other postsynaptic substrates for ubiquitylation whose levels are highly dynamic in response to neuronal activity. These are the multidomain scaffolding proteins Shank, GKAP, and AKAP79/150. Shank and GKAP act as adaptors for a variety of postsynaptic proteins, while AKAP79/150 brings signaling molecules to the complex of glutamate receptor and PSD-95.[59] Selective removal of these multivalent adaptor proteins by activity-induced ubiquitylation may cause a profound rearrangement of postsynaptic proteins by enforcing some signaling pathways and destabilizing others. Interestingly, the CREB and ERK-MAPK pathways are reciprocally regulated by activity-dependent ubiquitylation.[30] Selective activation of these latter signaling pathways has been linked to specific plasticity and functional responses.[60–62]

CONCLUDING REMARKS

Identification of E3s, DUBs, and substrates for ubiquitylation at the synapse is at the very beginning. However, some specific functions for ubiquitin, besides the proteasome/degradation pathway, are beginning to be delineated. Especially intriguing is the field of membrane traffic at both the pre- and postsynaptic side where several connections between clathrin-mediated endocytosis and ubiquitylation have emerged. Future directions include a systematic proteasome inventory of ubiquitin substrates and enzymes at the synapse and *in vivo* studies, including genetic studies in rodents, to test the contribution of the various components of the ubiquitin pathway to synaptic function. These analyses will certainly unravel novel and unexpected networks of interactions at the synapse, especially in the signaling field.

The ubiquitylation era of synaptic studies has just begun.

ACKNOWLEDGMENTS

We thank Pietro De Camilli for suggestions and helpful comments. Work in our laboratory is supported by Telethon (Project D.111), MIUR COFIN2001, and FIRB grants.

REFERENCES

1. LANSBURY, P.T., JR. & A. BRICE. 2002. Genetics of Parkinson's disease and biochemical studies of implicated gene products. Curr. Opin. Cell Biol. **14:** 653–660.
2. SKINNER, P.J. *et al.* 1997. Ataxin-1 with an expanded glutamine tract alters nuclear matrix–associated structures. Nature **389:** 971–974.
3. SAIGOH, K. *et al.* 1999. Intragenic deletion in the gene encoding ubiquitin carboxy-terminal hydrolase in gad mice. Nat. Genet. **23:** 47–51.
4. HOCHSTRASSER, M. 1996. Ubiquitin-dependent protein degradation. Annu. Rev. Genet. **30:** 405–439.
5. HICKE, L. 2001. A new ticket for entry into budding vesicles—ubiquitin. Cell **106:** 527–530.
6. PICKART, C.M. 2001. Mechanisms underlying ubiquitination. Annu. Rev. Biochem. **70:** 503–533.
7. WEISSMAN, A.M. 2001. Themes and variations on ubiquitylation. Nat. Rev. Mol. Cell Biol. **2:** 169–178.
8. HICKE, L. 2001. Protein regulation by monoubiquitin. Nat. Rev. Mol. Cell Biol. **2:** 195–201.
9. PICKART, C.M. 2000. Ubiquitin in chains. Trends Biochem. Sci. **25:** 544–548.
10. GLICKMAN, M.H. & A. CIECHANOVER. 2002. The ubiquitin-proteasome proteolytic pathway: destruction for the sake of construction. Physiol. Rev. **82:** 373–428.
11. HEGDE, A.N. & A. DIANTONIO. 2002. Ubiquitin and the synapse. Nat. Rev. Neurosci. **3:** 854–861.
12. MURATANI, M. & W.P. TANSEY. 2003. How the ubiquitin-proteasome system controls transcription. Nat. Rev. Mol. Cell Biol. **4:** 192–201.
13. SKOWYRA, D. *et al.* 1997. F-box proteins are receptors that recruit phosphorylated substrates to the SCF ubiquitin-ligase complex. Cell **91:** 209–219.
14. HENRY, P.C. *et al.* 2003. Affinity and specificity of interactions between Nedd4 isoforms and the epithelial Na^+ channel. J. Biol. Chem. **278:** 20019–20028.
15. PAGE, A.M. & P. HIETER. 1999. The anaphase-promoting complex: new subunits and regulators. Annu. Rev. Biochem. **68:** 583–609.
16. BUSCH, H. & I.L. GOLDKNOPF. 1981. Ubiquitin-protein conjugates. Mol. Cell. Biochem. **40:** 173–187.
17. HOFMANN, K. & P. BUCHER. 1996. The UBA domain: a sequence motif present in multiple enzyme classes of the ubiquitination pathway. Trends Biochem. Sci. **21:** 172–173.
18. DONALDSON, K.M. *et al.* 2003. Ubiquitin signals protein trafficking via interaction with a novel ubiquitin binding domain in the membrane fusion regulator, Vps9p. Curr. Biol. **13:** 258–262.
19. SHIH, S.C. *et al.* 2003. A ubiquitin-binding motif required for intramolecular monoubiquitylation, the CUE domain. EMBO J. **22:** 1273–1281.
20. KANG, R.S. *et al.* 2003. Solution structure of a CUE-ubiquitin complex reveals a conserved mode of ubiquitin binding. Cell **113:** 621–630.
21. PRAG, G. *et al.* 2003. Mechanism of ubiquitin recognition by the CUE domain of Vps9p. Cell **113:** 609–620.
22. HOFMANN, K. & L. FALQUET. 2001. A ubiquitin-interacting motif conserved in components of the proteasomal and lysosomal protein degradation systems. Trends Biochem. Sci. **26:** 347–350.
23. KLAPISZ, E. *et al.* 2002. A ubiquitin-interacting motif (UIM) is essential for Eps15 and Eps15R ubiquitination. J. Biol. Chem. **277:** 30746–30753.

24. OLDHAM, C.E. *et al.* 2002. The ubiquitin-interacting motifs target the endocytic adaptor protein epsin for ubiquitination. Curr. Biol. **12:** 1112–1116.
25. POLO, S. *et al.* 2002. A single motif responsible for ubiquitin recognition and mono-ubiquitination in endocytic proteins. Nature **416:** 451–455.
26. WILKINSON, K.D. 1997. Regulation of ubiquitin-dependent processes by deubiquitinating enzymes. FASEB J. **11:** 1245–1256.
27. CHUNG, C.H. & S.H. BAEK. 1999. Deubiquitinating enzymes: their diversity and emerging roles. Biochem. Biophys. Res. Commun. **266:** 633–640.
28. CHAPMAN, A.P. *et al.* 1992. Ubiquitin immunoreactivity of multiple polypeptides in rat brain synaptic membranes. Biochem. Soc. Trans. **20:** 155S.
29. CHAPMAN, A.P. *et al.* 1994. Multiple ubiquitin conjugates are present in rat brain synaptic membranes and postsynaptic densities. Neurosci. Lett. **168:** 238–242.
30. EHLERS, M.D. 2003. Activity level controls postsynaptic composition and signaling via the ubiquitin-proteasome system. Nat. Neurosci. **6:** 231–242.
31. FISCHER-VIZE, J.A., G.M. RUBIN & R. LEHMANN. 1992. The *fat facets* gene is required for *Drosophila* eye and embryo development. Development **116:** 985–1000.
32. DIANTONIO, A. *et al.* 2001. Ubiquitination-dependent mechanisms regulate synaptic growth and function. Nature **412:** 449–452.
33. WAN, H.I. *et al.* 2000. *Highwire* regulates synaptic growth in *Drosophila*. Neuron **26:** 313–329.
34. ZHEN, M. *et al.* 2000. Regulation of presynaptic terminal organization by *C. elegans* RPM-1, a putative guanine nucleotide exchanger with a RING-H2 finger domain. Neuron **26:** 331–343.
35. WILSON, S.M. *et al.* 2002. Synaptic defects in ataxia mice result from a mutation in Usp14, encoding a ubiquitin-specific protease. Nat. Genet. **32:** 420–425.
36. YIN, L. *et al.* 2000. Nonhydrolyzable diubiquitin analogues are inhibitors of ubiquitin conjugation and deconjugation. Biochemistry **39:** 10001–10010.
37. CADAVID, A.L., A. GINZEL & J.A. FISCHER. 2000. The function of the *Drosophila* fat facets deubiquitinating enzyme in limiting photoreceptor cell number is intimately associated with endocytosis. Development **127:** 1727–1736.
38. CHEN, X., B. ZHANG & J.A. FISCHER. 2002. A specific protein substrate for a deubiquitinating enzyme: liquid facets is the substrate of fat facets. Genes Dev. **16:** 289–294.
39. CARBONE, R. *et al.* 1997. eps15 and eps15R are essential components of the endocytic pathway. Cancer Res. **57:** 5498–5504.
40. CHEN, H., *et al.* 1998. Epsin is an EH-domain-binding protein implicated in clathrin-mediated endocytosis. Nature **394:** 793–797.
41. CREMONA, O. & P. DE CAMILLI. 1997. Synaptic vesicle endocytosis. Curr. Opin. Neurobiol. **7:** 323–330.
42. DE CAMILLI, P. *et al.* 2000. Synaptic Vesicle Endocytosis. Johns Hopkins Press. Baltimore.
43. SLEPNEV, V.I. & P. DE CAMILLI. 2000. Accessory factors in clathrin-dependent synaptic vesicle endocytosis. Nat. Neurosci. Rev. **1:** 161–172.
44. ITOH, T. *et al.* 2001. Role of the ENTH domain in phosphatidylinositol-4,5-bis-phosphate binding and endocytosis. Science **291:** 1047–1051.
45. FORD, M.G. *et al.* 2002. Curvature of clathrin-coated pits driven by epsin. Nature **419:** 361–366.
46. WENDLAND, B. 2002. Epsins: adaptors in endocytosis? Nat. Rev. Mol. Cell Biol. **3:** 971–977.
47. DAVIDSSON, P. *et al.* 2001. Proteome studies of human cerebrospinal fluid and brain tissue using a preparative two-dimensional electrophoresis approach prior to mass spectrometry. Proteomics **1:** 444–452.
48. WHEELER, T.C. *et al.* 2002. Regulation of synaptophysin degradation by mammalian homologues of seven in absentia. J. Biol. Chem. **277:** 10273–10282.
49. CHIN, L.S., J.P. VAVALLE & L. LI. 2002. Staring, a novel E3 ubiquitin-protein ligase that targets syntaxin 1 for degradation. J. Biol. Chem. **277:** 35071–35079.
50. SUSINI, L. *et al.* 2001. Siah-1 binds and regulates the function of Numb. Proc. Natl. Acad. Sci. USA **98:** 15067–15072.
51. SANTOLINI, E. *et al.* 2000. Numb is an endocytic protein. J. Cell Biol. **151:** 1345–1352.

52. CARTHEW, R.W. & G.M. RUBIN. 1990. Seven in absentia, a gene required for specification of R7 cell fate in the *Drosophila* eye. Cell **63:** 561–577.
53. HAGLUND, K. *et al.* 2003. Multiple monoubiquitination of RTKs is sufficient for their endocytosis and degradation. Nat. Cell Biol. **5:** 461–466.
54. MOSESSON, Y. *et al.* 2003. Endocytosis of receptor tyrosine kinases is driven by monoubiquitylation, not polyubiquitylation. J. Biol. Chem. **278:** 21323–21326.
55. BUTTNER, C. *et al.* 2001. Ubiquitination precedes internalization and proteolytic cleavage of plasma membrane–bound glycine receptors. J. Biol. Chem. **276:** 42978–42985.
56. LLEDO, P.M. *et al.* 1998. Postsynaptic membrane fusion and long-term potentiation. Science **279:** 399–403.
57. LUTHI, A. *et al.* 1999. Hippocampal LTD expression involves a pool of AMPARs regulated by the NSF-GluR2 interaction. Neuron **24:** 389–399.
58. BURBEA, M. *et al.* 2002. Ubiquitin and AP180 regulate the abundance of GLR-1 glutamate receptors at postsynaptic elements in *C. elegans*. Neuron **35:** 107–120.
59. SHENG, M. & M.J. KIM. 2002. Postsynaptic signaling and plasticity mechanisms. Science **298:** 776–780.
60. HARDINGHAM, G.E., Y. FUKUNAGA & H. BADING. 2002. Extrasynaptic NMDARs oppose synaptic NMDARs by triggering CREB shut-off and cell death pathways. Nat. Neurosci. **5:** 405–414.
61. MINICHIELLO, L. *et al.* 2002. Mechanism of TrkB-mediated hippocampal long-term potentiation. Neuron **36:** 121–137.
62. WU, G.Y., K. DEISSEROTH & R.W. TSIEN. 2001. Spaced stimuli stabilize MAPK pathway activation and its effects on dendritic morphology. Nat. Neurosci. **4:** 151–158.

Nicotinic Acetylcholine Receptors of Muscles and Nerves

Comparison of Their Structures, Functional Roles, and Vulnerability to Pathology

JON M. LINDSTROM

Medical School of the University of Pennsylvania, Philadelphia, Pennsylvania, USA

ABSTRACT: There are fetal and adult subtypes of muscle nicotinic receptors (AChRs), whose structures and functional roles are reasonably well known. Mutations of their subunits cause congenital myasthenic syndromes. An autoimmune response to them causes myasthenia gravis (MG). The main immunogenic region (MIR) on muscle AChRs accounts for many aspects of the pathological mechanisms by which the autoimmune response impairs neuromuscular transmission. There are many other AChR subtypes, each defined by a different combination of subunits, some of which are transiently expressed in muscle during development, others of which are expressed in keratinocytes, vascular and bronchial epithelia, and other nonneuronal cells, as well as in a wide variety of neurons. Their varied structures and functional roles are much less well known. Mutations in subunits of some of these AChRs have thus far been associated with rare forms of epilepsy and dysautonomia, but other genetic diseases associated with them probably remain to be discovered. Autoimmune responses to some of these subunits are associated with rare dysautonomias and a skin disease. The pathological mechanisms by which these autoimmune responses impair function are much less well known than in the case of MG. AChRs may provide useful drug targets in several neurological diseases. By far, the biggest direct medical impact of AChRs is addiction to tobacco, which is mediated by nicotine acting on a variety of neuronal AChRs.

KEYWORDS: AChR; nicotine; neuron; muscle; myasthenia gravis (MG)

ACHR STRUCTURES

AChRs are part of a superfamily of ligand-gated ion channel neurotransmitter receptors comprising five homologous subunits organized around a central ion channel.[1–3] Other superfamily members include receptors for γ amino butyric acid, glycine, and one type of serotonin receptor.

Address for correspondence: Jon M. Lindstrom, Medical School of the University of Pennsylvania, 217 Stemmler Hall, Philadelphia, PA 19104-6074. Voice: 215-573-2859; fax: 215-573-2858.

JSLKK@mail.med.upenn.edu

Ann. N.Y. Acad. Sci. 998: 41–52 (2003). © 2003 New York Academy of Sciences.
doi: 10.1196/annals.1254.007

The primordial AChR is thought to have been homomeric.[1–3] AChR α7, α8, and α9 subunits can form homomeric ACh-gated cation channel AChRs. α7 AChRs are the predominant form of homomeric AChR in mammals. ACh binding sites are formed at the interfaces between the extracellular domains of the five α7 subunits. An ACh-binding protein secreted by molluscan glial cells is a water-soluble protein whose structure corresponds to the extracellular domain of the α7 AChR.[4] The high-resolution crystal structure of this binding protein provides a model for the basic extracellular domain features of all AChRs.[5] Both α7–10 AChRs and muscle AChRs bind the snake venom toxin, α-bungarotoxin, as a competitive inhibitor. A model based on the crystal structure of a complex of an α1 peptide with α-bungarotoxin and the structure of the ACh-binding protein depicts a structure composed of a ring of five subunits with five toxin molecules sticking out of the ACh-binding sites like vanes of a windmill.[6] α7 is sometimes found with α8 in heteromeric AChRs in chickens, and α9 is usually found with α10 in heteromeric AChRs in mammals.[1–3]

The structure of muscle-type AChRs is typified by those in the electric organs of *Torpedo californica*.[1,2] The subunits are organized around the central cation channel in the order α1, γ, α1, δ, β1.[1] Two ACh-binding sites are formed at the interfaces between α1 and γ or δ subunits. The γ subunit of the fetal form of muscle AChR is replaced by ε in the adult form.

There are many potential heteromeric neuronal AChR subtypes formed from combinations of α2–α5 subunits with β2–β4 subunits.[3] There are a few predominant subtypes, but some minor subtypes are important medically. A single neuron often expresses several subtypes, but only in rare cases is the particular location or functional role of each subtype known. The primary brain AChR subtype with high affinity for nicotine contains α4 and β2 subunits, which are thought to be organized around the cation channel in the order α4, β2, α4, β2, β2. Two ACh-binding sites are thought to be formed at interfaces between α4 and β2. The β2 in the position corresponding to β1 of muscle AChRs does not take part in forming ACh-binding sites. This subunit can be replaced by α5 or β3 subunits, neither of which is thought to be able to participate in forming ACh-binding sites. α5 and β3 can influence channel properties because they contribute one-fifth of the channel lining, and they can influence agonist potency and efficacy because they participate in the conformation changes of the whole AChR protein associated with activation and desensitization. The primary autonomic ganglion AChR subtype contains α3 and β4 subunits, but β2 or α5 subunits may also be associated. Interesting minor subtypes found in brain dopaminergic and adrenergic neurons contain α6 subunits in combination with β2, β3, and often α3 or α4 subunits.

All AChR subunits share some structural features.[1–3] An N-terminal signal sequence is cleaved during translation. The N-terminal ~210 amino acids of the mature protein form a large extracellular domain whose fundamental features probably resemble those of the snail ACh-binding protein.[5] The N-terminus of the binding protein is at the extracellular tip of the subunit. A disulfide-linked loop corresponding to amino acids 128–142 of α1 subunits is characteristic of all subunits in the superfamily. In most AChR subunits, there is an N-glycosylation site in this loop at 141, and many subunits are also glycosylated at additional sites. In the binding protein, this loop is oriented near what would be the membrane surface,[5] but this may not usually be true. The loop sequence is highly conserved in most AChR subunits, but the binding protein loop sequence is substantially different and much more hydrophilic. This may be an adaptation of the binding protein to permit efficient assembly without transmembrane domains and high water solubility. Mutagenesis evidence suggests that the loop is normally involved in subunit assembly.[7] Truncated human α7 extracellular domain constructs assemble into pentamers very inefficiently unless there is at least one transmembrane domain, and the extracellular domain constructs are not secreted.[8] In all AChR subunits, immediately following the large extracellular domain, there are three closely spaced transmembrane domains, M1–M3, which comprise about 90 rather conserved amino acids. The N-terminal third of M1 and all of one side of M2 contribute to the lining of the cation channel.[1,2] M1 links sequences in the extracellular domain that contribute to the ACh-binding site with a short sequence near the cytoplasmic surface between M1 and M2 that forms the channel gate.[1] Between the M3 and M4 transmembrane domains is a large cytoplasmic domain of 150–280 amino acids whose sequence is not well conserved among subunits.[1–3] This region forms the "fingers" observed by low-resolution electron crystallography of *Torpedo* AChRs to contact rapsyn,[9] the 43,000-dalton extrinsic membrane protein that links muscle AChRs to the cytoskeleton,[10] thereby helping to localize them at the tips of junctional folds adjacent to active zones in the presynaptic membrane. Probably several proteins similar to rapsyn associate with neuronal AChRs, but they have yet to be identified. Sequences in the large cytoplasmic domain target AChRs for transport to particular parts of the cell.[11] At the C-terminus of the large cytoplasmic domain is the M4 transmembrane domain, which leads to a short (3–27 amino acid) C-terminal extracellular domain. Surprisingly, the C-terminus of neuronal AChR α4 subunits forms a binding site through which estrogenic steroids potentiate function.[12] There are likely other extracellular sites through which AChRs are allosterically regulated (e.g., through the prototoxin, lynx 1, which is structurally homologous with α-bungarotoxin),[13] in addition to regulation through phosphorylation on the large cytoplasmic domain.[14]

AChR subunits are rod-like in structures oriented around the central cation channel like barrel staves.[9] AChRs extend about 65 Å above the membrane, 40 Å across it, and 35 Å beneath it. Viewed from the top, they are about 80 Å in diameter with 25-Å-thick walls surrounding a 30-Å-diameter vestibule to the channel. The ACh-binding sites are located about 30 Å above the membrane surface.[5]

ACh-binding sites are accessible from the outside surface and formed at the interface between the "positive" side of α subunits and the "minus" side of adjacent subunits.[1,2,5] The structure of the ACh-binding protein shows that the positive side of α subunits is characterized by a projecting loop tipped by the disulfide-linked cysteine pair that characterizes α subunits and corresponds to amino acids 192 and 193 of muscle AChR α1 subunits.[5] Affinity labeling and mutagenesis studies of AChRs[1,2] agree with structural studies of the ACh-binding protein[5] in showing that the ACh-binding site is formed from amino acids from three parts of the α extracellular domain sequence and three parts of the sequence of the adjacent subunit. Thus, the ACh-binding sites are well positioned to produce or stabilize subtle conformation changes involving shifts along subunit interfaces. Mutagenesis and labeling studies reveal that conformation differences between resting, activated, and desensitized states of AChRs involve both the ACh-binding site and the channel, and probably involve the whole protein, allowing influence from points quite distant from the binding site or channel (e.g., the cytoplasmic domain or C-terminus).[1,2]

AChR FUNCTIONS

AChRs in the postsynaptic membrane of muscle are part of very large synapses containing tens of millions of AChRs. The neuromuscular junction is designed to greatly amplify the small currents involved in the motor neuron axon action potential more than sufficiently to trigger an action potential in a large muscle fiber, thereby insuring a large safety factor for neuromuscular transmission.[15] An excess of ACh is released from active zones in the presynaptic membrane directly onto an excess of AChRs. Despite all this redundancy, neuromuscular transmission is vulnerable to toxins that evolved to stop prey in its tracks (e.g., cobra toxins and conotoxins).[16] It is also vulnerable to man-made toxins designed for a quick kill (e.g., nerve gases[17] directed at ACh esterase that use excess ACh to produce desensitization and excito-toxicity). Genetic[18] and autoimmune diseases[19] can also overcome this robust system.

Properties of AChRs are not uniquely required for neuromuscular transmission. Insects use glutamate receptors for this purpose, while using AChRs as the principal excitatory receptor in their central nervous system (the opposite of vertebrates). These insect neuronal AChRs are also vulnerable to plant insecticides (e.g., nicotine) as well as man-made insecticides (both esterase inhibitors and agonists).[20]

By contrast with the ohmic conductance properties and low calcium permeability of muscle AChRs, most neuronal AChRs exhibit strong inward rectification (resulting in low currents at depolarized membrane potentials), and several neuronal AChR subtypes (especially α7) exhibit high calcium permeability.[3]

Although some neuronal AChR subtypes have postsynaptic roles in neurotransmission, for example, the α3β4 AChRs of autonomic ganglia,[21] the majority of brain AChRs are thought to act presynaptically or preterminally to modulate the release of many different transmitters.[22] For example, both α4β2 and α3β2 AChRs are thought to modulate release of γ amino butyric acid in the hippocampus,[23] and both α4β2 and α6β2β3 AChRs are thought to modulate dopamine release in the striatum and substantia nigra.[24] Some AChRs may be extrasynaptic and play a trophic role (e.g., α7 AChRs in chicken ciliary ganglia).[25] The high affinity α4β2 AChRs may respond to low levels of ACh released at a distance in a process of volume transmission.[26] In keratinocytes, both ACh synthesis and secretion and a variety of AChRs modulating cell motility have been reported, but morphologically identifiable synapses have not.[27] Cholinergic signaling has also been reported between lymphocytes.[28]

Muscle, prior to innervation or after denervation, expresses not only the fetal form of muscle AChR, but also some α7.[29] Presumably, the ACh affinity, channel properties, or turnover rates of these AChR subtypes are more suitable during synapse formation. Adult muscle expresses only adult muscle AChRs. α7 knockout mice exhibit no obvious muscle defects, so the contribution of α7 to neuromuscular development is probably small.[30]

Several neuronal AChR subtypes are often expressed by individual neurons. Autonomic ganglionic neurons typically express α3, β2, β4, α5, and α7 subunits.[31] In chicken ciliary ganglion, the differences in transport of the α3 AChRs and α7 AChRs have been shown to be due to their particular large cytoplasmic domains.[11] In locus ceruleus, there are two types of neurons, one expressing α3, β2, β4, and often α6, β3, α5, and α4, and the other expressing α6, β2, β3, and often α4.[32] Thus far, it is unclear which AChR subtypes are expressed in which parts of the locus ceruleus neurons or why.

CONGENITAL MYASTHENIC SYNDROMES

Congenital myasthenic syndromes (CMS) can be caused by mutations in muscle AChR subunits and other synapse components.[18] These AChR mutations have provided novel insights on both AChR structure and function. Whereas ε subunit knockout mice are perinatal lethal,[33] many CMS involve mutations in ε subunits apparently because γ subunits of fetal muscle AChRs can in part substitute for the loss of ε.[18]

Genetic defects in muscle AChR subunits predictably cause a myasthenic syndrome, and it is relatively easy (though still elegant) to explain the patients' pathology in terms of the altered functional properties of mutant muscle AChRs. Thus, more than 60 different muscle AChR mutations have been found to cause CMS.[18] These studies provide a model to which studies of mutations in human neuronal AChRs can now aspire only with great difficulty.

GENETIC DEFECTS IN NEURONAL AChRs

The major problem in identifying diseases resulting from mutations in neuronal AChRs is that our ignorance of their normal functional roles makes it difficult to know what symptoms to expect from neuronal AChR mutations. Further, the complexity of central neuronal pathways and the many possible pathways for compensation further complicate identifying syndromes resulting from mutations in neuronal AChRs. Nonetheless, some diseases resulting from mutations in neuronal AChRs have been identified, and neuronal AChR subunit knockout and knock-in mice have provided useful insights.

Autosomal dominant nocturnal frontal lobe epilepsy (ADNFLE) is associated with mutations in both α4[34] and β2[35,36] AChR subunits. The symptoms of this rare epilepsy resemble night terrors. The pathological mechanisms by which these mutations produce their effects are not clear. The mutations are in the M2 channel domain. Those in the α4 subunit tend to reduce function through slowing activation, increasing desensitization, and reducing calcium permeability,[37] but the β2 subunit mutations increase function through increased sensitivity to ACh and decreased desensitization.[35,36] Knockout of either α4 or β2 subunits in mice does not produce behavior resembling ADNFLE.[38]

The rare neonatal lethal human genetic disorder, megacystis-microcolon-intestinal hypoperistalsis syndrome, resembles the complete dysautonomia that results in mice from knockout of either AChR α3[21] subunits or both β2 and β4 subunits.[39] There is some evidence that the human disease may result from a null mutation of α3.[40] Interestingly, although α3β4 AChRs are thought to be the predominant form involved in autonomic ganglionic transmission, knockout of β4 does not produce profound dysautonomia.[38,39] Evidently, sufficient α3β2 AChRs are present or inducible to compensate for loss of β4. This is reminiscent of the substitution of γ for null ε mutations in CMS.[18]

Knockout mice reveal that α3 is the one neuronal AChR subunit whose loss is lethal because of the resulting dysautonomia.[21] Similarly, one would expect a null mutation of α1 to be lethal as a result of complete loss of all neuromuscular transmission.[18] Knockout of α4 results in reduced nicotine-induced antinociception.[38]

Although this causes loss of most AChRs with high affinity for nicotine, the effect on nicotine dependence has not been reported. Knockout of β2 subunits causes even more extensive loss of brain high-affinity binding sites, abolishes nicotine- and ACh-evoked dopamine release, prevents development of nicotine dependence, alters learning, and causes increased cholinergic neuron loss with age.[38] Knockout of β4 is compensated by β2, but knockout of both prevents autonomic ganglion neurotransmission as does knockout of α3. Knockout of α6 subunits causes no gross neurological or behavioral defects, but reduces cholinergic ligand binding in the aminergic neurons in which it is found.[41] Pharmacological evidence indicates that 40% of nicotine-induced dopamine release from brain synaptosomes is mediated by α6 AChRs. Nicotine-dependence studies of α6 knockout mice have not yet been reported. Despite the relatively large numbers of α7 AChRs in the central and peripheral nervous systems, and transient expression in muscle during development, α7 knockout mice exhibit very little obvious impairment.[30,38] Knockout of α9 subunits impairs innervation of cochlear outer hair cells.[42] α9α10 AChRs are responsible for transmission on hair cells in which influx of calcium ions through AChRs triggers a net inhibitory response through activating a calcium-sensitive potassium channel.[43,44] This process is involved in tuning the frequency sensitivity of the cochlea, which is important in the "cocktail party effect", which permits one to focus on a particular voice or sound. Overall, these studies illustrate how AChRs can be involved in forming and maintaining proper synaptic contacts, as they are in muscle, and how they can be involved in synaptic mechanisms quite different from those of muscle.

Knock-in mice expressing α4[45] or α7[46] M2 mutations that destabilize the resting state, promote activation, and reduce desensitization suffer from excitotoxicity. The knock-in AChRs resemble some of the excitotoxic long-channel CMS mutations,[18] but some neurons are less robust in tolerating the excitotoxicity than are muscle cells. Highly expressed hyperactive α4 and α7 knock-ins were neonatal lethal.[45,46] When expressed less efficiently, the α4 knock-in gradually destroyed the substantia nigra, inhibited learning, and increased the anxiety level.[45] Cytotoxic knock-in mutations of neuronal AChR subunits can exaggerate the normal physiological importance of the subunit by killing a neuron that expresses many AChR subunits.

MYASTHENIA GRAVIS

Myasthenia gravis (MG) is caused by an antibody-mediated autoimmune response to muscle AChRs.[19] What initiates and sustains this autoimmune response is unknown. Dogs with MG usually recover within 6 months, unless they also have a tumor.[47] This result, as well as the transience (when not fatal) of neonatal MG, penicillamine-induced MG, and passive or active experimental autoimmune MG (EAMG), all emphasize that the prolonged nature of human MG depends on mechanisms beyond input to the immune system of AChRs from damaged neuromuscular junctions to sustain the autoimmune response.

The immune response in MG and EAMG impairs neuromuscular transmission by several mechanisms.[19] Antibodies bound to AChRs target the postsynaptic membrane for focal lysis by complement. This both causes loss of AChRs and disrupts the folded architecture of the postsynaptic membrane that normally positions AChRs

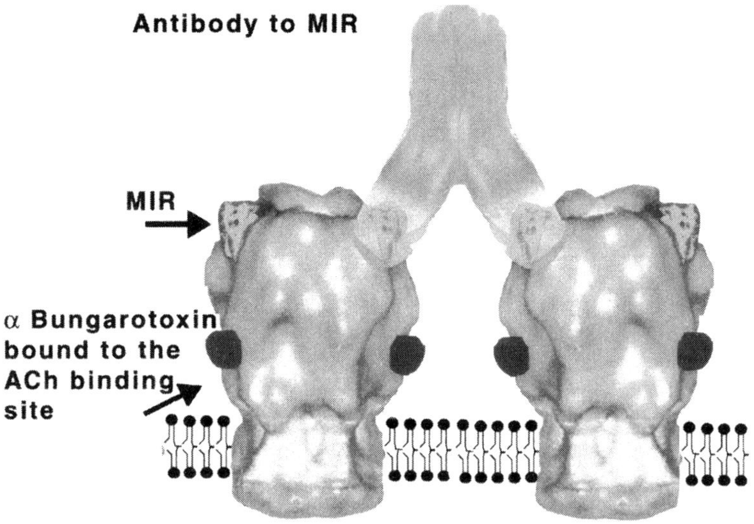

FIGURE 1. Structural basis of the pathological significance of the MIR. As detailed in the text and depicted in this cartoon, the structure of the MIR accounts for the characteristic pathological properties of mAbs to the MIR and typical serum autoantibodies.

at the tips of folds next to active zones of ACh release in the presynaptic membrane. Antibodies also cross-link AChRs, thereby increasing their rate of internalization and further reducing the amount of AChR by antigenic modulation. In most patients, inhibition of AChR function by competitive or noncompetitive mechanisms contributes relatively little to impairment of transmission.

Half or more of the autoantibodies to AChR in human or canine MG or in EAMG are directed at the main immunogenic region (MIR).[19,48] The MIR is defined by the ability of single mAbs, prepared from rats with EAMG, to inhibit the binding of MG patient autoantibodies to muscle AChRs. This is a conformation-dependent region on α1 subunits whose corresponding sequence is located at the extracellular tip of the ACh-binding protein.[5] Amino acids within the sequence 66–76 contribute to the MIR.[48] Mutation of *Torpedo* α1 amino acid 68 or 71 inhibits the binding of rat mAbs to the MIR raised against α1 AChRs from humans, rodents, *Electrophorus*, or *Torpedo*.[49] Thus, despite different origins and affinities for AChRs from various species, all of these Abs to the MIR overlap in their binding to a critical part of the MIR sequence.

The structure of the MIR accounts for major aspects of the pathological mechanisms by which autoantibodies impair neuromuscular transmission in MG (FIG. 1).[19] The MIR is on the top of the extracellular surface of AChRs, which are packed into the postsynaptic membrane in a semicrystalline array.[50] Thus, a high density of antibodies are easily bound *in vivo*, readily permitting complement fixation on focal lysis. The MIR is angled away from the central axis of the AChR so that a single antibody cannot cross-link the two α1 subunits in an AChR molecule; instead, the antibodies are ideally positioned to cross-link adjacent AChRs and induce antigenic modulation. The MIR is located far from the ACh-binding site;[5] thus, antibodies bound to it do not competitively inhibit AChR function. Also, antibodies bound to the MIR do not inhibit the binding of ^{125}I-α-bungarotoxin used to identify the AChR in immunodiagnostic assays. The MIR is located away from subunit interfaces; hence, it does not allosterically inhibit function by interfering with movements along these axes, which may be involved in activation or desensitization.

What accounts for the particular immunogenicity of the MIR is less clear. To judge from the corresponding sequence of the ACh-binding protein,[5] it is a prominent loop on the top surface of the AChR. The loop conformation may contribute to the conformation dependence of its antigenicity. The presence of two MIRs per AChR may contribute to cross-linking of immune receptors on B cells leading to the activation of these cells.

AUTOIMMUNE RESPONSES TO NEURONAL AChRs

Autoantibodies to α3 AChRs have been detected in patients with dysautonomia.[51] One might expect that transmission at autonomic ganglia might be inhibited by mechanisms similar to those that inhibit neuromuscular transmission in MG.[19] These antibodies to α3 AChRs are not directed at the MIR.[51] Thus, subunit-specific immune induction mechanisms differentially account for MG and these dysautonomias. Autoantibodies from patients with dysautonomia do not bind to muscle α1 AChRs, nor do antisera from patients with MG bind to α3 AChRs. Autoantibodies specific for β2, β4, or α5 AChRs could bind to α3 AChRs without reacting with α1 AChRs. Lack of reaction of antibodies from patients with MG with α3 AChRs would not be remarkable were it not for the fact that some rat mAbs to the MIR on α1 react very well with human α3 and α5 subunits.[19,52] α1, α3, α5, and β3 subunits are quite similar in their sequences in the 66–76 region.[3] Rats and humans must recognize slightly different epitopes or features of epitopes within the MIR. The identity or orientation of a single antigen amino acid can greatly influence the affinity of an antibody for an antigen, even though the contact area between antibody and antigen includes dozens of amino acids over a large area.[53] The crystal structures of Fab fragments from two rat mAbs to the MIR of human muscle have been determined.[54,55] It is interesting that the shapes of their two binding sites are quite different and do not reveal a clear negative image of the MIR.

Pemphigus is an antibody-mediated autoimmune disease in which keratinocytes become detached from one another. Autoantibodies to several proteins, including AChR α9 subunits, have been identified.[56]

NICOTINE ADDICTION THROUGH NEURONAL NICOTINIC AChRs

Addiction to tobacco is by far the largest medical effect mediated directly through AChRs. In developed countries, smoking is the largest single cause of premature death and is responsible for 20% of all premature deaths and more than 30% of all deaths in men aged 35–69. In the United States, there are ~25,000 patients with MG[57] and ~500,000 deaths[58] per year due to smoking-related illnesses.

Addiction to tobacco is mediated by nicotine through nicotinic AChRs.[3,59] The mechanisms are thought to involve dopamine-mediated pathways for reinforcement and learning that are also involved in addiction to cocaine and other abused drugs. The precise mechanisms are not known and may be more extensive. Addiction to tobacco is a strongly learned behavior that, although it carries with it a death threat through cancer and other diseases while offering no obvious euphoric reward, provides smokers with many nicotine-mediated benefits including relief of anxiety, enhanced attention and memory, and weight loss.[60] Nicotine facilitates dopamine release through several AChR subtypes, and it also facilitates the release of several other transmitters and hormones. Whereas ACh is released in a neuromuscular junction for a millisecond, nicotine is present for many hours. Nicotine is a time-averaged antagonist because desensitized AChRs accumulate. Accumulation of desensitized muscle AChRs is usually only encountered intentionally during surgical muscle relaxation with succinylcholine or inadvertently during overdose of MG patients with inhibitors of ACh esterase. The pattern of tobacco use allows for both acute activation of low-affinity AChRs immediately following inhaling smoke and chronic desensitization of high-affinity AChRs. Chronic exposure to nicotine causes up-regulation in the amount of AChRs. Tolerance to some of nicotine's adverse effects may reflect desensitization of AChRs. However, the total pattern of activation and desensitization of various AChR subtypes in various regions that accounts for addiction and other nicotine effects on behavior is not clear.

Muscle AChRs are largely spared the effects of nicotine in smoking because, although these nicotinic AChRs are the namesake for this ligand, nicotine has very low affinity for muscle AChRs. The EC_{50} for nicotine on α1 AChRs is $\geq 10^{-4}$ M (10^2-fold less than ACh), on α3 AChRs it is 5×10^{-5} M, and on α4 AChRs it is ~2×10^{-7} M.[61] The sustained serum nicotine concentration in smokers is ~2×10^{-7} M.[62] After inhaling smoke, the brain nicotine concentration may transiently reach ~1×10^{-6} M.

INDIRECT AChR ASSOCIATIONS WITH DISEASES

AChR effects have been associated with several diseases.[60] Substantial α4β2 AChR losses occur in Alzheimer's disease, and nicotine provides some benefit on memory. The amyloid Aβ fragment is very potent as an allosteric inhibitor of α7 AChRs,[63] and α7 mediates internalization of Aβ.[64] Schizophrenia and bipolar disorder exhibit some genetic linkage to α7, suggesting that α7 anomalies might be a predisposing factor for these diseases.[65] Nicotine and mecamylamine have been used to greatly reduce tics in children with Tourette's syndrome.[60] Other disease associations have been found as well, although in none are AChRs thought to be protagonists as they are in MG or some types of CMS.

Nicotinic agonists and antagonists are being investigated for possible use in these diseases and others, as well as for use in smoking cessation therapy.[60] Nicotine has a strong antinociceptive effect. The high-affinity agonist, epibatidine, discovered as an arrow frog toxin, is 100-fold more potent on certain kinds of pain than morphine (but its therapeutic index is low). In animal studies, nicotine has shown neuroprotective effects. Nicotine has strong anxiolytic effects and it is argued that 25% of U.S. smokers do so in part to self-medicate for depression.[65] Thus, there is significant interest in neuronal nicotinic AChRs as potential drug targets, but no new nicotinic drug has been approved yet.

REFERENCES

1. KARLIN, A. 2002. Emerging structure of the nicotinic acetylcholine receptors. Nat. Rev. Neurosci. **3:** 102–114.
2. GUTTER, T. & J-P. CHANGEUX. 2001. Nicotinic receptors in wonderland. Trends Biochem. Sci. **26:** 459–463.
3. LINDSTROM, J. 2000. The structures of neuronal nicotinic receptors. Handb. Exp. Pharmacol. **144:** 101–162.
4. SMIT, A., N. SYED, D. SCHAAP *et al.* 2001. A glia-derived acetylcholine-binding protein that modulates synaptic transmission. Nature **411:** 261–268.
5. BREJC, K., W. VAN DIJK, R. KLAASSEN *et al.* 2001. Crystal structure of an ACh-binding protein reveals the ligand-binding domain of nicotinic receptors. Nature **411:** 269–276.
6. HAREL, M., R. KASHER, A. NICHOLAS *et al.* 2001. The binding site of acetylcholine receptor as visualized in the X-ray structure of a complex peptide between α bungarotoxin and a mimotope. Neuron **32:** 265–275.
7. FU, D-X. & S. SINE. 1996. Asymmetric contribution of the conserved disulfide loop to subunit oligomerization and assembly of the nicotinic acetylcholine receptor. J. Biol. Chem. **271:** 31479–31484.
8. WELLS, G., R. ANAND, F. WANG *et al.* 1998. Water soluble nicotinic acetylcholine receptor formed by α7 subunit extracellular domains. J. Biol. Chem. **273:** 964–973.
9. MIYAZAWA, A., Y. FUJIYOSHI, M. STOWELL *et al.* 1999. Nicotinic acetylcholine receptor at 4.6 Å resolution: transverse tunnels in the channel wall. J. Mol. Biol. **288:** 765–786.
10. MAIMONE, M. & J. MERLIE. 1993. Interaction of the 43 kd postsynaptic protein with all subunits of the muscle nicotinic acetylcholine receptor. Neuron **11:** 53–66.
11. WILLIAMS, B., M. TEMBURNI, M. LEVY *et al.* 1998. The long internal loop of the α3 subunit targets in AChRs to subdomains within individual synapses on neurons *in vivo*. Nat. Neurosci. **1:** 557–562.
12. PARADISO, K., J. ZHANG, S. STEINBACH *et al.* 2001. The C-terminus of the human nicotinic α4β2 receptor forms a binding site required for potentiation by an estrogenic steroid. J. Neurosci. **21:** 6561–6568.
13. IBANEZ-TALLON, I., J. MIWA, H-L. WANG *et al.* 2002. Novel modulation of neuronal nicotinic acetylcholine receptors by association with endogenous prototoxin lynx 1. Neuron **33:** 893–903.
14. FENSTER, C., M. BECKMAN, J. PARKER *et al.* 1999. Regulation of α4β2 nicotinic receptor desensitization by calcium and protein kinase C. Mol. Pharmacol. **55:** 432–443.
15. ENGEL, A. 1994. The neuromuscular junction. *In* Myology. Second edition. Vol. 1, pp. 261–302. McGraw–Hill. New York.
16. MCINTOSH, J.M. 2000. Toxin antagonists of the neuronal nicotinic acetylcholine receptor. Handb. Exp. Pharmacol. **144:** 455–476.
17. GUNDERSON, C., C. LEHMANN, F. SIDELL *et al.* 1992. Nerve agents: a review. Neurology **42:** 946–950.
18. ENGEL, A., K. OHNO & S. SINE. 2002. The spectrum of congenital myasthenic syndromes. Mol. Neurobiol. In press.
19. LINDSTROM, J. 2000. Acetylcholine receptors and myasthenia. Muscle Nerve **23:** 453–477.
20. MATSUDA, K., S. BUCKINGHAM, D. KLEIER *et al.* 2001. Neonicotinoids: insecticides acting on nicotinic acetylcholine receptors. Trends Pharmacol. Sci. **22:** 573–580.
21. XU, W., S. GELBER, A. ORR-URTREGER *et al.* 1999. Megacystis, mydriasis, and ion channel defect in mice lacking the α3 neuronal nicotinic receptor. Proc. Natl. Acad. Sci. USA **96:** 5746–5751.
22. JONES, S., J. BOLAN & S. WONNACOTT. 2001. Presynaptic localization of the nicotinic acetylcholine receptor β2 subunit immunoreactivity in rat nigrostriatal dopaminergic neurons. J. Comp. Neurol. **439:** 235–247.
23. ALKONDON, M., E. PEREIRA, H. EISENBERG *et al.* 1999. Choline and selective antagonists identify two subtypes of nicotinic acetylcholine receptors that modulate GABA release from CAI interneurons in rat hippocampal slices. J. Neurosci. **19:** 2693–2705.
24. KULAK, J., J. MCINTOSH & M. QUIK. 2002. Loss of nicotinic receptors in monkey striatum after 1-methyl-4-phenyl-1,2,3,6-tetrahydropyridine treatment is due to a decline in α conotoxin M11 sites. Mol. Pharmacol. **61:** 230–238.

25. Shoop, R., E. Esquinazi, N. Yamada *et al.* 2002. Ultrastructure of a somatic spine mat for nicotinic signaling in neurons. J. Neurosci. **22:** 748–756.
26. Zoli, M., A. Jansson, E. Sykova *et al.* 1999. Volume transmission in the CNS and its relevance for neuropsychopharmacology. Trends Pharmacol. Sci. **20:** 142–150.
27. Grando, S. 2001. Receptor mediated action of nicotine in human skin. Int. J. Dermatol. **40:** 691–693.
28. Kawashima, K. & T. Fujii. 2000. Extraneuronal cholinergic system in lymphocytes. Pharmacol. Ther. **86:** 29–48.
29. Fischer, V., S. Reinhardt, E. Albuquerque *et al.* 1999. Expression of functional alpha 7 nicotinic acetylcholine receptor during mammalian muscle development and denervation. Eur. J. Neurosci. **11:** 2856–2864.
30. Orr-Urtreger, A., F. Goldner, M. Saeki *et al.* 1997. Mice deficient in the $\alpha7$ neuronal nicotinic acetylcholine receptor lack α bungarotoxin binding sites and hippocampal fast nicotinic currents. J. Neurosci. **17:** 9165–9171.
31. Conroy, W. & D. Berg. 1995. Neurons can maintain multiple classes of nicotinic acetylcholine receptors distinguished by different subunit compositions. J. Biol. Chem. **270:** 4424–4431.
32. Lena, C., M. de Kerchove d'Exaerde, M. Cordero-Erausquin *et al.* 1999. Diversity and distribution of nicotinic acetylcholine receptors in the locus ceruleus neurons. Proc. Natl. Acad. Sci. USA **96:** 12126–12131.
33. Missias, A., J. Mudd, J. Cunningham *et al.* 1997. Deficient development and maintenance of postsynaptic specializations in mutant mice lacking an "adult" acetylcholine receptor subunit. Development **124:** 5075–5086.
34. Steinlein, O. 2000. Neuronal nicotinic receptors in human epilepsy. Eur. J. Pharmacol. **393:** 243–247.
35. De Fusco, M., A. Becchetti, A. Patrignani *et al.* 2000. The nicotinic receptor $\beta2$ subunit is mutant in nocturnal frontal lobe epilepsy. Nat. Genet. **26:** 275–276.
36. Phillips, H., I. Favre, M. Kirkpatrick *et al.* 2001. CHRNB2 is the second acetylcholine receptor subunit associated with autosomal dominant nocturnal frontal lobe epilepsy. Am. J. Hum. Genet. **68:** 225–231.
37. Kuryatov, A., V. Gerzanich, M. Nelson *et al.* 1997. Mutation causing autosomal dominant nocturnal frontal lobe epilepsy alters Ca^{2+} permeability, conductance, and gating of human $\alpha4\beta2$ nicotinic acetylcholine receptors. J. Neurosci. **17:** 9035–9047.
38. Picciotto, M., B. Caldarone, S. King *et al.* 2002. Nicotinic receptors in the brain: links between molecular biology and behavior. Neuropsychopharmacology **22:** 451–465.
39. Xu, W., A. Orr-Urtreger, F. Nigro *et al.* 1999. Multiorgan autonomic dysfunction in mice lacking the $\beta2$ and $\beta4$ subunits of neuronal nicotinic acetylcholine receptors. J. Neurosci. **19:** 9298–9305.
40. Richardson, C., J. Morgan, B. Jasani *et al.* 2001. Megacystis-microcolon-intestinal hypoperistalsis syndrome and the absence of the $\alpha3$ nicotinic acetylcholine receptor subunit. Gastroenterology **121:** 350–357.
41. Champtiaux, N., Z-Y. Han, A. Bessis *et al.* 2002. Distribution and pharmacology of $\alpha6$-containing nicotinic acetylcholine receptors analyzed with mutant mice. J. Neurosci. **22:** 1207–1208.
42. Vetter, D., M. Liberman, J. Mann *et al.* 1999. Role of $\alpha9$ nicotinic ACh receptor subunits in the development and function of cochlear efferent innervation. Neuron **23:** 93–103.
43. Lustig, L., H. Peng, H. Hiel *et al.* 2001. Molecular cloning and mapping of the human nicotinic acetylcholine receptor $\alpha10$(CHRNA10). Genomics **73:** 272–283.
44. Elgoyhen, A., D. Vetter, E. Katz *et al.* 2001. Alpha 10: a determinant of nicotinic cholinergic receptor function in mammalian vestibular and cochlear mechanosensory hair cells. Proc. Natl. Acad. Sci. USA **98:** 3501–3506.
45. Labarca, C., J. Schwartz, P. Deshpande *et al.* 2001. Point mutant mice with hypersensitive $\alpha4$ nicotinic receptors show dopaminergic deficits and increased anxiety. Proc. Natl. Acad. Sci. USA **98:** 2786–2791.
46. Orr-Urtreger, A., R. Broide, M. Kasten *et al.* 2000. Mice homozygous for the L250T mutation in the $\alpha7$ nicotinic acetylcholine receptor show increased neuronal apoptosis and die within 1 day of birth. J. Neurochem. **74:** 2154–2166.

47. SHELTON, G. & J. LINDSTROM. 2001. Spontaneous remission in canine myasthenia gravis: implications for assessing human therapies. Neurology **57:** 2139–2141.
48. TZARTOS, S., T. BARKAS, M. CUNG *et al.* 1998. Anatomy of the antigenic structure of a large membrane autoantigen, the muscle-type nicotinic acetylcholine receptor. Immunol. Rev. **163:** 89–120.
49. SAEDI, M., R. ANAND, W. CONROY *et al.* 1990. Determination of amino acids critical to the main immunogenic region of intact acetylcholine receptors by *in vitro* mutagenesis. FEBS Lett. **267:** 55–59.
50. BEROUKHIM, R. & N. UNWIN. 1995. Three dimensional location of the main immunogenic region of the acetylcholine receptor. Neuron **15:** 323–331.
51. VERNINO, S., P. LOW, R. FEALEY *et al.* 2000. Autoantibodies to ganglionic acetylcholine receptors in autoimmune autonomic neuropathies. N. Engl. J. Med. **343:** 847–855.
52. WANG, F., M. NELSON, A. KURYATOV *et al.* 1998. Chronic nicotine treatment upregulates human α3β2, but not α3β4 AChRs stably transfected in human embryonic kidney cells. J. Biol. Chem. **273:** 28721–28732.
53. LAVER, W., G. AIR, R. WEBSTER *et al.* 1990. Epitopes on protein antigens: misconceptions and realities. Cell **61:** 553–556.
54. KONTON, M., D. LEONIDAS, E. VATZAKI *et al.* 2000. The crystal structure of the Fab fragment of a rat monoclonal antibody against the main immunogenic region of the human muscle acetylcholine receptor. Eur. J. Biochem. **267:** 2389–2396.
55. POULAS, K., E. ELIOPOULAS, E. VATZAKI *et al.* 2001. Crystal structure of Fab 198, an efficient protector of the acetylcholine receptor against myasthenogenic antibodies. Eur. J. Biochem. **268:** 3685–3693.
56. GRANDO, S. 2000. Autoimmunity to keratinocyte acetylcholine receptors in pemphigus. Dermatology **201:** 290–295.
57. DRACHMAN, D. 1994. Myasthenia gravis. N. Engl. J. Med. **330:** 1791–1810.
58. PETO, R., A. LOPEZ, J. BOUHAM *et al.* 1992. Mortality from tobacco in developed countries: indirect estimation from national vital statistics. Lancet **389:** 1268–1278.
59. DANI, J., D. JI & F-M. ZHOU. 2001. Synaptic plasticity and nicotine addiction. Neuron **31:** 349–352.
60. LLOYD, K. & M. WILLIAMS. 2000. Neuronal nicotinic acetylcholine receptors as novel drug targets. J. Pharmacol. Exp. Ther. **292:** 461–467.
61. LEUTJE, C. & J. PATRICK. 1991. Both α and β subunits contribute to the agonist sensitivity of neuronal nicotinic acetylcholine receptors. J. Neurosci. **11:** 837–845.
62. BENOWITZ, N. 1996. Pharmacology of nicotine: addiction and therapeutics. Annu. Rev. Pharmacol. Toxicol. **36:** 597–613.
63. LIU, Q., H. KAWAL & D. BERG. 2001. β amyloid peptide blocks the response of α7-containing nicotinic receptors on hippocampal neurons. Proc. Natl. Acad. Sci. USA **98:** 4734–4739.
64. NAGELE, R., M. D'ANDREA, W. ANDERSON *et al.* 2002. Intracellular accumulation of β-amyloid$_{1-42}$ in neurons is facilitated by the α7 nicotinic acetylcholine receptor in Alzheimer's disease. Neuroscience **110:** 199–211.
65. LEONARD, S., L. ADLER, K. BENHAMMOU *et al.* 2001. Smoking and mental illness. Pharmacol. Biochem. Behav. **70:** 561–570.

Synapse-Specific Gene Expression at the Neuromuscular Junction

ALEXANDRE MÉJAT, AYMERIC RAVEL-CHAPUIS, MARIE VANDROMME, AND LAURENT SCHAEFFER

Equipe Différenciation Neuromusculaire, UMR 5161 CNRS/ENS, Ecole Normale Supérieure de Lyon, Lyon, France

ABSTRACT: Agrin is the key neural factor that controls muscle postsynaptic differentiation, including the induction of synapse-specific transcription via neuregulins. In 1995, the promoter element responsible for the targeting of AChR δ and ϵ gene transcription to the skeletal muscle subsynaptic area was identified. This element, named N-box, recruits the Ets-related transcription factor GABP to AChR δ and ϵ promoters, and both the N-box and GABP are required to obtain transcriptional stimulation by neuregulins. The physiological importance of the N-box has been definitively established with the discovery of myasthenic families carrying single-point mutations in the N-box of the AChR ϵ gene promoter and showing reduced levels of AChR ϵ subunit expression. The control of synapse-specific transcription by agrin and neuregulins through the N-box and GABP is not restricted to the case of AChR genes. The same regulation holds true for the ACh esterase and utrophin genes, thus showing that nerve-induced transcriptional activation of several synapse-specific genes is triggered by a common mechanism involving agrin, neuregulins, and ultimately the N-box and Ets-related transcription factors.

KEYWORDS: neuromuscular junction (NMJ); acetylcholine receptor (AChR); transcription; neuregulins; GABP

INTRODUCTION

Multinucleated muscle fibers form by fusion of precursor myoblasts and are innervated shortly after by the axons of motor neurons. Concomitant to innervation, the proteins that will constitute the postsynaptic scaffold become highly concentrated in the central region of the myotubes in order to create a highly specialized structure entirely dedicated to the communication between the nerve and the muscle. Among the proteins that accumulate at the neuromuscular junction (NMJ), the nicotinic acetylcholine receptor (AChR) plays a particular role because it allows the transmission of the nerve influx to the muscle. The fetal AChR is a heteropentameric cationic

Address for correspondence: Laurent Schaeffer, Equipe Différenciation Neuromusculaire, UMR 5161 CNRS/ENS, Ecole Normale Supérieure de Lyon, 46 allée d'Italie, 69364 Lyon cedex 07, France. Voice: +33-472-728-573; fax: +33-472-728-080.
lschaeff@ens-lyon.fr

Ann. N.Y. Acad. Sci. 998: 53–65 (2003). **© 2003 New York Academy of Sciences.**
doi: 10.1196/annals.1254.008

ion-gated channel composed of four subunits, $\alpha_2\beta\gamma\delta$. In mammals, after birth, the γ subunit is replaced by the ε subunit in order to modify the electrophysiological properties of the receptor. (See FIG. 1.)

The AChR is an excellent marker of synaptic differentiation. Indeed, before innervation, it is uniformly distributed at the surface of the myotubes to an average density of 100 molecules/μm^2. After the NMJ has formed, the AChR density increases to 10,000 molecules/μm^2 at the synapse, whereas it drops to less than 10 molecules/μm^2 in the remainder of the fiber. This redistribution of the AChR originates from two distinct processes: first, the physical clustering of AChRs at the NMJ (along with the other components of the subneural network); second, the restriction of the AChR gene transcription to a few nuclei, the fundamental nuclei, located directly under the synapse. This compartmentalization of expression also results from the combined action of two regulation pathways.

On the one hand, the muscle electrical activity, triggered by the binding of the ACh released by the nerve terminal to the AChR accumulated at the NMJ, represses AChR gene transcription in extrasynaptic nuclei.[1] This repression is calcium-dependent and involves calcium-dependent kinases.[2] The best-described targets of this pathway are the bHLH myogenic factors.[3] Indeed, the blockade of electrical activity (by denervation or sodium channel blockade by tetrodotoxin) results in the reexpression of the fetal form of AChR in the extrasynaptic nuclei.[4–7] This reexpression can be blocked by mutating the myogenic factor binding sites, the E-boxes, in AChR gene promoters.[8,9] However, E-boxes are not sufficient and must cooperate with other promoter elements for the regulation of AChR gene expression by electrical activity.[10]

On the other hand, specific signals located at the NMJ stimulate the expression of synapse-specific genes, including AChR genes, in subsynaptic nuclei. This review will primarily focus on the recent advances that have been made in the characterization of the mechanisms leading to synapse-specific gene activation. The recent finding that these mechanisms preexist in the muscle independently of innervation will also be discussed.

FIGURE 1. A model for postsynaptic scaffold formation at the neuromuscular junction. Activation of the tyrosine kinase receptor MuSK, reinforced by z-agrin, induces the formation of the postsynaptic scaffold, which includes the clustering of AChR and rapsyn via Src kinases. MuSK and z-agrin also activate the transcription of synaptic genes in subsynaptic nuclei via neuregulins. The binding of neuregulins to their erbB2/3/4 receptors triggers both the MAPK and JNK kinase pathways via Ras and finally leads to the activation of the Ets-related transcription factor GABP, probably by phosphorylation. Phosphorylated GABPα/β then activates the expression of synapse-specific genes upon binding to the N-box. In extrasynaptic nuclei, nerve-evoked electrical activity leads to the repression of many synapse-specific genes via the activation of calcium-dependent serine/threonine kinases and the subsequent inhibition of the bHLH myogenic factors (for review, see ref. 1). *Terms*: AChR, acetylcholine receptor; MuSK, muscle-specific kinase; DGC, dystrophin glycoprotein complex; GABP, GA binding protein.

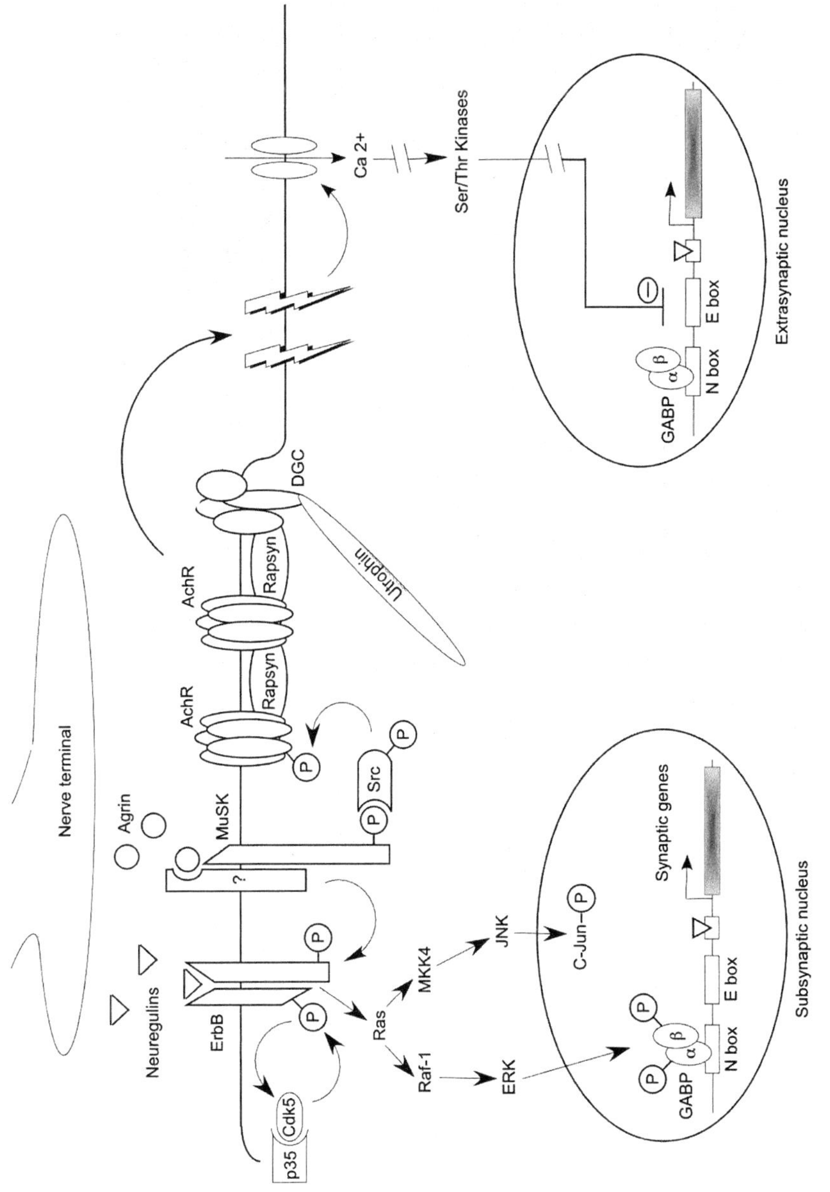

FIGURE 1. *See previous page for legend.*

THE AGRIN/MuSK PATHWAY AND MUSCLE PREPATTERNING

Among the nerve-derived signals produced by the motor neuron, agrin is undoubtfully the one that plays the most important role in NMJ formation. Agrin is a heparan sulfate proteoglycan first identified in the *Torpedo californica* electric organ basement membrane as an activity that promotes aggregation of AChRs in muscle cells.[11] Both the muscles and the motor nerve transcribe the agrin gene, but they differentially splice the resulting RNA. The nerve-specific spliced isoform z-agrin is 1000- to 10,000-fold more active than the muscle isoforms in inducing AChR clustering in cultured myotubes.[12]

The analysis of agrin knockout mice initially suggested that neural agrin was the starting point of the whole postsynaptic differentiation program.[13] Indeed, in these mice, very few NMJs were present at birth and both AChR clustering and synapse-specific gene expression were abolished, thus demonstrating that *in vivo* neural agrin is necessary for both the clustering of the subneural protein network and the activation of synaptic gene transcription in subsynaptic nuclei.

Over the past few years, several components of the muscle cell surface, including α-dystroglycan and MuSK, have been identified as potential candidate receptors for agrin.[14] The muscle-specific kinase, MuSK, has been shown to be an essential part of such an agrin receptor even if no direct interaction between agrin and MuSK has been demonstrable. Indeed, myotubes lacking MuSK are not responsive to agrin and, in C2C12 myotubes, agrin can be cross-linked to MuSK and triggers its phosphorylation.[15,16] The phenotype of MuSK knockout mice is reminiscent of what was observed in agrin-deficient mice because both synapse-specific transcription and clustering of synaptic gene products are abolished.[17] The MuSK-induced AChR clustering is mediated by the 43K/rapsyn protein, most likely through direct protein-protein interactions.[1] The Src-related family kinases, Src, Fyn, and Fyk, have been proposed to participate in the MuSK- and rapsyn-dependent AChR clustering. Indeed, they phosphorylate MuSK, rapsyn, and AChR, and their inhibition reduces the agrin-induced AChR clustering in cultured myotubes.[18–20]

Additional evidence of the pivotal role of agrin and MuSK came from the finding that the introduction in muscle extrasynaptic areas of expression constructs coding for either agrin or a constitutively active form of MuSK induces formation of ectopic pseudosynapses in the absence of any nerve terminal.[21,22] These ectopic pseudosynapses possess almost all the hallmarks of the postsynaptic region of the NMJ. In addition, fundamental nuclei having the same morphology and transcript expression program as the classical subsynaptic nuclei form under these pseudosynapses.[22]

From these numerous results, a model has emerged in which agrin-stimulated activation of MuSK triggers postsynaptic organization and activates the expression of synaptic genes at the onset of innervation. However, recent studies have demonstrated that both the expression of synaptic genes and the clustering of postsynaptic proteins are somehow prepatterned in the central region of the muscle fiber before innervation.[23] Indeed, the analysis of mutant mice with aneural diaphragm[24,25] revealed that AChR proteins were clustered in the central part of the diaphragm muscle fibers, although the motor nerve and thus neural agrin were absent. Moreover, the mRNAs coding for the AChR α and δ subunits were also enriched in this central region. These results demonstrate that both AChR distribution and gene expression are prepatterned in skeletal muscle in the absence of motor innervation. The roles of agrin and MuSK in this nerve-independent control of AChR expression were investigated by a double knockout mice approach. As expected, AChR clusters were also confined to the central region of the diaphragm in double mutants with aneural diaphragm and a deficiency in neural agrin. Conversely, no evidence of AChR clustering or preferential expression was observed in double mutants with aneural diaphragm and a deficiency in MuSK, thus demonstrating that MuSK, but not neural agrin, is required to pattern AChR expression in the absence of motor innervation.

In agrin-deficient mice, muscle self-patterning is very transient, whereas it persists up to birth in aneural muscles. This suggests that the nerve produces an agrin-independent negative signal that abolishes synaptic protein clustering and gene expression in the absence of agrin. This repressive signal could be acetylcholine, which triggers muscle electrical activity upon binding to muscle AChRs. This self-patterning ability of the muscle is not just a "default program" activated by the absence of motor innervation because, in wild-type mice, muscle fibers with central AChR accumulation can be detected.

From these results, we raised a model in which the muscle postsynaptic scaffold is prepatterned in a MuSK-dependent, agrin-independent fashion. Motor innervation would then refine the postsynaptic area by both destabilizing AChR clusters that are not directly in apposition to the nerve terminal and reinforcing the MuSK-dependent pathways with neural agrin at the site of innervation. However, this leaves open the questions of both the necessity and the role of such a prepatterning mechanism. Indeed, in MuSK heterozygote mice, AChR prepatterning is weaker than in wild-type animals, whereas NMJ formation does not seem to be affected.

NMJ formation was very recently analyzed carefully in various skeletal muscles in mouse embryos.[26] This study surprisingly revealed that skeletal muscles, independent of their fast or slow type, could be classified in two distinct categories, respectively named fast and delayed synapsing muscles, by function of the sharpness of AChR prepatterning and the speed of presynaptic maturation. In fast synapsing muscles, the clustering of AChRs as well as the alignment of nerve terminals and Schwann cells to AChR clusters are achieved in less than one day. In contrast, in delayed synapsing muscles such as the diaphragm, the completion of this process requires up to five days. The fast or delayed synapsing character is an intrinsic property of the muscle because the absence of motor innervation does not affect the fast or delayed AChR clustering phenotype of a given muscle. At birth, the NMJs formed by these two muscle classes are indistinguishable, but in young adult mice differences persist regarding their response to destabilizing treatments such as denervation or chronic blockade of neurotransmission. Such treatments induce in one month a nearly complete disassembly of the original AChR clusters together with the formation of ectopic AChR clusters in delayed synapsing muscles, whereas in fast synapsing muscles the original AChR clusters are still present and ectopic AChR clusters do not form. Interestingly, although the two classes of muscles seem to have equivalent distributions of MuSK, the fast and delayed synapsing phenotypes seem to be somehow correlated to a respectively low or high sensitivity of AChR clusters to the lack of agrin.

The existence of two classes of muscles exhibiting different sensitivities to NMJ destabilizing conditions suggests that delayed synapsing muscles could be more affected than fast synapsing muscles in diseases of either the NMJ or the motor neuron, such as myasthenia or spinal muscular atrophy. In addition, the finding that AChR clusters can be protected from destabilization by neural agrin could be of interest for new therapeutic investigations.

THE NEUREGULIN/ERBB PATHWAY AND THE ACTIVATION OF ACHR GENE EXPRESSION

In both innervated and aneural contexts, the local activation of AChR expression is dependent on MuSK, whose action is greatly potentiated by neural agrin. Synaptic gene activation by agrin and MuSK is probably an indirect mechanism involving the erbB tyrosine kinase receptors and their peptidic ligands, neuregulins. Indeed, in cultured myotubes, transcriptional activation of the AChR ε subunit gene by agrin can be prevented by a dominant negative mutant of erbB2.[27] In addition, *in vivo*, ectopic expression of either agrin or a constitutively active form of MuSK causes synaptic gene ectopic expression, together with the clustering of neuregulins and their receptors.[22,27] Neuregulins and their receptors thus likely act as second messengers to agrin and MuSK for the local activation of synaptic gene expression.

Neuregulins are produced both by nerve and muscle.[28] In the nervous system, they were first identified as ARIA (acetylcholine receptor–inducing activity), a 42-kDa polypeptide purified from chick brain that stimulates AChR expression in cultured myotubes.[29,30] ARIA, also known as heregulin β, neu-differentiation factor, or neuregulin β1, is encoded by the neuregulin 1 gene that codes for 14 members generated by alternative splicing.[31] Neuregulins are ligands for the transmembrane receptor tyrosine kinases of the erbB family.

Several lines of evidence support the idea that *in vivo* neuregulins and their receptors activate synaptic gene transcription in subsynaptic nuclei. First, ARIA is concentrated at synaptic sites in the synaptic basal lamina.[32] In addition, erbB2, erbB3, and erbB4 are also concentrated at the NMJ.[1,33,34] Although erbB2 and erbB3 are enriched at agrin-induced ectopic synapses in muscle,[22,32,35] a recent analysis of erbB receptor distribution at the NMJ in confocal microscopy shows that erbB2 and erbB4 would be localized in the postsynaptic muscle membrane, whereas erbB3 would rather be located in the terminal Schwann cells, thus suggesting that erbB2 and erbB4 constitute the muscle postsynaptic receptor for neuregulins.[1] Second, a promoter element required for synapse-specific expression, the N-box, has been identified in several synaptic genes,[36–38] and this element has also been shown to be essential for the transcriptional activation by neuregulins in cultured myotubes.[39–42]

Gene inactivation strategies in mice have not allowed a clear confirmation of the importance of neuregulins and erbB receptors in the control of synaptic gene expression. Indeed, mice lacking ARIA, erbB2, or erbB4 die at embryonic day 10.5 because of cardiac defects, 4 days prior to NMJ formation.[1] Nevertheless, mice heterozygous for ARIA are myasthenic because of a 50% reduction in AChR molecules compared to wild-type animals.[30] The cardiac defect has been corrected in erbB2-deficient mice by the cardiac expression of an erbB2 transgene, thus allowing the embryos to develop up to birth.[43,44] However, the major phenotype of these animals was a lack of Schwann cells and Schwann cell precursors, which resulted in the death of most motor and sensory neurons, thus rendering difficult the interpretation of gene expression perturbations at the NMJ. The muscle postsynaptic phenotype of these animals has nevertheless been analyzed in detail before axon withdrawal, and it appears that the formation of junctional folds is perturbed.[45] Given the new data obtained concerning muscle prepatterning of AChR gene expression, the reexamination of neuregulins or erbB genes in knockout mice to analyze this prepatterning (which is not affected by the motor neuron or Schwann cells) would probably yield new insight on the role of neuregulins and their receptors in the *in vivo* activation of synaptic gene expression.

SIGNAL TRANSDUCTION PATHWAYS ACTIVATED BY NEUREGULINS

The binding of neuregulins to their receptors results in the phosphorylation of tyrosine residues in the intracellular domains of the erbB proteins that create binding sites for various intracellular proteins. Such recruited factors and the downstream activated pathways have been intensively investigated in muscle.

The small G protein Ras and the subsequent mitogen-activated protein (MAP) kinase transduction pathway play a pivotal role in neuregulin-induced gene activation.[46–48] Indeed, ARIA induces a rapid activation of ERK1 and ERK2 in cultured myotubes, and inhibition of ERK2 abolishes the activation of AChR expression by ARIA.[46,47] Moreover, expression of constitutively active Ras or Raf mimics the ARIA-induced activation of AChR genes.[46] Finally, the expression of dominant negative mutants of Ras, Raf, or MEK *in vivo* greatly reduces the ARIA-induced activation of the AChR ε subunit expression.[48]

In addition to the requirement of ERK2, dominant negative mutants of MKK4, JNK, or c-jun have been shown to block the AChR ε subunit gene by ARIA. The JNK pathway and the transcription factor c-jun that it phosphorylates thus seem to be involved in the activation of synaptic genes by ARIA.[49] The kinetics of activation by ARIA suggests that it could be achieved by a multistep process. Indeed, the treatment of C2C12 myotubes with ARIA results in the activation of the immediate early genes c-fos and c-jun within a few minutes, whereas activation of the AChR ε subunit gene becomes detectable only five hours later.[49]

Recently, the cyclin-dependent kinase cdk5 and its activator p35 were shown to accumulate at the NMJ and to interact with phosphorylated erbB subunits. They are activated by erbB and seem to be themselves involved in erbB activation in C2C12 myotubes.[50]

Finally, another kinase, the phosphatidylinositol-3-kinase (PI3K), has been shown to be recruited and activated by erbB receptors.[46] In this initial work, inhibition of the PI3K abolished the activation of a reporter gene placed downstream of the AChR ε subunit promoter. Moreover, a constitutively active form of the PI3K could mimic the effect of ARIA on the reporter gene expression, thus suggesting that the PI3K pathway is required for synapse-specific gene activation. However, opposite results have been obtained since then. In one case, the inhibition of the PI3K by wortmannin failed to antagonize the stimulation of the AChR α subunit expression by ARIA, but conversely increased the AChR α subunit mRNA level in chick primary myotubes.[47] In the second case, wortmannin had no effect on the activation of the AChR α and ε gene expression by ARIA in C2C12 myotubes.[48] The physiological significance of such contradictory results is not currently clear, but could reflect intrinsic species and/or cell line specificities or could originate from the various protocols used to measure activation by ARIA (reporter genes transiently or stably transfected, or endogenous mRNA quantification).

IDENTIFICATION OF THE N-BOX

The ultimate targets of the signal transduction pathways triggered by neuregulins are specific transcription factors that activate the transcription of synapse-specific genes upon binding to defined promoter elements. The major promoter element involved in the transcriptional response to neuregulins in muscle was initially identified as the N-box, a 6-base-pair element indispensable for the synapse-specific expression of the AChR δ and ε subunit genes.[36,37] Subsequently, this element was demonstrated to be also required for the neuregulin-induced activation of several synaptic genes.

To identify promoter elements involved in the targeting of synapse-specific gene transcription to the NMJ, an *in vivo* DNA injection technique was used. A large number of constructs containing the β-galactosidase gene placed downstream of AChR δ and ε mutated promoters were injected, and the synaptic expression of the reporter gene was evaluated for each mutant.[36,37] This approach allowed the identification of a critical Ets-binding site, which was named the N-box. In addition, when fused to a minimal promoter, the N-box can confer preferential synaptic expression to a reporter gene.[36]

The critical role of the N-box in synapse-specific expression of the AChR δ subunit was subsequently confirmed in transgenic mice.[40] Indeed, in such mice, a 1848-bp fragment of the mouse AChR δ subunit promoter confers synapse-specific expression to a reporter gene, whereas the mutation of the N-box in this context totally abolishes the expression of the transgene in innervated muscle. Conversely, in response to denervation, the transgene is expressed all along the muscle fiber, and the mutation of the N-box does not affect this pattern. Since the mutation of the N-box in the AChR δ subunit promoter neither induces extrasynaptic expression in innervated muscle nor affects the derepression of transcription after denervation, the N-box is probably not involved in the control of gene expression by electrical activity.

The most convincing demonstration of the physiological importance of the N-box came from the genetic characterization of myasthenic patients. Single-point mutations were identified in the N-box of the AChR ε promoter of three unrelated patients suffering from mild congenital myasthenia.[51–53] The mutations identified in the patients were previously shown to produce an 80% decrease in the synaptic expression specificity of a reporter gene placed downstream of the mouse AChR ε subunit promoter.[37] Consistently, the muscle content in AChR ε subunit gene mRNA was found to be reduced in two of the patients.[51,53]

The function of the N-box does not seem to be restricted to AChR genes because, using the *in vivo* DNA injection technique, it has been shown to control the synaptic expression of the utrophin and ACh esterase genes.[38,41,54] Besides its central role in the synapse-specific expression of several genes, the N-box has also been shown to be required for the ARIA-induced transcriptional activation of either the AChR ε subunit or utrophin promoters in cultured myotubes.[38,42]

The critical role of the N-box for both synaptic expression and response to ARIA of several genes strengthens the notion that neuregulins are probably responsible for the transcriptional activation of synaptic genes initiated by MuSK.

N-BOX BINDS THE ETS-RELATED TRANSCRIPTION FACTOR GABPα/β

The fact that several genes depend on the same promoter element for their activation in subsynaptic nuclei suggests that a common transcription factor could regulate their transcription. The N-box contains the GGAA core binding sequence for transcription factors of the Ets family,[55] and a general Ets transdominant negative mutant has been shown to efficiently block the N-box-dependent response to neuregulins in cultured myotubes.[42] Moreover, overexpression of the rat muscle Ets-2 transcription factor resulted in an N-box-dependent activation of the AChR ε subunit promoter.[42] At the same time, a DNA affinity chromatography strategy allowed the purification of the transcription factor previously shown to bind the N-box in gel retardation experiments.[36,37,39] This transcription factor is the heterodimer GABP (GA binding protein) α/β.[39] The 58-kDa GABP α subunit contains a characteristic Ets DNA-binding domain, while the 43-kDa GABP β subunit does not contact DNA, but dimerizes with GABPα via ankyrin repeats and thus induces the nuclear translocation of the heterodimer and strengthens the binding of the α subunit to DNA.[56,57]

Given the role of the N-box in regulating the expression of the utrophin, AChE, and AChR δ and ε subunit genes, the implication of GABP in the transcriptional control of these genes was investigated *in vitro* and *in vivo*. In cultured myotubes, GABP activates the expression of the utrophin gene by binding to the N-box,[38,41] and the expression of a dominant negative mutant of either GABP α or β inhibits the expression of reporter genes controlled by the AChR δ and ε promoters.[39] *In vivo*, overexpression of a GABPβ dominant negative mutant was shown to reduce the expression of a coinjected reporter gene controlled by the AChR ε subunit promoter.[58] Transcriptional activation via the N-box is thus most likely due to the recruitment of GABP on N-box-containing promoters. This observation implies that GABP must participate in the transcriptional activation by agrin and neuregulins and in the synapse-specific expression of synaptic genes. Indeed, the GABP α and β dominant negative mutants inhibit the ARIA-induced stimulation of the AChR δ and ε promoters in cultured myotubes.[39] In addition, *in vivo*, the GABP dominant negative mutant inhibits the formation of agrin-induced postsynaptic structures in innervated muscle fibers and reduces the local activation of the utrophin and AChE genes by agrin.[58]

The determination of the expression pattern of GABP by *in situ* hybridization revealed that the expression of GABPα and β is not restricted to the neuromuscular region, but takes place all along the muscle fiber, although GABPα mRNA is enriched in the synaptic area.[39] These observations suggest that, in order to specifically obtain activation by GABP in subsynaptic nuclei, the nerve must provide signals that confer local competence to GABP. This could be obtained by phosphorylation because neuregulins were shown to induce the phosphorylation of both GABP subunits in cultured myotubes.[39,59] However, the effects of these phosphorylations on the transactivating potential of GABP remains to be determined.

Some synaptic genes, like the AChR α subunit gene, do not contain a canonical N-box in their promoter, although all of them most likely contain at least one core Ets-binding sequence, GGAA. Since the binding site specificity of Ets transcription factors, including GABP, is quite large, it will be interesting to determine whether these genes are regulated by GABP or whether an additional mechanism exists to obtain muscle synapse-specific expression in vertebrates. The results obtained with the GABP β mutant on the induction of synaptic genes by ectopic expression of agrin suggest that the expression of some synaptic genes, including MuSK and rapsyn, is not dependent on GABP[58] and thus that such an additional mechanism, which could be transcriptional or posttranscriptional, probably does exist.

CONCLUSIONS

Because of its large size and accessibility, the NMJ provides a favorable model to investigate the factors and mechanisms involved in synapse formation. Even if many aspects of NMJ formation still remain to be elucidated, the numerous results obtained during the last few decades permit a detailed scheme of the different neural and muscular factors leading to the formation of this highly specialized structure. The current model includes at least two major postsynaptic programs initiated by MuSK and leading respectively to synaptic protein clustering (e.g., agrin-MuSK/Src/rapsyn) and to synapse-specific gene expression (e.g., agrin-MuSK/ARIA-ErbB/MAPK/GABP). Although the N-box and GABP are essential for synaptic expression of several genes, they most likely cooperate with other promoter elements and transcription factors, such as Sp1 and Sp3, to activate transcription in subsynaptic nuclei.[60] In addition, the expression of some synaptic genes does not seem to be controlled by an N-box, and it will be interesting to determine which mechanisms confer synapse-specific expression to them.

Recent analysis of the respective roles of the muscle and the motoneuron in the control of these programs has shown that the muscle can autonomously initiate the formation of the postsynaptic region. The action of the nerve terminal would then be dual. On the one hand, the nerve would locally strengthen and stabilize synaptic gene activation and synaptic protein clustering through the activation of MuSK with neural agrin. On the other hand, the nerve would downregulate both of these processes in extrasynaptic areas according to an agrin-independent mechanism, possibly triggered by electrical activity.

Many factors involved in the induction, formation, or maintenance of the NMJ are also implicated in human diseases. The recent finding that synaptic expression of the utrophin gene is controlled by an N-box and ARIA has conferred a direct medical interest to this field of research. Indeed, when expressed all along the dystrophic muscle fibers, utrophin has been proposed to compensate for the lack of dystrophin in patients with Duchenne muscular dystrophy (DMD).[61,62] Hence, the demonstration that ARIA and GABP could stimulate utrophin expression *in vivo* has direct implications for the treatment of DMD and defines new pharmacological targets for the stimulation of utrophin expression in patients with DMD.[38,41] Progress made in the study of muscle synaptic genes and their regulation thus opens new approaches to therapeutic investigations for neuromuscular diseases such as DMD[38] or myasthenia.[51,52]

REFERENCES

1. SANES, J.R. & J.W. LICHTMAN. 1999. Development of the vertebrate neuromuscular junction. Annu. Rev. Neurosci. **22:** 389–442.
2. ALTIOK, N. & J.P. CHANGEUX. 2001. Electrical activity regulates AChR gene expression via JNK, PKCzeta, and Sp1 in skeletal chick muscle. FEBS Lett. **487:** 333–338.
3. DUCLERT, A. *et al.* 1991. Influence of innervation of myogenic factors and acetylcholine receptor alpha-subunit mRNAs. Neuroreport **2:** 25–28.
4. FONTAINE, B. *et al.* 1988. Detection of the nicotinic acetylcholine receptor alpha-subunit mRNA by *in situ* hybridization at neuromuscular junctions of 15-day-old chick striated muscles. EMBO J. **7:** 603–609.
5. GOLDMAN, D. *et al.* 1988. Acetylcholine receptor alpha-, beta-, gamma-, and delta-subunit mRNA levels are regulated by muscle activity. Neuron **1:** 329–333.
6. FONTAINE, B. & J.P. CHANGEUX. 1989. Localization of nicotinic acetylcholine receptor alpha-subunit transcripts during myogenesis and motor endplate development in the chick. J. Cell Biol. **108:** 1025–1037.
7. TSAY, H.J. & J. SCHMIDT. 1989. Skeletal muscle denervation activates acetylcholine receptor genes. J. Cell Biol. **108:** 1523–1526.
8. BESSEREAU, J.L. *et al.* 1994. *In vivo* and *in vitro* analysis of electrical activity–dependent expression of muscle acetylcholine receptor genes using adenovirus. Proc. Natl. Acad. Sci. USA **91:** 1304–1308.
9. TANG, J. *et al.* 1994. Separate pathways for synapse-specific and electrical activity–dependent gene expression in skeletal muscle. Development **120:** 1799–1804.
10. BESSEREAU, J.L. *et al.* 1998. Nonmyogenic factors bind nicotinic acetylcholine receptor promoter elements required for response to denervation. J. Biol. Chem. **273:** 12786–12793.
11. NITKIN, R.M. *et al.* 1987. Identification of agrin, a synaptic organizing protein from *Torpedo* electric organ. J. Cell Biol. **105:** 2471–2478.
12. BURGESS, R.W. *et al.* 1999. Alternatively spliced isoforms of nerve- and muscle-derived agrin: their roles at the neuromuscular junction. Neuron **23:** 33–44.
13. RUEGG, M.A. & J.L. BIXBY. 1998. Agrin orchestrates synaptic differentiation at the vertebrate neuromuscular junction. Trends Neurosci. **21:** 22–27.
14. SANES, J.R. *et al.* 1998. Agrin receptors at the skeletal neuromuscular junction. Ann. N.Y. Acad. Sci. **841:** 1–13.
15. GLASS, D. *et al.* 1996. Agrin acts via a MuSK receptor complex. Cell **85:** 513–523.
16. GLASS, D. *et al.* 1997. MuSK kinase domain is sufficient for phosphorylation, but not clustering of acetylcholine receptors. Proc. Natl. Acad. Sci. USA **94:** 8848–8853.
17. DECHIARA, T.M. *et al.* 1996. The receptor tyrosine kinase MuSK is required for neuromuscular junction formation *in vivo*. Cell **85:** 501–512.
18. FUHRER, C. & Z.W. HALL. 1996. Functional interaction of Src family kinases with the acetylcholine receptor in C2 myotubes. J. Biol. Chem. **271:** 32474–32481.
19. MITTAUD, P. *et al.* 2001. Agrin-induced activation of acetylcholine receptor–bound Src family kinases requires rapsyn and correlates with acetylcholine receptor clustering. J. Biol. Chem. **276:** 14505–14513.
20. MOHAMED, A.S. *et al.* 2001. Src-class kinases act within the agrin/MuSK pathway to regulate acetylcholine receptor phosphorylation, cytoskeletal anchoring, and clustering. J. Neurosci. **21:** 3806–3818.
21. JONES, G. *et al.* 1997. Induction by agrin of ectopic and functional postsynaptic-like membrane in innervated muscle. Proc. Natl. Acad. Sci. USA **94:** 2654–2659.
22. JONES, G. *et al.* 1999. Constitutively active MuSK is clustered in the absence of agrin and induces ectopic postsynaptic-like membranes in skeletal muscle fibers. J. Neurosci. **19:** 3376–3383.
23. FERNS, M. & S. CARBONETTO. 2001. Challenging the neurocentric view of neuromuscular synapse formation. Neuron **30:** 311–314.
24. LIN, W. *et al.* 2001. Distinct roles of nerve and muscle in postsynaptic differentiation of the neuromuscular synapse. Nature **410:** 1057–1064.
25. YANG, X. *et al.* 2001 Patterning of muscle acetylcholine receptor gene expression in the absence of motor innervation. Neuron **30:** 399–410.

26. Pun, S. *et al.* 2002. An intrinsic distinction in neuromuscular junction assembly and maintenance in different skeletal muscles. Neuron **34:** 357–370.
27. Meier, T. *et al.* 1998. Agrin can mediate acetylcholine receptor gene expression in muscle by aggregation of muscle-derived neuregulins. J. Cell Biol. **141:** 715–726.
28. Jo, S.A. *et al.* 1995. Neuregulins are concentrated at nerve-muscle synapses and activate ACh-receptor gene expression. Nature **373:** 158–161.
29. Falls, D.L. *et al.* 1993. ARIA, a protein that stimulates acetylcholine receptor synthesis, is a member of the neu ligand family. Cell **72:** 801–815.
30. Sandrock, A.W. *et al.* 1997. Maintenance of acetylcholine receptor number by neuregulins at the neuromuscular junction *in vivo*. Science **276:** 599–603.
31. Fischbach, G.D. & K.M. Rosen. 1997. ARIA: a neuromuscular junction neuregulin. Annu. Rev. Neurosci. **20:** 429–458.
32. Rimer, M. *et al.* 1998. Neuregulins and erbB receptors at neuromuscular junctions and at agrin-induced postsynaptic-like apparatus in skeletal muscle. Mol. Cell. Neurosci. **12:** 1–15.
33. Moscoso, L.M. *et al.* 1995. Synapse-associated expression of an acetylcholine receptor–inducing protein, ARIA/heregulin, and its putative receptors, ErbB2 and ErbB3, in developing mammalian muscle. Dev. Biol. **172:** 158–169.
34. Altiok, N. *et al.* 1995. ErbB3 and ErbB2/neu mediate the effect of heregulin on acetylcholine receptor gene expression in muscle: differential expression at the endplate. EMBO J. **14:** 4258–4266.
35. Meier, T. *et al.* 1997. Neural agrin induces ectopic postsynaptic specializations in innervated muscle fibers. J. Neurosci. **17:** 6534–6544.
36. Koike, S. *et al.* 1995. Identification of a DNA element determining synaptic expression of the mouse acetylcholine receptor delta-subunit gene. Proc. Natl. Acad. Sci. USA **92:** 10624–10628.
37. Duclert, A. *et al.* 1996. Identification of an element crucial for the sub-synaptic expression of the acetylcholine receptor epsilon-subunit gene. J. Biol. Chem. **271:** 17433–17438.
38. Gramolini, A.O. *et al.* 1999. Induction of utrophin gene expression by heregulin in skeletal muscle cells: role of the N-box motif and GA binding protein. Proc. Natl. Acad. Sci. USA **96:** 3223–3227.
39. Schaeffer, L. *et al.* 1998. Implication of a multisubunit Ets-related transcription factor in synaptic expression of the nicotinic acetylcholine receptor. EMBO J. **17:** 3078–3090.
40. Fromm, L. & S.J. Burden. 1998. Synapse-specific and neuregulin-induced transcription require an ets site that binds GABPalpha/GABPbeta. Genes Dev. **12:** 3074–3083.
41. Khurana, T.S. *et al.* 1999. Activation of utrophin promoter by heregulin via the ets-related transcription factor complex GA-binding protein alpha/beta. Mol. Biol. Cell **10:** 2075–2086.
42. Sapru, M.K. *et al.* 1998. Identification of a neuregulin and protein-tyrosine phosphatase response element in the nicotinic acetylcholine receptor epsilon subunit gene: regulatory role of an Ets transcription factor. Proc. Natl. Acad. Sci. USA **95:** 1289–1294.
43. Woldeyesus, M.T. *et al.* 1999. Peripheral nervous system defects in erbB2 mutants following genetic rescue of heart development. Genes Dev. **13:** 2538–2548.
44. Morris, J.K. *et al.* 1999. Rescue of the cardiac defect in ErbB2 mutant mice reveals essential roles of ErbB2 in peripheral nervous system development. Neuron **23:** 273–283.
45. Lin, W. *et al.* 2001. Distinct roles of nerve and muscle in postsynaptic differentiation of the neuromuscular synapse. Nature **410:** 1057–1064.
46. Tansey, M.G. *et al.* 1996. ARIA/HRG regulates AChR epsilon subunit gene expression at the neuromuscular synapse via activation of phosphatidylinositol 3-kinase and Ras/MAPK pathway. J. Cell Biol. **134:** 465–476.
47. Altiok, N. *et al.* 1997. Heregulin-stimulated acetylcholine receptor gene expression in muscle: requirement for MAP kinase and evidence for a parallel inhibitory pathway independent of electrical activity. EMBO J. **16:** 717–725.
48. Si, J. & L. Mei. 1999. ERK MAP kinase activation is required for acetylcholine receptor inducing activity–induced increase in all five acetylcholine receptor subunit

mRNAs as well as synapse-specific expression of acetylcholine receptor epsilon-transgene. Mol. Brain Res. **67:** 18–27.
49. Si, J. *et al.* 1999. Essential roles of c-JUN and c-JUN N-terminal kinase (JNK) in neuregulin-increased expression of the acetylcholine receptor epsilon-subunit. J. Neurosci. **19:** 8498–8508.
50. Fu, A.K. *et al.* 2001. Cdk5 is involved in neuregulin-induced AChR expression at the neuromuscular junction. Nat. Neurosci. **4:** 374–381.
51. Nichols, P. *et al.* 1999. Mutation of the acetylcholine receptor epsilon-subunit promoter in congenital myasthenic syndrome. Ann. Neurol. **45:** 439–443.
52. Ohno, K. *et al.* 1999. Congenital myasthenic syndrome caused by a mutation in the Ets-binding site of the promoter region of the acetylcholine receptor epsilon subunit gene. Neuromuscul. Disord. **9:** 131–135.
53. Abicht, A. *et al.* 2002. A newly identified chromosomal microdeletion and an N-box mutation of the AChR epsilon gene cause a congenital myasthenic syndrome. Brain **125:** 1005–1013.
54. Chan, R.Y. *et al.* 1999. An intronic enhancer containing an N-box motif is required for synapse- and tissue-specific expression of the acetylcholinesterase gene in skeletal muscle fibers. Proc. Natl. Acad. Sci. USA **96:** 4627–4632.
55. Sharrocks, A.D. 2001. The ETS-domain transcription factor family. Rev. Mol. Cell. Biol. **2:** 827–837.
56. Batchelor, A.H. *et al.* 1998. The structure of GABPalpha/beta: an ETS domain–ankyrin repeat heterodimer bound to DNA. Science **279:** 1037–1041.
57. Sawa, C. *et al.* 1996. Functional domains of transcription factor hGABP beta1/E4TF1-53 required for nuclear localization and transcription activation. Nucleic Acids Res. **24:** 4954–4961.
58. Briguet, A. & M.A. Ruegg. 2000. The Ets transcription factor GABP is required for postsynaptic differentiation *in vivo*. J. Neurosci. **20:** 5989–5996.
59. Fromm, L. & S.J. Burden. 2001. Neuregulin-1-stimulated phosphorylation of GABP in skeletal muscle cells. Biochemistry **40:** 5306–5312.
60. Galvagni, F. *et al.* 2001. Sp1 and Sp3 physically interact and co-operate with GABP for the activation of the utrophin promoter. J. Mol. Biol. **306:** 985–996.
61. Tinsley, J.M. *et al.* 1996. Amelioration of the dystrophic phenotype of mdx mice using a truncated utrophin transgene. Nature **384:** 349–353.
62. Rafael, J.A. *et al.* 1998. Skeletal muscle-specific expression of a utrophin transgene rescues utrophin-dystrophin deficient mice. Nat. Genet. **19:** 79–82.

Regulation of Nicotinic Acetylcholine Receptor Assembly

CHRISTIAN P. WANAMAKER, JOHN C. CHRISTIANSON,[a] AND WILLIAM N. GREEN

Department of Neurobiology, Pharmacology, and Physiology, University of Chicago, Chicago, Illinois 60637, USA

ABSTRACT: The four muscle-type nicotinic acetylcholine receptor (AChR) subunits, α, β, γ, and δ, assemble into functional $\alpha_2\beta\gamma\delta$ pentamers in the endoplasmic reticulum (ER) through a series of interdependent folding and oligomerization events. The first stable assembly intermediate is a trimer composed of α, β, and γ subunits. The formation of αβγ trimers initiates a series of subunit folding and processing events that allow addition of δ subunits to form αβγδ tetramers. Subunit folding and processing continue with formation of the ligand-binding sites on the α subunit of αβγδ tetramers and the second α subunit added to assemble $\alpha_2\beta\gamma\delta$ pentamers. AChR assembly is inefficient. Only 20–30% of synthesized subunits assemble into mature receptors in the ER, while the remaining unassembled subunits are degraded. However, the efficiency of subunit assembly can be regulated under certain conditions leading to higher AChR expression. Increased intracellular cAMP levels cause a 2- to 3-fold increase in AChR assembly efficiency and a comparable increase in surface expression. Additionally, block of ubiquitin-proteasome degradation appears to enhance AChR assembly and expression. Thus, the regulation of AChR assembly through posttranslational mechanisms is a potential therapeutic target for increasing AChR expression in diseases in which expression is compromised.

KEYWORDS: nicotinic acetylcholine receptor (AChR); endoplasmic reticulum (ER); ubiquitin proteasome system (UPS); assembly; degradation

INTRODUCTION

Among the earliest conditions identified as ion-channel diseases or channelopathies were those involving the muscle nicotinic acetylcholine receptor (AChR). The early connection made between myasthenia gravis (MG) and the AChR[1] occurred with the purification of the AChR, the first ion channel to be purified. Because the AChR was the first ion channel cloned, the mutations in its subunits that cause congenital myasthenic syndromes (CMSs) have been well characterized (e.g., see

Address for correspondence: William N. Green, Department of Neurobiology, Pharmacology, and Physiology, University of Chicago, Chicago, IL 60637. Voice: 773-702-1763; fax: 773-702-3774. wgreen@midway.uchicago.edu

[a]Present address: John C. Christianson, Department of Biological Sciences, Stanford University, Stanford, CA 94305-5020.

Ann. N.Y. Acad. Sci. 998: 66–80 (2003). © 2003 New York Academy of Sciences. doi: 10.1196/annals.1254.009

ref. 2). CMS research has primarily focused on AChR subunit mutations that have normal levels of AChR expression, but with altered channel properties, such as the mutations that result in the fast- and slow-channel types of the disease. However, many mutations cause a reduction in AChR expression and suggest an alteration of some step in either AChR subunit assembly or trafficking. Indeed, recent experiments suggest that a 3-codon deletion in the β subunit (β426delEQE) impairs receptor assembly by disrupting interaction with the δ subunit.[3] Similarly, little attention has been paid with respect to AChR subunit assembly or trafficking and possible therapies for MG. AChR subunit folding, assembly, and trafficking pathways are all potential targets for increasing AChR expression and overcoming the decrease in AChRs at the neuromuscular junction (NMJ) that occurs with MG.

The precise mechanisms by which any protein folds and assembles are unknown, and the question of how proteins fold remains a major challenge in biology. The correct folding and assembly of the muscle AChR is critical for the formation and maintenance of the NMJ. Because single AChRs control the flow of $\sim 10^7$ ions per second, the malfunction or improper targeting of even a few AChRs can be disastrous for a muscle fiber. To avoid this, AChR assembly and targeting must occur with almost perfect fidelity. Several diseases result from the misfolding/misassembly of other ion channels, the best known being cystic fibrosis. Most cases of cystic fibrosis are caused by the ΔF508 mutation of the cystic fibrosis transmembrane regulator (CFTR). The disease results from misfolding of the protein, which prevents CFTR delivery to the cell surface.[4] The events that fold and assemble ion channels are also significant because they are usually the rate-limiting steps leading to surface membrane expression. Little is known about the mechanisms that control the insertion of ion channels at the cell surface, even though it is evident that regulation of the number of ion channels underlies numerous physiological changes. As the rate-limiting steps in expression, ion-channel folding, and assembly are likely to be points at which ion-channel expression can be regulated. We and others have found that both muscle and neuronal AChR assembly can be regulated by increasing intracellular cAMP levels,[5,6] as described in more detail below.

With advances in recombinant DNA, structural, and electrophysiological techniques, much progress has been made in understanding the structure and, in particular, the function of ion channels such as the AChR. Less progress has been made in resolving the cell biological events that guide the assembly and trafficking of these proteins. For muscle AChR receptors, these processes include the following. To start, mRNAs are selectively targeted to the endoplasmic reticulum (ER) membrane where subunit synthesis occurs. The initial events are cotranslational. These events include (1) membrane insertion of subunits, (2) a set of different processing events such as attachment of the core N-linked glycan and signal sequence cleavage, and (3) initial rapid folding and oligomerization. Because these events are cotranslational, they proceed from the N-terminus to the C-terminus and establish a vectoral order to the assembly. The rapid cotranslational events are followed by slower folding reactions where different domains can interact, and other types of processing occur, such as disulfide bond formation and proline isomerization, as well as further subunit oligomerization. Posttranslational folding, processing, and ultimately oligomerization of all membrane proteins occur in the ER, which provides "quality control" by identifying and degrading any misassembled proteins[7,8] (see below). After subunit folding and assembly, AChRs are specifically targeted and transported to the synapse or are clustered during synaptogenesis at the NMJ. The following will focus on studies examining how the ER quality control machinery for folding and degradation ensures that only correctly folded and assembled AChRs enter the secretory pathway.

STRUCTURE OF THE ACHR

The muscle AChR is a member of the family of neurotransmitter-gated ion channels that includes the neuronal nicotinic ACh, $GABA_A$, glycine, and $5HT_3$ receptors. The AChR resides in the postsynaptic membrane of the NMJ and is the mediator of synaptic input from motor neurons. The receptor functions similarly in the electric organ of the marine ray *Torpedo*, where huge numbers of AChRs generate large voltages to stun prey. These organs have been a rich source of AChRs. Consequently, the *Torpedo* AChR was the first family member to be purified, characterized, and cloned. It also remains the only member of the family to be characterized structurally and much of what is assumed about the structure of the other members of the family is based on *Torpedo* AChR structural data.[9] The recent structural model derived from the homopentameric ACh binding protein has led to a further understanding of the ligand-binding domain.[10,11]

The AChR is an integral membrane protein composed of four different, yet homologous subunits (α, β, γ, and δ) that form a pentamer with a stoichiometry of $\alpha_2\beta\gamma\delta$ and a molecular weight of ~270 kDa. A combination of biochemical, electrophysiological, immunochemical, and sequence analyses have led to a consensus structure for all four subunits (FIG. 1). Both amino- and carboxy-termini are extracellular, with the amino-terminus forming a large domain where ACh binds. In between, each subunit spans the membrane four times (M1–M4), with a large cytoplasmic domain between the two membrane-spanning regions M3 and M4. The subunits are arranged like barrel staves, with each subunit contributing membrane-

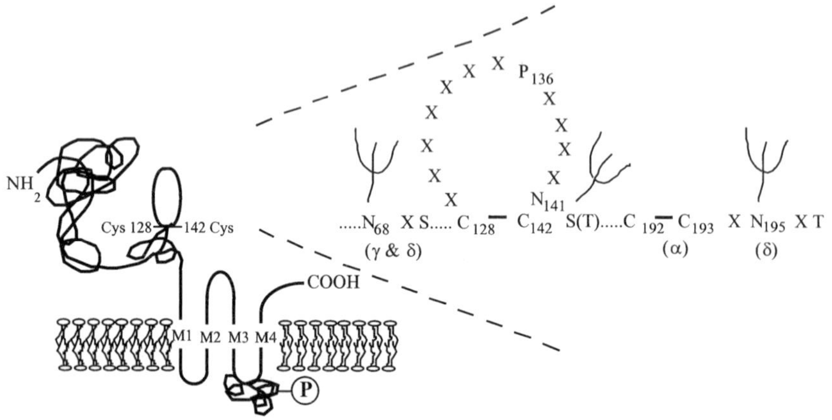

FIGURE 1. Consensus structure for the AChR subunits. Depicted are the extracellular domain at the N-terminus, the membrane-spanning regions (M1–M4), the cytoplasmic domain between M3 and M4, and some of the subunit processing events. Enlarged to show more detail are the glycosylation sites (ψ) and disulfides (Cx–Cx) found on each of the four subunits.

spanning regions to form an ion channel along the central axis of the pentamer. The ion channel opens only when two ACh molecules bind to both α subunits on sites distant from the ion channel. These structural features, the subunit membrane topology and the pentameric quaternary structure, along with the functional features, the ligand-binding sites and the ligand-gated ion channel, appear to be common features of the whole family of neurotransmitter-gated ion channels.[9,12] Because of these common structural features, it is likely that features of the biogenesis of the AChR are also common to the whole family. The mammalian AChR is highly homologous to *Torpedo*, and the receptor is structurally identical, with an exception being the interchangeable subunits γ and ε, which distinguish the fetal and adult forms of the receptor.

ASSEMBLY OF THE ACHR

The best-characterized eukaryotic membrane proteins (e.g., the T cell receptor, insulin receptor, and AChR) are large hetero-oligomers and their folding and oligomerization are more complex than soluble proteins.[13,14] The AChR is particularly complex, not only because of its size and its 20 membrane-spanning domains, but also because the finished product must have the correct oligomeric arrangement as well as subunit stoichiometry for proper function. Consequently, AChR assembly is both slow and inefficient. AChR subunits assemble into pentamers with a $t_{1/2}$ of more than 90 min and only ~30% of the synthesized α subunits are assembled.[15] This is in contrast to influenza hemagglutinin (HA) where most of the subunits form homotrimers with a $t_{1/2}$ of 7–10 min.[16,17] AChR biogenesis thus represents an extreme case in the general cell biological problem of how membrane proteins fold and assemble. The inefficiency of AChR assembly also illustrates the interplay between subunit folding and degradation that ensures receptor fidelity.

As shown schematically in FIGURE 2, there are currently two models that describe the assembly in the ER of α, β, γ, and δ subunits into the native AChR. In both models, assembly occurs along a pathway where defined subsets of the four subunits oligomerize into intermediates, which then assemble into the $\alpha_2\beta\gamma\delta$ pentamer. In the first model (FIG. 2A), the "heterodimer" model,[18–21] the assembly is similar to that of HA in that most subunit folding is completed before oligomerization can occur. Posttranslationally, the subunits undergo a series of slow-folding reactions before oligomerization, the best characterized being the formation of the α-bungarotoxin (Bgt) binding site and the mAb 35 epitope on the α subunit. Afterwards, the "mature" α subunit associates with γ or δ subunits to assemble αγ or αδ heterodimers, and the heterodimers assemble with β subunits into $\alpha_2\beta\gamma\delta$ pentamers. In this model, the two ACh binding sites, distinguishable by a difference in affinity for ligands such as *d*-tubocurare (dTC), form on the αδ and αγ heterodimers. The evidence for αγ and αδ intermediates comes from studies where α and either γ or δ subunits were expressed in the absence of the other two subunits. Using steady-state protocols, it was shown that heterodimeric complexes bind Bgt and that binding is blocked appropriately by agonists and antagonists. However, kinetic measurements in which subunits were pulse-labeled and followed were not consistent with the heterodimer model (see below). Further, all experiments were performed using Triton X-100 to solubilize the AChR subunits, which has been shown subsequently to cause the dissociation of complexes formed as intermediates in the assembly process.[22]

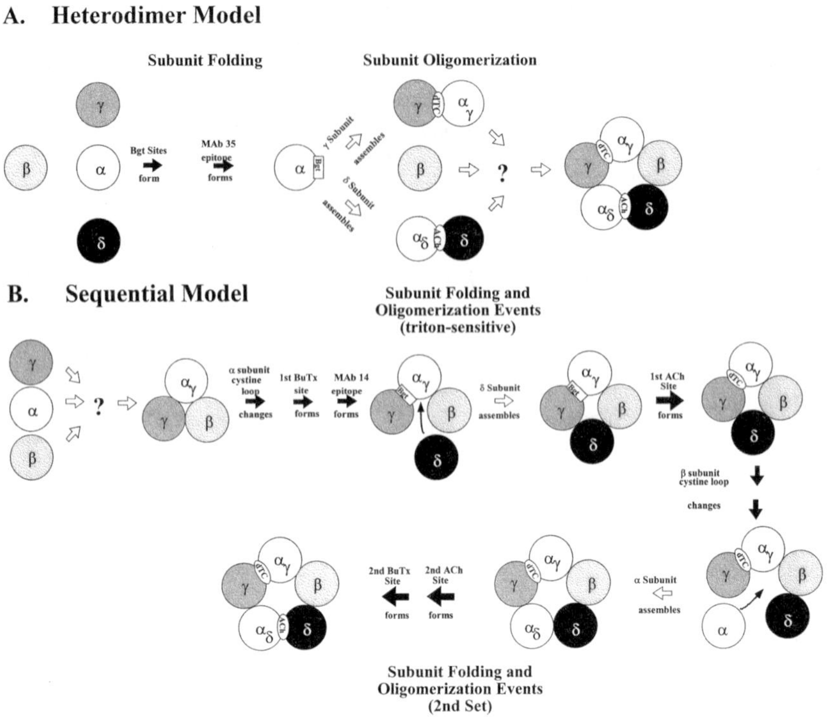

FIGURE 2. Two models of AChR assembly. Subunit folding reactions are denoted by the *solid arrows* and oligomerization events by the *open arrows*. **(A)** Formation of the Bgt binding sites and the mAb 35 epitope precede all subunit associations. The two different ACh binding sites, the high-affinity *d*-tubocurare site (marked as dTC) and the low-affinity dTC site (marked as ACh), appear on $\alpha\gamma$ or $\alpha\delta$ heterodimers, respectively. **(B)** A conformational change in the α subunit cystine loop region and the formation of the first Bgt binding site and mAb 14 epitope occur on $\alpha\beta\gamma$ trimers. A conformational change in the β subunit cystine loop region and formation of the first ACh binding site, the high-affinity dTC site, occur on $\alpha\beta\gamma\delta$ tetramers. Finally, the second Bgt and ACh binding sites appear on $\alpha_2\beta\gamma\delta$ pentamers. Note that we are not proposing that subunits in the trimers and tetramers reposition to allow the insertion of unassembled δ and α subunits. This is only shown to illustrate the possible links between the subunit additions and the conformational changes on the trimers and tetramers.

In the second model (FIG. 2B), the "sequential" model,[22–26] α, β, and γ subunits rapidly assemble into trimers. The slow posttranslational folding of the α subunit occurs only after trimers are assembled. Soon after the Bgt binding site forms, the δ subunit joins the complex to make $\alpha\beta\gamma\delta$ tetramers. The first ACh binding appears on tetramers, after which the second α subunit is added to make $\alpha_2\beta\gamma\delta$ pentamers, and the second Bgt and ACh sites form on the pentamer. The evidence for this model is based on pulse-chase protocols in which assembly intermediates were identified by coimmunoprecipitation using subunit-specific antibodies, by immunoprecipitation with conformation-dependent antibodies, or by precipitation with affinity resin. Once they are formed, most αβγ trimers could be "chased" into αβγδ tetramers, then into $\alpha_2\beta\gamma\delta$ pentamers, and finally onto the cell surface as $\alpha_2\beta\gamma\delta$ pentamers that demonstrated a precursor-product relation between each intermediate and the surface pentamers.[24] Another laboratory has expressed different combinations of the rat AChR subunits and analyzed their assembly using nondenaturing gels.[27] Their results support the sequential model.

One difference between the two models is that, in the sequential model, subunits rapidly associate into trimers before most of the posttranslational folding occurs. The associations are so fast that they could be cotranslational.[22,25] K^+-channel subunits similarly associate rapidly, perhaps cotranslationally.[28,29] If subunit associations occur cotranslationally, it is likely that the associating regions are at the N-terminal end of the subunits. This is consistent with studies that have shown that regions at the N-terminus of AChR subunits[25,30–32] and K^+-channel subunits[33,34] mediate subunit associations. One reason why subunits might associate so rapidly is to protect

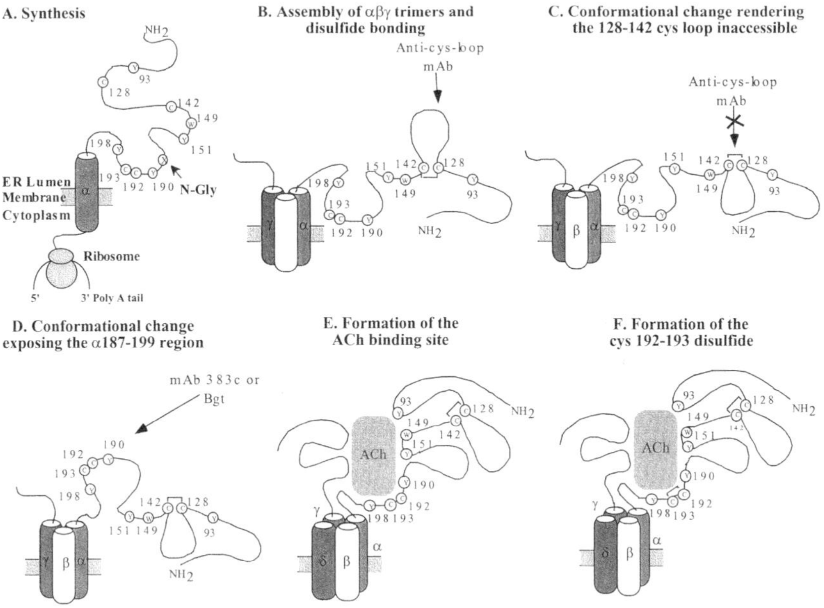

FIGURE 3. A sequential set of α subunit conformational changes and processing events that occur during formation of the ligand binding sites. **(A)** As the α subunit folds during synthesis, the 187–199 region rapidly becomes aqueous-inaccessible, while the 128–142 region becomes accessible. **(B)** αβγ (or ε) trimers assemble and the 128–142 cystine loop forms. **(C)** A conformational change causes the 128–142 cystine loop to become aqueous-inaccessible. **(D)** A conformational change exposes the 187–199 region during formation of the Bgt binding site so that Bgt and mAb 383c can bind. **(E)** The ACh binding site forms as the δ subunit assembles at the interface between the β and γ (or ε) subunits, and the α and γ (or ε) subunits fold, bringing together all of the residues lining the ACh binding site. **(F)** In the final step, cysteines 192 and 193 form a disulfide bond.

critical domains from exposure to either the membrane or the aqueous environment, which should help to prevent misfolding of these domains.

Another feature of the sequential model is that subunits continue to fold during subunit assembly, even after all of the subunits have assembled together into pentamers. The picture that has emerged from work in our lab is that subunit associations and folding during assembly are continuous and interdependent processes. Based on a number of studies,[23,24,26] we have obtained a detailed picture of the first set of folding and oligomerization steps that follow the assembly of $\alpha\beta\gamma$ trimers and result in the formation of the first of two Bgt and ACh binding sites (FIG. 3). As depicted in FIGURE 3B, an intramolecular disulfide bond first forms between α subunit cysteines 128 and 142 as $\alpha\beta\gamma$ trimers assemble. The next step is a conformational change that causes the disulfide loop created by the disulfide bond to be no longer accessible to a monoclonal antibody (mAb) that specifically recognizes the disulfide loop (FIG. 3C). Soon after, another mAb specific for α subunit residues 187–199 becomes accessible to this region, contributing to both the Bgt and ACh binding site. At the same time, the Bgt binding site forms and ^{125}I-Bgt can bind to the $\alpha\beta\gamma$ trimer (FIG. 3D). Next, δ subunits associate with $\alpha\beta\gamma$ trimers and the ACh binding site forms (FIG. 3E). Finally, the disulfide bond is formed between cysteines 192 and 193. Thus, Bgt and ACh binding site formation involves a rearrangement of the α subunit that exposes the 187–199 region to the ER lumen and determines when cysteines 192 and 193 disulfide-bond.

AChR ASSEMBLY AND ER-RESIDENT CHAPERONE PROTEINS

Unfortunately, ion channels do not assemble in a test tube or by use of *in vitro* translation methods (see ref. 35 for an exception). Presently, ion channels only assemble within the environment of a cell. For the AChR, this is likely due to the fact that AChR subunits exit the ER only as fully assembled pentamers.[36–39] Therefore, all subunit folding and oligomerization necessary to achieve AChR quaternary structure occur in or on the surface of the ER membrane. Further, some nicotinic receptors are properly assembled only in cells of neuronal origin and appear to require additional unidentified factors for proper assembly.[40–42] ER chaperone proteins are likely to be some of the unidentified cellular factors required for AChR assembly.

Studies with chaperone proteins are just beginning. ER-resident chaperone proteins include (but are not limited to) immunoglobulin heavy-chain binding protein (BiP),[43] calnexin (CN),[44] and ERp57.[45] These chaperones are not only responsible for helping nascent polypeptides fold, but they are also important in retaining the immature polypeptides within the ER. This retention increases the probability that the immature polypeptide will be correctly folded and that it does not prematurely enter the secretory pathway. At some stage, the prolonged retention of the misfolded or incompletely assembled polypeptide leads to its degradation.[46] It is unclear how the cell determines that a polypeptide is to be degraded, but it remains a possibility that the folding machinery is also intimately involved in degradation signaling. A small number of studies have recently begun to look at the association of chaperones with AChR subunits. These studies have found that CN associates with each of the unassembled subunits[39,47,48] (Wanamaker and Green, unpublished data). BiP also associates with unassembled α and β subunits[49–51]

(Wanamaker and Green, unpublished data). In contrast, ERp57 and calreticulin, a soluble homologue of CN, have been reported not to associate with the α subunit.[48] Among these studies, there are a number of disagreements. One study concluded that the association between CN and the subunit was dependent on the glycans,[52] while another concluded that, in addition to the lectin association, polypeptide associations also occurred.[48] These reports also differ on the effect glucose trimming has on α subunit folding and assembly; in one finding, it disrupted folding and assembly,[52] while the other observed no effect.[48] It is also unclear whether CN is associated with only immature unassembled α subunits[39] or with a more mature unassembled α subunit.[47] In addition, we have found that ERp57 associates with each of the unassembled subunits (Wanamaker and Green, unpublished data), in contrast to the finding of Keller *et al.*[48] Because of these discrepancies, further studies are needed to resolve these differences and to begin to understand the role of ER chaperones in AChR subunit folding and assembly.

Studies characterizing the associations of BiP with other proteins indicate that BiP can associate in the first 50 amino acids of proteins as they are synthesized.[53] Thus, each AChR subunit may associate rapidly and possibly cotranslationally with BiP. As discussed above, the subunit also appears to interact with CN and ERp57, possibly in tandem. Because ERp57 is a protein disulfide isomerase,[54–57] it may serve to promote the formation of critical disulfide bonds within the subunit in the ER. The interactions between the chaperones and the AChR subunits may be one reason for the slow kinetics of AChR assembly. This suggests that the chaperones may not actively fold subunits, but act as protectors of early folding intermediates to ensure and likely increase the fidelity of assembly. Thus, the rate-limiting steps in AChR assembly would not be subunit folding and oligomerization; rather, assembly is dependent on when ER chaperone proteins associate and dissociate from assembling subunits.

ER-ASSOCIATED DEGRADATION OF MEMBRANE PROTEINS

ER-associated degradation (ERAD) in concert with chaperone-assisted protein folding comprises the secretory pathway's ER quality control mechanism. These processes ensure the fidelity of secreted and membrane protein folding and assembly in eukaryotic cells.[7] ERAD is a specialized function of the ubiquitin-proteasome system (UPS), which prevents the accumulation of misfolded, extraneous, and potentially toxic proteins from the ER by degrading them cytosolically.[46,58] In the current model for ERAD, misfolded and/or unassembled proteins in the ER are recognized and retrotranslocated via the Sec61 translocon to the cytosol for degradation. During this process, ubiquitin is covalently and repeatedly attached to a substrate's lysine residues by components of an ATP-dependent, ubiquitin-conjugating enzyme cascade (E1, E2, and E3) that reside in or are recruited to the cytosolic face of the ER (reviewed in ref. 59). The "polyubiquitin" chains attached to degradation-bound proteins are recognized by the AAA-ATPase p97/cdc48, whose ratcheting action is sufficient to dislocate membrane proteins from the ER.[60–62] The 26S proteasome can also provide the energy for retrotranslocation, but may do so only for dislocation of larger, polytopic proteins[63,64] such as AChR subunits. Polyubiquitin chains are recognized by 19S cap subunits of the 26S proteasome complex, which then degrades the substrate and recycles the ubiquitin.

Two particular features of AChRs suggest that ERAD might have a critical role in receptor assembly. As mentioned above, only ~30% of the subunits synthesized become incorporated into mature pentamers,[15] indicating that the assembly of AChRs is an inefficient process. Second, the residual unassembled subunits remain in the ER[20,65–67] and are degraded by mechanisms as yet unidentified.[65,66] Unassembled subunits are degraded much more rapidly ($t_{1/2} < 1$ h) than their oligomerized counterparts ($t_{1/2} = 11–16$ h).[68] Thus, degradation rather than assembly is the fate for most synthesized AChR subunits. It is likely that degradation of unassembled AChR subunits mimics that of unassembled subunits of other hetero-oligomeric receptors, such as the T cell receptor, which are targets of ERAD.[69–71]

Recently, we have investigated the fate of AChR subunits that fail to assemble in the ER. To study unassembled AChR subunits, each of the mouse subunits (α, β, γ, ε, or δ) was stably transfected into HEK cells. Degradation rates of all four subunits were slowed by treatment with the proteasome inhibitor, lactacystin (LACT), a finding consistent with subunit degradation, at least in part, by a UPS-dependent ERAD mechanism (Christianson and Green, unpublished data). How might subunit degradation affect assembly of AChRs? Applying LACT to C_2C_{12} myotubes surprisingly increased the expression of mature AChRs on the cell surface (Christianson and Green, unpublished data). This finding is consistent with examples where detection of mature, wild-type protein is increased in the presence of proteasome inhibitors, including ENaC,[72,73] connexins,[74] CFTR,[75] and rhodopsin.[76] Since blocking degradation by proteasomes does not enhance maturation of folding-defective proteins,[77] our findings suggest that the suboptimal efficiency of AChR assembly is due to degradation of unassembled, yet assembly-competent subunits by ERAD. Moreover, while folding and oligomerization limit the rate of AChR assembly, ERAD appears to be a factor limiting the overall number of receptors being assembled.

If ERAD indeed limits subunit availability, the UPS may represent a novel therapeutic target for conditions with inadequate receptor expression such as MG. Increasing the percentage of subunits assembled would likely result in a net increase in AChRs expressed and could increase synaptic efficacy at the NMJ. Blocking ERAD by inhibiting UPS-mediated degradation represents a means to posttranslationally enhance receptor expression. Proteasome inhibitors are highly specific and often cell-permeable,[78] and recent studies have explored their therapeutic potential in cancer[79] and neuropathic pain.[80] However, the 26S proteasome is the major degradation mechanism for intracellular proteins.[81,82] As such, there is likely to be a substantial number of pleiotropic cellular consequences of using inhibitors that prevent general proteasome-mediated degradation, and concerns have been raised regarding their therapeutic usefulness.[83] A more appealing target for disrupting ERAD is the ubiquitin-ligase (E3), which (together with an E2 ubiquitin-conjugating enzyme) is responsible for specifically polyubiquitinating unassembled AChR subunits. E3s are believed to provide the specificity for ubiquitin conjugation, but our understanding of this recognition is only in its infancy. Based on searches for consensus domains, the number of putative E3s in the human genome is likely to be around 800, but so far only 6 have been implicated in ERAD.[84–88] Given the plethora of substrates, there are likely to be many more ERAD-associated E3s identified in the coming years. Drug or small-molecule screens may provide candidates that disrupt particular E3s and the ubiquitination reaction they mediate, but this possibility has not yet been realized. Nevertheless, our findings suggest that the capacity to upregulate ion channel expression posttranslationally does exist and inhibiting UPS-mediated degradation of unassembled subunits could prove useful for treatment of conditions exhibiting deficient receptor expression.

CONCLUSIONS AND FUTURE DIRECTIONS

What is not clear from our results is why AChRs (and other complex oligomeric membrane proteins) take so long to assemble? The folding and oligomerization events required for assembly typically occur over a time scale of seconds to a few minutes for most proteins. For the *Torpedo* subunits assembling at 20°C, the first Bgt and ACh binding sites take 6 to 12 h to form;[24] for the mouse subunits at 37°C, the sites take 45 to 60 min to form.[15,22] Our working hypothesis is that AChR assembly is greatly slowed because of the involvement of ER chaperone proteins that associate with assembling subunits and prevent much of subunit folding from rapidly occurring. Thus, the rate-limiting steps in assembly would not be subunit folding and oligomerization. Instead, we suggest that the timing of AChR assembly is controlled by when ER chaperone proteins associate and dislodge from assembling subunits.

Another issue of interest for future studies is the identity of signals within the AChR subunits that provide a signal for the transport of correctly folded AChRs from the ER to the cell surface. For instance, RXR motifs in K^+-channels prevent the subunits from exiting the ER while they are exposed.[89] In the AChR, a dibasic motif (Arg-Lys) in the cytoplasmic loop of the α subunit can regulate ER to Golgi trafficking.[90] These signals could act in conjunction with ER chaperones to keep immature proteins in the ER. Another point of trafficking control could be from the trans-Golgi to the synapse. This may include understanding the role of the clustering (and scaffolding) protein, rapsyn, on the transport and trafficking of the AChR. Rapsyn is critical for the clustering of the AChR at the NMJ and, as a result, signaling at the synapse. It is unclear when during the maturation process rapsyn interacts with the AChR. However, recent results suggest that rapsyn and AChRs interact in the trans-Golgi network and that lipid raft domains could play a role in the correct sorting and targeting of the rapsyn/AChR complex.[91] In addition, there are now reported cases of CMS that are a result of rapsyn mutations.[92]

A question relevant to MG and CMS is whether the efficiency of AChR assembly can be regulated. Previously, we have found that any agents that increase the cytoplasmic concentration of cAMP increase the surface expression of AChRs (FIG. 4). As shown in FIGURE 4, this effect of increasing cAMP levels was found in rat myotubes expressing endogenous rat AChRs (FIG. 4A, lane 2), transfected rat myotubes expressing endogenous rat AChRs plus hybrid AChRs containing the *Torpedo* α subunit (FIG. 4A, lane 3), or mouse fibroblasts expressing full *Torpedo* AChRs (FIG. 4B). The cAMP effect on AChR expression is posttranslational[93] and results in an increase in the efficiency of AChR assembly in the ER as large as threefold.[22,38] Thus, the efficiency of AChR can be upregulated from ~30% to close to 100% under certain conditions. Recently, we have found that other agents can act to increase the efficiency of AChR assembly. Agents that block the proteasome and the degradation of unassembled AChR subunits also increase surface AChR expression. Like the

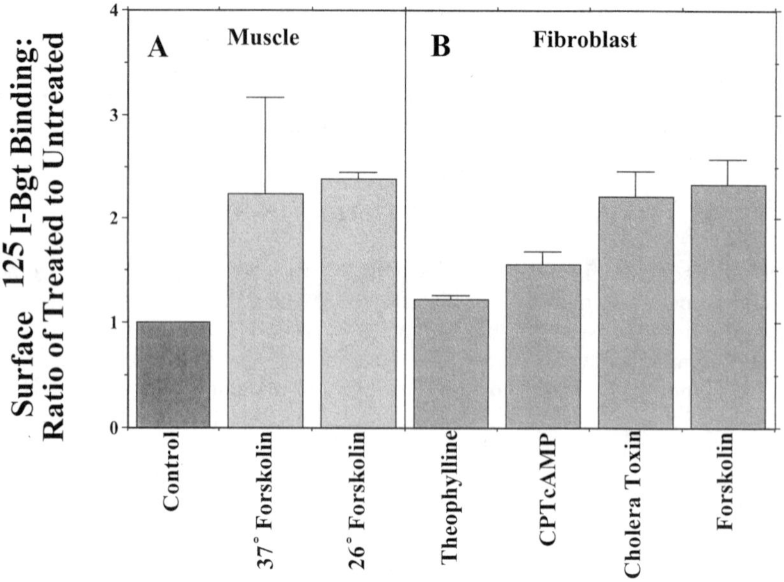

FIGURE 4. **(A)** Effect on the number of cell surface AChRs expressed in rat muscle L6 (L6-DOL-α) cells by forskolin. The bars are ratios of the number of cell surface AChRs, agent to control, as determined by ^{125}I-Bgt binding. Values are expressed as mean ± SD. Confluent cultures of L6-DOL-α cells expressing only endogenous rat AChRs were treated with 100 μM forskolin (lane 2). L6-DOL-α cells expressing 50% endogenous rat and 50% *Torpedo*-rat hybrid AChRs were treated with 100 μM forskolin (lane 3). The control bar in lane 1 represents untreated L6-DOL-α cells. **(B)** Effect on the number of cell surface *Torpedo* AChRs expressed in mouse fibroblast (L) cells by agents that increase intracellular cAMP. As in panel A, the bars are ratios of the number of cell surface AChRs, agent to control, as determined by ^{125}I-Bgt binding and are expressed as mean ± SD. Confluent cultures of cells stably expressing *Torpedo* AChRs were treated with 1 mM theophylline (lane 1), 1 mM CPTcAMP (lane 2), 100 nM cholera toxin (lane 3), or 100 μM forskolin (lane 4). (Adapted from ref. 93.)

effects of cAMP, inhibition of proteasomes increases the efficiency of AChR assembly in the ER (Christianson and Green, unpublished data). It is unknown whether the mechanism or mechanisms underlying the effect of cAMP and proteasome inhibitors overlap or are independent, although the phosphorylation state of a substrate can regulate its ubiquitination by an appropriate E3 ubiquitin ligase (e.g., see ref. 94). Clearly, much work needs to be done to fully characterize and understand the myriad cellular factors regulating the assembly efficiency of AChRs.

ACKNOWLEDGMENTS

We thank the National Institutes of Health and the Alzheimer's Association for their support.

REFERENCES

1. PATRICK, J. & J. LINDSTROM. 1973. Autoimmune response to acetylcholine receptor. Science **180:** 871–872.
2. SINE, S. *et al.* 1995. Mutation of the acetylcholine receptor alpha subunit causes a slow-channel myasthenic syndrome by enhancing agonist binding affinity. Neuron **15:** 229–239.
3. QUIRAM, P.A. *et al.* 1999. Mutation causing congenital myasthenia reveals acetylcholine receptor beta/delta subunit interaction essential for assembly. J. Clin. Invest. **104:** 1403–1410.
4. CHENG, S.H. *et al.* 1990. Defective intracellular transport and processing of CFTR is the molecular basis of most cystic fibrosis. Cell **63:** 827–834.
5. GREEN, W.N., A.F. ROSS & T. CLAUDIO. 199. Acetylcholine receptor assembly is stimulated by phosphorylation of its γ subunit. Neuron **7:** 659–666.
6. ROTHHUT, B. *et al.* 1996. Post-translational regulation of neuronal acetylcholine receptors stably expressed in a mouse fibroblast cell line. J. Neurobiol. **29:** 115–125.
7. ELLGAARD, L., M. MOLINARI & A. HELENIUS. 1999. Setting the standards: quality control in the secretory pathway. Science **286:** 1882–1888.
8. KOPITO, R.R. 1997. ER quality control: the cytoplasmic connection. Cell **88:** 427–430.
9. UNWIN, N. 1993. Neurotransmitter action: opening of ligand-gated ion channels. Cell (Suppl.) **72:** 31–41.
10. BREJC, K. *et al.* 2001. Crystal structure of an ACh-binding protein reveals the ligand-binding domain of nicotinic receptors. Nature **411:** 269–276.
11. SINE, S.M. 2002. The nicotinic receptor ligand binding domain. J. Neurobiol. **53:** 431–446.
12. KARLIN, A. & M.H. AKABAS. 1995. Towards a structural basis for the function of nicotinic acetylcholine receptors and their cousins. Neuron **15:** 1231–1244.
13. KLAUSNER, R.D., J. LIPPINCOTT-SCHWARTZ & J.S. BONIFACINO. 1990. The T cell antigen receptor: insights into organelle biology. Annu. Rev. Cell Biol. **6:** 403–431.
14. OLSON, T.S., M.J. BAMBERGER & M.D. LANE. 1988. Post-translational changes in tertiary and quaternary structure of the insulin proreceptor. J. Biol. Chem. **263:** 7342–7351.
15. MERLIE, J.P. & J. LINDSTROM. 1983. Assembly *in vivo* of mouse muscle acetylcholine receptor: identification of an alpha subunit species that may be an assembly intermediate. Cell **34:** 747–757.
16. COPELAND, C.S. *et al.* 1986. Assembly of influenza hemagglutinin trimers and its role in intracellular transport. J. Cell Biol. **103:** 1179–1191.
17. GETHING, M-J., K. MCKANNON & J. SAMBROOK. 1986. Expression of wildtype and mutant forms of influenza hemagglutinin: the role of folding in transport. Cell **46:** 939–950.
18. BLOUNT, P., M.M. SMITH & J.P. MERLIE. 1990. Assembly intermediates of the mouse muscle nicotinic acetylcholine receptor in stably transfected fibroblasts. J. Cell Biol. **111:** 2601–2611.
19. SAEDI, M.S., W.G. CONROY & J. LINDSTROM. 1991. Assembly of *Torpedo* acetylcholine receptors in *Xenopus* oocytes. J. Cell Biol. **112:** 1007–1015.
20. GU, Y. *et al.* 1991. Assembly of mammalian muscle acetylcholine receptors in transfected COS cells. J. Cell Biol. **114:** 799–807.
21. KREIENKAMP, H.J. *et al.* 1995. Intersubunit contacts governing assembly of the mammalian nicotinic acetylcholine receptor. Neuron **14:** 635–644.
22. GREEN, W.N. & T. CLAUDIO. 1993. Acetylcholine receptor assembly: subunit folding and oligomerization occur sequentially. Cell **74:** 57–69.
23. GREEN, W.N. & C.P. WANAMAKER. 1997. The role of the cystine loop in acetylcholine receptor assembly. J. Biol. Chem. **272:** 20945–20953.
24. GREEN, W.N. & C.P. WANAMAKER. 1998. Formation of the nicotinic acetylcholine receptor binding sites. J. Neurosci. **18:** 5555–5564.
25. EERTMOED, A.L. & W.N. GREEN. 1999. Nicotinic receptor assembly requires multiple regions throughout the gamma subunit. J. Neurosci. **19:** 6298–6308.
26. MITRA, M., C.P. WANAMAKER & W.N. GREEN. 2001. Rearrangement of nicotinic receptor alpha subunits during formation of the ligand binding sites. J. Neurosci. **21:** 3000–3008.

27. NICKE, A. *et al.* 1999. Blue native PAGE as a useful method for the analysis of the assembly of distinct combinations of nicotinic acetylcholine receptor subunits. J. Recept. Signal. Transduct. Res. **19:** 493–507.
28. DEAL, K.K., D.M. LOVINGER & M.M. TAMKUN. 1994. The brain Kv1.1 potassium channel: *in vitro* and *in vivo* studies on subunit assembly and posttranslational processing. J. Neurosci. **14:** 1666–1676.
29. SHI, G. *et al.* 1996. Beta subunits promote K^+ channel surface expression through effects early in biosynthesis. Neuron **16:** 843–852.
30. GU, Y. *et al.* 1991. Identification of two amino acid residues in the ε subunit that promote mammalian muscle acetylcholine recptor asssembly in COS cells. Neuron **6:** 879–887.
31. YU, X-M. & Z.W. HALL. 1991. Extracellular domains mediating ε subunit interactions of muscle acetylcholine receptor. Nature **352:** 64–67.
32. SUMIKAWA, K. & T. NISHIZAKI. 1994. The amino acid residues 1–128 in the alpha subunit of the nicotinic acetylcholine receptor contain assembly signals. Brain Res. Mol. Brain Res. **25:** 257–264.
33. LI, M., Y.N. JAN & L.Y. JAN. 1992. Specification of subunit assembly by the hydrophilic amino-terminal domain of the Shaker potassium channel. Science **257:** 1225–1230.
34. SHEN, N.V. *et al.* 1993. Deletion analysis of K^+ channel assembly. Neuron **11:** 67–76.
35. ROSENBERG, R.L. & J.E. EAST. 1992. Cell-free expression of functional Shaker potassium channels. Nature **360:** 166–169.
36. SMITH, M.M., J. LINDSTROM & J.P. MERLIE. 1987. Formation of the α-bungarotoxin binding site and assembly of the acetylcholine receptor subunits occur in the endoplasmic reticulum. J. Biol. Chem. **262:** 4367–4376.
37. GU, Y. *et al.* 1989. Acetylcholine receptors in a C2 muscle cell variant is retained in the endoplasmic reticulum. J. Cell Biol. **109:** 729–738.
38. ROSS, A.F. *et al.* 1991. Efficiency of acetylcholine receptor subunit assembly and its regulation by cAMP. J. Cell Biol. **113:** 623–636.
39. GELMAN, M.S. *et al.* 1995. Role of the endoplasmic reticulum chaperone calnexin in subunit folding and assembly of nicotinic acetylcholine receptors. J. Biol. Chem. **270:** 15085–15092.
40. COOPER, S.T. & N.S. MILLAR. 1997. Host cell-specific folding and assembly of the neuronal nicotinic acetylcholine receptor alpha7 subunit. J. Neurochem. **68:** 2140–2151.
41. RANGWALA, F. *et al.* 1997. Neuronal alpha-bungarotoxin receptors differ structurally from other nicotinic acetylcholine receptors. J. Neurosci. **17:** 8201–8212.
42. COOPER, S.T. & N.S. MILLAR. 1998. Host cell-specific folding of the neuronal nicotinic receptor alpha8 subunit. J. Neurochem. **70:** 2585–2593.
43. GETHING, M.J. 1999. Role and regulation of the ER chaperone BiP. Semin. Cell Dev. Biol. **10:** 465–472.
44. ELLGAARD, L. & A. HELENIUS. 2001. ER quality control: towards an understanding at the molecular level. Curr. Opin. Cell Biol. **13:** 431–437.
45. HIGH, S. *et al.* 2000. Glycoprotein folding in the endoplasmic reticulum: a tale of three chaperones? FEBS Lett. **476:** 38–41.
46. BRODSKY, J.L. & A.A. MCCRACKEN. 1999. ER protein quality control and proteasome-mediated protein degradation. Semin. Cell Dev. Biol. **10:** 507–513.
47. KELLER, S.H., J. LINDSTROM & P. TAYLOR. 1996. Involvement of the chaperone protein calnexin and the acetylcholine receptor beta-subunit in the assembly and cell surface expression of the receptor. J. Biol. Chem. **271:** 22871–22877.
48. KELLER, S.H., J. LINDSTROM & P. TAYLOR. 1998. Inhibition of glucose trimming with castanospermine reduces calnexin association and promotes proteasome degradation of the alpha-subunit of the nicotinic acetylcholine receptor. J. Biol. Chem. **273:** 17064–17072.
49. BLOUNT, P. & J.P. MERLIE. 1991. BIP associates with newly synthesized subunits of the mouse muscle nicotinic receptor. J. Cell Biol. **113:** 1125–1132.
50. PAULSON, H.L. *et al.* 1991. Analysis of early events in acetycholine receptor assembly. J. Cell Biol. **113:** 1371–1384.

51. FORSAYETH, J.R., Y. GU & Z.W. HALL. 1992. BiP forms stable complexes with unassembled subunits of the acetylcholine receptor in transfected COS cells and in C2 muscle cells. J. Cell Biol. **117:** 841–847.
52. CHANG, W., M.S. GELMAN & J.M. PRIVES. 1997. Calnexin-dependent enhancement of nicotinic acetylcholine receptor assembly and surface expression. J. Biol. Chem. **272:** 28925–28932.
53. MOLINARI, M. & A. HELENIUS. 2000. Chaperone selection during glycoprotein translocation into the endoplasmic reticulum. Science **288:** 331–333.
54. SRIVASTAVA, S.P., J.A. FUCHS & J.L. HOLTZMAN. 1993. The reported cDNA sequence for phospholipase C alpha encodes protein disulfide isomerase, isozyme Q-2, and not phospholipase-C. Biochem. Biophys. Res. Commun. **193:** 971–978.
55. BOURDI, M. *et al.* 1995. cDNA cloning and baculovirus expression of the human liver endoplasmic reticulum P58: characterization as a protein disulfide isomerase isoform, but not as a protease or a carnitine acyltransferase. Arch. Biochem. Biophys. **323:** 397–403.
56. HIRANO, N. *et al.* 1995. Molecular cloning of the human glucose-regulated protein ERp57/GRP58, a thiol-dependent reductase: identification of its secretory form and inducible expression by the oncogenic transformation. Eur. J. Biochem. **234:** 336-342.
57. MOLINARI, M. & A. HELENIUS. 1999. Glycoproteins form mixed disulphides with oxidoreductases during folding in living cells. Nature **402:** 90–93.
58. PLEMPER, R.K. & D.H. WOLF. 1999. Retrograde protein translocation: ERADication of secretory proteins in health and disease. Trends Biochem. Sci. **24:** 266–270.
59. GLICKMAN, M.H. & A. CIECHANOVER. 2002. The ubiquitin-proteasome proteolytic pathway: destruction for the sake of construction. Physiol. Rev. **82:** 373–428.
60. RABINOVICH, E. 2001. AAA-ATPase p97/Cdc48p, a cytosolic chaperone required for endoplasmic reticulum-associated protein degradation. Nature **414:** 652–656.
61. YE, Y. 2001. The AAA ATPase Cdc48/p97 and its partners transport proteins from the ER into the cytosol. Cell **107:** 667–677.
62. JAROSCH, E. *et al.* 2002. Protein dislocation from the ER requires polyubiquitination and the AAA-ATPase Cdc48. Nat. Cell Biol. **4:** 134–139.
63. XIONG, X., E. CHONG & W.R. SKACH. 1999. Evidence that endoplasmic reticulum (ER)–associated degradation of cystic fibrosis transmembrane conductance regulator is linked to retrograde translocation from the ER membrane. J. Biol. Chem. **274:** 2616–2624.
64. PLEMPER, R.K. *et al.* 1998. Endoplasmic reticulum degradation of a mutated ATP-binding cassette transporter Pdr5 proceeds in a concerted action of Sec61 and the proteasome. J. Biol. Chem. **273:** 32848–32856.
65. CLAUDIO, T. *et al.* 1989. Fibroblasts transfected with *Torpedo* acetylcholine receptor beta, gamma, and delta subunit cDNA's express functional receptors when infected with a retroviral alpha recombinant. J. Cell Biol. **108:** 2277–2290.
66. BLOUNT, P. & J.P. MERLIE. 1988. Native folding of an acetylcholine receptor alpha subunit expressed in the absence of other receptor subunits. J. Biol. Chem. **263:** 1072–1080.
67. SUMIKAWA, K. & R. MILEDI. 1989. Assembly and N-glycosylation of all ACh receptor subunits are required for their efficient insertion into plasma membranes. Mol. Brain Res. **5:** 183–192.
68. HYMAN, C. & S.C. FROEHNER. 1983. Degradation of acetylcholine receptors in muscle cells: effect of leupeptin on turnover rate, intracellular pool sizes, and receptor properties. J. Cell Biol. **96:** 1316–1324.
69. YANG, M. *et al.* 1998. Novel aspects of degradation of T cell receptor subunits from the endoplasmic reticulum (ER) in T cells: importance of oligosaccharide processing, ubiquitination, and proteasome-dependent removal from ER membranes. J. Exp. Med. **187:** 835–846.
70. YU, H. *et al.* 1997. Cytosolic degradation of T-cell receptor alpha chains by the proteasome. J. Biol. Chem. **272:** 20800–20804.
71. TIWARI, S. 2001. Endoplasmic reticulum (ER)–associated degradation of T cell receptor subunits: involvement of ER-associated ubiquitin-conjugating enzymes (E2s). J. Biol. Chem. **276:** 16193–16200.

72. STAUB, O. *et al.* 1997. Regulation of stability and function of the epithelial Na^+ channel (ENaC) by ubiquitination. EMBO J. **16:** 6325–6336.
73. MALIK, B. *et al.* 2001. Enac degradation in A6 cells by the ubiquitin-proteosome proteolytic pathway. J. Biol. Chem. **276:** 12903–12910.
74. MUSIL, L.S. *et al.* 2000. Regulation of connexin degradation as a mechanism to increase gap junction assembly and function. J. Biol. Chem. **275:** 25207–25215.
75. JENSEN, T.J. *et al.* 1995. Multiple proteolytic systems, including the proteasome, contribute to CFTR processing. Cell **83:** 129–135.
76. ILLING, M.E. *et al.* 2002. A rhodopsin mutant linked to autosomal dominant retinitis pigmentosa is prone to aggregate and interacts with the ubiquitin proteasome system. J. Biol. Chem. **277:** 34150–34160.
77. WARD, C.L., S. OMURA & R.R. KOPITO. 1995. Degradation of CFTR by the ubiquitin-proteasome pathway. Cell **83:** 121–127.
78. LEE, D.H. & A.L. GOLDBERG. 1998. Proteasome inhibitors: valuable new tools for cell biologists. Trends Cell Biol. **8:** 397–403.
79. ELLIOTT, P.J. & J.S. ROSS. 2001. The proteasome: a new target for novel drug therapies. Am. J. Clin. Pathol. **116:** 637–646.
80. MOSS, A. *et al.* 2002. A role of the ubiquitin-proteasome system in neuropathic pain. J. Neurosci. **22:** 1363–1372.
81. CIECHANOVER, A. & A.L. SCHWARTZ. 1998. The ubiquitin-proteasome pathway: the complexity and myriad functions of proteins death [comment]. Proc. Natl. Acad. Sci. USA **95:** 2727–2730.
82. HILT, W. & D.H. WOLF. 1996. Proteasomes: destruction as a programme. Trends Biochem. Sci. **21:** 96–102.
83. HALLIWELL, B. 2002. Hypothesis: proteasomal dysfunction—a primary event in neurogeneration that leads to nitrative and oxidative stress and subsequent cell death. Ann. N.Y. Acad. Sci. **962:** 182–194.
84. IMAI, Y. *et al.* 2002. CHIP is associated with Parkin, a gene responsible for familial Parkinson's disease, and enhances its ubiquitin ligase activity. Mol. Cell **10:** 55–67.
85. SHAN, H. *et al.* 2001. HRD gene dependence of endoplasmic reticulum–associated degradation. J. Biol. Chem. **276:** 8681–8694.
86. YOSHIDA, Y. *et al.* 2002. E3 ubiquitin ligase that recognizes sugar chains. Nature **418:** 438–442.
87. SWANSON, R., M. LOCHER & M. HOCHSTRASSER. 2001. A conserved ubiquitin ligase of the nuclear envelope/endoplasmic reticulum that functions in both ER-associated and Matalpha2 repressor degradation. Genes Dev. **15:** 2660–2674.
88. FANG, S. *et al.* 2001. The tumor autocrine motility factor receptor, gp78, is a ubiquitin protein ligase implicated in degradation from the endoplasmic reticulum. Proc. Natl. Acad. Sci. USA **98:** 14422–14427.
89. ZERANGUE, N. *et al.* 1999. A new ER trafficking signal regulates the subunit stoichiometry of plasma membrane K(ATP) channels. Neuron **22:** 537–548.
90. KELLER, S.H. *et al.* 2001. Adjacent basic amino acid residues recognized by the COP I complex and ubiquitination govern endoplasmic reticulum to cell surface trafficking of the nicotinic acetylcholine receptor alpha-subunit. J. Biol. Chem. **276:** 18384–18391.
91. MARCHAND, S. *et al.* 2002. Rapsyn escorts the nicotinic acetylcholine receptor along the exocytic pathway via association with lipid rafts. J. Neurosci. **22:** 8891–8901.
92. OHNO, K. *et al.* 2002. Rapsyn mutations in humans cause endplate acetylcholine-receptor deficiency and myasthenic syndrome. Am. J. Hum. Genet. **70:** 875–885.
93. GREEN, W.N., A.F. ROSS & T. CLAUDIO. 1991. cAMP stimulation of acetylcholine receptor expression is mediated through posttranslational mechanisms. Proc. Natl. Acad. Sci. USA **88:** 854–858.
94. BERCOVICH, B. *et al.* 1999. Ubiquitin ligase activity and tyrosine phosphorylation underlie suppression of growth factor signaling by c-Cbl/Sli-1. J. Biol. Chem. **274:** 14823–14830.

Structure and Function of AChBP, Homologue of the Ligand-Binding Domain of the Nicotinic Acetylcholine Receptor

AUGUST B. SMIT,[a] KATJUŠA BREJC,[b,c] NAWEED SYED,[d] AND TITIA K. SIXMA[b]

[a]*Department of Molecular and Cellular Neurobiology, Faculty of Biology, Research Institute Neurosciences Vrije Universiteit, Amsterdam, the Netherlands*

[b]*Division of Molecular Carcinogenesis, Netherlands Cancer Institute, Amsterdam, the Netherlands*

[d]*Department of Cell Biology and Anatomy, University of Calgary, T2N4N1 Calgary, Canada*

ABSTRACT: Acetylcholine-binding protein (AChBP) is a novel protein with high similarity to the extracellular domain of the nicotinic acetylcholine receptor. AChBP lacks the transmembrane domains and intracellular loops typical for the nAChRs. AChBP is secreted from glia cells in the central nervous system of the freshwater snail, *Lymnaea stagnalis*, where it modulates synaptic transmission. AChBP forms homopentamers with pharmacology that resembles the α_7-type of nicotinic receptors. As such, AChBP is a good model for the ligand-binding domain of the nAChRs. In the crystal structure of AChBP at 2.7 Å, each protomer has a modified immunoglobulin fold. Almost all residues previously shown to be involved in ligand binding in the nicotinic receptor are found in a pocket at the subunit interface, which is lined with aromatic residues. The AChBP crystal structure explains many of the biochemical studies on the nicotinic acetylcholine receptors. Surprisingly, the interface between protomers is relatively weakly conserved between families in the superfamily of pentameric ligand-gated ion channels. The lack of conservation has implications for the mechanism of gating of the ion channels.

KEYWORDS: nicotinic acetylcholine receptor; ligand-gated ion channel; crystal structure; AChBP; glia; acetylcholine-binding site; modulating synaptic transmission

IDENTIFICATION OF ACETYLCHOLINE-BINDING PROTEIN (AChBP)

The central nervous system of the freshwater snail, *Lymnaea stagnalis*, has been studied as a model in neurobiology for many years. The reason for this is that it con-

Address for correspondence: August B. Smit, Department of Molecular and Cellular Neurobiology, Faculty of Biology, Research Institute Neurosciences Vrije Universiteit, De Boelelaan 1087, 1081 HV Amsterdam, the Netherlands. Voice: +31-20-4447003.
absmit@bio.vu.nl
[c]Present address: Cytokinetics Inc., 280 East Grand Avenue, South San Francisco, CA 94080.

Ann. N.Y. Acad. Sci. 998: 81–92 (2003). © 2003 New York Academy of Sciences.
doi: 10.1196/annals.1254.010

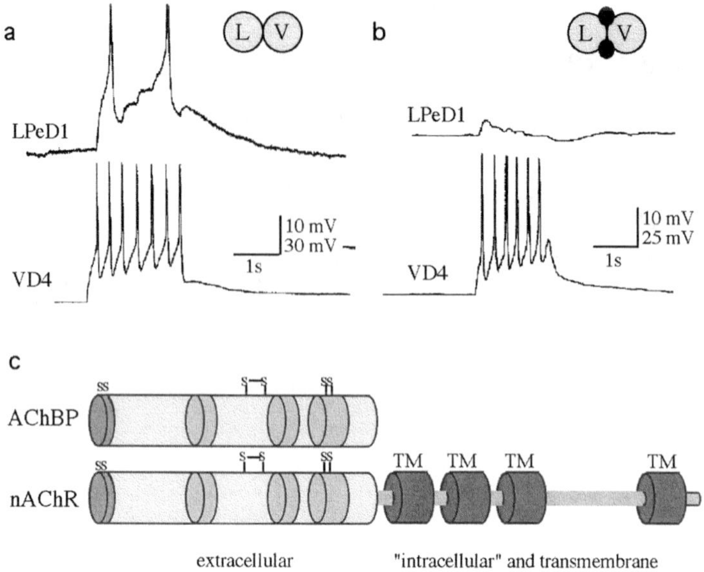

FIGURE 1. Glial cells cocultured with synaptically paired neurons specifically inhibit cholinergic synaptic transmission. Schematic representation of synapse pairs is given (V, VD4; L, LPeD1; R, RPeD1). Black circles: glial cells. **(a)** VD4-LPeD1 pairs formed a characteristic cholinergic excitatory synapse. Action potentials induced in the presynaptic cholinergic neuron VD4 generate EPSP and action potentials in LPeD1 (n = 13 cell pairs). **(b)** Same as above, but now with cocultured glial cells that suppress synaptic transmission between VD4 and LPeD1 (n = 13). **(c)** Schematic overall structure of AChBP and the α_7 nAChR subunit. Three ligand-binding loop regions, A, B, C (as described for the nAChRs), are indicated. TM, transmembrane domain.

tains large, well-identifiable neurons, which can be analyzed at the molecular level, at the level of the synapse, or as part of a neuronal network. In recent years, we explored the existence of mechanisms of glia-mediated modulation of neurotransmission, in which glial cells residing at tripartite synapses (consisting of pre- and postsynaptic element and glia) would directly modulate synaptic transmision. In these studies, we turned to individually identifiable neurons isolated from the *Lymnaea* central nervous system, which readily form cholinergic excitatory synapses *in vitro* and can be cocultured with or without glial cells. Synapses between a presynaptic cholinergic neuron and its postsynaptic partner were reconstructed.[1–3] It was found that, in the absence of glial cells, a train of induced action potentials in the cholinergic presynaptic neuron produced facilitatory excitatory postsynaptic potentials (EPSP) in the postsynaptic cell, which often led to spiking activity (FIG. 1a). In the presence of glial cells, however, the presynaptically induced action potentials failed to elicit facilitatory EPSP and action potentials in the postsynaptic cell (FIG. 1b). These data demonstrate that the glial cells specifically modulated the efficacy of cholinergic synaptic transmission. After an extensive series of experiments, we were able to show that suppression of neurotransmission is caused by secretion of a novel glia-derived protein.[4] For its acetylcholine-binding properties, we named it acetylcholine-binding protein (AChBP).

Subsequent biochemical purification and molecular cloning identified AChBP as a 210-residue protein (FIG. 1c). The protein has a moderate sequence identity with subunits of the Cys-loop family of ligand-gated ion channels, that is, the nicotinic acetylcholine receptors (nAChRs), $GABA_A$-, $GABA_C$-, glycine-, and $5HT_3$-receptors.[5–10] These receptors comprise 5 subunits, each consisting of an N-terminal, extracellular domain, which is involved in ligand binding, and a C-terminal half-containing 4 transmembrane segments, M1–M4, which make up the channel pore. AChBP is much shorter than these subunits and aligns only with the extracellular part, lacking pore-forming transmembrane regions altogether.[4] Homologous proteins of this size have at present not been found in sequence databases.

ACHBP ACTS AS A MODULATOR OF SYNAPTIC TRANSMISSION

On the basis of our *in vitro* data, we postulated a model of synaptic function for AChBP (FIG. 2). In short, the release experiments of AChBP from glial cells *in vitro*

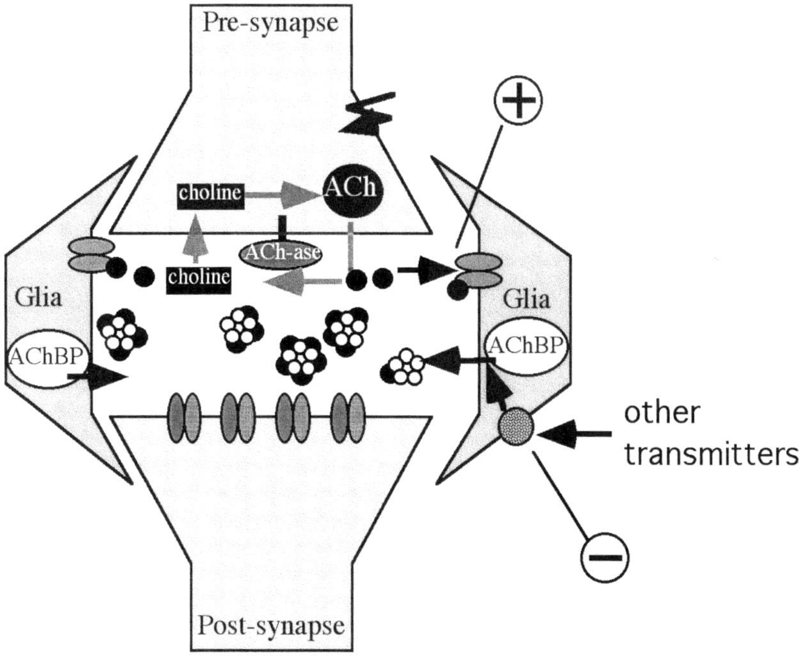

FIGURE 2. Model of the role of AChBP in neurotransmission. A basal level of AChBP is present in the synaptic cleft. Presynaptic ACh release can lead to activation of post-synaptic receptors and to EPSP. In parallel, nAChRs on glia are activated, causing increased release of AChBP into the synapse, which subsequently leads to suppression of cholinergic transmission (see text).

suggest that there is a basal level of AChBP in the synaptic cleft, set by continuous release from the synaptic glial cells. Under conditions of active presynaptic transmitter release, high millimolar concentrations of free ACh[11] will probably activate both postsynaptic receptors and the nAChRs on the synaptic glial cells (EC_{50} is in µM range), which would enhance the release of AChBP, thereby increasing its concentration in the synaptic cleft. The increase in AChBP levels may either diminish or terminate the ongoing ACh response, or raise the concentration of basal AChBP to the extent that subsequent responses to ACh are decreased.[4] Accurate models of the kinetics of AChBP in synaptic modulation will require data on concentrations of ACh, AChE, and postsynaptic nAChRs, on the localization and individual affinities of these components, as well as on diffusion characteristics of ACh.[12–14] Also, it must incorporate the effect of the ultrastructure of the synapse that determines the kinetic properties of these constituents, that is, small processes of synapse-invaginating glial cells that locally release AChBP. However, in a simplified example of various concentrations of ACh and AChBP, one can calculate that, if AChBP release would bring down the free ACh concentration to values below the EC_{50}, the postsynaptic response would be substantially affected.[4] As such, the concentration of AChBP in the synapse might critically determine whether transmission is either fully active or suppressed.

When in the synaptic cleft ACh is bound to AChBP, acetylcholinesterase will only hydrolyze the free ACh, thereby keeping the ACh concentration minimal and draining it from the AChBP buffer. Thus, ACh that is bound to AChBP is physically removed from the volume communication channel, unable to activate other receptor sites. Interestingly, molluscan glial cells are found throughout the brain; however, their density and subtype differ regionally, leaving the possibility that there are also local differences in the involvement of AChBP in neurotransmission. Also, different type of glial cells may integrate diverse inputs, which might selectively determine AChBP release and the strength of cholinergic transmission at specific synapses. Taken together, glial cells in the *Lymnaea* CNS are able to directly modulate cholinergic synaptic transmission and can do so via the release and buffering capacity of AChBP.

TOWARD A STRUCTURAL MODEL OF THE nACHRs

The nicotinic acetylcholine receptor (nAChR) has long been the prototype of ligand-gated ion channels, also known as Cys-loop receptors. This superfamily also includes the $GABA_A$ and $GABA_C$, the glycine, and the $5HT_3$ serotonin receptors.[10] These transmembrane receptors form pentamers of related subunits, in which each subunit consists of an N-terminal ligand-binding domain, 4 membrane-spanning regions (M1–M4), and a short intracellular region.[10] Extensive biochemical studies have defined the complexly organized ligand-binding sites that are found at the subunit interface. The binding of ligands goes through a complicated cycle of activation and desensitization.[7,15] Structurally, the proteins are well defined by the work of Nigel Unwin and colleagues, who have studied the *Torpedo* receptor up to a resolution of 4.6 Å,[16,17] but an atomic model has been lacking.

AChBP IS A HOMOLOGUE OF THE LIGAND-BINDING DOMAIN OF nAChRs

As discussed above, AChBP has a moderate sequence identity with subunits of the Cys-loop family of ligand-gated ion channels, that is, the nAChRs, $GABA_A$-, $GABA_C$-, glycine-, and $5HT_3$-receptors (cf. FIG. 1c). The conserved regions are the hallmarks of the superfamily of ligand-gated ion channels. The recombinant AChBP protein, expressed in yeast *Pichia pastoris*, assembles into stable homopentamers. Furthermore, AChBP contains all the amino acid residues needed for the ligand binding, showing pharmacology that is similar to a homopentameric nAChR, such as the neuronal α_7 receptor.[18] Thus, it binds better to nicotine than to ACh, and it binds very well to epibatidine. Nicotinic antagonists bind as expected, but some of

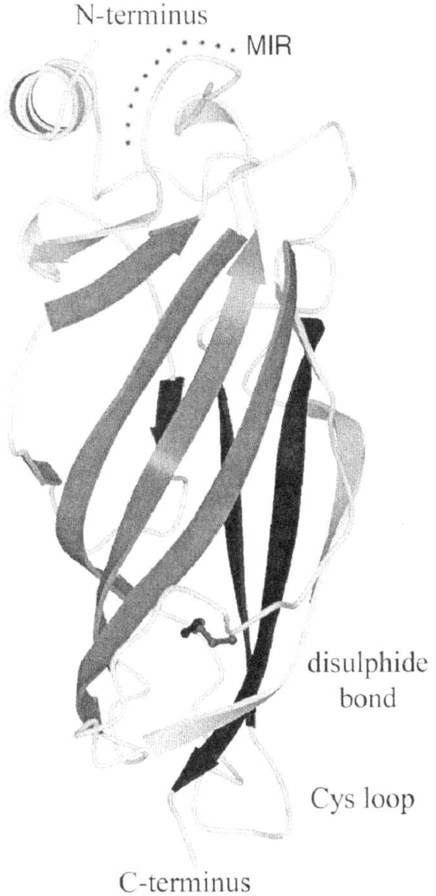

FIGURE 3a. Protomer fold of AChBP. The protein has an N-terminal helix followed by a β-sandwich. The C-terminal residue would be the start of the transmembrane receptor in nAChRs. Indicated is the approximate position of the MIR in the nAChR.

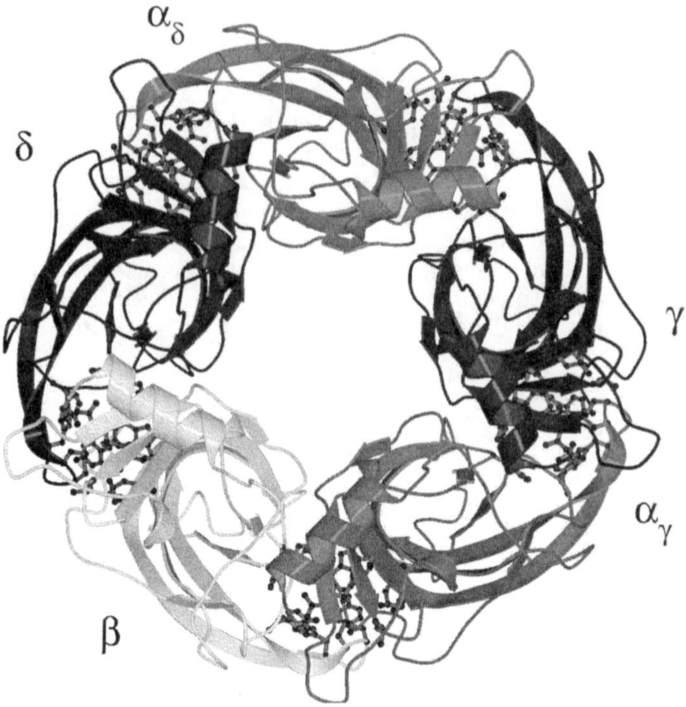

FIGURE 3b. Pentamer of AChBP, viewed along the fivefold axis. Possible subunit organization for the *Torpedo* nAChR is indicated.

the muscarinic antagonists also bind,[4] an effect that has also been observed for the homopentameric α_9 receptor.[19] In conclusion, AChBP is a soluble homologue of a ligand-binding domain of the nicotinic receptors. Revealing its structure is therefore relevant to the structure of the nAChRs.

STRUCTURE OF AChBP

The recombinant AChBP has been crystallized and its structure was determined with phases from multiwavelength anomalous diffraction on a Pb-derivative in two different crystal forms.[20] The electron density was improved by noncrystallographic and multicrystal averaging across three different crystal forms. The AChBP model was refined in the $P4_22_12$ crystal form, with one pentamer per asymmetric unit at 2.7 Å resolution.

The AChBP homopentamer (FIG. 3a) is composed of five protomers. It forms a doughnut-like structure with a radius of 80 Å and height of 62 Å (FIG. 3b), conforming to the electron microscopy data for the nAChR.[16] Each AChBP protomer has a modified immunoglobulin (Ig topology) with relatively long and twisted strands. Both β-sheets have at least one extra β-strand compared to the standard Ig-fold

TABLE 1. Numbering of ligand-binding residues in AChBP compared to *Torpedo* and muscle α_1, γ, and δ and human α_7 subunits

Loop	AChBP	α_1	γ	δ	α_7
A	Tyr89	Tyr93			Tyr93
B	Trp143	Trp149			Trp149
C	Tyr185	Tyr190			Tyr188
	Cys187	Cys192			Cys190
	Cys188	Cys193			Cys191
	Tyr192	Tyr198			Tyr195
D	Trp53		Trp55	Trp57	Trp55
	Gln55		Glu57	Thr59	Gln57
E	Arg104		Leu109	Leu111	Leu109
	Val106		Tyr111	Arg113	Asn111
	Leu112		Tyr117	Thr119	Gln117
	Met114		Leu119	Leu121	Leu119
F	Tyr164				
			Asp174	Asp180	Asp164

(FIG. 3b). An Ig-fold was predicted by Le Novère[21] and Corringer,[10] but the additional strands were not predicted, and the binding site is in a different place.

A disulfide bridge (Cys123–Cys136) is found in AChBP. This disulfide bond is absolutely conserved in the superfamily of pentameric ligand-gated ion channels and has importance for the stabilization of the fold as shown by Blount and Merlie[22] and Green and Wanamaker.[23] Its structural similarity to the Ig "tyrosine cornerstone", stabilizing the Ig-fold, may indicate that this disulfide bond has a structural role in keeping the two β-sheets together.

THE LIGAND-BINDING SITE OF ACHBP

The residues involved in ligand binding in the muscle and *Torpedo* nAChR subtypes have been extensively investigated and are found at the interface between an α-subunit and a neighboring subunit, forming the primary and complementary parts of the binding pocket, respectively.[10] The α-subunit residues important for binding are clustered in "loop" regions A,[24] B,[25] and C.[25–27] The neighboring subunit, γ or δ, contributes loops D,[28] E,[28–30] and F[31] (TABLE 1); in homopentamers, the equivalent loops will be contributed by α-subunits.

In the AChBP structure, all of these loop regions are indeed found to form a single pocket region at the subunit interface (FIG. 4), with loops A–C contributed from one subunit and D–F from another. Loops A, B, C, and F are indeed structural loops in the structure, but the residues contributed from loops D and E are found on β-strands. The pocket is lined by aromatic residues of loop A–D, while the hydrophobic components of the residues in loop E form the lid of the pocket. The Tyr164 that is contributed from the loop F region is not conserved, and the variation in length and

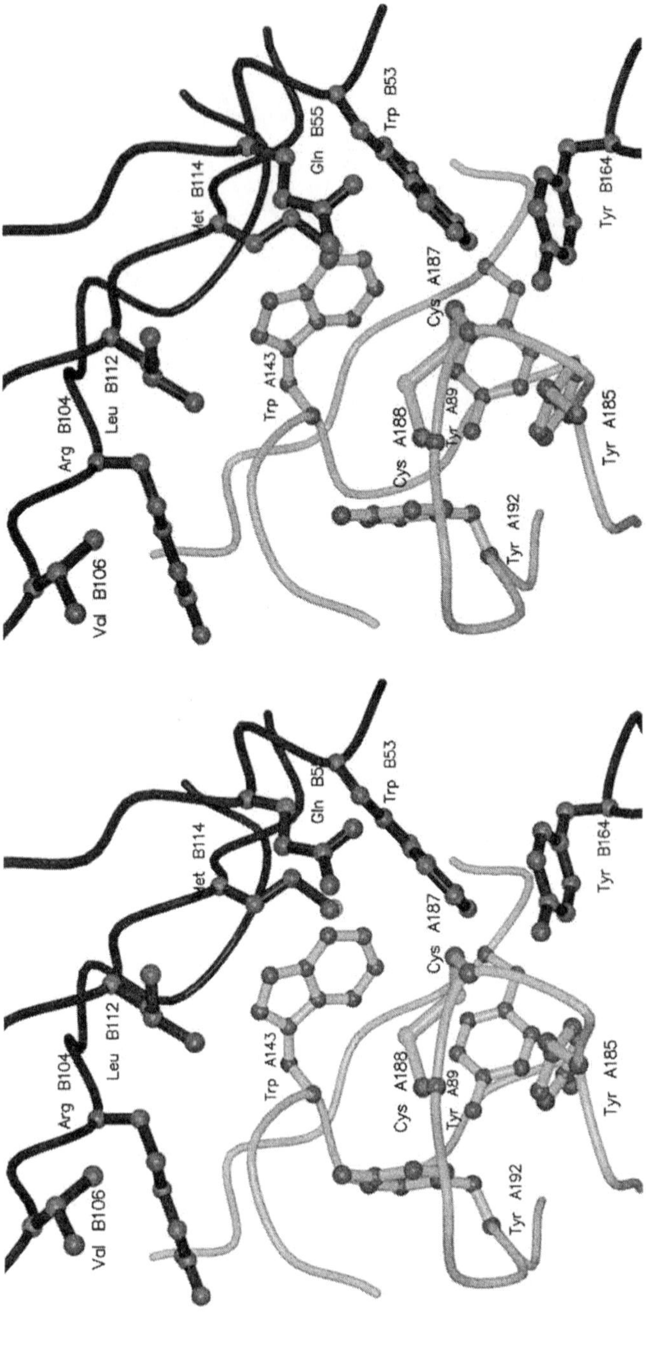

FIGURE 4. Stereo representation of the ligand-binding site of AChBP: principal side in light gray, complementary side in dark gray. For the equivalent residues in other receptors, see TABLE 1.

sequence in this area indicates that the region may form a somewhat different fold in other family members, contributing another residue to the binding site.

In the experimental electron density, extra features were observed in the ligand-binding site. This density was attributed to a HEPES buffer molecule that was used in crystallization. HEPES was found to bind with an IC_{50} of 100 mM, which could cause partial occupancy at the concentrations used. The HEPES buffer has a positive charged nitrogen atom, similar to ACh. This atom stacks on Trp143 in a similar fashion as expected for ACh stacking on the equivalent Trp149 in nAChR.[32] Initially, the position of the HEPES molecule could not be unambiguously revealed, but in recent 2.0 resolution data of AChBP (unpublished) the position of the molecule was refined to show that the sulfate group points down and toward the solvent. However, the position of the charged ammonium group is not changed in this updated model.

POSITION OF (NON-)CONSERVED SEQUENCES IN THE STRUCTURE

There is considerable sequence conservation in the superfamily of ligand-gated ion channels (LGICs). The conserved residues are mostly found within the protomer, contributing hydrophobic residues to the core and hydrophilic residues to structurally important sites. This conserved core structure indicates that the overall fold of the other family members will greatly resemble the AChBP fold.

The residues that form the so-called Cys-loop are a conserved region that is lacking in AChBP. This region, connecting the absolutely conserved cysteines (123–136 in AChBP, 128–142 in *Torpedo* receptor), is a conserved hydrophobic region in the LGIC superfamily, but in AChBP it is one residue shorter and mostly hydrophilic. The loop is found on the membrane-facing side of AChBP and probably interacts with the transmembrane domain in the receptor, a region that is absent in AChBP.

A major surprise in the structure is the lack of conservation of the subunit interface across the superfamily of LGICs. The residues that are forming the subunit interface in AChBP vary between superfamily members, including changes in character from charged to hydrophobic and vice versa, without the necessary complementary changes. Thus, it can be concluded that the precise interactions in the interface are not very important for preserving the pentamer formation. Moreover, they are apparently not essential for maintaining the mechanism of opening a channel in response to a ligand binding.

THE MIR REGION

In muscle-type nAChRs, the main immunogenic region (MIR), comprising residues $\alpha_1 67$–$\alpha_1 76$, acts as an epitope in the autoimmune disease, myasthenia gravis.[33] Although the MIR-related region in AChBP (residues 65–72) shows no sequence homology to the α_1-subunit, its location in a highly accessible position in loop L3 at the "top" of the pentamer agrees well with the expected accessibility for this region. It also fits with EM studies that located the MIR at the distal end of the receptor relative to the membrane.[16] The NMR structure of the MIR peptide[34] is different from the equivalent region in AChBP. The largest region that can be superimposed will be residues 68–72 of the receptor peptide onto residues 66–70 of AChBP. Such

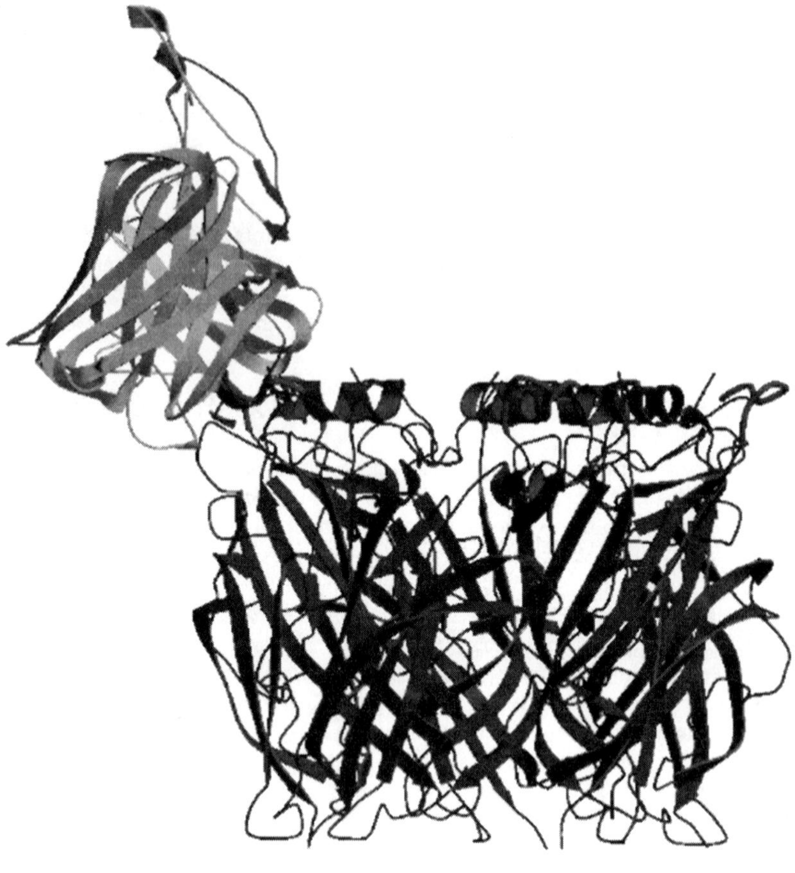

FIGURE 5. A model of the complex formed between the antibody and the MIR peptide was superposed on AChBP, yielding a very interesting impression of the antibody binding to AChBP.

a superposition yields an rms deviation of 1.0 Å. A model of the complex formed between the antibody and the MIR peptide was published.[35] Combination of that model and the superposition described above yields a very interesting impression of the antibody binding to AChBP, in which no major clashes occur (FIG. 5).

MECHANISM OF GATING

Once a ligand is bound to the extracellular domain of the receptor, this will cause a signal that is relayed to the transmembrane domain. One possible mechanism is a pivoting motion about the ligand-binding site of the entire protomer. Such a rigid body motion would presumably cause a rearrangement in the transmembrane domain. Other mechanisms can be imagined, but the lack of conservation of the subunit interface would seem to imply that they have to be looked for in the protomer. Possibilities involve a movement of the loop C β-hairpin and a rearrangement of the β-sandwich structure. It will be interesting to see whether AChBP itself will be useful as a model to study such ligand-dependent movements. It does not have a transmembrane domain and presumably would not need such a movement for its function. Further studies have to show whether this will be the case. However, the crystal structure of AChBP undoubtedly will be a starting point for studying such movements since it shows what regions of the sequence are found at what sites in the structure and thus will provide new ideas for experiments.

REFERENCES

1. Feng, Z.P., J. Klumperman, K. Lukowiak & N.I. Syed. 1997. *In vitro* synaptogenesis between the somata of identified *Lymnaea* neurons requires protein synthesis, but not extrinsic growth factors or substrate adhesion molecules. J. Neurosci. **17:** 7839–7849.
2. Hamakawa, T. *et al.* 1999. Excitatory synaptogenesis between identified *Lymnaea* neurons requires extrinsic trophic factors and is mediated by receptor tyrosine kinases. J. Neurosci. **19:** 9306–9312.
3. Woodin, M.A., T. Hamakawa, M. Takasaki *et al.* 1999. Trophic factor–induced plasticity of synaptic connections between identified *Lymnaea* neurons. Learn. Mem. **6:** 307–316.
4. Smit, A.B., N.I. Syed, D. Schaap *et al.* 2001. A glia-derived acetylcholine-binding protein that modulates synaptic transmission. Nature **411:** 261–268.
5. Le Novère, N. & J.P. Changeux. 1995. Molecular evolution of the nicotinic acetylcholine receptor: an example of multigene family in excitable cells. J. Mol. Evol. **40:** 155–172.
6. Devillers-Thiery, A., J.L. Galzi, J.L. Eiselé *et al.* 1993. Functional architecture of the nicotinic acetylcholine receptor: a prototype of ligand-gated ion channels. J. Membr. Biol. **136:** 97–112.
7. Karlin, A. & M.H. Akabas. 1995. Toward a structural basis for the function of nicotinic acetylcholine receptors and their cousins. Neuron **15:** 1231–1244.
8. Mehta, A.K. & M.K. Ticku. 1999. An update on $GABA_A$ receptors. Brain Res. Rev. **2/3:** 196–217.
9. Betz, H., J. Kuhse, V. Schmieden *et al.* 1999. Structure and functions of inhibitory and excitatory glycine receptors. Ann. N.Y. Acad. Sci. **868:** 667–676.
10. Corringer, P.J., N. Le Novère & J.P. Changeux. 2000. Nicotinic receptors at the amino-acid level. Annu. Rev. Pharmacol. Toxicol. **40:** 431–458.
11. Kuffler, S.W. & D. Yoshikama. 1975. The number of transmitter molecules in a quantum: an estimate from iontophoretic application of acetylcholine at the neuromuscular synapse. J. Physiol. **1:** 465–482.
12. Whatey, J.C., M.M. Nass & H.A. Lester. 1979. Numerical reconstruction of the quantal event at nicotinic synapses. Biophys. J. **27:** 145–164.
13. Land, B.R., E.E. Salpeter & M.M. Salpeter. 1981. Kinetic parameters for acetylcholine interaction in intact neuromuscular junction. Proc. Natl. Acad. Sci. USA **78:** 7200–7204.
14. Katz, B. & R. Miledi. 1973. The binding of acetylcholine to receptors and its removal from the synaptic cleft. J. Physiol. **231:** 549–574.
15. Changeux, J.P. & S.J. Edelstein. 2001. Allosteric mechanism in normal and pathological nicotinic acetylcholine receptors. Curr. Opin. Neurobiol. **11:** 369–377.
16. Miyazawa, A., Y. Fujiyoshi, M. Stowell & N. Unwin. 1999. Nicotinic acetylcholine receptor at 4.6 Å resolution: transverse tunnels in the channel wall. J. Mol. Biol. **288:** 765–786.
17. Unwin, N. 2000. The Croonian Lecture 2000: Nicotinic acetylcholine receptor and the structural basis of fast synaptic transmission. Philos. Trans. R. Soc. Lond. **B355:** 1813–1829.

18. ANAND, R., X. PENG & J. LINDSTROM. 1993. Homomeric and native α7 acetylcholine receptors exhibit remarkably similar, but non-identical pharmacological properties, suggesting that the native receptor is a heteromeric protein complex. FEBS Lett. **327:** 241–246.
19. ELGOYHEN, A.B., D.S. JOHNSON, J. BOULTER *et al.* 1994. Alpha 9: an acetylcholine receptor with novel pharmacological properties expressed in rat cochlear hair cells. Cell **79:** 705–715.
20. BREJC, K., W.J. VAN DIJK, R.V. KLAASSEN *et al.* 2001. Crystal structure of an ACh-binding protein reveals the ligand-binding domain of nicotinic receptors. Nature **411:** 269–276.
21. LE NOVÈRE, N., P.J. CORRINGER & J.P. CHANGEUX. 1999. Improved secondary structure predictions for a nicotinic receptor subunit: incorporation of solvent accessibility and experimental data into a two-dimensional representation. Biophys. J. **76:** 2329–2345.
22. BLOUNT, P. & J.P. MERLIE. 1990. Mutational analysis of muscle nicotinic acetylcholine receptor subunit assembly. J. Cell Biol. **111:** 2613–2622.
23. GREEN, W.N. & C.P. WANAMAKER. 1997. The role of the cysteine loop in acetylcholine receptor assembly. J. Biol. Chem. **272:** 20945–20953.
24. GALZI, J.L., F. REVAH, D. BLACK *et al.* 1990. Identification of a novel amino acid alpha-tyrosine 93 within the cholinergic ligands-binding sites of the acetylcholine receptor by photoaffinity labeling: additional evidence for a three-loop model of the cholinergic ligands-binding sites. J. Biol. Chem. **265:** 10430–10437.
25. DENNIS, M., J. GIRAUDAT, F. KOTZYBA-HIBERT *et al.* 1988. Amino acids of the *Torpedo marmorata* acetylcholine receptor alpha subunit labeled by a photoaffinity ligand for the acetylcholine binding site. Biochemistry **27:** 2346–2357.
26. KAO, P.N., A.J. DWORK, R.R. KALDANY *et al.* 1984. Identification of the alpha subunit half-cystine specifically labeled by an affinity reagent for the acetylcholine receptor binding site. J. Biol. Chem. **259:** 11662–11665.
27. SINE, S.M., P. QUIRAM, F. PAPANIKOLAOU *et al.* 1994. Conserved tyrosines in the alpha subunit of the nicotinic acetylcholine receptor stabilize quaternary ammonium groups of agonists and curariform antagonists. J. Biol. Chem. **269:** 8808–8816.
28. CHIARA, D.C. & J.B. COHEN. 1997. Identification of amino acids contributing to high and low affinity *d*-tubocurarine sites in *Torpedo* nicotinic acetylcholine receptor. J. Biol. Chem. **272:** 32940–32950.
29. CHIARA, D.C., Y. XIE & J.B. COHEN. 1999. Structure of the agonist-binding sites of the *Torpedo* nicotinic acetylcholine receptor: affinity-labeling and mutational analyses identify γTyr-111/δArg-113 as antagonist affinity determinants. Biochemistry **38:** 6689–6698.
30. SINE, S.M. 1997. Identification of equivalent residues in the γ, δ, and ε subunits of the nicotinic receptor that contribute to α-bungarotoxin binding. J. Biol. Chem. **272:** 23521–23527.
31. CZAJKOWSKI, C. & A. KARLIN. 1995. Structure of the nicotinic receptor acetylcholine-binding site: identification of acidic residues in the δ subunit within 0.9 nm of the α subunit-binding site disulfide. J. Biol. Chem. **270:** 3160–3164.
32. ZHONG, W., J.P. GALLIVAN, Y. ZHANG *et al.* 1998. From ab initio quantum mechanics to molecular neurobiology: a cation-pi binding site in the nicotinic receptor. Proc. Natl. Acad. Sci. USA **90:** 9031–9035.
33. FERNANDO VALENZUELA, C., P. WEIGN, J. YGUERABIDE & D.A. JOHNSON. 1994. Transverse distance between the membrane and the agonist binding sites on the *Torpedo* acetylcholine receptor: a fluorescence study. Biophys. J. **66:** 674–682.
34. CUNG, M.T., P. DEMANGE, M. MARRAUD *et al.* 1991. Two-dimensional 1H-NMR study of antigen-antibody interactions: binding of synthetic decapeptides to an anti-acetylcholine receptor monoclonal antibody. Biopolymers **6:** 769–776.
35. KLEINJUNG, J., M.C. PETIT, P. ORLEWSKI *et al.* 2000. The third-dimensional structure of the complex between an Fv antibody fragment and an analogue of the main immunogenic region of the acetylcholine receptor: a combined two-dimensional homology, and molecular modeling approach. Biopolymers **53:** 113–128.

The Binding Site of Acetylcholine Receptor

From Synthetic Peptides to Solution and Crystal Structure

SARA FUCHS,[a,b] RONI KASHER,[c] MOSHE BALASS,[c] TALI SCHERF,[d] MICHAL HAREL,[e] MATI FRIDKIN,[e] JOEL L. SUSSMAN,[e] AND EPHRAIM KATCHALSKI-KATZIR[c]

Departments of [a]Immunology, [b]Biological Chemistry, [c]Chemical Services, [d]Structural Biology, and [e]Organic Chemistry, The Weizmann Institute of Science, Rehovot 76100, Israel

ABSTRACT: Our group has been employing short synthetic peptides, encompassing sequences from the acetylcholine receptor (AChR) α-subunit for the analysis of the binding site of the AChR. A 13-mer peptide mimotope, with similar structural motifs to the AChR binding region, was selected by α-bungarotoxin (α-BTX) from a phage-display peptide library. The solution structure of a complex between this library-lead peptide and α-BTX was solved by NMR spectroscopy. On the basis of this NMR study and on structure-function analysis of the AChR binding site, and in order to obtain peptides with higher affinity to α-BTX, additional peptides resulting from systematic residue replacement in the lead peptide were designed and characterized. Of these, four peptides, designated high-affinity peptides (HAPs), homologous to the binding region of the AChR, inhibited the binding of α-BTX to the AChR with an IC_{50} of 2 nM. The solution and crystal structures of complexes of α-BTX with HAP were solved, demonstrating that the HAP fits snugly to α-BTX and adopts a β-hairpin conformation. The X-ray structures of the bound HAP and the homologous loop of the acetylcholine binding protein (AChBP) are remarkably similar. Their superposition results in a model indicating that α-BTX wraps around the receptor binding-site loop and, in addition, binds tightly at the interface of two of the receptor subunits, where it inserts a finger into the ligand-binding site. Our proposed model explains the strong antagonistic activity of α-BTX and accommodates much of the biochemical data on the mode of interaction of α-BTX with the AChR.

KEYWORDS: acetylcholine receptor (AChR); α-bungarotoxin (α-BTX); binding site; NMR structure; X-ray structure

The binding site of the AChR has been a subject of intensive research over the years. α-BTX binds the AChR with very high affinity and, specifically, has been most instrumental in the analysis of the structure of the ligand-binding site of this

Address for correspondence: Dr. Sara Fuchs, Department of Immunology, The Weizmann Institute of Science, Rehovot 76100, Israel. Voice: +972-8-9342618; fax: +972-8-9344141. sara.fuchs@weizmann.ac.il

Ann. N.Y. Acad. Sci. 998: 93–100 (2003). © 2003 New York Academy of Sciences. doi: 10.1196/annals.1254.011

receptor. Various strategies for mapping and characterizing the binding site of the AChR have been employed in our lab, mainly by using short synthetic peptides.

SYNTHETIC PEPTIDES AND THEIR ANTIBODIES FOR MAPPING THE α-BTX BINDING SITE

Antibodies to short synthetic peptides from the α-subunit of the AChR were first employed to map the α-BTX binding site.[1,2] We demonstrated that the binding site is within a 15-kDa proteolytic fragment of the α-subunit that includes the two adjacent cysteine residues 192 and 193, and that have been reported by Karlin's group[3] to be at the binding site. We have then shown that a synthetic dodecapeptide within this fragment, KHWVYYTCCPAT, corresponding to residues 185–196 of the α-subunit of *Torpedo* AChR and including cys 192 and 193, contains the essential elements for α-BTX binding.[2,4] This peptide binds α-BTX directly, and the binding is inhibited by *d*-tubocurarine. The binding of the peptide to toxin is rather low, with an IC_{50} of about 10^{-5} M, which is about six orders of magnitude weaker than the binding of toxin to the entire AChR. At this point, we realized that changes in this region may be associated with changes in binding specificity. Interestingly, the homologous dodecapeptide of human AChR failed to bind α-BTX.[4]

THE BINDING SITE IN ANIMAL SPECIES THAT IS RESISTANT TO α-BTX

In an attempt to elucidate the molecular basis for the ligand-binding site of the AChR, we chose to study muscle AChRs from animal species exhibiting various degrees of resistance to α-BTX, in particular the snake and the mongoose.[5–8] Sequence comparison of the binding site domains between species indicates that substitutions at positions 187, 189, 194, and 197 of the AChR α-subunit are important in determining the resistance to α-BTX.[5–7] In addition, the snake as well as the mongoose AChR both have a glycosylation site at the binding-site domain.[5,6] Such a glycosylation may provide additional protection against the toxin. Site-directed mutagenesis on the ligand-binding domain of the mongoose AChR α-subunit, obtained by exchanging residues 187, 189, 194, and 197 with those present in the mouse α-subunit, led us to propose two subsites in the binding domain for α-BTX:[8] (1) the proline subsite that includes proline residues 194 and 197 and is critical for α-BTX binding and (2) the aromatic subsite that includes amino acid residues 187 and 189 and determines the extent of α-BTX binding.

A LEAD PEPTIDE SELECTED BY α-BTX FROM A RANDOM PHAGE-DISPLAY PEPTIDE LIBRARY

Studies on the AChR binding site by various groups revealed that additional segments in the α-subunit as well as residues from neighboring subunits participate in the binding site. Thus, linear sequences from the protein by themselves may not be good enough to design short peptides that bind α-BTX with high affinity. We have therefore turned to random combinatorial libraries and employed phage-display peptide libraries to select peptides that interact specifically with α-BTX. A library-derived lead peptide (MRYYESSLKSYPD) that binds specifically α-BTX and inhibits its binding to the AChR with an IC_{50} value in the low-micromolar range has been defined.[9] This peptide contains the motif YYXSS that is homologous to the AChR consensus motif YYXCC, located at the putative ligand-binding site of muscle AChRs as well as of neuronal AChRs that bind α-BTX.

The structure of the complex between α-BTX and the library-lead peptide was determined using 2-D ^{1}H-NMR spectroscopy.[10] The bound peptide was found to adopt an almost globular conformation around a hydrophobic core created by a side chain of Tyr11 of the peptide, whereas the free peptide in solution was characterized by a rather random conformation. The amino acid residues that were shown to bind tightly with α-BTX, or whose side chains interact internally with other residues in the peptide, were identified. These are Arg2, Tyr3, Tyr4, Glu5, Ser7, Leu8, and Tyr11.[10]

HIGH-AFFINITY PEPTIDES (HAPs) DESIGNED BY SYSTEMATIC RESIDUE REPLACEMENT

The affinity of the library-lead peptide to α-BTX was still about four orders of magnitude weaker than the affinity of α-BTX to the AChR. We therefore attempted to design peptides with higher affinity that would have biological activity *in vivo* and that could be cocrystallized with α-BTX for X-ray analysis. We first designed and prepared a new peptide library based on systematic single amino acid replacement of some of the residues of the library-lead peptide.[11] In order to reduce the number of prepared peptides, the natural amino acids were categorized into six groups according to the chemical nature of their side chains: amino acids with hydrophobic side chains (Ile, Val, Leu), amino acids with aromatic side chains (Phe, Trp, Tyr), amino acids with positively charged side chains (Lys, Arg, His), amino acids with negatively charged side chains or their corresponding amides capable of hydrogen bonding (Asp, Glu, Asn, Gln), amino acids with the smallest side chain (Gly and Ala), and proline as a group by itself since it affects the backbone conformation in a unique way. Cysteine, serine, threonine, and methionine were excluded in most cases. Taking into consideration the structural data from the NMR analysis of the complex of α-BTX with the library-lead peptide,[10] replacements were introduced only at positions that did not contribute to α-BTX binding or to intrapeptide interactions. Thus, in this new library of peptides, replacements were carried out at positions 1, 6, 9, 10, 12, and 13 of the lead peptide. Each of these positions was systematically replaced by six different amino acid residues, one at a time, representing each one of the categories of amino acids (e.g., hydrophobic, aromatic, and acidic).[11] The inhibition of the binding of α-BTX to *Torpedo* AChR by the newly synthesized peptides was measured, and the IC_{50} values were compared with that of the original library-lead peptide that exhibited an IC_{50} value of 3.3×10^{-7} M. Differences in inhibitory potencies of some of the peptides were observed, although all of them differ from each other by only one residue. One peptide in this series (MRYYESS-LKPYPD) exhibited an increase of one order of magnitude in the inhibitory activity (IC_{50} of 3.2×10^{-8} M) as compared with that of the library-lead peptide. Interestingly, this peptide represents a replacement of Ser10 by Pro, which is the residue present at this corresponding position in the AChR (see TABLE 1).

In addition to this series of peptides, we have also replaced Met1 in the lead peptide by Trp (W), corresponding to Trp187 of the α-subunit of muscle AChR. This residue has been reported to be important for α-BTX binding.[5–8] Indeed, a peptide with this replacement (peptide 39 in TABLE 1) exhibited an IC_{50} of 3.5×10^{-8} M, which is one order of magnitude better than that of the original library-lead peptide.[11]

In an attempt to further increase the inhibitory potency of the peptides, we designed a new series of peptides having two or more replacements (TABLE 1).[11] Some of these peptides, designated high-affinity peptides (HAPs), inhibited the binding of α-BTX to the AChR with IC_{50} values of $2–4 \times 10^{-9}$ M. The inhibitory potency of the HAPs is stronger by at least two orders of magnitude than the inhibitions obtained by the original phage library-lead peptide (TABLE 1) and is also stronger than the inhibition obtained by any 13- or 14-mer peptide derived from sequences at the binding-site domain of the AChR.[11] Moreover, the HAPs exhibit inhibitory potency that is equal to that of the entire α-subunit of the AChR.[11,12] Thus, the systematic residue replacement approach yielded peptides with high affinities that could not have been achieved by the preparation of peptides corresponding to the amino acid sequences of the α-BTX binding site of the AChR. The increased affinity of the HAPs could be explained by the NMR and crystal structures of the peptides complexed with α-BTX (see below).

It should be noted that, in preliminary *in vivo* studies, we have observed that under appropriate experimental conditions, when HAP1 (see TABLE 1) is injected into mice, it is capable of neutralizing the toxic effect of α-BTX.[11]

NMR STRUCTURE OF THE HAP/α-BTX COMPLEX IN SOLUTION

The structure of the complex between α-BTX and HAP1 (TABLE 1) has been solved by ^{1}H-NMR spectroscopy.[13] A schematic ribbon diagram of the NMR-derived structure of the bound toxin in its complex with HAP1 is shown in FIGURE 1. As observed earlier for the complex with the library-lead peptide, the HAP interacts mainly with fingers 1 and 2 and the C-terminus of α-BTX.[13] However, whereas the library peptide folded into nearly a round shape conformation,[10] the HAP folds into an elongated β-hairpin conformation. The β-hairpin structure of the peptide is created by two antiparallel β-strands, which combine with the already existing triple-stranded β-sheet of the toxin to form a five-stranded intermolecular, antiparallel β-sheet.[13] The fact that a short peptide (HAP1) in its bound form has such a well-organized and well-defined structural element, which exists both intra- and intermolecularly, seems to be a unique phenomenon. The formation of a short stretch of antiparallel β-sheet, not only within the bound peptide, but also between the peptide and the protein, represents a novel structural motif as previously reported.[14] This unique structure accounts for most of the increased binding affinity of HAP1 to α-BTX. Trp1 of the HAP that corresponds to position 187 of muscle AChR contributes, through its side chain, to the formation of both intermolecular contacts (hydrophobic interactions and hydrogen bonding with A7, T8, and S9 of α-BTX) as well as intrapeptide interactions. The presence of Pro10 and Pro12 seems to represent the proline subsite of muscle AChR that was shown to be of critical importance in estab-

TABLE 1. HAPs and their IC_{50} values

Peptide	1	2	3	4	5	6	7	8	9	10	11	12	13	IC_{50} (M)
Library	M	R	Y	Y	E	S	S	L	K	S	Y	P	D	$3.3x10^{-7}$
39[a]	W	R	Y	Y	E	S	S	L	K	S	Y	P	D	$3.5x10^{-8}$
29	M	R	Y	Y	E	S	S	L	K	P	Y	P	D	$3.2x10^{-8}$
48	W	R	Y	Y	E	S	S	L	K	P	Y	P	D	$1.0x10^{-8}$
49	W	R	Y	Y	E	S	S	L	D	P	Y	P	D	$3.8x10^{-9}$
50 HAP1	W	R	Y	Y	E	S	S	L	E	P	Y	P	D	$2.0x10^{-9}$
51	W	R	Y	Y	E	S	S	K	E	P	Y	P	D	$5.8x10^{-8}$
52	W	R	Y	Y	E	Y	S	L	D	P	Y	P	D	$1.6x10^{-9}$
53	W	R	Y	Y	E	S	S	L	D	P	Y	P	E	$4.8x10^{-9}$
54 HAP2	W	R	Y	Y	E	S	S	L	L	P	Y	P	D	$1.9x10^{-9}$
55	M	R	Y	Y	E	C	C	L	K	S	Y	P	D	$3.3x10^{-8}$
56	W	R	Y	Y	E	C	C	L	D	P	Y	P	D	$1.9x10^{-9}$

[a]Numbers of peptides are as given in ref. 11.

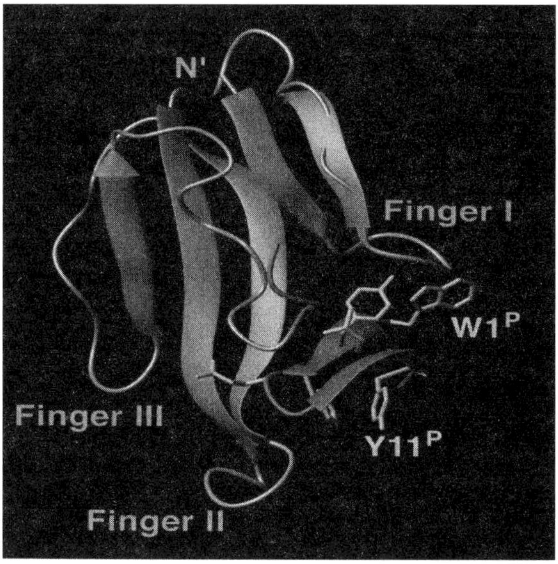

FIGURE 1. Solution structure of the HAP1/α-BTX complex (a ribbon diagram). Adapted from ref. 13.

lishing the affinity of the receptor to the toxin.[8] Hydrophobic interactions of Trp1 and Pro10 provide further stabilization of the bound peptide by holding together the two peptide ends.[13]

CRYSTAL STRUCTURE OF THE HAP/α-BTX COMPLEX

Attempts were made to obtain well-diffracting crystals of a complex between HAP and α-BTX and to elucidate its 3-D structure by X-ray crystallography. We were successful in obtaining such crystals of the complex of α-BTX with HAP2 (WRYYESSLLPYPD, TABLE 1) and have determined the crystal structure at 1.8 Å resolution.[15] The structure obtained (FIG. 2) agreed well with the NMR findings described above. The 13-mer HAP2 assumes an antiparallel β-hairpin structure and is held snugly between fingers 1, 2, and 4 of α-BTX. Out of a total of 1552 $Å^2$ of accessible surface area of HAP, approximately 45% (682 $Å^2$) became inaccessible upon its binding to α-BTX.

The detailed X-ray analysis of the HAP2/α-BTX complex reveals the importance of Trp1 and Pro10 (Trp187 and Pro196 in AChR) in determining the high affinity of HAP2 toward the toxin. Trp1 at the N-terminus of the peptide adds two side-chain interactions with the toxin between the indole N^{ε} atom and the carbonyl oxygen of residues 6 and 7 of α-BTX. The substitution of Ser10 of the lead peptide to Pro in HAP2 adds to the stability of the binding conformation of the peptide. Proline fits well in a hydrophobic pocket. It is situated at the core of the HAP2 intramolecular β-sheet and makes stacking interactions with Tyr3 and edge-on interactions with Trp1.

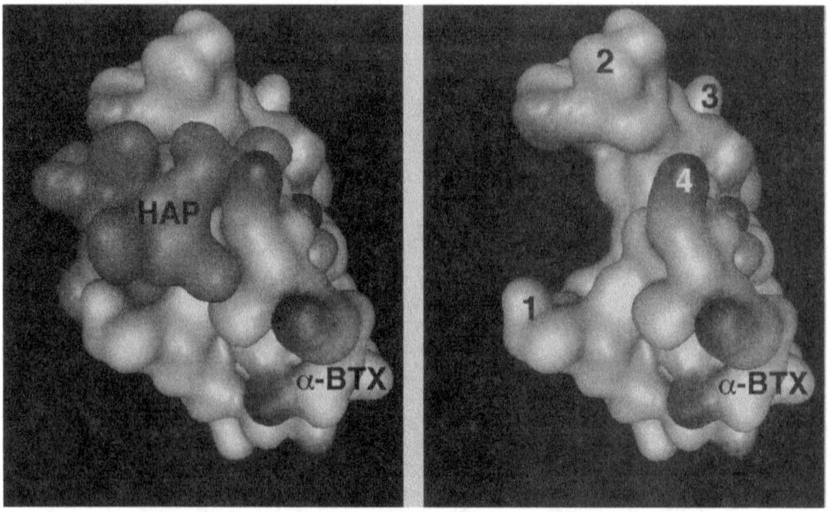

FIGURE 2. A 3-D surface drawing of the crystal structure of the HAP2/α-BTX complex (space-filling model): (*left*) HAP2/α-BTX complex; (*right*) α-BTX with HAP2 removed. Adapted from ref. 15.

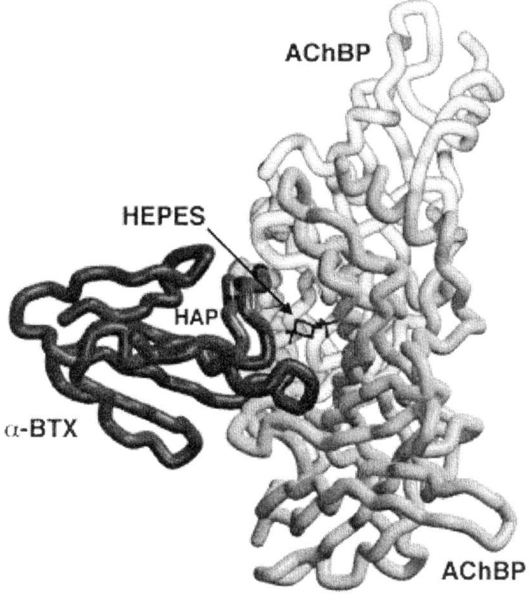

FIGURE 3. The combined model of HAP2/α-BTX complex and AChBP structure. Adapted from ref. 15.

Of particular interest was the finding that the structures of the bound peptide and the homologous loop of acetylcholine binding protein (AChBP)[16] (an analogue of the soluble extracellular domain of the AChR) are remarkably similar.[15] This is in spite of the fact that the sequence of HAP2 has only three residues identical to residues in the 182–194 loop of the AChBP.[15] It thus seems that even the short 13-mer binding HAP assumes a structure similar to the corresponding region of the AChR upon binding to α-BTX.

On the basis of the superposition of the bound peptide and the corresponding loop of the AChBP, it was possible to build a molecular model of the interaction of α-BTX with the AChBP and, by analogy, to visualize the interaction of α-BTX with the AChR (FIG. 3). In this detailed model complex, α-BTX wraps around the receptor binding-site loop and, in addition, binds tightly at the interface of two of the receptor subunits, where it inserts a finger into the ligand-binding site, thus blocking access to the acetylcholine binding site, explaining its strong antagonistic activity.[15]

In conclusion, our continuing efforts to study the binding site of the AChR by employing synthetic peptides have resulted in the elucidation of the 3-D structure of the peptide that forms the binding-site loop of the AChR for α-BTX, as well as of the mode of interaction of α-BTX with the AChR. The structural knowledge gained may prove a powerful tool in the development of antivenom drugs and in the design of therapies for disorders in which the AChR is involved.

ACKNOWLEDGMENTS

Research in the laboratory of S. Fuchs was supported by grants from the Muscular Dystrophy Association of America and by the Association Française contre les Myopathies.

REFERENCES

1. NEUMANN, D., G.M. GERSHONI, M. FRIDKIN & S. FUCHS. 1985. Antibodies to synthetic peptides as probes for the binding site on the α-subunit of the acetylcholine receptor. Proc. Natl. Acad. Sci. USA **82:** 3490–3493.
2. NEUMANN, D., D. BARCHAN, A. SAFRAN *et al.* 1986. Mapping of the α-bungarotoxin binding site within the α-subunit of the acetylcholine receptor. Proc. Natl. Acad. Sci. USA **83:** 3008–3011.
3. KAO, P., A. DWORK, R. KALDANY *et al.* 1984. Identification of the α-subunit half-cysteine specifically labeled by an affinity reagent for the acetylcholine receptor binding site. J. Biol. Chem. **259:** 11662–11665.
4. NEUMANN, D., D. BARCHAN, M. FRIDKIN & S. FUCHS. 1986. Analysis of ligand binding to the synthetic dodecapeptide 185–196 of the acetylcholine receptor α-subunit. Proc. Natl. Acad. Sci. USA **83:** 9250–9253.
5. NEUMANN, D., D. BARCHAN, M. HOROWITZ *et al.* 1989. Snake acetylcholine receptor: cloning of the domain containing the four extracellular cysteines of the α-subunit. Proc. Natl. Acad. Sci. USA **86:** 7255–7259.
6. BARCHAN, D., S. KACHALSKY, D. NEUMANN *et al.* 1992. How the mongoose can fight the snake: the binding site of the mongoose acetylcholine receptor. Proc. Natl. Acad. Sci. USA **89:** 7717–7721.
7. BARCHAN, D., M. OVADIA, E. KOCHVA & S. FUCHS. 1995. The binding site of the nicotinic acetylcholine receptor in animal species resistant to α-bungarotoxin. Biochemistry **34:** 9172–9176.
8. KACHALSKY, S.G., B.S. JENSEN, D. BARCHAN & S. FUCHS. 1995. Two subsites in the binding domain of the acetylcholine receptor: an aromatic subsite and a proline subsite. Proc. Natl. Acad. Sci. USA **92:** 10801–10805.
9. BALASS, M., E. KATCHALSKI-KATZIR & S. FUCHS. 1997. The α-bungarotoxin binding site on the nicotinic acetylcholine receptor: analysis using a phage-epitope library. Proc. Natl. Acad Sci USA **94:** 6054–6058.
10. SCHERF, T., M. BALASS, S. FUCHS *et al.* 1997. Three-dimensional solution structure of the complex of α-bungarotoxin with a library-derived peptide. Proc. Natl. Acad. Sci. USA **94:** 6059–6064.
11. KASHER, R., M. BALASS, T. SCHERF *et al.* 2001. Design and synthesis of peptides that bind alpha-bungarotoxin with high affinity. Chem. Biol. **8:** 147–155.
12. TZARTOS, S.J. & J.P. CHANGEUX. 1984. Lipid-dependent recovery of alpha-bungarotoxin and monoclonal antibody binding to the purified alpha-subunit from *Torpedo marmorata* acetylcholine receptor: enhancement by noncompetitive channel blockers. J. Biol. Chem. **259:** 11512–11519.
13. SCHERF, T., R. KASHER, M. BALASS *et al.* 2001. A β-hairpin structure in a 13-mer peptide that binds α-bungarotoxin with high affinity and neutralizes its toxicity. Proc. Natl. Acad. Sci. USA **98:** 6629–6634.
14. LESCAR, J., R. STOURACOVA, M.M. RIOTTOT *et al.* 1997. Three-dimensional structure of an Fab-peptide complex: structural basis of HIV-1 protease inhibition by a monoclonal antibody. J. Mol. Biol. **267:** 1207–1222.
15. HAREL, M., R. KASHER, A. NICOLAS *et al.* 2001. The binding site of acetylcholine receptor as visualized in the X-ray structure of a complex between α-bungarotoxin and a mimotope peptide. Neuron **32:** 265–275.
16. BREJC, K., W.J. VAN DIJK, R.V. KLAASSEN *et al.* 2001. Crystal structure of an ACh-binding protein reveals the ligand-binding domain of nicotinic receptors. Nature **411:** 269–276.

Agonist-Induced Transitions of the Acetylcholine Receptor

ROBERT H. FAIRCLOUGH, MARK A. AGIUS, ESWARI GUDIPATI, LAURA SILVIAN, BRENT HAMAOKA, CHRISTOPHER C. BELTZNER, MIKE Y. LIN, ANTHONY R. CHUANG, AND DAVID P. RICHMAN

Department of Neurology, University of California, Davis, Davis, California 95616, USA

ABSTRACT: Anti-acetylcholine receptor (AChR) monoclonal antibody 383C binds to the β-hairpin loop α(187–199) of only one of the two *Torpedo* AChR α subunits. The loop recognized is associated with the α subunit corresponding to the high-affinity *d*-tubocurarine (dTC) binding site. Desensitization of the receptor with carbamylcholine completely blocks the binding of 383C. Mild reduction of AChR α subunit cys 192–193 disulfide with DTT and subsequent reaction with 5-iodoacetamidofluorescein label only the high-affinity dTC α subunit. Rhodamine-labeled α-bungarotoxin (R-Btx) binds to the unlabeled AChR α subunit as monitored by fluorescence resonance energy transfer between the fluorescein and rhodamine dyes. A 10-Å contraction of the distance between the dyes is observed following the addition of carbamylcholine. In a small angle X-ray diffraction experiment exploiting anomalous X-ray scattering from Tb(III) ions titrated into AChR Ca(II) binding sites, we find evidence for a change in the Tb(III) ion distribution in the region of the ion channel following addition of carbamylcholine to the AChR. The carbamylcholine-induced loss of the 383C epitope, the 10-Å contraction of the β-hairpin loop, and the loss of multivalent cations from the channel likely represent the first molecular transitions leading to AChR channel opening.

KEYWORDS: acetylcholine receptor (AChR); *d*-tubocurarine (dTC); ELISA; FRET; X-ray scattering; X-ray diffraction; agonist; carbamylcholine

INTRODUCTION

Using three different experimental techniques, we have examined structural changes in different parts of the AChR in response to binding the nicotinic agonist, carbamylcholine. The first technique is an enzyme-linked immunosorbent assay (ELISA) antibody binding titration; the second is a fluorescence resonance energy transfer (FRET) experiment designed to measure critical distances on the receptor; and the third is an anomalous X-ray scattering experiment designed to "observe" multivalent cations bound to the AChR. The results of these experiments suggest a possible mechanism for the agonist-induced channel activation of the AChR.

Address for correspondence: Robert H. Fairclough, Neurosciences Building, University of California, Davis, 1515 Newton Court, Room 510, Davis, CA 95616. Voice: 530-754-5005; fax: 530-754-5036.
rhfairclough@ucdavis.edu

Ann. N.Y. Acad. Sci. 998: 101–113 (2003). © 2003 New York Academy of Sciences.
doi: 10.1196/annals.1254.012

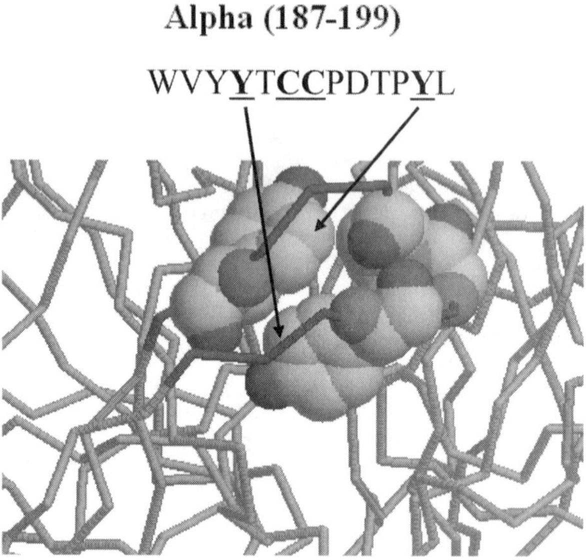

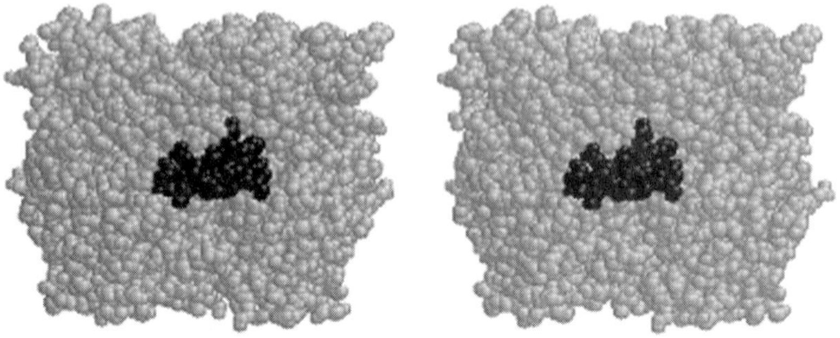

FIGURE 1. (Top) Cα trace of the acetylcholine binding protein (gray) in the region of an acetylcholine-binding site. Shown in dark gray is the homologous β-hairpin loop of the *Torpedo* α(187–199) with the four affinity-labeled amino acids, Y190, C192, C193, and Y198, displayed in space-filling format. **(Bottom)** Stereo view of the *Torpedo* α(187–199) β-hairpin peptide (black) highlighted on the AChBP (gray) in the relaxed-eyed view format.

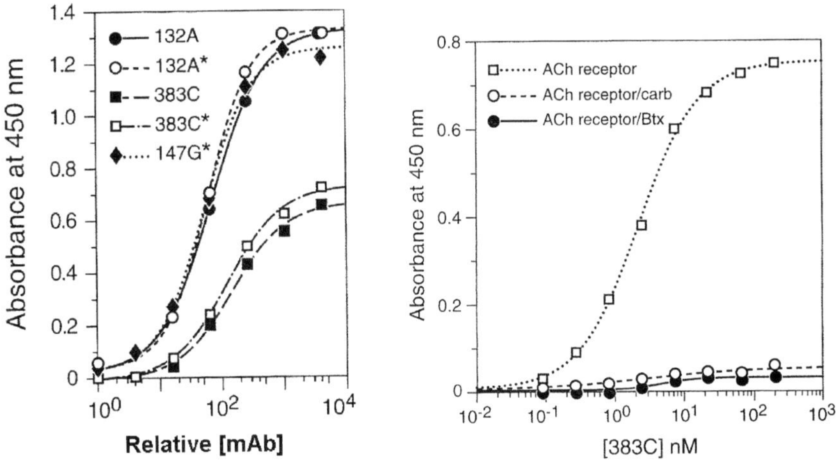

FIGURE 2. (Left) Titrations of *Torpedo* AChR and fluorescein-labeled AChR (*) with anti-AChR mAb 132A (*circles*), 383C (*squares*), and an antifluorescein mAb 147G (*diamonds*). Note the plateau of the 383C titrations is one-half that of the 132A titrations. **(Right)** Titration of *Torpedo* AChR untreated (*squares*), 10^{-7} M α-Btx-treated AChR (*closed circles*), and 10^{-4} M carbamylcholine-treated AChR (*open circles*) with purified mAb 383C.

RESULTS

ELISA Monitoring of Antibody Binding

Anti-AChR monoclonal antibody (mAb) 383C binds to the β-hairpin loop, α(187–199), of the *Torpedo* AChR.[1] This loop is illustrated in FIGURE 1 (top) with a Cα trace highlighted on the gray Cα backbone of the acetylcholine binding protein (AChBP) of Brejc *et al.*[2] The space-filling side chains of Y190, C192/193, and Y198 are the four amino acids of this peptide that have been affinity-labeled with cholinergic agonist and antagonist analogues.[3–7] The location of this loop on the AChBP is illustrated in FIGURE 1 (bottom), a stereo pair representation of the AChBP that corresponds to the synaptic head of the *Torpedo* AChR.

The stoichiometry of 383C binding to the AChR is one antibody per receptor, as determined by the ELISA titration of the AChR with 383C compared to the titration with mAb 132A directed to the AChR main immunogenic region (FIG. 2, left). Note that the plateau of the β-hairpin-binding 383C is half the value of the plateau of the MIR-directed 132A, suggesting 383C binds to only one of the two α subunit β-hairpin loops. Further studies have marked the 383C-binding α subunit β-hairpin loop as one associated with the high-affinity *d*-tubocurarine (dTC) binding site.[8] Upon addition of carbamylcholine, the β-hairpin loop epitope disappears (FIG. 2, right). We have hypothesized that, in the closed resting state, the β-hairpin loop associated with the high-affinity dTC binding site is more extended from the body of the receptor than the other (FIG. 3, left). In the presence of carbamylcholine, both loops are pulled tight to the body of the receptor, much as a bird's wings at perch (FIG. 3, right).

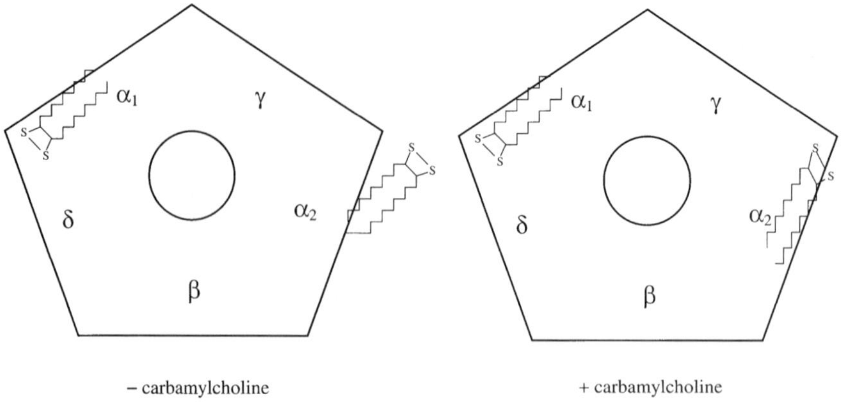

FIGURE 3. **(Left)** Diagram of the surface accessibility of α(187–199) in the two α subunits of the *Torpedo* AChR in the closed resting state. The α_2 β-hairpin is more readily accessible to binding mAb 383C than the α_1 hairpin. **(Right)** In the presence of carbamylcholine, both hairpin loops are occluded from binding mAb 383C, and hence we hypothesize that the α_2 loop is pulled closely into the body of the AChR much as we envision α_1 in the absence of carbamylcholine.

FRET Experiment to Measure Intramolecular Distances

To test this hypothesis, we measured the distance between the tip of the β-hairpin loop of one α subunit and the α-bungarotoxin bound to the β-hairpin on the other α subunit via FRET as outlined in FIGURE 4.

We first label the cys 192–193 disulfide of the high-affinity tubocurarine binding α subunit by mild DTT reduction followed by reaction with iodoacetamidofluorescein to produce fluorescein-labeled AChR (F-AChR).[9] We then label the lysines of α-Btx with rhodamine and HPLC, purify the R-Btx modified at lys 70 and lys 51/52,[9] and combine these singly labeled isomers. We titrate F-AChR with R-Btx in parallel with a second F-AChR sample with unlabeled Btx, followed by a comparison of the fluorescein emission in the two samples (FIG. 5). The decrease in fluorescein emission (at 520 nm) in the presence of the rhodamine dye is the result of resonance energy transfer, and this decrease can be used to measure the distance between the fluorescein and rhodamine labels.[10] In this energy transfer experiment, the titration of F-AChR with increasing concentrations of R-Btx gives a plateau in the measured distance of 74 Å.[9] Adding carbamylcholine to the samples, remeasuring the emission spectra, and recalculating the fluorescein to rhodamine distance reveals a contraction of 9–10 Å from 74 Å to 65 Å[9] This new distance closely approximates the width across the AChBP. This result is clearly consistent with the bird wing at perch hypothesis for the carbamylcholine-bound state of the AChR (FIG. 3, right).

Small Angle X-ray Diffraction from AChR-Enriched Membranes

Thus, how does pulling the β-hairpin loop to the side of the body of the receptor activate the ion channel? From the C-terminal end of the β-hairpin loop at α199, the

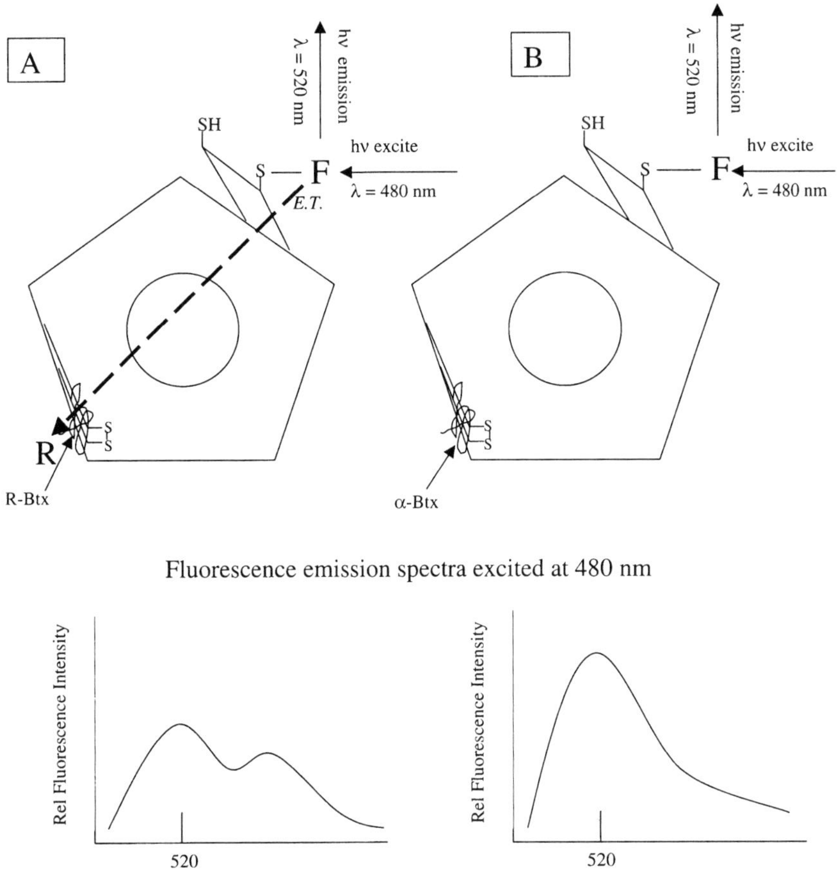

FIGURE 4. Diagram of the FRET experiment. Two identical samples, A and B, of AChR labeled with iodoacetamidofluorescein (F), the energy donor, are titrated with rhodamine (R)–labeled α-Btx and unlabeled α-Btx, respectively. Quantitatively comparing the fluorescence emission of F at 520 nm in the two samples is the heart of the experiment. Sample A with the energy transfer acceptor, R, has some of the energy of excitation of F nonradiatively transferred to R (*dashed arrow*), resulting in a decrease in the fluorescence emission of F at 520 nm compared to the emission from sample B without rhodamine attached to the Btx. Using the relative fluorescence (RF) at 520 nm of F emission in samples A and B, one calculates the efficiency of energy transfer from the relation, $E = 1 - RF_{520}(A)/RF_{520}(B)$. The distance, R, between F and R is found using $E = R_0^6/(R_0^6 + R^6)$, where R_0 is a characteristic distance for a donor/acceptor pair called the "R-zero", which for the fluorescein/rhodamine pair is 55 Å. This is the distance at which the efficiency of energy transfer is 50%, that is, 50% of excitation energy is transferred to rhodamine with a concomitant 50% decrease of fluorescein emission. Hence, from the measurement of E, one can measure the distance between F and R.

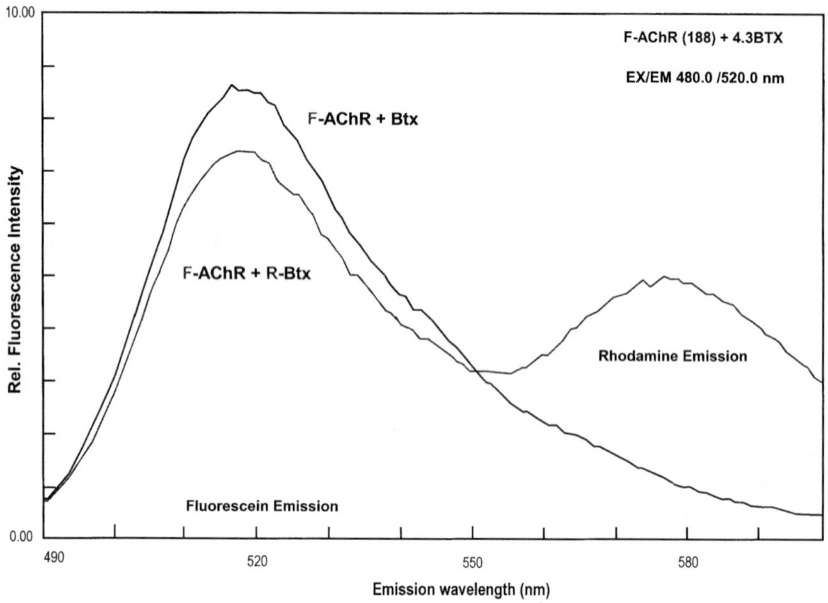

FIGURE 5. Raw emission scans of samples A and B prepared as described in the legend for FIGURE 4. The rhodamine emission is well to the red of the fluorescein emission, leaving much of the fluorescein emission uncontaminated with that of the rhodamine. Thus, fluorescein emission is the choice emission to monitor for measuring the efficiency of energy transfer.

α subunit continues in an extended β-strand to the top of the first transmembrane segment at α211. The "closing of the door" by the β-hairpin swing may directly affect α subunit amino acids at the beginning of the first transmembrane segment that are important for stabilizing the closed resting state of the ion channel. To examine this possibility, we are studying Tb(III) occupation of Ca^{2+} binding sites before and after agonist treatment. We "see" the Tb(III) ions using small angle X-ray diffraction from receptor-enriched membranes along with anomalous X-ray scattering from the Tb(III) ions. What is small angle X-ray diffraction (SAXD)? As applied to AChR-enriched membranes, one irradiates a pellet of centrifugally oriented membranes with an X-ray beam parallel to the average orientation of the lipid bilayer planes[11] (FIG. 6). The intensity of X rays diffracted along an axis parallel to the centrifugal field (meridian axis in FIG. 6) derives from the electron density distribution in the membranes normal to the bilayer plane. This electron density distribution is obtained by a constrained iterative refinement procedure,[12] starting with the membrane electron density of Klymkowsky and Stroud[13] using the diffracted amplitudes from the SAXD experiment. The results of such an experiment are presented in FIGURE 7, with the diffracted amplitudes in panel "a" and the corresponding electron density derived from this in panel "b". The horizontal axis (Z) is the normal to the bilayer plane. The electron density of the membrane relative to that of the buffer is plotted

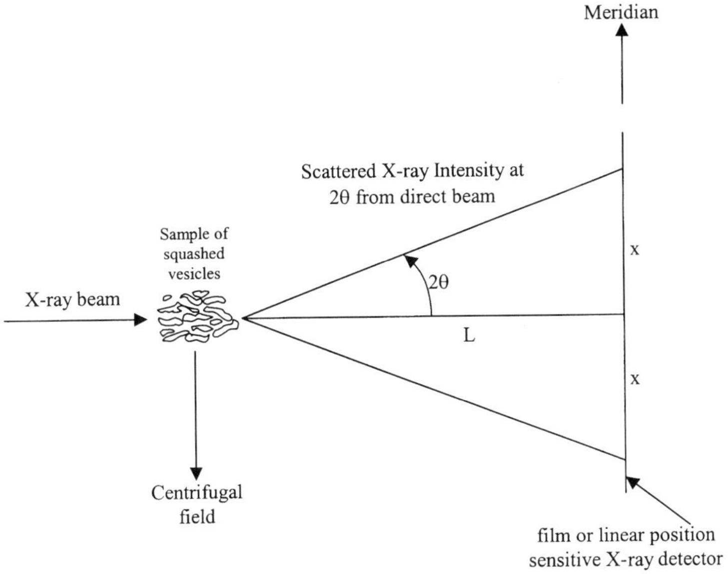

FIGURE 6. Geometry of the small angle X-ray diffraction experiment. The intensity of diffracted X rays, I(x), at an angle 2θ from the direct beam is recorded on film or a linear position sensitive detector at distance, L, from the sample. All diffracted intensities are presented as a function of the scattering variable, S, which is related to the distance, x, on the X-ray detector from the direct beam and the wavelength of the X rays, $\lambda = 1.65$ Å, through the following relations: $S = (2 \sin \theta)/\lambda$, where $\tan 2\theta = x/L$. Diffraction amplitudes, $|F(S)|$, and intensities, I(S), along the meridian (axis of diffraction parallel to the orienting gravitational field) are derived from the electron density distribution in the membranes along an axis perpendicular to the membrane planes. Finally, amplitude is related to intensity by $|F(S)| = [I(S)]^{1/2}$.

along this axis. The largest peak of this plot corresponds to the electron-rich phosphate groups of the extracellular side of the bilayer, and the major trough in this profile corresponds to the electron-poor hydrocarbon center of the bilayer. Also evident is the asymmetric distribution of electron density to the left of the extracellular phosphate groups, whose density corresponds to the synaptic head of the receptor.

Anomalous X-ray Scattering from Tb(III) Ions

Calcium-depleted AChR-enriched membranes titrate with 45 Tb(III) ions per receptor.[14] Using the small angle X-ray experimental format just described with Tb(III)-titrated membranes, we tune the Tb(III) into and out of the diffraction profile by very small changes in the energy of the incident X-ray beam such that only the scattering power of Tb(III) changes. For example, using X-ray beam energies of 7505 eV and 7515 eV and subtracting the measured scattering amplitudes, we obtain the differences in scattering amplitude as displayed in FIGURE 8. Applying difference Fourier analysis and heavy atom refinement to these scattering amplitudes produces the six narrow regions of Tb(III) density displayed in FIGURE 8, seen as the dashed curve relative to the electron density of the entire membrane normal to the bilayer in

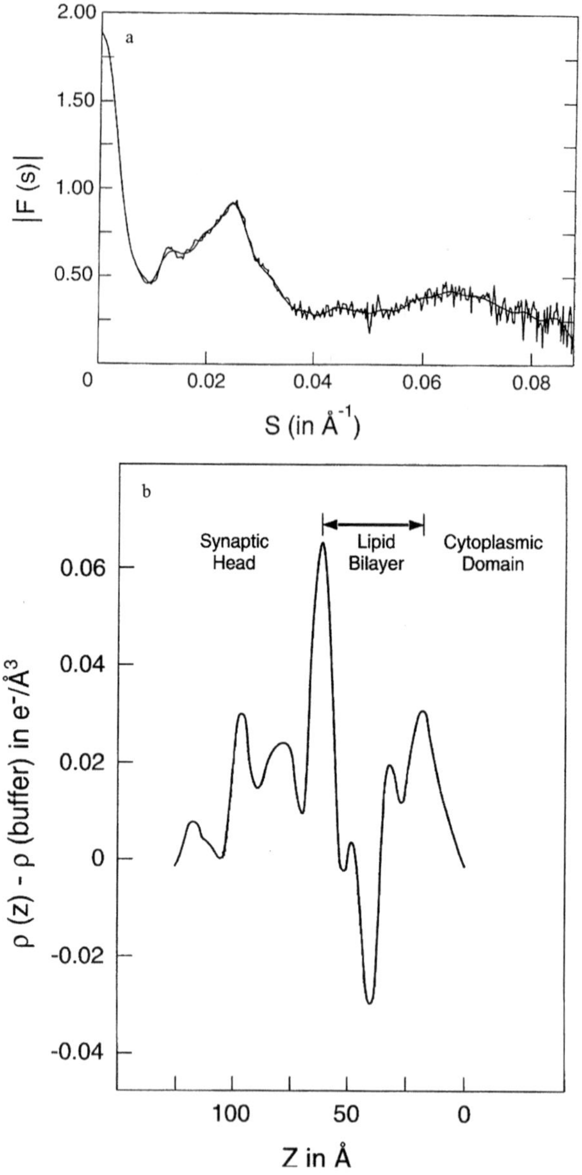

FIGURE 7. **(a)** Diffracted amplitude of X rays at S from AChR membrane vesicles that have been oriented in a 100,000*g* centrifugal field for 18 h. The noisy curve represents the raw data, and the smooth curve through the noisy data represents the diffraction predicted from the refined electron density profile, presented in **(b)**. The first peak of electron density, as Z increases from 0.0, derives from the electron-rich cytoplasmic phosphate head groups of the lipid bilayer; the large trough at 40 Å derives from the electron-poor region at the center of the lipid bilayer; and the large peak at 65 Å derives from the synaptic-side phosphate head groups.

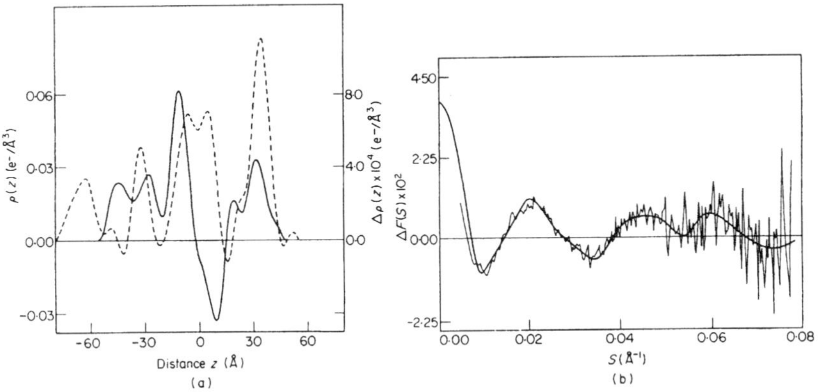

FIGURE 8. **(a)** Heavy atom refinement results in the Tb(III) distribution (*dashed line*), which is overlaid on the electron density distribution of the entire membrane (*solid line*). **(b)** Refinement is based on the fit of the anomalous scattering difference amplitude data (7505–7515 eV) from Tb(III) (*noisy data*) with the model-predicted fit (*smooth line through the noisy data*).

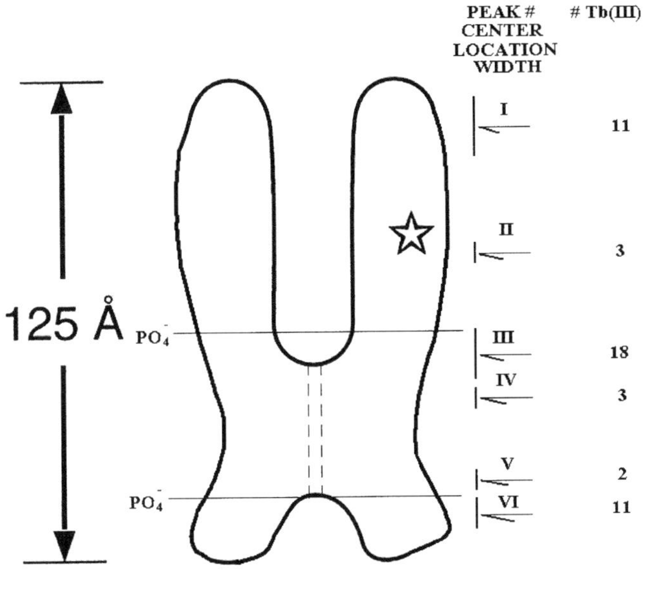

FIGURE 9. Distribution of Tb(III) on a side-view cartoon of the AChR.

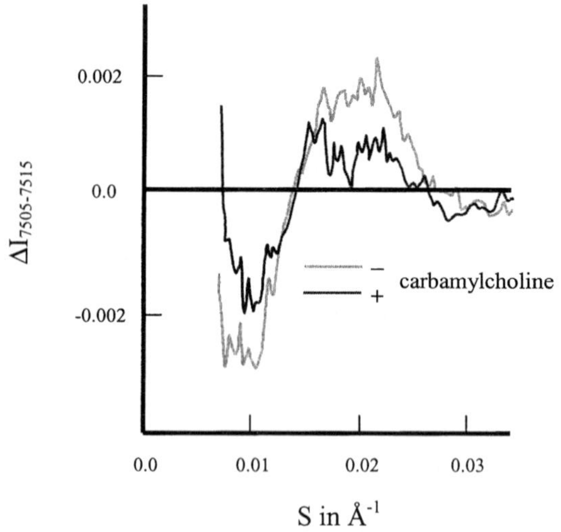

FIGURE 10. Anomalous intensity differences for AChR treated with (dark gray) and without (light gray) carbamylcholine, both titrated with Tb(III).

the solid curve.[14] FIGURE 9 illustrates the distribution of the six narrow Tb(III) domains across the side view of the AChR. In region I at the top of the AChR, we find 11 Tb(III); in region II just below the β-hairpin indicated by the star, we find 2–3 Tb(III); then 18 Tb(III) in a broad region III near the synaptic side phosphates and the floor of the synaptic side receptor well; then 3 Tb(III) in region IV at the synaptic neck of the ion channel; then 2 Tb in region V, a second ion channel region near the cytoplasmic side of the bilayer; and finally 11 Tb in region VI that includes the cytoplasmic side phosphates as well as the floor of the cytoplasmic well. Most significantly, based on the refined Tb(III) distribution relative to the overall membrane electron density, we find 47 Tb(III) ions bound per receptor compared to the 45 determined via a Scatchard analysis of a spectrofluorometric Tb(III) titration.[14]

What happens when we add carbamylcholine to this system? FIGURE 10 presents the energy-dependent difference intensities of scattering for AChR samples plus and minus carbamylcholine. Note the frequency of the oscillations in the difference intensities in the presence of carbamylcholine compared to the difference intensities just discussed in the absence of carbamylcholine. Between 0.01 and 0.03 S, the curve obtained in the absence of carbamylcholine has just one major broad peak, whereas the curve obtained in the presence of carbamylcholine has two narrower peaks. What does this indicate? Here is a quick lesson in Fourier analysis. If one moves scattering centers further apart in a Young two-slit experiment, the interference fringes (the minima) move closer together (FIG. 11).[15] The anomalous (energy-dependent) scattering differences in the presence of carbamylcholine have the minima closer together than those in the absence of carbamylcholine, suggesting the Tb(III) scattering centers are further apart in the carbamylcholine-treated sample. This is exactly

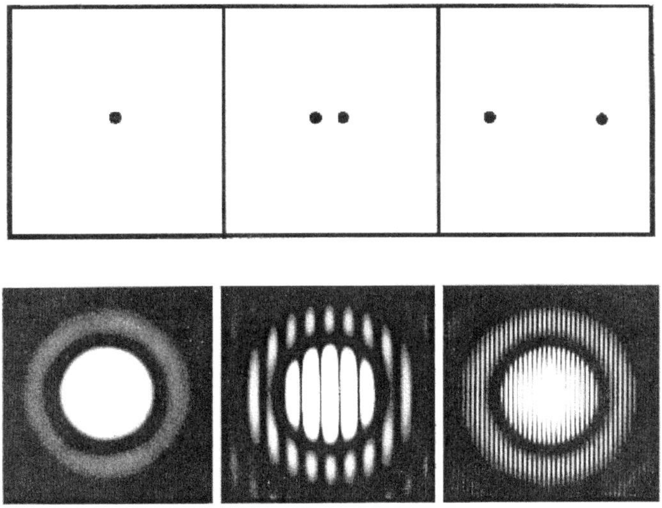

FIGURE 11. The effect of moving scattering centers further apart in a Young two-slit experiment. The *top row* represents the spacing of pinholes in a mask through which laser light shines, with the resulting diffraction patterns displayed below each mask. Note that the fringes (minima) move closer together as the pinholes move further apart.

what one would expect if the ion channel Tb(III) ions are released upon the binding of carbamylcholine. One would expect that the number released should be 5. When Chang and Neumann treated Ca-titrated receptors with agonist, they found 4–6 Ca ions released.[16] This corresponds to the number of Tb(III) ions localized in the ion channel domains of the AChR (regions IV and V of FIG. 9). Whether the domain in the synaptic head is also released will have to await the difference Fourier analysis of the data. However, these data provide strong evidence for a role for multivalent cations in stabilizing the closed resting state of the ion channel. The molecular gymnastics of the β-hairpins, connected by an extended β-strand to amino acids exposed to the cation-restrictive environment of the ion channel,[17] likely serves to disrupt the positioning of chelating side chains that with multivalent cations stabilize the closed resting state of the AChR ion channel. This disruption stimulates the release of the multivalent cations, leading to the mutual rotation and expansion of this negatively charged chelating region of the ion channel pore[18] and thus opening the channel to the flow of sodium and potassium down their electrochemical gradients.

SUMMARY

The AChR in the closed resting state exhibits one of the two acetylcholine binding β-hairpin loops more extended from the body of the receptor. Upon addition of carbamylcholine, this extended β-hairpin loop retracts into the body of the AChR. We measure a contraction of 9–10 Å in the distance between the tip of this loop and the α-Btx on the other side upon the addition of carbamylcholine. The resulting new

AChR conformation binds fewer Ca/Tb ions than that of the closed resting state conformation, with Tb(III) density differences suspected in the region of the ion channel.

ACKNOWLEDGMENTS

Robert H. Fairclough thanks Sebastian Doniach, Keith O. Hodgson, and Robert M. Stroud for directing attention to the role of multivalent cations in AChR function and thanks many collaborators at the Stanford synchrotron radiation lab that made the collection of the small angle X-ray data possible. Included in this group of investigators is Richard Miake-Lye, Stevan Hubbard, Soichi Wakatski, and Jean-Luc Ranck, as well as the beam line staff at SSRL that make collecting data at SSRL possible, fun, and humorous. Additional thanks go to Janet Finer-Moore for the extensive help and advice in modifying the crystallographic heavy atom refinement program to analyze membrane small angle anomalous scattering data, and also to Tom Lee and Tsung-Yu Chen for their encouragement and inspiration in pursuing the role of Ca/Tb in regulating AChR channel activity. Funding for this work has come from the NIH, several Viets fellowships to students from the Myasthenia Gravis Foundation of America, an Osserman fellowship to Eswari Gudipati from this same foundation, and the Myasthenia Gravis Foundation of California.

FIGURES 2, 7, and 8 are reprinted from references 8, 1, and 14, respectively, with permission from Elsevier. FIGURE 11 is reprinted from plate 1 found in reference 15.

REFERENCES

1. FAIRCLOUGH, R.H., G.M. TWADDLE, E. GUDIPATI *et al.* 1998. Mapping the mAb 383C epitope to α_2 (187–199) of the *Torpedo* acetylcholine receptor on the three dimensional model. J. Mol. Biol. **282:** 301–315.
2. BREJC, K., W.J. VAN DIJK, R.V. KLAASSEN *et al.* 2001. Crystal structure of an ACh-binding protein reveals the ligand-binding domain of nicotinic receptors. Nature **411:** 269–276.
3. DENNIS, M., J. GIRAUDAT, F. KOTZYBA-HIBERT *et al.* 1988. Amino acids of the *Torpedo marmorata* acetylcholine receptor subunit labeled by a photoaffinity ligand for the acetylcholine binding site. Biochemistry **27:** 2346–2357.
4. ABRAMSON, S.N., Y. LI, P. CULVER & P. TAYLOR. 1989. An analogue of lophotoxin reacts covalently with tyr^{190} in the α-subunit of the nicotinic acetylcholine receptor. J. Biol. Chem. **264:** 12666–12672.
5. KAO, P.N., A.J. DWORK, R.J. KALDANY *et al.* 1984. Identification of the α subunit half-cystine specifically labeled by an affinity reagent for the acetylcholine receptor binding site. J. Biol. Chem. **259:** 11662–11665.
6. KAO, P.N. & A. KARLIN. 1989. Acetylcholine receptor binding site contains a disulfide cross-link between adjacent half-cystinyl residues. J. Biol. Chem. **264:** 8085–8088.
7. MIDDLETON, R.E. & J.B. COHEN. 1991. Mapping of the acetylcholine binding site of the nicotinic acetylcholine receptor: [^{3}H]nicotine as an agonist photoaffinity label. Biochemistry **30:** 6987–6997.
8. FAIRCLOUGH, R.H., G.M. TWADDLE, E. GUDIPATI *et al.* 1998. Differential surface accessibility of α(187–199) in the *Torpedo* acetylcholine receptor α subunits. J. Mol. Biol. **282:** 317–330.
9. FAIRCLOUGH, R.H. *et al.* 2003. In preparation.
10. FAIRCLOUGH, R.H. & C.R. CANTOR. 1978. The use of singlet-singlet energy transfer to study macromolecular assemblies. Methods Enzymol. **XLVIII:** 347–379.

11. Ross, M.J., M.W. Klymkowsky, D.A. Agard & R.M. Stroud. 1977. Structural studies of a membrane bound acetylcholine receptor from *Torpedo californica*. J. Mol. Biol. **116:** 635–659.
12. Stroud, R.M. & D.A. Agard. 1979. Structure determination of asymmetric membrane profiles using an iterative Fourier method. Biophys. J. **25:** 495–512.
13. Klymkowsky, M.W. & R.M. Stroud. 1979. Immunospecific identification and three-dimensional structure of a membrane-bound acetylcholine receptor from *Torpedo californica*. J. Mol. Biol. **128:** 319–334.
14. Fairclough, R.H., R.C. Miake-Lye, R.M. Stroud *et al.* 1986. Location of terbium binding sites on acetylcholine receptor-enriched membranes. J. Mol. Biol. **189:** 673–680.
15. Harburn, G., C.A. Taylor & T.R. Welberry. 1975. Atlas of Optical Transforms. Cornell University Press. Ithaca, New York.
16. Chang, H.W. & E. Neumann. 1976. Dynamic properties of isolated acetylcholine receptor proteins: release of calcium ions caused by acetylcholine binding. Proc. Natl. Acad. Sci. USA **73:** 3994–3998.
17. Akabas, M.H. & A. Karlin. 1995. Identification of acetylcholine receptor channel-lining residues in the M1 segment of the α-subunit. Biochemistry **334:** 12496–12500.
18. Imoto, K., C. Busch, B. Sakmann *et al.* 1988. Rings of negatively charged amino acids determine the acetylcholine receptor channel conductance. Nature **335:** 645–648.

Structural Abnormalities of the AChR Caused by Mutations Underlying Congenital Myasthenic Syndromes

DAVID BEESON,[a] RICHARD WEBSTER,[a] JOHN EALING,[a] REBECCA CROXEN,[a] SHARON BROWNLOW,[a] MARTIN BRYDSON,[a] JOHN NEWSOM-DAVIS,[a] CLARKE SLATER,[b] CHRIS HATTON,[c] CHRIS SHELLEY,[c] DAVID COLQUHOUN,[c] AND ANGELA VINCENT[a]

[a]*Neurosciences Group, Weatherall Institute of Molecular Medicine, The John Radcliffe, Headington, Oxford OX3 9DS, United Kingdom*

[b]*Department of Neurobiology, University of Newcastle, Newcastle, United Kingdom*

[c]*Department of Pharmacology, University College London, London, United Kingdom*

ABSTRACT: The objective was to define the molecular mechanisms underlying congenital myasthenic syndromes (CMS) by studying mutations within genes encoding the acetylcholine receptor (AChR) and related proteins at the neuromuscular junction. It was found that mutations within muscle AChRs are the most common cause of CMS. The majority are located within the ε-subunit gene and result in AChR deficiency.

KEYWORDS: congenital myasthenic syndromes (CMS); acetylcholine receptor (AChR); mutations; AChR deficiency; green fluorescent protein; fast channel; slow channel; *in situ* hybridization

INTRODUCTION

The congenital myasthenic syndromes (CMS) are a heterogeneous group of inherited disorders of neuromuscular transmission. They share the characteristic clinical feature of fatigable muscle weakness. Differential diagnosis may be important since different syndromes require different treatment strategies. However, except in specialist centers, a definitive diagnosis based on clinical examination may prove difficult. Over the last two decades, defects in postsynaptic, synaptic, and presynaptic proteins have been defined and the underlying genetic basis determined.[1] Mutations in the muscle acetylcholine receptor (AChR) underlie AChR deficiency,[2–10] slow channel, and fast channel syndromes;[11–20] mutations in rapsyn can also cause AChR deficiency syndrome;[21] mutations in ColQ cause endplate acetylcholinesterase deficiency;[22,23] and mutations in choline acetyltransferase (ChAT) underlie CMS

Address for correspondence: David Beeson, Neurosciences Group, Weatherall Institute of Molecular Medicine, The John Radcliffe, Headington, Oxford OX3 9DS, United Kingdom. Voice: +44 (0)1865 222311; fax: +44 (0)1865 222402.
dbeeson@hammer.imm.ox.ac.uk

Ann. N.Y. Acad. Sci. 998: 114–124 (2003). © 2003 New York Academy of Sciences.
doi: 10.1196/annals.1254.013

TABLE 1A. CMS kinships where the specific diagnosis of the syndrome has been defined or confirmed by molecular genetic studies

Syndrome	Kinships
Slow channel	14
Fast channel	6
AChR deficiency	60
AChR deficiency (rapsyn)	9
Acetylcholinesterase deficiency[a]	6
CMS with episodic apnea[a]	5
	100

[a]Functional studies have not been performed for the DNA changes in these disorders.

TABLE 1B. Location of the CMS mutations in DNA samples analyzed at the Weatherall Institute of Molecular Medicine

Protein	Subunit	Mutations	Kinships
AChR	α	6	8
	β	2	2
	δ	4	4
	ε	38	66
Rapsyn		5	9
ColQ		7	6
ChAT		6	5
Total		68	100

with episodic apnea.[24] Although it is likely that mutations will be identified in additional candidate proteins located at the neuromuscular junction,[25,26] it is now possible to use genetic screening combined with functional studies to provide definitive diagnosis for the majority of affected families.

Here, we highlight the results of the genetic screen that we have performed on suspected cases of CMS and discuss some of our studies of the molecular mechanisms that underlie these disorders.

SCREENING FOR MUTATIONS IN SUSPECTED CASES OF CMS

Exons within the genes encoding the human AChR α, β, δ, and ε subunits, ColQ, ChAT, and rapsyn were screened using single-strand conformation polymorphism analysis (SSCP). Amplicons in which abnormal conformers were detected were subjected to direct DNA sequencing. Restriction endonuclease digestions were used to confirm DNA sequence changes and to track the segregation of mutant alleles within pedigrees. In cases where no abnormal conformers were detected, but the clinical

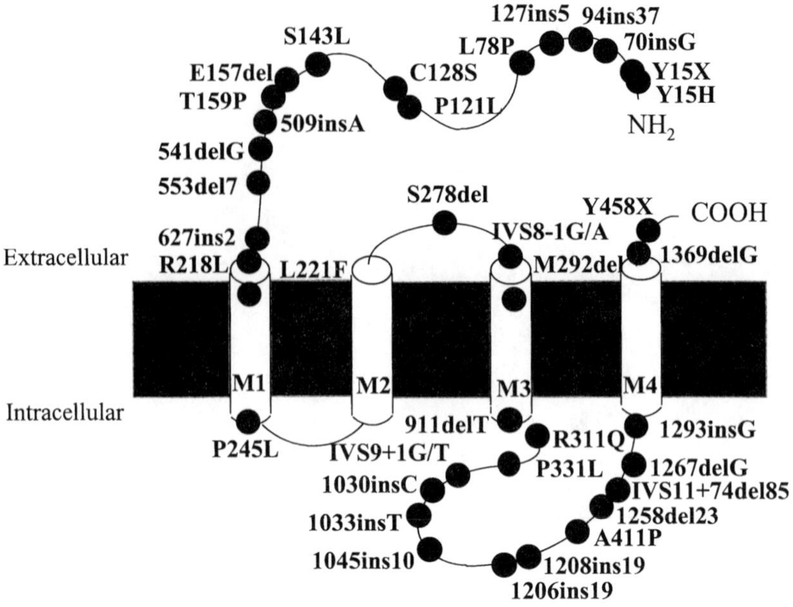

FIGURE 1. Schematic representation of the AChR ε-subunit showing the different mutations identified at the Weatherall Institute of Molecular Medicine.

diagnosis strongly implicated one particular gene, all the exons within that gene were subject to direct DNA sequencing. Functional effects of mutations were investigated by biochemical or electrophysiological analysis of mutant AChR or AChR/rapsyn expressed in HEK 293 cells.

TABLE 1A shows the subdivision of diagnosed syndromes based upon clinical features and mutational analysis. TABLE 1B shows the proteins/AChR subunits in which the mutations are located. Our screening has tended to focus on the AChR subunit genes; thus, the proportion of patients with ColQ and ChAT mutations may be underrepresented. Nevertheless, it is clear that AChR deficiency is the most common CMS and that, in the majority of cases, it is due to mutations in the AChR ε-subunit gene. The mutations that we have identified in the ε-subunit gene are shown in FIGURE 1. εL78P and εL221F underlie slow channel syndromes,[25] εL121P underlies a fast channel syndrome,[15] and the remaining 34 are either low expression or null alleles that underlie AChR deficiency syndromes or unmask the phenotype of fast channel syndromes. The majority are "private", and ε1267delG, which is common in the Romany Gypsy population of Southeast Europe,[6] is the only clear-cut example of a founder effect. ε1369delG, εR311Q, and ε553del7 are the most common mutations identified in Caucasians from northern Europe or the United Kingdom. In addition, we and others have detected mutations in the N-box, an ets-binding element in the ε-subunit promoter region.[27–29] In CMS cases where ε-subunit null mutations are present on both alleles, it is thought that maintenance of low-level expression of the γ-subunit enables fetal AChR to partially compensate for loss of adult AChR.[2]

We have been unable to detect mutations within the genes encoding the AChR in around 25% of AChR deficiency cases defined by the analysis of muscle biopsies. Recently, it has been demonstrated that mutations in rapsyn, which plays an essential role in clustering of the AChR on the postsynaptic membrane, underlie some of these cases.[21] Thus far, we have identified rapsyn mutations in nine unrelated kinships. Each harbors the missense mutation, N88K. In three kinships, N88K is present on both alleles and, in the remaining six kinships, the mutations are heteroallelic. Thus, by contrast with the many private mutations identified in other CMS, preliminary results suggest that N88K will be identified in the majority of AChR deficiencies due to rapsyn mutations.

CMS WITH UNUSUAL PATTERNS OF INHERITANCE

The mode of inheritance within a pedigree may often give clues for diagnosis. For mutations of the AChR, the slow channel syndrome usually shows dominant inheritance, whereas AChR deficiency and fast channel syndromes show recessive inheritance. Recently, recessive inheritance and variable penetrance of slow channel

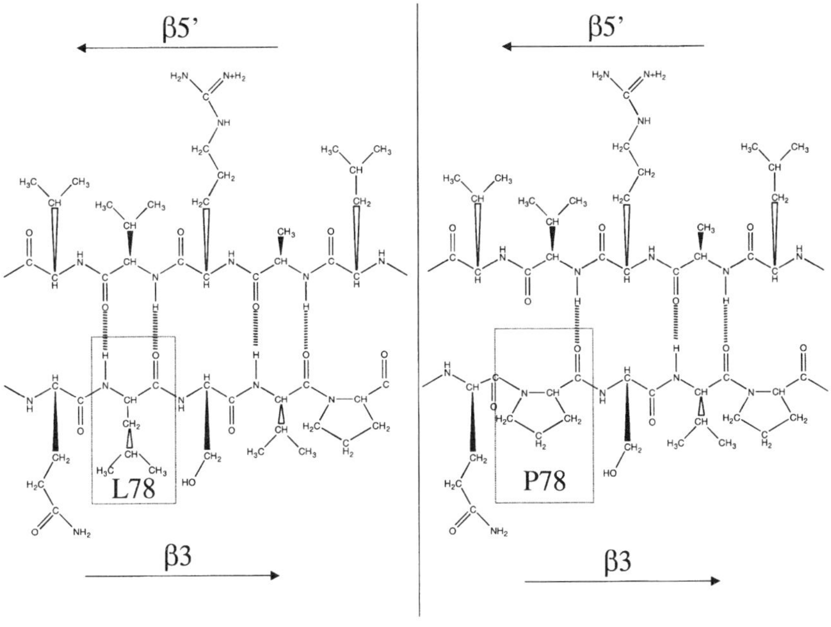

FIGURE 2. Diagram of the β-sheets from the ε-subunit, located above the putative ACh-binding site, showing the possible disruptive molecular effect of the εL78P amino acid substitution.

syndrome mutations have been reported.[30] The index case presented following difficulty recovering from anesthesia and is a member of a consanguineous pedigree that harbors the slow channel mutation εL78P. Although all family members analyzed harbored the εL78P mutation, weakness was only apparent on clinical examination in cases where the mutation is present on both alleles. The crystal structure of the snail (*Lymnaea*) ACh-binding protein places εL78 at the α-ε interface.[31] In the snail protein, this position is occupied by valine, and the backbone at this position is hydrogen-bonded to a β-strand that lines the ACh-binding region (FIG. 2). Substitution of a proline for leucine at this position will disrupt the hydrogen bond formation at this position and thus affect ACh binding.

We have also noted considerable variation of disease severity within other slow channel syndrome pedigrees. εL221F has been identified in two kinships. In one, there is normal dominant inheritance through three generations; in the second kinship, there is variable inheritance of the phenotype, with the males (in three generations) yet to present with symptoms. Factors other than the AChR mutation must influence phenotype, and an understanding of the mechanisms that underlie this phenotypic variability may help in investigations of other excitotoxic disorders and in devising new treatments.

Since each AChR pentamer contains two α-subunits, then, theoretically, mutations of the α subunit that cause a loss of function could have a dominant-negative effect. We studied a family, described previously,[32,33] in which we believe this occurs. A muscle biopsy from the index patient showed very small miniature endplate potentials (MEPPs), but otherwise normal ACh content and receptor numbers. A biopsy from the patient's father demonstrated similar small MEPPs, although he did not present with clinical symptoms.

Mutational analysis of DNA from family members detected a single missense mutation, αF256L, which was present in father and son (FIGS. 3A and 3B). Direct sequencing of the α-subunit gene coding and promoter regions (and screening of other subunit genes) from the patient failed to detect an additional mutation. Single channel recordings show AChRs containing αF256L with fast channel characteristics (FIG. 3C, TABLE 2). The phenylalanine at position 256 maps to the M2 region. Interestingly, as shown in FIGURE 3D, several slow channel kinetic mutations have been

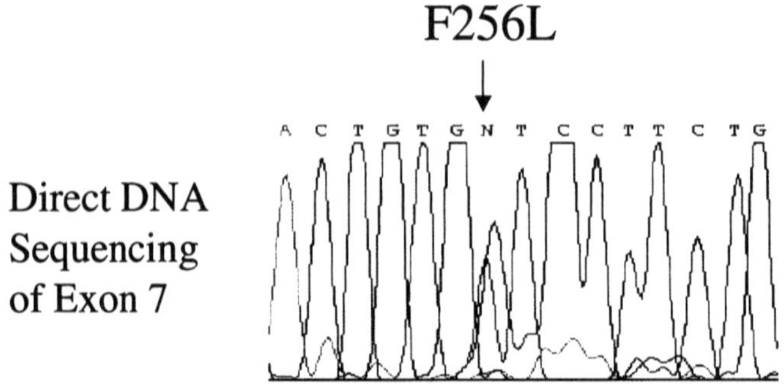

FIGURE 3A. DNA sequence analysis shows a T to C transition in exon 7, mutating a phenylalanine to a leucine.

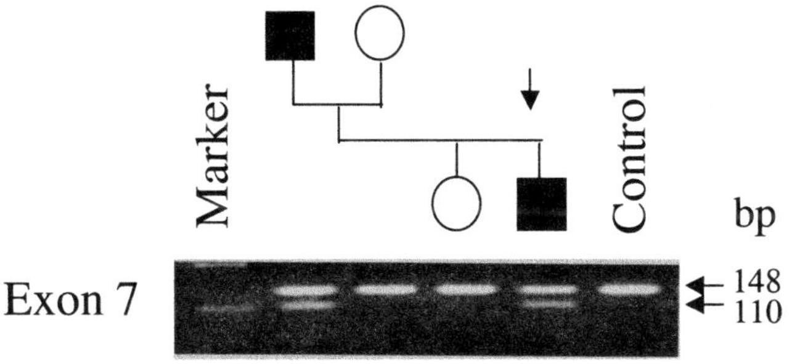

FIGURE 3B. Digestion of PCR amplicons with restriction enzyme *Bsi*HKAI showed the presence of the mutation in the index patient (↓) and his father, but not in his mother or sister.

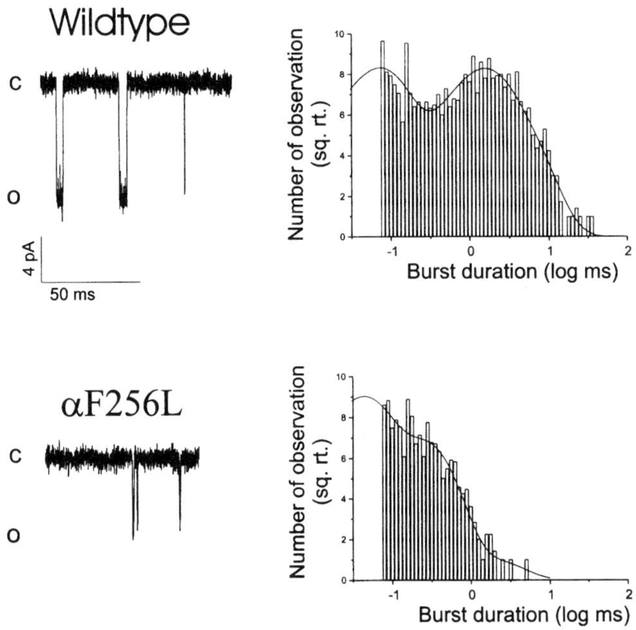

FIGURE 3C. Single channel activity recorded at low ACh concentration (100 nM) of wild-type and αF256L-AChR transfected HEK 293 cells: channel openings are downward deflections. Burst activity was fitted to the sum of three exponentials (*right of figure*); the duration of the longest population of burst activity was significantly reduced in αF256L-AChR. The proportion of bursts in the longest population was also significantly reduced.

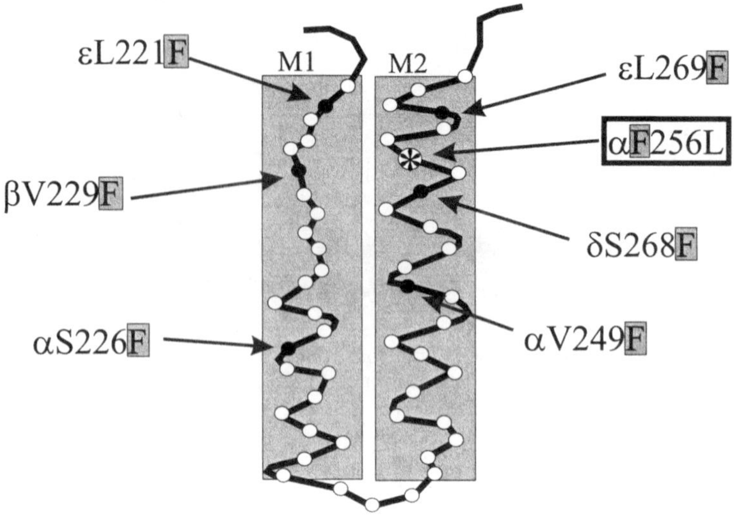

FIGURE 3D. Diagrammatic representation of the location of published slow channel phenylalanine missense mutations and the αF256L fast channel mutation in the M1-M2 pore region of AChR. Slow channel conversions to phenylalanine are highlighted, as well as the fast channel αF256L conversion from phenylalanine to leucine.

reported in this region in which residues have been mutated to a phenylalanine. It is tempting to speculate that bulky phenylalanine residues in this region might have a steric influence on channel gating, leading to stabilization of the open state and giving the characteristics of a slow channel; conversely, loss of this residue would destabilize the open state, leading to a fast channel kinetic profile.

This study implies that there are normal numbers of AChRs on the postsynaptic membrane, but a dominant-negative effect of the α-subunit mutation results in only 25% of the AChRs, those made up of normal α-subunits, being fully functional. However, a dominant inheritance pattern has not been reported for other α-subunit fast channel syndrome mutations.[34]

TABLE 2. AChR burst durations

	τ_1 (ms)	α_1 (x/1)	τ_2	α_2	τ_3	α_3	n
Wild-type	0.07	0.40	1.25	0.31	3.62	0.28	3
(SEM)	(0.01)	(0.01)	(0.25)	(0.03)	(0.61)	(0.04)	
αF256L	0.06	0.44	0.30*	0.54*	1.87*	0.02*	5
(SEM)	(0.01)	(0.03)	(0.01)	(0.03)	(0.49)	(0.01)	

NOTE: AChR burst durations were fitted to the sum of three exponential functions. The time constant (τ_n) and fractional proportion (α_n) were compared by Student's t test. *Indicates a significant difference; n indicates the number of patches studied.

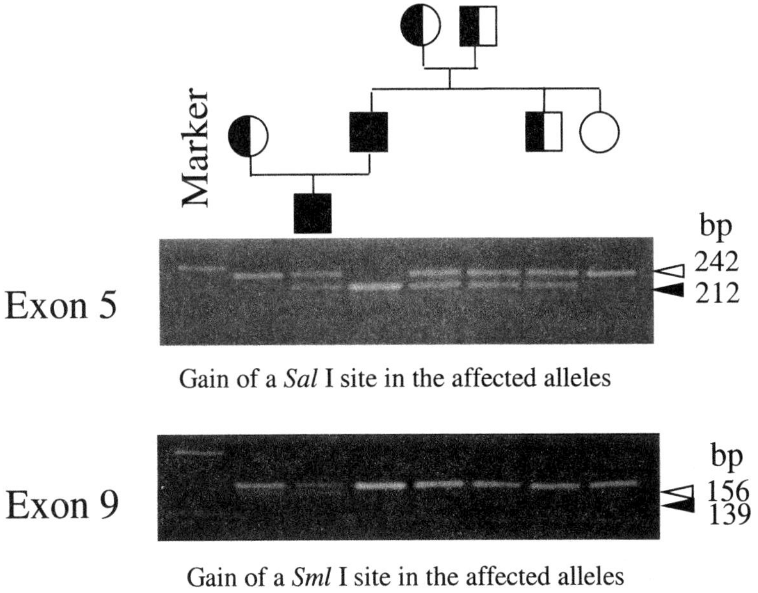

FIGURE 4. Restriction digests of PCR amplicons from family members confirming the presence of alleles harboring ε553del7 (exon 5) and εIVS8-1G→A (exon 9). Shaded symbols indicate affected individuals; half-shaded symbols indicate one mutant allele.

In consanguineous kinships or in communities where a founder effect is evident, recessive disorders sometimes occur in more than one generation. We recently analyzed a family in which the index case had difficulty in feeding from birth, ptosis, and delayed motor milestones. Myasthenia was diagnosed at the age of 3 on the basis of a systemic neostigmine injection. On examination at 29 years of age, external ophthalmoplegia, bilateral ptosis, facial weakness, and some proximal upper limb weakness were apparent. Electromyography showed increased decrement and jitter. Antibodies against the AChR were absent, and his condition has remained stable on anticholinesterase medication. The son of the index case presented at 11 weeks of age with failure to thrive and dysphagia. He had a positive response to a tensilon test, and a CMS, thought to be dominantly inherited, was diagnosed. Mutational analysis of DNA samples from family members (FIG. 4) revealed that the family harbors two mutations in the AChR ε-subunit gene. Although there was no consanguinity, the index case is homozygous for a seven-nucleotide deletion in exon 7, ε553del7.

This mutation has been reported previously,[3] and we have identified it in five other kinships: in three, the index case is homozygous for ε553del7; in two, the index case is heteroallelic. As expected, the patient's son harbors the ε553del7 mutation, but strikingly he also harbors an ε-subunit gene splice site mutation, IVS8-1G→A, which was inherited from his mother. Both mutations are predicted to cause truncation of the ε-subunit polypeptide prior to the M3 transmembrane domain and thus will be null alleles. In both father and son, the residual expression of the γ-subunit is likely to rescue the phenotype.

STUDIES OF THE MOLECULAR MECHANISMS UNDERLYING AChR DEFICIENCY SYNDROME

While some mutations in the ε-subunit gene give rise to low-expressing alleles, the majority are null mutations. Premature nonsense mutations within an RNA transcript may be recognized by RNA surveillance systems and lead to the rapid degradation of transcript. *In vitro* hybridization with ^{35}S-labeled antisense cRNA was used to study the steady state levels of mRNA in subsynaptic regions of muscle biopsies from AChR deficiency patients with defined ε-subunit mutations. Biopsies from patients with mutations located between the ε-subunit M3 and M4 transmembrane domains showed robust signal for ε mRNA transcripts, comparable to the signal from control samples. Thus, the mutations we identified and studied in the ε-subunit coding region did not have a severe effect on ε-subunit mRNA levels. It is likely that the AChR deficiency in these patients is caused by retention of misfolded mutant ε-subunits within the endoplasmic reticulum (ER) and the failure of mutant pentamers to insert into the surface membrane.

Two of the mutations in the ε-subunit gene, εY458X and ε1369delG, are located in the short extracellular tail C-terminal to the M4 transmembrane domain. We were interested in investigating the molecular mechanism underlying AChR deficiency in these cases since ε-subunits expressed from these mutant alleles contain all the domains thought to be essential for AChR function. In order to visualize wild-type and mutant subunits, we created a cDNA construct that integrates a green fluorescent (GFP) tag between M3 and M4. Biochemical and electrophysiological analyses show the functional properties of AChRε-GFP and wild-type AChR to be almost indistinguishable. AChRε-GFP was expressed in HEK 293 cells or in the RD muscle cell line and viewed using confocal microscopy. AChRε-GFP could be visualized in the plasma membrane, whereas AChRε1369delG-GFP was restricted to intercellular compartments. Coexpression of AChRε1369delG-GFP with a blue fluorescent marker for the ER shows precise colocalization of the blue and green fluorescence to give a "cyano" staining of the ER. Similar results were obtained with the ε458X mutation, indicating that these mutant subunits are being retained within the ER.

To investigate further, deletion mutations were constructed spanning the 18-amino-acid C-terminal extracellular tail, and surface expression of AChR was analyzed by immunoprecipitation with ε-subunit specific antisera. Robust surface expression of adult AChR was seen only when the ε-subunit contained C470, which is conserved between mammalian species and is located just 4 amino acids from the C-terminus. This surface adult AChR expression was lost if C470 was mutated to serine, indicating that it is likely to form a disulfide bond. The results suggest that a previously unidentified disulfide-bonded cystine plays a crucial role in the assembly of adult AChR and suggest a mechanism by which frameshift or nonsense mutations in the ε-subunit C-terminal region cause AChR deficiency.

PERSPECTIVES

Coincident with increased knowledge about these disorders, it has become apparent that they are more common than previously estimated. The availability of genetic screens for mutations underlying CMS should allow a definitive diagnosis in many more cases. From the data obtained thus far, it is clear that individuals sharing the same mutations may show a wide variation in disease severity. Understanding the factors underlying this phenotypic variation may provide potential targets for new therapies.

As reported for mouse AChR,[35] insertion of the GFP tag in the cytoplasmic domain between M3 and M4 (avoiding the amphipathic region, MA) can generate tagged human AChR that is expressed on the cell surface with functional properties almost indistinguishable from wild type. Initial studies indicate that the presence of the GFP tag does not interfere with rapsyn-induced clustering of the AChR. These GFP-tagged AChRs should provide a powerful tool for the study of disorders of the localization, assembly, and trafficking of the AChR.

ACKNOWLEDGMENTS

This work was supported by the MRC, the Wellcome Trust, and the Muscular Dystrophy Campaign/Myasthenia Gravis Association.

REFERENCES

1. Ohno, K. & A.G. Engel. 2002. Congenital myasthenic syndromes: genetic defects of the neuromuscular junction. Curr. Neurol. Neurosci. Rep. **2:** 78–88.
2. Engel, A.G. *et al.* 1996. End-plate acetylcholine receptor deficiency due to nonsense mutations in the epsilon subunit. Ann. Neurol. **40:** 810–817.
3. Ohno, K. *et al.* 1997. Congenital myasthenic syndromes due to heteroallelic nonsense/missense mutations in the acetylcholine receptor epsilon subunit gene: identification and functional characterization of six new mutations. Hum. Mol. Genet. **6:** 753–766.
4. Middleton, L. *et al.* 1999. Chromosome 17p–linked myasthenias stem from defects in the acetylcholine receptor epsilon-subunit gene. Neurology **53:** 1076–1082.
5. Ohno, K. *et al.* 1998. Myasthenic syndromes in Turkish kinships due to mutations in the acetylcholine receptor. Ann. Neurol. **44:** 234–241.
6. Abicht, A. *et al.* 1999. A common mutation (epsilon1267delG) in congenital myasthenic patients of Gypsy ethnic origin. Neurology **53:** 1564–1569.
7. Quiram, P.A. *et al.* 1999. Mutation causing congenital myasthenia reveals acetylcholine receptor beta/delta subunit interaction essential for assembly. J. Clin. Invest. **104:** 1403–1410.
8. Croxen, R. *et al.* 1999. Novel functional epsilon-subunit polypeptide generated by a single nucleotide deletion in acetylcholine receptor deficiency congenital myasthenic syndrome. Ann. Neurol. **46:** 639–647.
9. Sieb, J.P. *et al.* 2000. Immature end-plates and utrophin deficiency in congenital myasthenic syndrome caused by epsilon-AChR subunit truncating mutations. Hum. Genet. **107:** 160–164.
10. Croxen, R. *et al.* 2001. End-plate gamma- and epsilon-subunit mRNA levels in AChR deficiency syndrome due to epsilon-subunit null mutations. Brain **124:** 1362–1372.
11. Ohno, K. *et al.* 1995. Congenital myasthenic syndrome caused by prolonged acetylcholine receptor channel openings due to a mutation in the M2 domain of the epsilon subunit. Proc. Natl. Acad. Sci. USA **92:** 758–762.
12. Sine, S.M. *et al.* 1995. Mutation of the acetylcholine receptor alpha subunit causes a slow-channel myasthenic syndrome by enhancing agonist binding affinity. Neuron **15:** 229–239.
13. Engel, A.G. *et al.* 1996. New mutations in acetylcholine receptor subunit genes reveal heterogeneity in the slow-channel congenital myasthenic syndrome. Hum. Mol. Genet. **5:** 1217–1227.
14. Gomez, C.M. *et al.* 1996. A beta-subunit mutation in the acetylcholine receptor channel gate causes severe slow-channel syndrome. Ann. Neurol. **39:** 712–723.

15. OHNO, K. *et al.* 1996. Congenital myasthenic syndrome caused by decreased agonist binding affinity due to a mutation in the acetylcholine receptor epsilon subunit. Neuron **17:** 157–170.
16. CROXEN, R. *et al.* 1997. Mutations in different functional domains of the human muscle acetylcholine receptor alpha subunit in patients with the slow-channel congenital myasthenic syndrome. Hum. Mol. Genet. **6:** 767–774.
17. GOMEZ, C.M. *et al.* 1997. Slow-channel transgenic mice: a model of postsynaptic organellar degeneration at the neuromuscular junction. J. Neurosci. **17:** 4170–4179.
18. MILONE, M. *et al.* 1997. Slow-channel myasthenic syndrome caused by enhanced activation, desensitization, and agonist binding affinity attributable to mutation in the M2 domain of the acetylcholine receptor alpha subunit. J. Neurosci. **17:** 5651–5665.
19. GOMEZ, C.M. *et al.* 2002. Novel delta subunit mutation in slow-channel syndrome causes severe weakness by novel mechanisms. Ann. Neurol. **51:** 102–112.
20. BROWNLOW, S. *et al.* 2001. Acetylcholine receptor delta subunit mutations underlie a fast-channel myasthenic syndrome and arthrogryposis multiplex congenita. J. Clin. Invest. **108:** 125–130.
21. OHNO, K. *et al.* 2002. Rapsyn mutations in humans cause endplate acetylcholine-receptor deficiency and myasthenic syndrome. Am. J. Hum. Genet. **70:** 875–885.
22. OHNO, K. *et al.* 1998. Human endplate acetylcholinesterase deficiency caused by mutations in the collagen-like tail subunit (ColQ) of the asymmetric enzyme. Proc. Natl. Acad. Sci. USA **95:** 9654–9659.
23. DONGER, C. *et al.* 1998. Mutation in the human acetylcholinesterase-associated collagen gene, COLQ, is responsible for congenital myasthenic syndrome with end-plate acetylcholinesterase deficiency (type Ic). Am. J. Hum. Genet. **63:** 967–975.
24. OHNO, K. *et al.* 2001. Choline acetyltransferase mutations cause myasthenic syndrome associated with episodic apnea in humans. Proc. Natl. Acad. Sci. USA **98:** 2017–2022.
25. VINCENT, A., D. BEESON & B. LANG. 2000. Molecular targets for autoimmune and genetic disorders of neuromuscular transmission. Eur. J. Biochem. **267:** 6717–6728.
26. LIYANAGE, Y. *et al.* 2002. The agrin/muscle-specific kinase pathway: new targets for autoimmune and genetic disorders at the neuromuscular junction. Muscle Nerve **25:** 4–16.
27. NICHOLS, P. *et al.* 1999. Mutation of the acetylcholine receptor epsilon-subunit promoter in congenital myasthenic syndrome. Ann. Neurol. **45:** 439–443.
28. OHNO, K., B. ANLAR & A.G. ENGEL. 1999. Congenital myasthenic syndrome caused by a mutation in the Ets-binding site of the promoter region of the acetylcholine receptor epsilon subunit gene. Neuromuscul. Disord. **9:** 131–135.
29. ABICHT, A. *et al.* 2002. A newly identified chromosomal microdeletion and an N-box mutation of the AChRepsilon gene cause a congenital myasthenic syndrome. Brain **125:** 1005–1013.
30. CROXEN, R. *et al.* Recessive inheritance and variable penetrance in slow channel congenital myasthenic syndrome. Neurology. In press.
31. BREJC, K. *et al.* 2001. Crystal structure of an ACh-binding protein reveals the ligand-binding domain of nicotinic receptors. Nature **411:** 269–276.
32. VINCENT, A. *et al.* 1981. Congenital myasthenia: end-plate acetylcholine receptors and electrophysiology in five cases. Muscle Nerve **4:** 306–318.
33. VINCENT, A. *et al.* 1993. Clinical and experimental observations in patients with congenital myasthenic syndromes. Ann. N.Y. Acad. Sci. **681:** 451–460.
34. WANG, H.L. *et al.* 1999. Acetylcholine receptor M3 domain: stereochemical and volume contributions to channel gating. Nat. Neurosci. **2:** 226–233.
35. GENSLER, S. *et al.* 2001. Assembly and clustering of acetylcholine receptors containing GFP-tagged epsilon or gamma subunits: selective targeting to the neuromuscular junction *in vivo*. Eur. J. Biochem. **268:** 2209–2217.

Congenital Myasthenic Syndrome in Cattle due to Homozygosity for a Truncating Mutation in the Acetylcholine Receptor (AChR) Epsilon-Subunit Gene

JOERN P. SIEB,[a] SIMONE KRANER,[b] PETER N. THOMPSON,[c] AND ORTRUD K. STEINLEIN[b]

[a]*Max Planck Institute of Psychiatry, Clinical Neurogenetics, Munich, Germany*

[b]*Institute of Human Genetics, University Hospital Bonn, Rheinische Friedrich Wilhelms-University Bonn, Bonn, Germany*

[c]*Epidemiology Section, Department of Production Animal Studies, Faculty of Veterinary Science, University of Pretoria, Onderstepoort, South Africa*

KEYWORDS: South African Red-Brahman calves; domestic animals; sequence analysis; deletion; mutation

Autoimmune myasthenia has been described repeatedly in domestic animals. There are few reports of inherited myasthenic weakness in domestic animals, but so far the molecular basis of these syndromes is still elusive. We have elucidated the genetic defect of a severe congenital myasthenic syndrome in cattle.

The clinical phenotype of one of four South African Red-Brahman calves with suspected congenital myasthenic syndromes has been published in detail.[1,2] In summary, the affected animal developed progressive muscle weakness, beginning at three to four weeks of age. Within a week, it was no longer able to rise without assistance. High-frequency stimulation revealed decremental responses. Acetylcholinesterase inhibitors improved the condition transiently.

RESULTS

Genomic Structure of bovCHRNE

The bovine gene for the epsilon-subunit of the acetylcholine receptor (bov*CHRNE*) consists of 12 exons, coding for a predicted protein of 405 amino acid residues. *In silico* cloning and exon-exon PCR showed that the localizations of the

Address for correspondence: J. P. Sieb, M.D., Neurology, Max Planck Institute of Psychiatry, Kraepelinstr. 10, D-80804 Munich, Germany. Voice: +49-89-30622-374; fax: +49-89-30622-585. sieb@mpipsykl.mpg.de

Ann. N.Y. Acad. Sci. 998: 125–127 (2003). © 2003 New York Academy of Sciences. doi: 10.1196/annals.1254.014

exon boundaries are conserved compared to the human *CHRNE* gene structure. The gt/ag rule of conserved splice sites is followed in all introns. The sizes of bov*CHRNE* introns obtained by sequencing-through (introns 1–2, 4, 6–7, 9–12) or by estimation of fragment sizes from gel electrophoresis (intron 3) were comparable to the known intron sizes of the human *CHRNE* gene. The ATG-start codon is localized in exon 1, and the TAG-stop codon in exon 12. The four transmembrane regions are coded by exons 7, 8, 9, and 12, respectively. At the amino acid level, the human and bovine *CHRNE* genes have 89% identity and 91% similarity. The genomic bovine *CHRNE* sequences have been submitted to GenBank under accession number AF457656.

Detection of a 20-bp Deletion

PCR amplification and subsequent direct sequencing of bov*CHRNE* exons from the DNA of the myasthenic calf revealed a loss of 20 bp within the coding sequence of exon 5 between nucleotides 469 and 490 (nucleotide numbering refers to the cDNA sequence published under accession number X02597). The myasthenic calf was homozygous for the mutation 470del20. The sequence change was present in DNA samples extracted from two different tissues (skeletal muscle and spinal cord). It is therefore highly unlikely that the 20-bp deletion was artificially caused by DNA degradation during tissue fixation or DNA preparation. The 470del20 mutation was found neither in 46 chromosomes from German red or black-and-white control cattle, nor in 20 chromosomes from South African Red-Brahman or Gray-Brahman control animals. Thus, 470del20 is not part of the normal bov*CHRNE* gene sequence nor is it a variation typically found in Brahman genomes. Mutation screening showed that both the sire and the maternal grandsire shared by all four affected calves were heterozygous for the 470del20 mutation. The heterozygous deletion genotype was also detected in the dam of one of the calves, as well as in three healthy half-sisters. Another three half-sisters and a half-sister to the dam of an affected calf were tested and found to be homozygous for the bov*CHRNE* wild-type allele.

Confirmation of the bovCHRNE cDNA Sequence

The cDNA sequence obtained from the cattle control DNA and the affected Brahman calf differed at position bp317 from the published bov*CHRNE* sequence (accession number X02597). The observed A/C exchange did not affect the predicted amino acid sequence, but deleted a *Dde*I restriction site in our cDNA sequence. The expected fragment sizes of the 193-bp exon 4–PCR product were 105 bp and 88 bp for the published sequence. Only the 193-bp fragment was observed after *Dde*I digestion of amplification products from 90 chromosomes of red, black-and-white, Red-Brahman, and Gray-Brahman cattle. Thus, the published adenine in position bp317 is either a rare variant or a sequencing error.

DISCUSSION

We identified a homozygous 20-bp deletion within exon 5 of the bov*CHRNE* gene. The predicted bov*CHRNE* protein coded by the RNA carrying the 470del20 mutation would be truncated upstream from the four transmembrane domains. Sequence analysis showed that the 470del20 mutation causes a frameshift in the predicted bov*CHRNE* protein after 129 codons, substituting 342 wild-type amino acid residues by 40 aberrant amino acids followed by a stop codon. The frameshift occurs at 90 amino acid residues N-terminal of the first transmembrane region. Thus, the bov*CHRNE* mutation reported here leads to a nonfunctional allele, which is likely to be the primary cause for the myasthenic syndrome in the affected Brahman calves.[2]

ACKNOWLEDGMENTS

This work was supported by grants from the Deutsche Forschungsgemeinschaft (DFG) to O. K. Steinlein and J. P. Sieb (Nos. STE 769/3-2 and SI 472/3-1).

REFERENCES

1. THOMPSON, P.N. 1998. Suspected congenital myasthenia gravis in Brahman calves. Vet. Rec. **143:** 526–529.
2. KRANER, S. *et al.* 2002. Congenital myasthenia in Brahman calves caused by homozygosity for a *CHRNE* truncating mutation. Neurogenetics **4:** 87–91.

Mechanistic Diversity Underlying Fast Channel Congenital Myasthenic Syndromes

STEVEN M. SINE,[a] HAI-LONG WANG,[a] KINJI OHNO,[b] XIN-MING SHEN,[b] WON YONG LEE,[a] AND ANDREW G. ENGEL[b]

[a]*Receptor Biology Laboratory, Department of Physiology and Biophysics, Mayo Medical School, Rochester, Minnesota 55905, USA*

[b]*Muscle Research Laboratory, Department of Neurology and Mayo Foundation, Mayo Medical School, Rochester, Minnesota 55905, USA*

ABSTRACT: A host of missense mutations in muscle nicotinic receptor subunits have been identified as the cause of congenital myasthenic syndromes (CMS). Two classes of CMS phenotypes have been identified: slow channel myasthenic syndromes (SCCMSs) and fast channel myasthenic syndromes (FCCMSs). Although both have similar phenotypic consequences, they are physiologic opposites. Expression of the FCCMS phenotype requires the missense mutation to be accompanied by a second mutation, either a null or a missense mutation, in the second allele encoding the same receptor subunit. This seemingly rare scenario has arisen with surprisingly high incidence over the past few years, and analyses of the syndromes have revealed a diverse array of mechanisms underlying the pathology. This review focuses on new mechanisms underlying the FCCMS.

KEYWORDS: congenital myasthenic syndromes; fast channel myasthenic syndromes; slow channel myasthenic syndromes; transmembrane domain

INTRODUCTION

Since the mid-1990s, a host of missense mutations in muscle nicotinic receptor subunits have been identified as the cause of congenital myasthenic syndromes (CMS; reviewed by Engel *et al.*[1]). Two classes of CMS phenotypes have been identified: slow channel myasthenic syndromes (SCCMSs) and fast channel myasthenic syndromes (FCCMSs). The SCCMSs are dominant, gain-of-function mutations that increase activation of the receptor by speeding the rate of opening of the receptor channel, slowing the rate of closing of the channel, or allowing repeated opening during each ACh occupancy. The result is staircase summation of endplate potentials that cause depolarizing block of the muscle action potential and consequent failure to contract. The FCCMSs, by contrast, are recessive, gain-of-function mutations that decrease activity of the receptor by slowing the rate of opening of the receptor

Address for correspondence: Steven M. Sine, Receptor Biology Laboratory, Department of Physiology and Biophysics, Mayo Medical School, Rochester, MN 55905. Voice: 507-284-9404; fax: 507-284-9420.
sine@mayo.edu

Ann. N.Y. Acad. Sci. 998: 128–137 (2003). **© 2003 New York Academy of Sciences.**
doi: 10.1196/annals.1254.015

channel, speeding the rate of closing of the channel, or decreasing the number of openings of the channel during ACh occupancy. The result is failure to achieve threshold depolarization of the endplate and consequent failure to fire an action potential. Thus, although slow and fast channel CMS have similar phenotypic consequences, they are physiologic opposites.

Expression of the FCCMS phenotype requires the missense mutation to be accompanied by a second mutation, either a null or a missense mutation, in the second allele encoding the same receptor subunit. This seemingly rare scenario has arisen with surprisingly high incidence over the past few years, and analyses of the syndromes have revealed a diverse array of mechanisms underlying the pathology. Thus, the following review focuses on new mechanisms underlying the FCCMS.

STRUCTURAL COUNTERPARTS OF THE CMS

The muscle nicotinic receptor is a pentamer composed of four different types of subunits (α, β, ε, and γ) arranged as barrel staves around a central ion channel. Approximately half of the resulting cylindrical structure extends into the synaptic cleft and harbors the ACh binding sites, while the remaining structure comprises the transmembrane and cytoplasmic domains that form the ion channel and regulatory domains, respectively. Mutations that cause SCCMS predominantly localize to the second of four transmembrane domains (TMD), although two SCCMS mutations have been found at the ACh binding site (reviewed by Engel *et al.*[2]). Mutations that cause FCCMS, on the other hand, have not been found in TMD2, but localize predominantly to the ACh binding site, the cytoplasmic domain of the ε subunit, or TMD3. Because the ACh binding site is formed at αε and αδ subunit interfaces (reviewed by Sine[3]), the corresponding FCCMS mutations have been found in α, δ, or ε subunits.

OVERVIEW OF RECEPTOR ACTIVATION MECHANISMS

The following core mechanistic description emerged from early studies of receptor activation and still serves today as a starting point for quantitatively describing receptor activation kinetics:[4,5]

$$A + R \underset{k_{-1}}{\overset{k_{+1}}{\rightleftharpoons}} AR + A \underset{k_{-2}}{\overset{k_{+2}}{\rightleftharpoons}} A_2R \underset{\alpha}{\overset{\beta}{\rightleftharpoons}} A_2R^*$$

Scheme 1

where A is the agonist, R is the receptor in the resting state, and R* is the receptor in the open channel state. SCHEME 1 provides a useful framework for understanding receptor activation because it provides a formal description of events at the ACh binding site and couples them to activation of the ion channel. Inherent in SCHEME 1 and its expanded forms is the existence of stable ground states, R, AR, A_2R, and A_2R^*, which represent deep wells in the energy landscape of the receptor. The rate constants for each step provide a measure of the height of the energy barrier, or activated complex, between stable ground states. SCHEME 1 accounts for positive cooperativity in the ACh dose-response relationship and the dependence of single channel open and closed dwell times on ACh concentration. Thus, SCHEME 1 accounts for essential features of activation for AChRs from a variety of species. SCHEME 1 is a subset of the Monod-Wyman-Changeux (MWC) description of allosteric protein function:[6]

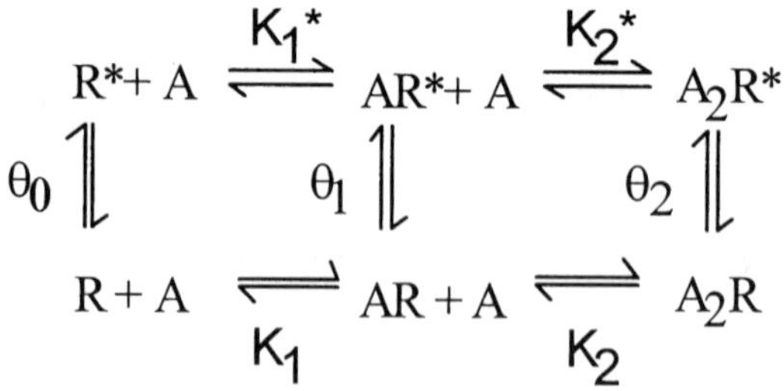

Scheme 2

which contains resting (R) and active (R*) states that interconvert in the absence of agonist and predict tighter binding of agonist to the active state than to the resting state (the equilibrium dissociation constants K* are much smaller than K). Given that ACh binds more tightly to the active state, the equilibrium constant θ between resting and active states increases progressively with increasing agonist occupancy so that $\theta_0 < \theta_1 < \theta_2$; for muscle AChR, θ_0 is approximately 10^{-6}, θ_1 is approximately 10^{-2}, and θ_2 is ~25. Thus, agonist activates the receptor by overcoming the unfavorable equilibrium constant θ_0 through tighter binding to the active state compared to the resting state.[7]

MECHANISTIC UNDERPINNINGS OF THE FCCMS

The end result of FCCMS mutations is reduced responsiveness to ACh, for which four fundamentally different mechanisms have been described to date. The first mechanism is decreased ACh affinity for the open state relative to the closed state of the receptor (i.e., increased K_2^*/K_2), which diminishes the energetic driving force for opening the channel. The second is increased ACh affinity for the closed state relative to the open state of the receptor, which again opposes opening of the channel. The third mechanism is diminished efficiency of gating of the channel without a change in open or closed state affinities for ACh (i.e., decreased θ_2). The fourth mechanism results from loss of fidelity in the kinetics of activation in which the receptor spends substantial time in multiple modes with markedly reduced probability of opening. As might be expected, the first two mechanisms have been established for mutations at the ACh binding site, whereas the third mechanism was uncovered for a mutation in TMD3. The fourth class of mechanism is associated with mutations in the cytoplasmic regulatory domain of the ε subunit. The overall studies show that even very small structural perturbations, if strategically placed, can have profound consequences for function.

EXPERIMENTAL DETERMINATION OF MECHANISTIC CONSEQUENCES

Heterologous expression systems are now widespread and allow studies of wild-type and mutant receptors under controlled *in vitro* conditions. A popular and convenient expression system is the clonal fibroblast system. Clonal fibroblasts, such as 293 human embryonic kidney cells,[8] can be readily transfected using calcium phosphate precipitation of the cDNAs encoding the receptor subunits. As soon as one day following transfection, standard patch-clamp techniques can be implemented to record the activity of individual receptor channels.[9] Typically, concentrations of ACh are employed that cause desensitization because this suppresses activation of most receptors, allowing ready identification of epochs during which only one channel is active. Subsequent analysis using Q-matrix techniques,[10] available as free software, allows fitting kinetic schemes such as SCHEME 1 to the single channel dwell times and estimation of rate constants for each state transition.[11] In many cases, comparison of rate constants between wild-type and mutant receptors provides a ready explanation of the pathogenesis.

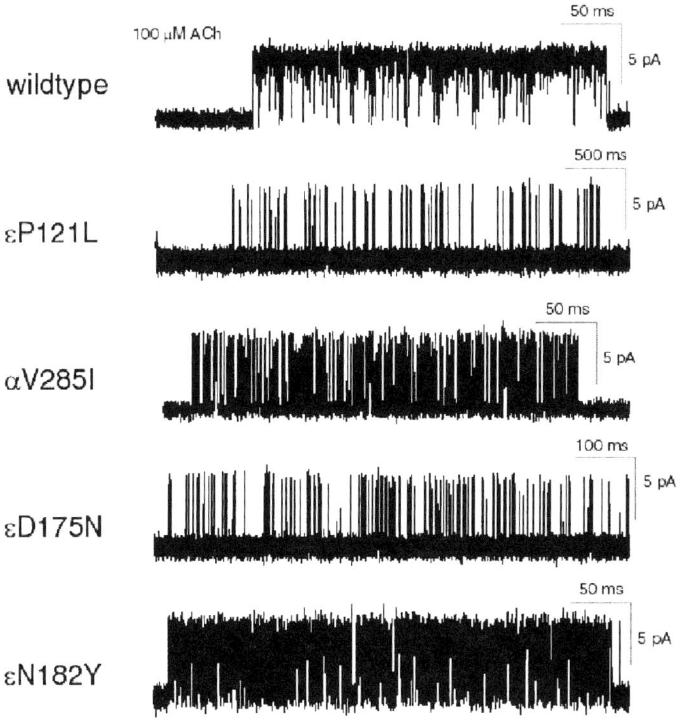

FIGURE 1. Single channel currents elicited by 100 μM ACh through receptor channels containing the indicated FCCMS mutations. Currents were recorded using previously described methods[12,14] and are displayed at a bandwidth of 10 kHz. Individual clusters of currents corresponding to a single receptor channel are displayed. Despite the high concentration of ACh, the various mutations reduce the probability that an individual channel opens.

THE FCCMS MUTATION εP121L

The FCCMS mutation, εP121L, localizes to one of four regions in the ε subunit that contributes to the ACh binding site.[12] Located at the C-terminal boundary of a series of residues that affect competitive antagonist binding, including εY111 and εT117,[8,13] εP121L does not affect ACh affinity for the resting state of the receptor, but instead markedly reduces probability of channel opening at saturating ACh concentrations (FIG. 1). Accompanying this reduced probability of opening, the rate at which doubly liganded receptors open slows by nearly 500-fold, while the rate of channel closing increases about 2-fold.

Kinetic analysis of currents through AChRs containing εP121L provided a complete set of rate constants underlying the activation process.[12] Thus, the conclusion of normal affinity of ACh for the resting state followed directly from the measured rate constants. Open state affinity was determined by applying the principle of microscopic reversibility to the second cycle in SCHEME 2, rate constants describing resting state affinity and gating steps for singly and doubly liganded receptors. Doubly liganded open state affinity, given by $K_2^* = K_2\theta_1/\theta_2$, decreased from 35 nM for wild type to 1.5 μM for εP121L. Hence, εP121 selectively stabilizes ACh bound to the open state of wild-type AChR. Additionally, the dramatic slowing of the rate of opening of the doubly liganded AChR, β_2, suggested that εP121 is critical in forming the transition state in the path toward the open state. Thus, the results from the εP121L mutation suggested that the proline at position 121 is critical in contributing to a structure at the binding site that better complements ACh bound to the open state relative to the resting state. The overall findings show that, in wild-type AChR, tighter binding of ACh to the active state is the fundamental driving force underlying agonist-induced activation.

THE FCCMS MUTATION εN182Y

Single channel kinetic analysis showed that εN182Y markedly increased ACh affinity for one of the two binding sites in the resting closed state of the receptor, but did not affect affinity for the second binding site.[3] The dissociation constant for the altered site decreased from 138 μM for wild-type AChR to 2 μM for the mutant, owing to a 30-fold slowing of the rate constant for ACh dissociation and a 2-fold increase of the rate constant for ACh association. Because the mutation was present in the ε subunit, the binding site with increased ACh affinity corresponded to the αε site. The increased affinity conferred by εN182Y defined the sequence in which ACh occupies the binding sites of the mutant receptor; the αε site is occupied first, whereas the αδ site is occupied second.

The εN182Y mutation not only altered ACh binding, but it also altered gating of the channel. The gating equilibrium constants for singly occupied (θ_1) and doubly occupied (θ_2) receptors were reduced by an order of magnitude. Reduction of θ_2 was a direct consequence of the reduction in θ_1; ACh occupancy of the second binding site began with a singly occupied receptor less prone to opening. Thus, although the second occupancy step in the mutant receptor promoted channel gating as well as the second occupancy step in wild type ($\theta_2/\theta_1 = 1080$ for the mutant; $\theta_2/\theta_1 = 1083$ for wild type), gating of the doubly occupied mutant receptor was reduced by an order of magnitude.

Mechanistic underpinnings for the reduced θ_1 could be understood by inspection of SCHEME 2 described above. According to SCHEME 2, θ_1 could decrease due to (1) a decrease of K_1 relative to K_1* or (2) a decrease of θ_0 without a change in K_1 relative to K_1*. Because neither K_1* nor θ_0 were defined by the data, both alternatives were formal possibilities.

Comparison of ACh binding steps for wild-type and εN182Y mutant receptors showed that the second binding site in the εN182Y receptor is similar to the first binding site in the wild-type receptor; the corresponding association and dissociation rate constants were similar between the two types of receptors. The most likely explanation is that εN182Y affects the αε binding site without altering the αδ binding site. Thus, the mutation at εN182 not only revealed a new determinant of ACh binding affinity, but it also provided independent estimates of the rate constants underlying ACh occupancy of the wild-type αδ site.

THE FCCMS MUTATION εD175N

Single channel kinetic analysis of currents through receptors containing εD175N revealed that the mutation slowed the rate of ACh association about 10-fold and accelerated the rate of ACh dissociation 2-fold.[3] Thus, the εD175N mutation increased the dissociation constant for ACh binding to the αε site by 20-fold. The analysis also revealed that εD175N reduced gating of singly and doubly occupied receptors by about an order of magnitude. The decrease of θ_2 was a direct consequence of the decrease of θ_1 because binding of the second ACh started with a singly occupied receptor less prone to opening. Therefore, although ACh occupancy of the mutant binding site promoted channel gating nearly as well as occupancy of the second binding site in wild type (θ_2/θ_1 = 677 for εD175N; θ_2/θ_1 = 1083 for wild type), gating of the doubly occupied mutant receptor was reduced by an order of magnitude.

If ACh promotes nearly normal gating when it occupies the mutant αε site, how does εD175N impair gating of the channel? The earliest discernable effect in SCHEME 1 was reduction of θ_1, but this observation led to the following paradox: how does a mutation at the αε site affect the gating equilibrium constant associated with ACh occupancy of the nonmutant αδ site? A likely explanation was that residues at the binding site not only mediate recognition of ACh, but also set the trigger point for opening the channel. Thus, the results suggested that residues at the binding site not only govern ACh affinity of the resting closed state of the receptor, but they also contribute to stability of closed states relative to open states of the channel even when agonist is not bound to the receptor.

THE FCCMS MUTATION αV285I

By simply adding a methyl group, the mutation αV285I impaired efficiency of channel gating.[14] The mutation slowed the rate of channel opening and increased the rate of channel closing, consequences opposite to those of mutations in TMD2. Agonist binding steps were largely unaffected by αV285I, indicating lack of allosteric effects at the remote binding site. Analysis of genetically engineered mutations of αV285 showed that effects on channel gating depended on the size of the side chain, with αV285L impairing gating beyond that of αV285I, and αV285A enhancing gating beyond that of wild type. Because the side chain of leucine has the same size as that of isoleucine, stereochemical considerations were required to explain the effects on channel gating. Gating depended on size of the moiety attached to the β-carbon, which is ethyl for isoleucine and isopropyl for leucine. Moreover, the volume of the β-carbon substitution altered free energy of the channel gating equilibrium in a linear fashion, spanning ranges of 4 kcal/mol and 110 $Å^3$, indicating both stereochemical and volume contributions to channel gating. The αV285I mutation exhibited two open states even at saturating concentrations of ACh, unlike wild type, which exhibited one open state.

Kinetic analysis of currents through AChRs containing αV285I provided a complete set of rate constants describing the activation process. The mutation impaired the channel gating step, most likely by destabilizing the doubly liganded open state. The possibility that ACh binds more tightly to the resting state could not explain the impaired gating because ACh affinity for this state was only minimally affected and did not correlate with changes in gating produced by other side chains placed at αV285. The presence of two distinct open states in the mutant was described better by open states connected in series rather than open states branching from a common closed state, as follows:

$$A + R \underset{k_{-1}}{\overset{k_{+1}}{\rightleftharpoons}} AR + A \underset{k_{-2}}{\overset{k_{+2}}{\rightleftharpoons}} A_2R \underset{\alpha}{\overset{\beta}{\rightleftharpoons}} A_2R^* \underset{\alpha'}{\overset{\beta'}{\rightleftharpoons}} A_2R^{**}$$

Scheme 3

Thus, αV285 appeared to unmask a metastable open state not normally detected in wild-type AChRs; the free energy profile for channel opening in the mutant thus contains a distinct well, which in wild type is much shallower and not detectable over the experimentally accessible bandwidth.

THE FCCMS DUE TO A SIX-RESIDUE DUPLICATION (STRDQE) IN THE ε SUBUNIT

The STRDQE duplication caused individual receptor channels to suddenly change kinetics in a phenomenon known as mode-switching (FIG. 2). Mode-switching is quite rare in wild-type AChR, but the fact that it occurs suggests that the STRDQE mutation amplifies a normal process. Mode-switches were readily observed during activation episodes elicited by high concentrations of ACh, which appeared as clusters of events in quick succession flanked by prolonged quiescent periods. Three distinct kinetic modes could be discerned within clusters, each with reduced probability of opening due to slower rates of channel opening and faster rates of channel closing. Also, kinetic analysis of the separated modes revealed two open states at saturating concentrations of ACh, rather than the single open state observed for wild-type AChR. Thus, the additional open state unmasked by the mutation may correspond to a metastable open state in the wild-type AChR, as suggested by the CMS mutation

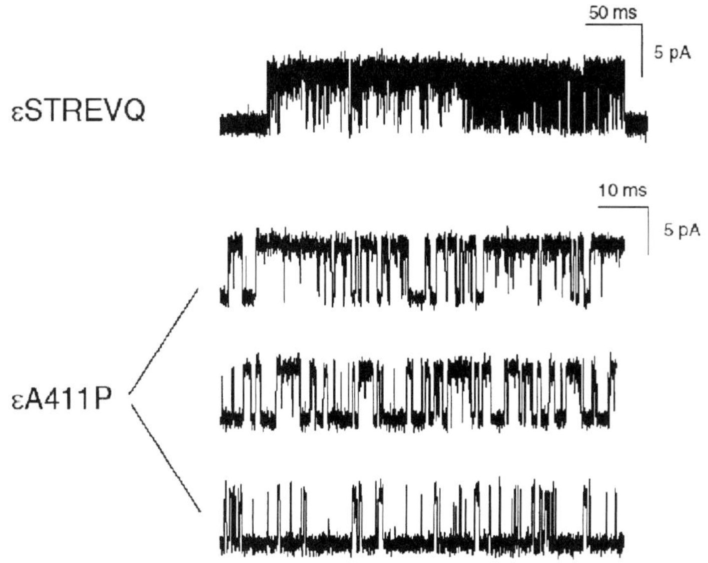

FIGURE 2. Single channel currents elicited by 100 μM ACh through receptor channels containing the indicated mutations that disrupt the fidelity of gating. An individual cluster of channel events is illustrated for the εSTREVQ insertion mutation, whereas segments of recording for three different clusters are shown for the εA411P mutation. Note the abrupt change in gating kinetics for the εSTREVQ insertion mutation and the very different probabilities of individual receptor channels for the εA411P mutation.

αV285I in TMD3. Therefore, the cytoplasmic domain emerges as a determinant of rates of opening and closing of the channel gate.

THE FCCMS MUTATION εA411P

Unlike the STRDQE duplication beginning at codon 413 of the ε subunit, the nearby mutation εA411P did not increase frequency of mode-switching within clusters, but instead caused individual clusters of activation episodes to span a wide spectrum of kinetics.[15] Current pulses through most individual mutant receptors appeared kinetically uniform, but each activation episode had a unique kinetic signature, spanning a wide range of open probability (FIG. 2). Hidden Markov modeling analysis of the kinetics of individual receptors revealed a Gaussian distribution for each rate constant in a kinetic description of receptor activation (i.e., SCHEME 1). The distributions for agonist binding rate constants were unaltered by the mutation, but those for channel opening and closing steps showed remarkable broadening. Proline mutations placed in positions flanking εA411 also produced a wide spectrum of kinetics similar to that produced by εA411P, whereas proline mutations placed in equivalent positions of β and δ subunits produced the usual narrow range of kinetics. The possibility of folding heterogeneity of individual receptors was considered unlikely because in a few activation episodes, several gating modes were readily detected. Thus, the ε subunit again emerged as specific for governing the kinetics of channel gating where residues flanking εA411 maintain fidelity of the opening and closing rate constants.

Analysis of the εA411P mutation provided a unifying explanation for the kinetic consequences of several structural changes in the cytoplasmic loop, including the fetal to adult kinetic switch (γ to ε subunit), mode-switching by the STRDQE duplication, and the wide spectrum of kinetics produced by εA411P. Each of these effects can be ascribed to a localized structural contribution of the cytoplasmic domain to the global energetics governing channel gating. The observation that both wild-type and mutant AChRs shuttle among multiple stable states indicates that the energy landscape underlying gating of the AChR is corrugated. Because the wild-type AChR gates in predominantly one mode, the corrugations superimpose upon a steep funnel-shaped foundation. Receptors containing the εA411P mutation are subject to a similar corrugated energy landscape, but the corrugations superimpose on a much shallower funnel-shaped foundation. Thus, the local region flanking εA411 can be viewed as shaping the broad foundation upon which the corrugations superimpose. In the εA411P mutant, barriers separating energy wells are relatively high, similar to wild type, so only rare mode-switches are detected during individual activation episodes. Hence, in addition to affecting absolute rates of gating, the cytoplasmic loop of the ε subunit controls fidelity of the gating rate constants.[16,17]

SUMMARY OF MECHANISMS UNDERLYING THE FCCMS

The FCCMSs described to date result from genetic alteration of key structural cornerstones governing activation of the nicotinic receptor found at the motor endplate. Although the underlying mechanisms are diverse, the functional end point of each alteration is reduced responsiveness of the postsynaptic membrane to ACh. The predominant location of these alterations is the ACh binding site formed at interfaces between subunits, αε or αδ, and the sites of the mutations have unmasked previously unknown residues critical for function. These functional hot spots include residues that stabilize ACh in a manner that depends on the functional state of the receptor, closed or open. Mechanistic analyses show that FCCMS mutations can cause disease by either increasing or decreasing affinity for ACh, but what is decisive is the state of the receptor that is affected. Increased affinity of the closed state and decreased affinity of the open state are equally deleterious. Additionally, structures that maintain fidelity of channel gating emerged from analyses of FCCMS, which should spur search for analogous structures in other channels or even enzymes as potential disease loci. Future studies will likely unmask new mechanistic classes of FCCMS due to mutation of the AChR, and their analyses will advance understanding of how this crucial neuromuscular signaling protein is activated, as well as allow improved clinical intervention.

REFERENCES

1. ENGEL, A.G., K. OHNO & S.M. SINE. 2001. Acetylcholine receptor channelopathies and other congenital myasthenic syndromes. *In* Channelopathies of the Nervous System, pp. 179–191. Butterworth-Heinemann. Oxford.

2. ENGEL, A.G., K. OHNO & S.M. SINE. 2002. The spectrum of congenital myasthenic syndromes. Mol. Neurobiol. **26:** 347–367.
3. SINE, S.M. 2003. The nicotinic receptor ligand binding domain. J. Neurobiol. **3:** 431–446.
4. ZHANG, Y., J. CHEN & A. AUERBACH. 1995. Activation of recombinant mouse acetylcholine receptors by acetylcholine, carbamylcholine, and tetramethylammonium. J. Physiol. **486:** 189–206.
5. SINE, S.M., T. CLAUDIO & F.J. SIGWORTH. 1990. Activation of *Torpedo* acetylcholine receptors expressed in mouse fibroblasts: single channel current kinetics reveal distinct agonist binding affinities. J. Gen. Physiol. **96:** 395–437.
6. MONOD, J., J. WYMAN & J.P. CHANGEUX. 1965. On the nature of allosteric transitions: a plausible model. J. Mol. Biol. **3:** 318–356.
7. JACKSON, M.B. 1989. Perfection of a synaptic receptor: kinetics and energetics of the acetylcholine receptor. Proc. Natl. Acad. Sci. USA **86:** 2199–2203.
8. SINE, S.M. 1993. Molecular dissection of subunit interfaces in the acetylcholine receptor: identification of residues that determine curare selectivity. Proc. Natl. Acad. Sci. USA **90:** 9436–9440.
9. HAMILL, O.P., A. MARTY, E. NEHER *et al.* 1981. Improved patch-clamp techniques for high-resolution current recording from cells and cell-free membrane patches. Pflüg. Archiv. **391:** 85–100.
10. COLQUHOUN, D. & A.G. HAWKES. 1981. On the stochastic properties of single ion channels. Proc. R. Soc. Lond. **211:** 205–235.
11. QIN, F., A. AUERBACH & F. SACHS. 1996. Estimating single-channel kinetic parameters from idealized patch-clamp data containing missed events. Biophys. J. **70:** 264–280.
12. OHNO, K., H-L. WANG, M. MILONE *et al.* 1996. Congential myasthenic syndrome caused by decreased agonist binding affinity due to a mutation in the acetylcholine receptor ε subunit. Neuron **17:** 157–170.
13. SINE, S.M., H.J. KREIENKAMP, N. BREN *et al.* 1995. Molecular dissection of subunit interfaces in the acetylcholine receptor: identification of determinants of α-conotoxin M1 selectivity. Neuron **15:** 205–211.
14. WANG, H-L., M. MILONE, K. OHNO *et al.* 1999. Acetylcholine receptor M3 domain: stereochemical and volume contributions to channel gating. Nat. Neurosci. **2:** 226–233.
15. WANG, H-L., K. OHNO, M. MILONE *et al.* 2000. Fundamental gating mechanism of nicotinic receptor channel gating revealed by mutation causing a congenital myasthenic syndrome. J. Gen. Physiol. **116:** 449–460.
16. SINE, S.M., X-M. SHEN, H-L. WANG *et al.* 2002. Naturally-occurring mutations at the acetylcholine receptor binding site independently alter ACh binding and channel gating. J. Gen. Physiol. **120:** 483–496.
17. WANG, H-L., M. MILONE, K. OHNO *et al.* 1998. Mode switching kinetics by a naturally occurring mutation in the cytoplasmic loop of the human acetylcholine receptor ε subunit. Neuron **20:** 575–588.

Congenital Myasthenic Syndromes: Multiple Molecular Targets at the Neuromuscular Junction

ANDREW G. ENGEL,[a] KINJI OHNO,[a] XIN-MING SHEN,[a] AND STEVEN M. SINE[b]

[a]*Neuromuscular Disease Research Laboratory, Department of Neurology, and* [b]*Receptor Biology Laboratory, Department of Physiology and Biophysics, Mayo Clinic, Rochester, Minnesota 55905, USA*

ABSTRACT: Congenital myasthenic syndromes (CMS) stem from defects in presynaptic, synaptic, and postsynaptic proteins. The presynaptic CMS are associated with defects that curtail the evoked release of acetylcholine (ACh) quanta or ACh resynthesis. Defects in ACh resynthesis have now been traced to mutations in choline acetyltransferase. A synaptic CMS is caused by mutations in the collagenic tail subunit (ColQ) of the endplate species of acetylcholinesterase that prevent the tail subunit from associating with catalytic subunits or from becoming inserted into the synaptic basal lamina. Most postsynaptic CMS are caused by mutations in subunits of the acetylcholine receptor (AChR) that alter the kinetic properties or decrease the expression of AChR. The kinetic mutations increase or decrease the synaptic response to ACh and result in slow- and fast-channel syndromes, respectively. Most low-expressor mutations reside in the AChR ϵ subunit and are partially compensated by residual expression of the fetal-type γ subunit. In a subset of CMS patients, endplate AChR deficiency is caused by mutations in rapsyn, a molecule that plays a critical role in concentrating AChR in the postsynaptic membrane.

KEYWORDS: acetylcholinesterase; acetylcholine receptor (AChR); choline acetyltransferase; congenital myasthenic syndromes (CMS); patch-clamp recordings; neuromuscular junction; rapsyn

INTRODUCTION

The past decade saw remarkable advances in defining the molecular and genetic basis of the congenital myasthenic syndromes (CMS). These advances would not have been possible without antecedent clinical observations, electrophysiologic analysis, and careful morphologic studies that pointed to candidate genes or proteins. For example, a kinetic abnormality of the acetylcholine receptor (AChR) detected at the single-channel level pointed to a kinetic mutation in an AChR subunit;[1] endplate (EP) AChR deficiency suggested mutations residing in an AChR subunit[2,3] or in rapsyn;[4] absence of acetylcholinesterase (AChE) from the EP predicted mutations in

Address for correspondence: Dr. Andrew G. Engel, Department of Neurology, Mayo Clinic, 200 First Street SW, Rochester, MN 55905. Voice: 507-284-5102; fax: 504-284-5831. age@mayo.edu

Ann. N.Y. Acad. Sci. 998: 138–160 (2003). © 2003 New York Academy of Sciences.
doi: 10.1196/annals.1254.016

TABLE 1. Classification of the CMS based on the site of defect[a]

Classification	Index cases
Presynaptic defects (8%)	
Choline acetyltransferase deficiency[b]	6
Paucity of synaptic vesicles and reduced quantal release	1
Lambert-Eaton syndrome–like	1
Other presynaptic defects	4
Synaptic basal lamina–associated defects (16%)	
Endplate AChE deficiency[b]	24
Postsynaptic defects (76%)	
Kinetic abnormality of AChR with/without AChR deficiency[b] (slow- and fast-channel syndromes)	37
AChR deficiency with/without minor kinetic abnormality[b]	67
Rapsyn deficiency[b]	6
Plectin deficiency	1
Total (100%)	147

[a]Classification based on cohort of CMS patients investigated at the Mayo Clinic between 1988 and 2002.
[b]Genetic defects identified.

the catalytic or collagen-tailed subunit of EP species of this enzyme;[5] and a history of abrupt episodes of apnea associated with a stimulation-dependent decrease of EP potentials and currents implicated proteins concerned with acetylcholine (ACh) resynthesis or vesicular filling.[6] Discovery of mutations in EP-specific proteins also prompted expression studies that afforded proof of pathogenicity, provided clues for rational therapy, led to precise structure function correlations, and highlighted functionally significant residues or molecular domains that previous systematic mutagenesis studies had failed to detect.

TABLE 1 shows a site-of-defect based classification of 147 CMS kinships investigated at the Mayo Clinic. We classify the presently recognized CMS into three major categories: presynaptic, synaptic basal lamina–associated, and postsynaptic. This classification is useful, but it is still tentative because additional types of CMS may exist and because in incompletely studied disorders, not listed in TABLE 1, for example, the limb-girdle CMS, or the CMS associated with facial malformation in Iranian Jews, the site of the defect[7a] was not identified until recently[7b] (see section below on DISCOVERY OF CMS CAUSED BY MUTATIONS IN RAPSYN). TABLE 1 indicates that about 10% of CMS cases are presynaptic, 15% are caused by AChE deficiency, and 75% are postsynaptic. The representation of the different types of CMS, however, could be affected by embryonic or perinatal lethality, reproductive capacity, geographic location, racial origin, or other factors. For example, the 1267delG mutation in the AChR ε subunit is a common cause of CMS among South-Eastern European Gypsies;[8] also, homozygous AChR ε subunit mutations are endemic in Mediterranean countries.[9,10]

This review focuses mainly on advances in CMS since 1997, when the last International Conference on Myasthenia Gravis was held.

DISCOVERY OF EP CHOLINE ACETYLTRANSFERASE DEFICIENCY

Clinical Features

The distinguishing clinical feature is *sudden* episodes of severe dyspnea and bulbar weakness leading to apnea precipitated by infections, fever, excitement, or no discernible cause. In some patients, the disease presents at birth with hypotonia and severe bulbar and respiratory weakness, requiring ventilatory support that gradually improves, but is followed by apneic attacks and bulbar paralysis in later life. Other patients are normal at birth and develop myasthenic symptoms and apneic attacks during infancy or childhood.[7a] Some children, following an acute episode, experience prolonged respiratory insufficiency that may last for weeks. Phenotypic heterogeneity may occur even within a given kinship. For example, in one kinship, two siblings died suddenly at 2 and 11 months of age during febrile episodes; one was asymptomatic and the other had mild ptosis prior to death. A third sibling began having abrupt episodes of dyspnea and cyanosis precipitated by fever or vaccination, or without antecedent cause, at age 14 months; at age 32 months, she developed ptosis and abnormal fatigue on exertion, which led to the diagnosis of a myasthenic disorder.[11]

Morphology and Clinical Electrophysiology Studies

Morphologic studies reveal no AChR deficiency and the postsynaptic region displays no structural abnormality. The synaptic vesicles are smaller than normal in rested muscle and increase or do not change in size after stimulation.[12] In clinical electrophysiology studies, a decremental response at 2-Hz stimulation and single fiber EMG (SFEMG) abnormalities are detected only when the tested muscles are weak. Weakness and a decremental response at 2-Hz stimulation can be induced in some, but not all, muscles by either exercise or a conditioning train of 10-Hz stimuli for 5 to 10 minutes.[12–16] This finding is helpful only if the induced abnormalities disappear slowly over several minutes: a rapid decline of the CMAP followed by rapid recovery (in <1 min) after a 10-Hz stimulation can occur in some patients with EP AChE or AChR deficiency.

In Vitro *Microelectrode Observations*

In vitro studies of intercostal muscle specimens reveal that the synaptic response to ACh, reflected by the amplitude of the miniature EP potential (MEPP) and EP potential (EPP), is normal in rested muscle, but decreases abnormally during a 10-Hz stimulation for 5 minutes and then recovers *slowly* over the next 10 to 15 minutes (FIG. 1A), while the quantal content of the EPP is essentially unaltered.[11,12] A rapid decline of the EPP followed by rapid recovery (in <1 min) of EPP after a 10-Hz stimulation is not a specific finding since it can also occur in other CMS, including EP AChE or AChR deficiency.

Genetic Analysis and Expression Studies

That the MEPP and EPP amplitudes decline abnormally when neuronal impulse flow is increased and then recover *slowly* points to a defect in resynthesis or vesicular packaging of ACh. According to current understanding, a defect in ACh resynthesis implicates four candidate genes: the presynaptic high-affinity choline transporter,[17,18]

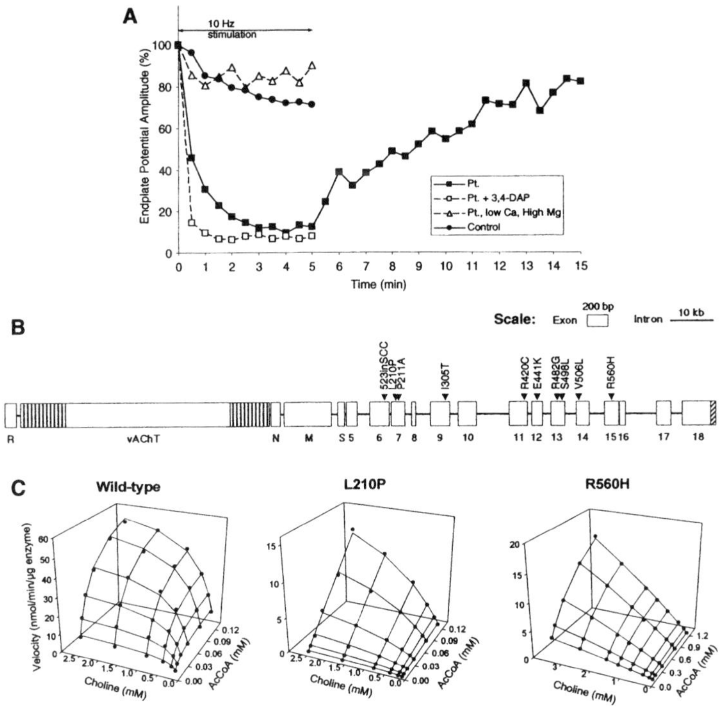

FIGURE 1. CMS with episodic apnea. **(A)** 10-Hz stimulation for 5 min results in a rapid abnormal decline of the endplate potential, which then recovers slowly over >10 min. 3,4-Diaminopyridine (3,4-DAP), which accelerates ACh release, enhances the defect, whereas a low Ca^{2+}/high Mg^{2+} solution, which reduces ACh release, prevents the abnormal decline of the endplate potential. **(B)** Genomic structure of *CHAT* and identified mutations. Note that the gene encoding the vesicular ACh transporter *VACHT* is located in the first *CHAT* intron. **(C)** Individually scaled kinetic landscapes of the wild-type and the L210P and R560H ChAT mutants. The L210P mutant shows no saturation over a practical range of acetyl-CoA (AcCoA) concentrations, indicating an extremely high K_m for AcCoA. Similarly, the R560H mutant does not saturate with increasing concentrations of choline, indicating a very high K_m for choline.

ChAT,[19] the vesicular ACh transporter (VAChT),[20] and the vesicular proton pump.[21] In the course of investigating five CMS-EA patients, we first searched for mutations in *VACHT*, but detected no mutations. We next searched for mutations in *CHAT* and uncovered ten different recessive mutations in the five patients[6] (FIG. 1B). One mutation (523insCC) was a null mutation; three others (I305T, R420C, and E441K) markedly reduced ChAT expression in COS cells. Kinetic studies of nine bacterially expressed and purified missense mutants revealed that one (E441K) lacked all catalytic activity, and eight (L210P, P211A, I305T, R420C, R482G, S498L, V506L, and R560H) had significantly impaired catalytic efficiencies (TABLE 2; FIG. 1C).

TABLE 2. Kinetic parameters of wild-type (WT) and mutant ChAT enzymes

	k_{cat}, s^{-1}	K_m^{AcCoA}, μM	K_m^{chol}, mM	k_{cat}/K_m^{AcCoA}	$k_{cat}/(K_m^{AcCoA} - K_m^{chol})$
WT	99.6 ± 3.5	26.8 ± 1.9	0.478 ± 0.036	1.00	1.00
L210P	35.0 ± 2.2[a]	n.d.[b]	2.693 ± 0.280[a]	0.09	0.02[a]
P211A	418.8 ± 15.9	287.9 ± 28.6	0.514 ± 0.046	0.39	0.36
I305T	60.4 ± 3.4	70.6 ± 6.5	0.590 ± 0.064	0.23	0.19
R420C	176.8 ± 42.9	461.8 ± 134.4	1.018 ± 0.389	0.10	0.05
R482G	99.0 ± 6.9	91.7 ± 10.7	0.500 ± 0.067	0.29	0.28
S498L	88.6 ± 1.5	94.6 ± 7.2	0.418 ± 0.018	0.25	0.29
V506L	125.8 ± 7.4	68.4 ± 7.7	0.370 ± 0.053	0.49	0.64
R560H	34.1 ± 1.3[c]	870.8 ± 62.4[c]	n.d.[d]	0.011[c]	0.002[c]

NOTE: Values indicate estimate ± SE of estimate. Catalytic efficiency (k_{cat}/K_m^{AcCoA}) and the overall catalytic efficiency [$k_{cat}/(K_m^{AcCoA} - K_m^{chol})$] are normalized with respect to wild type. In wild type, $k_{cat}/K_m^{AcCoA} = 3.72 \times 10^6\ s^{-1}M^{-1}$ and $k_{cat}/(K_m^{AcCoA} - K_m^{chol}) = 7.77 \times 10^9\ s^{-1}M^{-1}$.

[a]Apparent values calculated at 116 μM AcCoA.

[b]Not determined because K_m^{AcCoA} exceeds the practical concentration range of AcCoA. Catalytic efficiency was calculated from equation 3 in ref. 6.

[c]Apparent values calculated at 3.5 mM choline.

[d]Not determined because K_m^{chol} exceeds the practical concentration range of choline.

None of the observed CMS-EA patients had central or autonomic nervous system symptoms, indicating that the motor EP is selectively vulnerable to *CHAT* mutations. Tissue-specific isoforms of ChAT do not explain the selective vulnerability. Although there are five alternative *CHAT* transcripts with at least three different promoters in humans,[22] the observed mutations are in the shared coding region of the recognized ChAT isoforms. The selective neuromuscular involvement may exist because of ChAT's rate-limiting characteristics for ACh synthesis at the neuromuscular synapse, but not at other cholinergic synapses, when ACh release is stressed.

Genetic and Clinical Heterogeneity

Not all CMS patients who experience abrupt and unexpected episodes of apnea have mutations in *CHAT*. We have observed two patients who had no mutations in *CHAT* (or in AChR subunit genes), but their clinical histories, EMG findings, and *in vitro* microelectrode studies were indistinguishable from those of patients with mutations in *CHAT*. Analyses of other candidate genes in these patients are in progress. Second, some patients with *CHAT* mutations may not experience apneic episodes (personal communication from R. A. Maselli to A. G. Engel). In such patients, rigorous analysis of the kinetic properties of the mutant ChAT protein is of considerable interest. Finally, an *abrupt* onset of life-threatening or fatal apnea in a myasthenic patient could also arise by an as yet unidentified mechanism.

ENDPLATE ACETYLCHOLINESTERASE DEFICIENCY

This CMS is caused by the absence of AChE from the synaptic space.[23–25] AChE is the enzyme responsible for rapid hydrolysis of ACh released at cholinergic synapses. At the normal EP, AChE limits the number of collisions between ACh and AChR and, hence, the duration of the synaptic response.[26] Inhibition of the enzyme results in prolonged exposure of AChR to ACh, prolonged EPPs, desensitization of AChR[27] and a depolarization block at physiologic rates of stimulation,[28] and an EP myopathy with loss of AChR owing to cationic overloading of the postsynaptic region.[29]

Clinical Features

In most patients the disease presents in the neonatal period and is highly disabling, but in some patients it presents in childhood and becomes disabling only in the second decade[30] or later in life.[31] Moreover, patients in different kinships with identical homozygous mutations can show marked differences in phenotypic expressivity.[31] The following clinical clues point to the diagnosis: (1) a decremental EMG response; (2) a repetitive CMAP that is of smaller amplitude and decreases faster than the first CMAP; (3) no effect of AChE inhibitors on the decremental response, the repetitive CMAP, or the clinical state; and (4) a slow pupillary light response in some,[24] but not all,[31] patients.

The Endplate Species of AChE

The endplate species of AChE is a heteromeric asymmetric enzyme composed of 1, 2, or 3 homotetramers of globular catalytic subunits ($AChE_T$) attached to a triple-stranded collagenic tail (ColQ) (FIG. 2, right). ColQ has an N-terminal proline-rich region attachment domain (PRAD), a collagenic central domain, and a C-terminal region enriched in charged residues and cysteines (FIG. 2, left). Each ColQ strand can bind an $AChE_T$ tetramer to its PRAD, giving rise to A_4, A_8, and A_{12} species of asymmetric AChE.[32] Two groups of charged residues in the collagen domain (heparan sulfate proteoglycan binding domains, or HSPBD)[33] plus other residues in the C-terminal region[25,34] assure that the asymmetric enzyme is inserted into the synaptic basal lamina. The C-terminal region is also required for initiating the triple-helical assembly of ColQ that proceeds from a C- to an N-terminal direction in a zipper-like manner.[35]

Genetic Analysis and Expression Studies

In 1998, human *COLQ* cDNA was cloned,[5,30] the genomic structure of *COLQ* determined,[5] and the molecular basis of EP AChE deficiency traced to recessive mutations in *COLQ*.[5,30] Twenty-four *COLQ* mutations in 25 kinships have been identified to date[5,25,30,31,36,37] (FIG. 2, right). Density gradient ultracentrifugation can monitor the molecular species AChE at normal or patient EPs, or in COS cells that had been cotransfected with genetically engineered wild-type $AChE_T$ along with wild-type or mutant ColQ. These studies indicate that (1) mutations involving PRAD prevent attachment of $AChE_T$ to ColQ; (2) collagen domain mutations produce a truncated, single-stranded ColQ that binds a single $AChE_T$ tetramer and

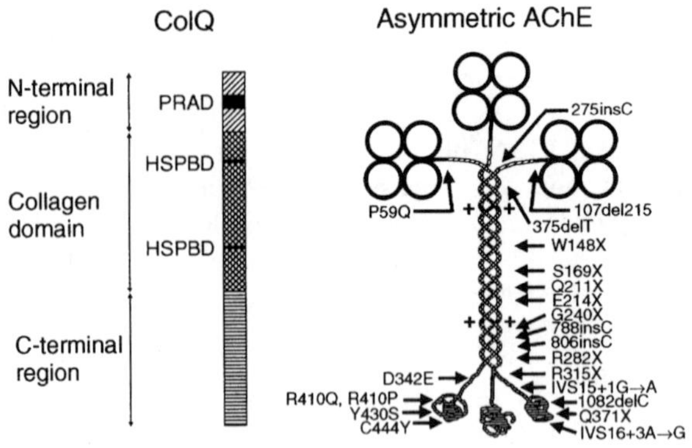

FIGURE 2. **Left**: Schematic diagram showing domains of a ColQ strand. **Right:** Components of the A_{12} species of asymmetric AChE and 24 identified ColQ mutations. AChE = acetylcholinesterase; HSPBD = heparan sulfate proteoglycan binding domain; PRAD = proline-rich attachment domain.

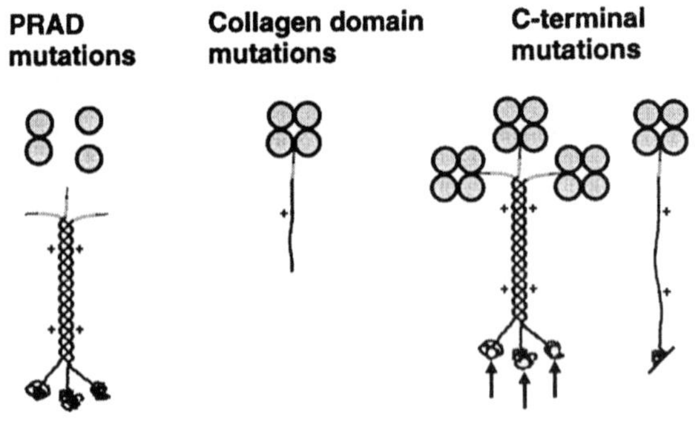

FIGURE 3. Schematic representation of the consequences of ColQ mutations. Mutations in the PRAD domain result in nonattachment of the catalytic subunits; frameshift or nonsense mutations in the collagen domain result in a truncated single-stranded ColQ that is insertion-incompetent; missense or truncation mutations in the C-terminal region result in triple-helical or single-stranded ColQ that are also insertion-incompetent.

is insertion-incompetent; (3) C-terminal mutations either hinder the triple-helical assembly of the collagen domain or produce asymmetric AChE that may or may not be insertion-incompetent (FIG. 3). That the asymmetric AChE species produced by some C-terminal ColQ mutations are insertion-incompetent was recently demonstrated by Kimbell and coworkers. They showed that purified wild-type asymmetric AChE was transplantable into the basal lamina of the frog EP, but C-terminal-mutant asymmetric AChEs were not.[34]

TABLE 3. Kinetic abnormalities of AChR

	Slow-channel syndromes	Fast-channel syndromes
Endplate currents	Slow decay	Fast decay
Channel opening events	Prolonged	Brief
Open states	Stabilized	Destabilized
Closed states	Destabilized	Stabilized
Mechanisms[a]	Increased affinity Increased β Decreased α	Decreased affinity Decreased β Increased α Mode-switching kinetics
Pathology	Endplate myopathy from cationic overloading	No anatomic footprint
Genetic background	Dominant gain-of-function mutations in most cases[b]	Recessive loss-of-function mutation
Response to therapy	Long-lived open channel blockade of AChR with quinidine or fluoxetine	3,4-DAP and AChE inhibitors

NOTE: β = channel opening rate; α = channel closing rate.
[a]Different combinations of mechanisms operate in the individual slow- and fast-channel syndromes.
[b]Three recessive slow-channel mutations, all located in the ε subunit, also exist: εP245L,[3] εL78P,[50] and εL221F.[50]

KINETIC MUTATIONS OF THE ACETYLCHOLINE RECEPTOR

Two major types of kinetic syndromes have emerged since 1995: the slow-channel syndromes and the fast-channel syndromes. The two syndromes represent physiological opposites. TABLE 3 lists reciprocal features of the two syndromes.

SLOW-CHANNEL SYNDROMES

Endplate Studies

The prolonged opening episodes of the AChR channel result in prolonged EP currents and potentials (FIGS. 4B and 4C), which in turn elicit one or more repetitive CMAPs. Repetitive stimulation reveals a decremental response that is present at low stimulation frequency and increases progressively in a frequency-dependent manner. The repetitive CMAP is of lower amplitude and decrements faster than the first CMAP.

The morphologic consequences stem from prolonged activation episodes of the AChR channel that cause cationic overloading of the postsynaptic region. In addition, some slow-channel mutations in transmembrane domains 1 and 2 render AChR leaky so that it opens even in the absence of ACh,[1,38,39] and some slow-channel mutants were reported to be opened by choline even at concentrations present in serum.[40] Excessive accumulation of Ca^{2+} can be demonstrated at some EPs with

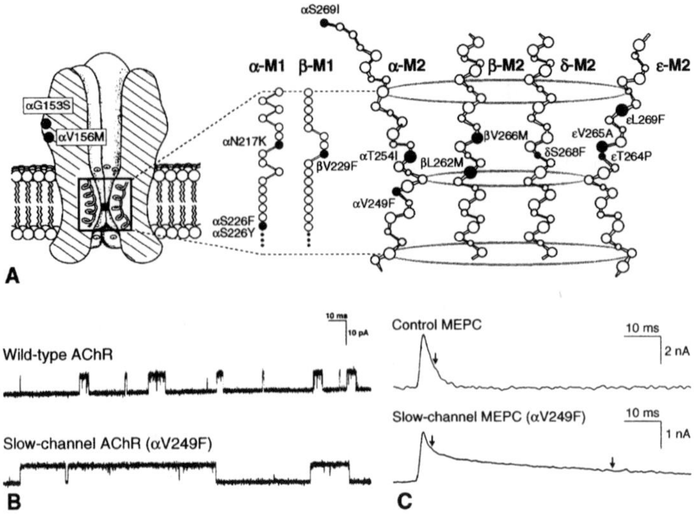

FIGURE 4. **(A)** Schematic diagram of slow-channel mutations. The drawing on the *left* shows a section through the AChR indicating approximate position of mutations that are not in transmembrane domains of the receptor. In the drawing on the *right*, dotted lines delimit transmembrane domains. Mutations appear in the TMD2 domains of the α, β, δ, and ε subunits, and in the TMD1 domain of the α subunit. The αS269I mutation above the dotted line is in the extracellular TMD2/TMD3 linker. **(B)** Examples of single-channel currents from wild-type and slow-channel (αV249F) AChRs expressed in HEK cells. **(C)** Miniature endplate currents (MEPC) recorded from EPs of a control subject and a patient harboring the αV249F slow-channel mutation. The slow-channel MEPC decays biexponentially due to expression of both wild-type and mutant AChRs at the EP, with one decay time constant that is normal and one that is markedly prolonged.

alizarin red, which detects millimolar concentrations of Ca^{2+}. The EP myopathy that develops is like that in EP AChE deficiency, but is even more severe, sometimes causing massive destruction of the junctional folds, nuclear apoptosis, and vacuolar degeneration near the EPs.[7a,38,39,41] The disease is progressive owing to structural damage to the EP.

In vitro microelectrode studies demonstrate markedly prolonged currents that decay biexponentially, owing to the presence of both wild-type and mutant receptors (Fig. 4C).[1,38,42] Single-channel patch-clamp recordings at the EP reveal a dual population of AChR channels, one with normal and one with prolonged opening episodes, again reflecting the presence of both wild-type and mutant channels (Fig. 4B). The safety margin of neuromuscular transmission is compromised by the altered EP geometry, loss of AChR from degenerating junctional folds, and a depolarization block during physiologic activity, owing to staircase summation of the markedly prolonged EPPs.

Genetic Analysis and Expression Studies

Altogether, 18 slow-channel mutations have been published to date.[1,3,38,39,42–49] Six of these mutations were reported since 1997: εV265A,[46] α226F,[47] α226Y,[47]

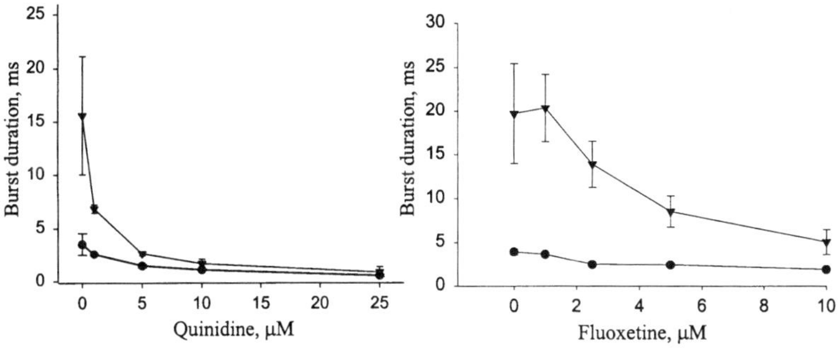

FIGURE 5. Effect of quinidine (*left panel*) and fluoxetine (*right panel*) on the duration of AChR channel opening bursts of five genetically engineered slow-channel mutants (*triangles*) and wild-type AChR (*circles*) expressed in HEK cells. *Vertical lines* indicate SD. Note that 5 μM quinidine normalizes and 10 μM fluoxetine nearly normalizes the duration of the slow-channel bursts. (*Left panel* reproduced from ref. 53 by permission.)

βV299F,[48] δS268F,[49] and εL221F.[50] Sixteen mutations are dominant, but two mutations in the ε subunit, one in its extracellular domain (εL78P[50]) and one in its first transmembrane domain (εP245L[3]), are recessive, and one mutation (εL221F[50]) is dominant, but shows variable penetrance. FIGURE 4A indicates positions of the 15 dominant mutations in the different AChR subunits. In general, mutations in transmembrane domains of subunits have more severe clinical consequences than mutations in an extracellular domain. From a mechanistic standpoint, the mutations exert their effect by increasing gating efficiency, affinity for ACh, or both, and variably enhance the extent of desensitization. Detailed accounts of the mechanistic consequences of the εT264P,[1] εP245L,[3] αG153S,[42] αN217K,[43] αV249F,[39] αS269I,[51] and δS268F[49] mutations were previously published.

Therapy

Quinidine is a long-lived open-channel blocker of AChR,[52] and clinically attainable levels of quinidine normalize the prolonged opening episodes of mutant slow-channels expressed in HEK cells (FIG. 5, left).[53] On the basis of these findings, Harper and Engel[54] treated slow-channel patients with quinidine sulfate, 200 mg three to four times daily, producing serum levels of 0.7–2.5 μg/mL (2.1–7.7 μM/L), and found that the patients improved gradually by clinical and EMG criteria. Fluoxetine, another long-lived open-channel blocker of AChR (FIG. 5, right), is also therapeutically effective, but relatively high doses of the medication (~80 mg/day in adults) are required to obtain a therapeutic effect.[55]

FAST-CHANNEL SYNDROMES

Fast-channel mutations have been observed in the AChR α, δ, and ε subunits (see FIG. 6). Mutations in extracellular domains of subunits diminish affinity for ACh, those in transmembrane domains impair gating efficiency, and those in the long

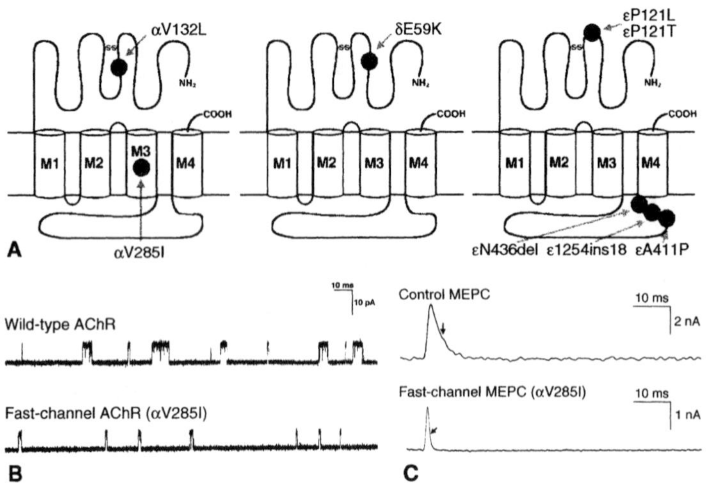

FIGURE 6. **(A)** Schematic diagram of fast-channel mutations in the AChR α, β, and δ subunits. **(B)** Examples of single-channel currents from wild-type and fast-channel (αV285I) AChRs expressed in HEK cells. **(C)** Miniature endplate currents (MEPC) recorded from EPs of a control subject and a patient harboring the αV285I fast-channel mutation. *Arrows* indicate decay time constants.

cytoplasmic loop of the ε subunit destabilize channel kinetics. The clinical features resemble those of autoimmune myasthenia gravis, but symptoms are mild when the main effect is on gating efficiency,[56] moderately severe when channel kinetics are unstable,[57,58] and severe when affinity for ACh or both affinity and gating efficiency are impaired.[59–62] The δE59K mutation in the extracellular domain of the δ subunit reported by Brownlow and coworkers[62] that reduces affinity for ACh is of special interest since it also causes multiple congenital joint contractures owing to fetal hypomotility *in utero*.[62]

Endplate Studies

EP morphology and AChR expression are normal in the low-affinity fast-channel syndrome caused by εP121L.[59,61] In contrast, AChR expression is reduced, EP regions are dispersed, and some postsynaptic regions are simplified, yet structurally intact with the αV285I mutation that reduces gating efficiency[56] and with the 18-bp insertion (ε1254ins18) in the long cytoplasmic loop of the ε subunit that destabilized channel kinetics.[57]

The common electrophysiologic features of the fast-channel CMS are abnormally brief channel activation episodes (FIG. 6B) and rapidly decaying low-amplitude EP currents (FIG. 6C). The reduced amplitude of the synaptic response results from reduced probability of channel opening and, in the case of ε1254ins18 and αV285I, from reduced expression of the mutant receptor.

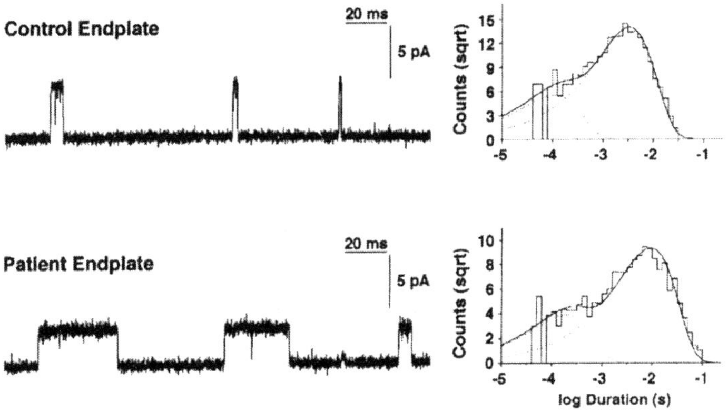

FIGURE 7. Single-channel currents (*left panels*) and burst open duration histograms (*right panels*) recorded from a control EP and from an EP of a patient with a homozygous null mutation in the extracellular domain of the ε subunit (ε553del7). At the patient's EP, the channel currents are longer and of lower amplitude than at the control EP, indicating the presence of the fetal AChR that harbors the γ instead of the ε subunit.

Genetic Analysis and Expression Studies

Eight fast-channel mutations have been identified to date[56–63] (FIG. 6A). In most cases, the mutated allele causing the kinetic abnormality is accompanied by a null mutation in the second allele so that the kinetic mutation dominates the clinical phenotype, but homozygous fast-channel mutations also exist. In a companion to this paper, Sine and coworkers[64] provide a detailed account of the mechanistic consequences of the fast-channel mutations deduced from expression studies.

Therapy

Fast-channel syndrome patients generally respond well to combined therapy with 3,4-diaminopyridine (3,4-DAP), which increases the number of quanta released by the nerve impulse, and cholinesterase inhibitors, which increase the number of receptors activated by each quantum. Patients with a normal density of AChR on the junctional folds respond best since a decreased density of receptors on the folds entails a proportionate reduction in the number of receptors that can be saturated by any given quantum.

ACHR DEFICIENCY CAUSED BY MUTATIONS IN ACHR SUBUNIT GENES

Clinical Features

These vary from mild to very severe. In general, patients harboring low-expressor or even homozygous null mutations in the ε subunit may have mild symptoms. Conversely, patients with low-expressor mutations in non-ε subunits are severely

TABLE 4. Low expressor mutations in AChR subunits

Subunit/effect	Mutation	Reference
α subunit		
Frameshift	α381delC	61
	α459insG	90
Missense	αG74C	91
	αF233V	56
	αI296L	90
	αV402F	91
β subunit		
Frameshift	β1276del9	70
	βdelEx8	70
δ subunit		
Frameshift	δ756ins2	62
Missense	δP250Q	92
ε subunit		
Chromosomal microdeletion	εΔ1290bp	69
Promoter point mutation	ε-156C→T	68
	ε-155G→A	67
	ε-154G→A	68
Signal peptide, missense	εV-13D	10
	εG-8R	59
Frameshift	ε59ins5	9
	ε67insG	93
	ε70insG	9
	ε127ins5	3
	ε553del7	3, 65, 94
	ε627ins2	95
	ε723delC	10
	ε734delC	96, 97
	ε760ins8	10
	ε911delT	96, 98
	ε1012del20	99
	ε1030insC	96
	ε1030delC	98
	ε1033delG	95, 100
	ε1101insT	2
	ε1197delG	93
	ε1206ins19	9, 95
	ε1208ins19	66
	ε1259del23	100
	ε1267delG	9, 71, 72, 93, 101

TABLE 4. Low expressor mutations in AChR subunits (*Continued*)

Subunit/effect	Mutation	Reference
	ε1276delG	9
	ε1293insG	2, 58, 66, 96, 102
	ε1369delG	93
Nonsense	εR64X	3, 98
	εE154X	96
	εQ310X	96
	εQ378X	93, 96
Splice-site	εIVS41G→A	98
	εIVS6-1G→C	96
	εIVS61G→T	103
	εIVS7-2A→G	93, 96
	εIVS72T→C	9, 93
	εIVS91G→T	66
	εIVS9-1G→C	63, 94
	εIVS102T→G	10
	εIVS10-9ins16	104
Missense	εR20W	60
	εT51P	10
	εC128S	57, 93
	εS143L	59
	εR147L	3
	εT159P	58
	εP245L	3
	εR311W	3, 10
	εP331L	66

affected, and no patients with null mutations in both alleles of a non-ε subunit have been observed to date.

Endplate Studies

Morphologic studies show an increased number of EP regions distributed over an increased span of the muscle fiber. The integrity of the junctional folds is preserved, but some EP regions are simplified and smaller than normal. The distribution of AChR on the junctional folds is patchy and the density of the reaction for AChR is attenuated. The immunocytochemical reaction for rapsyn, a molecule that cross-links AChRs, is decreased in proportion to the decrease of AChR expression.

The quantal response at the EP, indicated by the amplitude of MEPPs and currents, is reduced, but quantal release by nerve impulse is frequently higher than normal. In patients with low-expressor or null mutations of the ε subunit, single-channel patch-clamp recordings[3,65] (see FIG. 7) and immunocytochemical studies[2] reveal the presence of fetal γ-AChR at the EP.

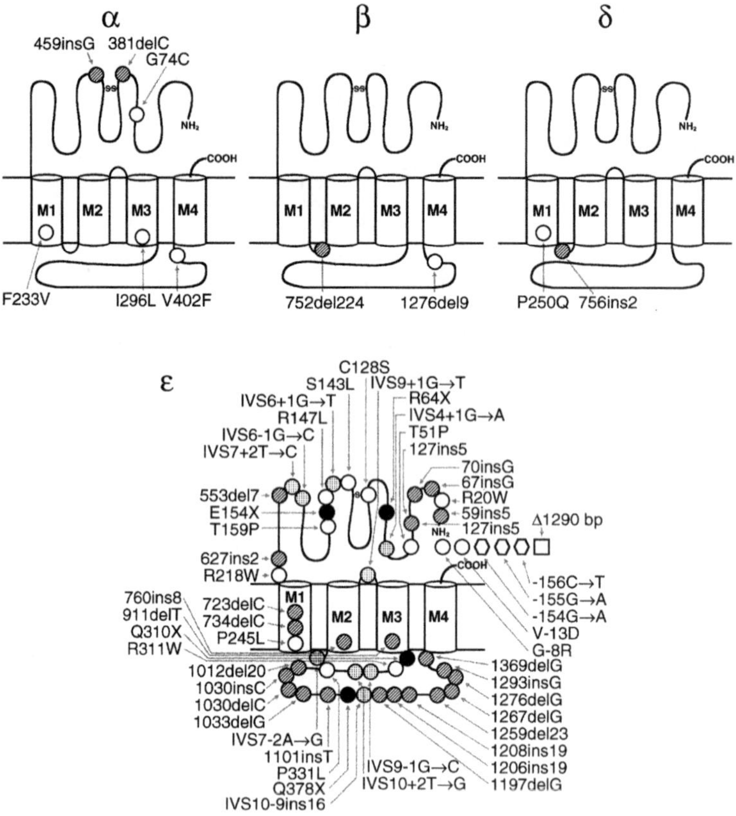

FIGURE 8. Schematic diagram of low-expressor and null mutations reported in the α, β, δ, and ε subunits of AChR. The *square* indicates a chromosomal microdeletion; *hexagons* are promoter mutations; *open circles* are missense mutations; *closed circles* are nonsense mutations; *shaded circles* are frameshifting mutations; and *dotted circles* are splice-site mutations. The most likely consequence of a splice-site mutation is skipping of a flanking exon; thus, the splice-site mutations point to N-terminal codons of the predicted skipped exons. TABLE 4 indicates references for each mutation.

Genetic Studies

CMS with severe EP AChR deficiency result from different types of homozygous or, more frequently, heterozygous recessive mutations in AChR subunit genes (TABLE 4; FIG. 8). The mutations are concentrated in the ε subunit. A likely reason for this is that persistent expression of the fetal-type γ subunit, although at a low level, may compensate for absence of the ε subunit,[2,3,57,66] whereas patients harboring null mutations in subunits other than ε might not survive for lack of a substituting subunit. In addition, the gene encoding the ε subunit, and especially exons encoding the long cytoplasmic loop, have a high GC content that could predispose to DNA rearrangements.

The AChR deficiency results from mutations that cause premature termination of the translational chain by frameshift, by being at a splice site, or by generating a stop codon directly; from point mutations in the promoter region;[67,68] from chromosomal microdeletion;[69] and from missense mutations. Some missense mutations appear in the signal peptide region.[10,59] Other missense mutations involve residues essential for assembly of the pentameric receptor; mutations of this type were observed in the ε subunit at an N-glycosylation site,[59] in cysteine 128,[57] in arginine 147 that lies between residues that contribute to subunit assembly,[3] and in threonine 51;[10] and with a 3-codon deletion in the long cytoplasmic loop of the β subunit.[70] Still other missense mutations affect both AChR expression and kinetics. For example, εR311W in the long cytoplasmic loop between transmembrane domains 3 and 4 has mild fast-channel properties,[3] whereas εP245L in the first transmembrane domain has mild slow-channel properties.[3]

Finally, it is noteworthy that the frameshifting ε1267delG mutation occurring at homozygosity is endemic in families of Gypsy or South-Eastern European origin,[9,71,72] where it derives from a Gypsy founder.[72]

Therapy

Most patients respond moderately well to anti-AChE drugs, and some derive additional benefit from 3,4-DAP.[73]

DISCOVERY OF CMS CAUSED BY MUTATIONS IN RAPSYN

EP AChR deficiency also could stem from defects in proteins that regulate the expression or concentration of AChR at the EP. These include agrin[74,75] and its signaling molecules, MuSK[76] and rapsyn;[77–79] neuregulin and its signaling molecules;[80–82] as well as α-dystrobrevin,[83] utrophin,[84] and α-syntrophin.[85] Thus far, however, only mutations in rapsyn have been shown to cause a CMS associated with EP AChR deficiency (see FIG. 9).[4]

The primary structure of rapsyn predicts distinct structural domains: a myristoylation signal at the N-terminus required for membrane association;[79] seven tetratrico peptide repeats (TPRs; codons 6–279) that subserve rapsyn self-association;[79,86] a coiled-coil domain (codons 298–331) whose hydrophobic surface can bind to determinants within the long cytoplasmic loop of each AChR subunit;[86,87] a cysteine-rich RING-H2 domain (codons 363–402) that binds to the cytoplasmic domain of β-dystroglycan[88] and to the synaptic nebulin-related anchoring protein (S-NRAP);[89] and a serine phosphorylation site at codon 406 (FIG. 9).

Genetic Analysis and Expression Studies

In four patients with EP AChR deficiency, but no mutations in AChR, we recently identified three recessive rapsyn mutations: one patient carries L14P in TPR1 and N88K in TPR3; two are homozygous for N88K; and one carries N88K and 553ins5 that frameshifts in TPR5.[4] EP studies in each case show decreased staining for rapsyn as well as AChR, and impaired postsynaptic morphologic development. Expression studies in HEK cells reveal that none of the mutations hinders rapsyn self-association, but all three diminish coclustering of AChR with rapsyn. That mis-

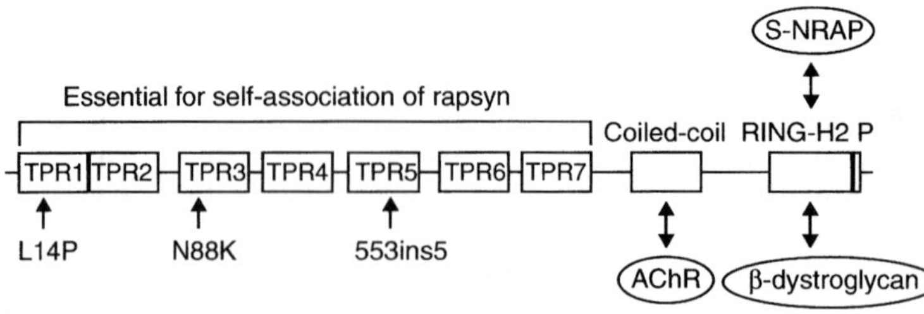

FIGURE 9. Schematic diagram showing domains of rapsyn and the first three identified mutations. Seven tetratricopeptide repeats (TPRs) are required for rapsyn self-association; the coiled-coil domain binds to the long cytoplasmic loop of AChR subunits; the RING-H2 domain links rapsyn to β-dystroglycan and to the actin-binding synaptic nebulin-related anchoring protein (S-NRAP).

sense mutations in TPR domains decrease coclustering of rapsyn with AChR implies that effects of these mutations propagate downstream to the coiled-coil domain, or that the mutations have an allosteric effect on the conformation of the coiled-coil or RING-H2 domains. Our rapsyn-deficient patients have responded well to combined therapy with anti-AChE drugs and 3,4-DAP.

Recently, we also identified two mutations in E-box elements of the *RAPSN* promoter (−38A→G and −27C→G) in CMS patients. The −38A→G was found to be homozygous in 7 Oriental Jewish kinships with characteristic facial malformations and was traced to a common founder. The pathogenicity of the E-box mutations was confirmed in a luciferase reporter assay that showed attenuated reporter gene expression in C2C12 myotubes.[7b] These mutations represent the first E-box mutations observed in humans.

DISCOVERY OF CMS CAUSED BY A DEFECT IN THE NA$_V$1.4 SODIUM CHANNEL

We recently observed a patient with myasthenic symptoms since birth consisting of eyelid ptosis, fatigable generalized weakness, and recurrent attacks of respiratory and bulbar paralysis since birth. Nerve stimulation at physiologic rates rapidly decremented the compound muscle action potential. Intercostal muscle studies revealed no abnormality of the resting membrane potential, evoked quantal release, synaptic potentials, AChR channel kinetics, or EP ultrastructure, but EP potentials depolarizing the resting potential to −40 mV failed to excite action potentials. Pursuing this clue, we sequenced *SCN4A* encoding the Na$_V$1.4 skeletal muscle sodium channel and detected two heteroallelic mutations involving conserved residues not present in 400 normal alleles: S246L in the S4/S5 cytoplasmic linker in domain I, and V1442E in the S3/S4 extracellular linker in domain IV. Expression studies on the observed mutations in HEK cells by Steve Cannon and Chantal Maertens revealed that the V1442E–Na channel showed marked enhancement of fast inactivation close to the resting potential, and enhanced use-dependent inactivation on high frequency stimulation; S246L showed only minor kinetic abnormalities, suggesting that it is a benign polymorphism. The V1442E mutation in *SCN4A* defines a novel disease mechanism and a novel phenotype with myasthenic features.[105]

FINAL COMMENTS

The past decade saw a rapid increase in our understanding of the clinical semiology, electrophysiological basis, and molecular biology of the CMS. Since discovery of the first mutations in AChR in 1995, the combined efforts of many investigators resulted in discovery of an avalanche of mutations in AChR. After 1998, other molecular targets of the CMS, namely ColQ, ChAT, rapsyn, and $Na_V1.4$, were identified, and the observed mutations were validated by appropriate expression studies. Yet still further molecular targets of the CMS likely exist and await discovery.

ACKNOWLEDGMENTS

This work was supported by National Institutes of Health grants to A. G. Engel (No. NS6277) and S. M. Sine (No. NS31744), and an MDA Research Grant to A. G. Engel.

REFERENCES

1. Ohno, K., D.O. Hutchinson, M. Milone *et al.* 1995. Congenital myasthenic syndrome caused by prolonged acetylcholine receptor channel openings due to a mutation in the M2 domain of the ε subunit. Proc. Natl. Acad. Sci. USA **92:** 758–762.
2. Engel, A.G., K. Ohno, C. Bouzat *et al.* 1996. End-plate acetylcholine receptor deficiency due to nonsense mutations in the ε subunit. Ann. Neurol. **40:** 810–817.
3. Ohno, K., P. Quiram, M. Milone *et al.* 1997. Congenital myasthenic syndromes due to heteroallelic nonsense/missense mutations in the acetylcholine receptor ε subunit gene: identification and functional characterization of six new mutations. Hum. Mol. Genet. **6:** 753–766.
4. Ohno, K., A.G. Engel, X-M. Shen *et al.* 2002. Rapsyn mutations in humans cause endplate acetylcholine receptor deficiency and myasthenic syndrome. Am. J. Hum. Genet. **70:** 875–885.
5. Ohno, K., J.M. Brengman, A. Tsujino & A.G. Engel. 1998. Human endplate acetylcholinesterase deficiency caused by mutations in the collagen-like tail subunit (ColQ) of the asymmetric enzyme. Proc. Natl. Acad. Sci. USA **95:** 9654–9659.
6. Ohno, K., A. Tsujino, J.M. Brengman *et al.* 2001. Choline acetyltransferase mutations cause myasthenic syndrome associated with episodic apnea in humans. Proc. Natl. Acad. Sci. USA **98:** 2017–2022.
7. (a) Engel, A.G., K. Ohno & S.M. Sine. 1999. Congenital myasthenic syndromes. *In* Myasthenia Gravis and Myasthenic Disorders, pp. 251–297. Oxford University Press. London/New York; (b) Ohno, K., M. Sadeh, I. Blatt *et al.* 2003. E-box mutations in *RAPSN* promoter region in eight cases with congenital myasthenic syndrome. Hum. Mol. Genet. **12:** 739–748.
8. Karcagi, V., I. Tournev, A. Hercegfalvi *et al.* 2001. Congenital myasthenic syndromes in South-Eastern European Roma (Gypsies). Acta Myol. **20:** 231–237.
9. Ohno, K., B. Anlar, E. Özdirim *et al.* 1998. Myasthenic syndromes in Turkish kinships due to mutations in the acetylcholine receptor. Ann. Neurol. **44:** 234–241.
10. Middleton, L., K. Ohno, K. Christodoulou *et al.* 1999. Congenital myasthenic syndromes linked to chromosome 17p are caused by defects in acetylcholine receptor ε subunit gene. Neurology **53:** 1076–1082.

11. Byring, R.F., H. Pihko, X-M. Shen *et al.* 2002. Congenital myasthenic syndrome associated with epsiodic apnea and sudden infant death. Neuromuscul. Disord. **12:** 548–553.
12. Mora, M., E.H. Lambert & A.G. Engel. 1987. Synaptic vesicle abnormality in familial infantile myasthenia. Neurology **37:** 206–214.
13. Hart, Z., K. Sahashi, E.H. Lambert *et al.* 1979. A congenital, familial, myasthenic syndrome caused by a presynaptic defect of transmitter resynthesis of mobilization [abstract]. Neurology **29:** 559.
14. Engel, A.G. & E.H. Lambert. 1987. Congenital myasthenic syndromes. Electroencephalogr. Clin. Neurophysiol. Suppl. **39:** 91–102.
15. Harper, C.M. 2002. Electrodiagnosis of endplate disease. *In* Myasthenia Gravis and Myasthenic Disorders, pp. 65–84. Oxford University Press. London/New York.
16. Robertson, W.C., R.W.M. Chun & S.E. Kornguth. 1980. Familial infantile myasthenia. Arch. Neurol. **37:** 117–119.
17. Okuda, T., T. Haga, Y. Kanai *et al.* 2000. Identification and characterization of the high-affinity choline transporter. Nat. Neurosci. **3:** 120–125.
18. Apparsundaram, S., S.M. Ferguson, A.L. George, Jr. & R.D. Blakely. 2000. Molecular cloning of a human, hemicholinium-3-sensitive choline transporter. Biochem. Biophys. Res. Commun. **276:** 862–867.
19. Oda, Y., I. Nakanishi & T. Deguchi. 1992. A complementary DNA for human choline acetyltransferase induces two forms of enzyme with different molecular weights in cultured cells. Brain Res. Mol. Brain Res. **16:** 287–294.
20. Erickson, J.D., H. Varoqui, L.E. Eiden *et al.* 1994. Functional identification of a vesicular acetylcholine transporter and its expression from a "cholinergic" gene locus. J. Biol. Chem. **269:** 21929–21932.
21. Reimer, R.J., A.E. Fon & R.H. Edwards. 1998. Vesicular neurotransmitter transport and the presynaptic regulation of quantal size. Curr. Opin. Neurobiol. **8:** 405–412.
22. Eiden, L.E. 1998. The cholinergic gene locus. J. Neurochem. **70:** 2227–2240.
23. Engel, A.G., E.H. Lambert & M.R. Gomez. 1977. A new myasthenic syndrome with end-plate acetylcholinesterase deficiency, small nerve terminals, and reduced acetylcholine release. Ann. Neurol. **1:** 315–330.
24. Hutchinson, D.O., T.J. Walls, S. Nakano *et al.* 1993. Congenital endplate acetylcholinesterase deficiency. Brain **116:** 633–653.
25. Ohno, K., A.G. Engel, J.M. Brengman *et al.* 2000. The spectrum of mutations causing endplate acetylcholinesterase deficiency. Ann. Neurol. **47:** 162–170.
26. Katz, B. & R. Miledi. 1973. The binding of acetylcholine to receptors and its removal from the synaptic cleft. J. Physiol. (Lond.) **231:** 549–574.
27. Katz, B. & S. Thesleff. 1957. A study of the "desensitization" produced by acetylcholine at the motor end-plate. J. Physiol. (Lond.) **138:** 63–80.
28. Maselli, R.A. & B.C. Soliven. 1991. Analysis of the organophosphate-induced electromyographic response to repetitive nerve stimulation: paradoxical response to edrophonium and *d*-tubocurarine. Muscle Nerve **14:** 1182–1188.
29. Salpeter, M.M., H. Kasprzak, H. Feng & H. Fertuck. 1979. End-plates after esterase inactivation *in vivo*: correlation between esterase concentration, functional response and fine structure. J. Neurocytol. **8:** 95–115.
30. Donger, C., E. Krejci, P. Serradell *et al.* 1998. Mutation in the human acetylcholinesterase-associated gene, *COLQ*, is responsible for congenital myasthenic syndrome with end-plate acetylcholinesterase deficiency. Am. J. Hum. Genet. **63:** 967–975.
31. Shapira, Y.A., M.E. Sadeh, M.P. Bergtraum *et al.* 2002. The novel *COLQ* mutations and variation of phenotypic expressivity due to G240X. Neurology **58:** 603–609.
32. Bon, S., F. Coussen & J. Massoulié. 1997. Quaternary associations of acetylcholinesterase. II. The polyproline attachment domain of the collagen tail. J. Biol. Chem. **272:** 3016–3021.
33. Deprez, P.N. & N.C. Inestrosa. 1995. Two heparin-binding domains are present on the collagenic tail of asymmetric acetylcholinesterase. J. Biol. Chem. **270:** 11043–11046.
34. Kimbell, L.M., K. Ohno, R.L. Rotundo & A.G. Engel. 2001. Transplanting mutant human collagenic tailed acetylcholinesterase onto the frog neuromuscular junction:

evidence for an attachment defect in a congenital myasthenic syndrome [abstract]. Mol. Biol. Cell (Suppl.) **12:** 161a.
35. PROCKOP, D.J. & K.I. KIVIRIKKO. 1995. Collagens: molecular biology, diseases, and potentials for therapy. Annu. Rev. Biochem. **64:** 403–434.
36. OHNO, K., J.M. BRENGMAN, K.J. FELICE *et al.* 1999. Congenital endplate acetylcholinesterase deficiency caused by a nonsense mutation and an A-to-G splice site mutation at position +3 of the collagen-like tail subunit gene (*COLQ*): how does G at position +3 result in aberrant splicing? Am. J. Hum. Genet. **65:** 635–644.
37. ISHIGAKI, K., D. NICOLLE, E. KREJCI *et al.* 2001. Two novel mutations in the ColQ gene causing endplate acetylcholinesterase deficiency [abstract]. Neuromuscul. Disord. **11:** 666–667.
38. ENGEL, A.G., K. OHNO, M. MILONE *et al.* 1996. New mutations in acetylcholine receptor subunit genes reveal heterogeneity in the slow-channel congenital myasthenic syndrome. Hum. Mol. Genet. **5:** 1217–1227.
39. MILONE, M., H-L. WANG, K. OHNO *et al.* 1997. Slow-channel syndrome caused by enhanced activation, desensitization, and agonist binding affinity due to mutation in the M2 domain of the acetylcholine receptor alpha subunit. J. Neurosci. **17:** 5651–5665.
40. ZHOU, M., A.G. ENGEL & A. AUERBACH. 1999. Serum choline activates mutant acetylcholine receptors that cause slow channel congenital myasthenic syndrome. Proc. Natl. Acad. Sci. USA **96:** 10466–10471.
41. ENGEL, A.G., E.H. LAMBERT, D.M. MULDER *et al.* 1982. A newly recognized congenital myasthenic syndrome attributed to a prolonged open time of the acetylcholine-induced ion channel. Ann. Neurol. **11:** 553–569.
42. SINE, S.M., K. OHNO, C. BOUZAT *et al.* 1995. Mutation of the acetylcholine receptor α subunit causes a slow-channel myasthenic syndrome by enhancing agonist binding affinity. Neuron **15:** 229–239.
43. WANG, H-L., A. AUERBACH, N. BREN *et al.* 1997. Mutation in the M1 domain of the acetylcholine receptor alpha subunit decreases the rate of agonist dissociation. J. Gen. Physiol. **109:** 757–766.
44. GOMEZ, C.M., R. MASELLI, J. GAMMACK *et al.* 1996. A beta-subunit mutation in the acetylcholine receptor gate causes severe slow-channel syndrome. Ann. Neurol. **39:** 712–723.
45. CROXEN, R., C. NEWLAND, D. BEESON *et al.* 1997. Mutations in different functional domains of the human muscle acetylcholine receptor α subunit in patients with the slow-channel congenital myasthenic syndrome. Hum. Mol. Genet. **6:** 767–774.
46. OHNO, K., M. MILONE, J.M. BRENGMAN *et al.* 1998. Slow-channel congenital myasthenic syndrome caused by a novel mutation in the acetylcholine receptor ε subunit [abstract]. Neurology **50:** A432.
47. OHNO, K., H-L. WANG, X-M. SHEN *et al.* 2000. Slow-channel mutations in the center of the M1 transmembrane domain of the acetylcholine receptor α subunit [abstract]. Neurology **54**(suppl. 3): A183.
48. GOMEZ, C.M., R. MASELLI, J. STAUB *et al.* 1998. Novel δ and β subunit acetylcholine receptor mutations in the slow-channel syndrome demonstrate phenotypic variability [abstract]. Soc. Neurosci. Abstr. **24:** 484.
49. GOMEZ, C.M., R. MASELLI, B.P.S. VOHRA *et al.* 2002. Novel delta subunit mutation in slow-channel syndrome causes severe weakness by novel mechanism. Ann. Neurol. **51:** 102–112.
50. CROXEN, R., C. HATTON, C. SHELLEY *et al.* 2002. Recessive inheritance and variable penetrance of slow-channel congenital myasthenic syndromes. Neurology **59:** 162–168.
51. GROSMAN, C., F.N. SALAMONE, S.M. SINE & A. AUERBACH. 2000. The extracellular linker of muscle acetylcholine receptor channels is a gating control element. J. Gen. Physiol. **116:** 327–339.
52. SIEB, J.P., M. MILONE & A.G. ENGEL. 1996. Effects of the quinoline derivatives quinine, quinidine, and chloroquine on neuromuscular transmission. Brain. Res. **712:** 179–189.
53. FUKUDOME, T., K. OHNO, J.M. BRENGMAN & A.G. ENGEL. 1998. Quinidine normalizes the open duration of slow-channel mutants of the acetylcholine receptor. Neuroreport **9:** 1907–1911.

54. HARPER, C.M. & A.G. ENGEL. 1998. Quinidine sulfate therapy for the slow-channel congenital myasthenic syndrome. Ann. Neurol. **43:** 480–484.
55. HARPER, C.M., A.G. ENGEL, T. FUKUDOME *et al.* 2003. Treatment of slow channel congenital myasthenic syndrome with fluoxetine. Neurology **60:** 1710–1713.
56. WANG, H-L., M. MILONE, K. OHNO *et al.* 1999. Acetylcholine receptor M3 domain: stereochemical and volume contributions to channel gating. Nat. Neurosci. **2:** 226–233.
57. MILONE, M., H-L. WANG, K. OHNO *et al.* 1998. Mode switching kinetics produced by a naturally occurring mutation in the cytoplasmic loop of the human acetylcholine receptor ε subunit. Neuron **20:** 575–588.
58. WANG, H-L., K. OHNO, M. MILONE *et al.* 2000. Fundamental gating mechanism of nicotinic receptor channel revealed by mutation causing a congenital myasthenic syndrome. J. Gen. Physiol. **116:** 449–460.
59. OHNO, K., H-L. WANG, M. MILONE *et al.* 1996. Congenital myasthenic syndrome caused by decreased agonist binding affinity due to a mutation in the acetylcholine receptor ε subunit. Neuron **17:** 157–170.
60. SHEN, X-M., K. OHNO, M. MILONE *et al.* 2001. Fast-channel syndrome [abstract]. Neurology **56**(suppl. 3)**:** A60.
61. SHEN, X-M., A. TSUJINO, K. OHNO *et al.* 2000. A novel fast-channel congenital myasthenic syndrome caused by a mutation in the Cys-loop domain of the acetylcholine receptor ε subunit [abstract]. Neurology **54**(suppl. 3)**:** A138.
62. BROWNLOW, S., R. WEBSTER, R. CROXEN *et al.* 2001. Acetylcholine receptor δ subunit mutations underlie a fast-channel myasthenic syndrome and arthrogryposis multiplex congenita. J. Clin. Invest. **108:** 125–130.
63. SHEN, X-M., K. OHNO, T. FUKUDOME *et al.* 1999. Deletion of a single codon from the long cytoplasmic loop of the nAChR subunit gene causes brief single channel currents [abstract]. Soc. Neurosci. Abstr. **25:** 1721.
64. SINE, S.M., H-L. WANG, K. OHNO *et al.* 2003. Mechanistic diversity underlying fast channel congenital myasthenic syndromes. This volume.
65. MILONE, M., K. OHNO, J.N. PRUITT *et al.* 1996. Congenital myasthenic syndrome due to frameshifting acetylcholine receptor epsilon subunit mutation. Soc. Neurosci. Abstr. **22:** 1942–1942.
66. CROXEN, R., C. YOUNG, C. SLATER *et al.* 2001. Endplate γ and ε subunit mRNA levels in AChR deficiency syndrome due to ε subunit null mutations. Brain **124:** 1362–1372.
67. OHNO, K., B. ANLAR & A.G. ENGEL. 1999. Congenital myasthenic syndrome caused by a mutation in the Ets-binding site of the promoter region of the acetylcholine receptor ε subunit gene. Neuromuscul. Disord. **9:** 131–135.
68. NICHOLS, P.R., R. CROXEN, A. VINCENT *et al.* 1999. Mutation of the acetylcholine receptor ε-subunit promoter in congenital myasthenic syndrome. Ann. Neurol. **45:** 439–443.
69. ABICHT, A., R. STUCKA, C. SCHMIDT *et al.* 2002. A newly identified chromosomal microdeletion and an N-box mutation of the AChRε gene cause a congenital myasthenic syndrome. Brain **125:** 1005–1013.
70. QUIRAM, P., K. OHNO, M. MILONE *et al.* 1999. Mutation causing congenital myasthenia reveals acetylcholine receptor β/δ subunit interaction essential for assembly. J. Clin. Invest. **104:** 1403–1410.
71. CROXEN, R., C. NEWLAND, M. BETTY *et al.* 1999. Novel functional ε-subunit polypeptide generated by a single nucleotide deletion in acetylcholine receptor deficiency congenital myasthenic syndrome. Ann. Neurol. **46:** 639–647.
72. ABICHT, A., R. STUCKA, V. KARCAGI *et al.* 1999. A common mutation (ε1267delG) in congenital myasthenic patients of Gipsy ethnic origin. Neurology **53:** 1564–1569.
73. HARPER, C.M. & A.G. ENGEL. 2000. Treatment of 31 congenital myasthenic syndrome patients with 3,4-diaminopyridine [abstract]. Neurology **54**(suppl. 3)**:** A395.
74. GAUTAM, M., P.G. NOAKES, L. MOSCOSO *et al.* 1996. Defective neuromuscular synaptogenesis in agrin-deficient mutant mice. Cell **85:** 525–535.
75. MITTAUD, P., A. MARANGI, S. ERB-VÖGTLI & C. FUHRER. 2001. Agrin-induced activation of acetylcholine receptor–bound Src family kinases requires rapsyn and correlates with acetylcholine receptor clustering. J. Biol. Chem. **276:** 14505–14513.

76. GLASS, D.J., D.C. BOWEN, T.N. STITT *et al.* 1996. Agrin acts via MuSK receptor complex. Cell **85:** 513–523.
77. GAUTAM, M., P.G. NOAKES, J. MUDD *et al.* 1995. Failure of postsynaptic specialization to develop at neuromuscular junctions of rapsyn-deficient mice. Nature **377:** 232–236.
78. APEL, E.D., D.J. GLASS, L.M. MOSCOSCO *et al.* 1997. Rapsyn is required for MuSK signaling and recruits synaptic components to a MuSK-containing scaffold. Neuron **18:** 623–625.
79. RAMARAO, M.K. & J.B. COHEN. 1998. Mechanism of nicotinic acetylcholine receptor cluster formation by rapsyn. Proc. Natl. Acad. Sci. USA **95:** 4007–4012.
80. SANDROCK, A.W., S.E. DRYER, K.M. ROSEN *et al.* 1997. Maintenance of acetylcholine receptor number by neuregulins at the neuromuscular junction *in vivo*. Science **276:** 599–603.
81. SI, J., Z. LUO & L. MEI. 1996. Induction of acetylcholine receptor gene expression by ARIA requires activation of mitogen-activated protein kinase. J. Biol. Chem. **271:** 19752–19759.
82. ALTIOK, N., K. ALTIOK & J-P. CHANGEUX. 1997. Heregulin-stimulated acetylcholine receptor gene expression in muscle—requirement for MAP kinase and evidence for parallel inhibitory pathway independent electrical activity. EMBO J. **16:** 717–725.
83. NEWEY, S.A., A.O. GRAMOLINI, J. WU, *et al.* 2001. A novel mechanism for modulating synaptic gene expression: differential localization of α-dystrobrevin transcripts in skeletal muscle. Mol. Cell. Neurosci. **17:** 127–140.
84. GRADY, R.M., J.P. MERLIE & J.R. SANES. 1997. Subtle neuromuscular defects in utrophin-deficient mice. J. Cell Biol. **136:** 871–882.
85. ADAMS, M.E., M. KRAMARCY, S.P. KRALL *et al.* 2000. Absence of α-syntrophin leads to structurally aberrant neuromuscular synapses deficient in utrophin. J. Cell Biol. **150:** 1385–1398.
86. RAMARAO, M.K., M.J. BIANCHETTA, J. LANKEN & J.B. COHEN. 2001. Role of rapsyn tetratrichopeptide repeat and coiled-coil domains in self-association and nicotinic acetylcholine receptor clustering. J. Biol. Chem. **276:** 7475–7483.
87. BARTOLI, M. & J.B. COHEN. 2001. Identification of the modular domains of rapsyn binding to nicotinic acetylcholine receptor (AChR) and to dystroglycan [abstract]. Soc. Neurosci. Abstr. **27:** 904.16.
88. BARTOLI, M., M.K. RAMARAO & J.B. COHEN. 2001. Interactions of the rapsyn RING-H2 domain with dystroglycan. J. Biol. Chem. **276:** 24911–24917.
89. TSENG, C.N., Y. YAO, J.M. WANG *et al.* 2001. A synaptic isoform of NRAP interacts with the postsynaptic 43K protein rapsyn and links it to the cytoskeleton at the neuromuscular junction. Soc. Neurosci. Abstr. **27:** 694.6.
90. MASELLI, R., M. CHEN, T-Y. CHEN *et al.* 2002. A heteroallelic nonsense/missense mutation in the acetylcholine receptor α-subunit causing severe endplate AChR deficiency [abstract]. Neurology **58**(suppl. 3)**:** A230.
91. MILONE, M., X-M. SHEN, K. OHNO *et al.* 1999. Unusual congenital myasthenic syndrome with endplate AChR deficiency caused by alpha subunit mutations and a remitting-relapsing course [abstract]. Neurology **52**(suppl. 2)**:** 185–186.
92. OHNO, K., X-M. SHEN, T. FUKUDOME *et al.* 2001. First report of acetylcholine receptor δ subunit mutation causing endplate AChR deficiency [abstract]. Neurology **56**(suppl. 3)**:** 232–233.
93. ABICHT, A., R. STUCKA, I-H. SONG *et al.* 2000. Genetic analysis of the entire AChR ε-subunit gene in 52 congenital myasthenic families. Acta Myol. **19:** 23–27.
94. OHNO, K., A.G. ENGEL, M. MILONE *et al.* 1995. A congenital myasthenic syndrome with severe acetylcholine receptor deficiency caused by heteroallelic frameshifting mutations in the epsilon subunit [abstract]. Neurology **45**(suppl. 4)**:** A283.
95. CROXEN, R., J. NEWSOM-DAVIS & D. BEESON. 2000. Endplate acetylcholine receptor deficiency syndrome: two new mutations. Acta Myol. **19:** 45–48.
96. BRENGMAN, J.M., K. OHNO, M. MILONE *et al.* 2000. Identification and functional characterization of eight novel acetylcholine receptor mutations in six congenital myasthenic syndrome kinships [abstract]. Neurology **54**(suppl. 3)**:** A182–A183.

97. MASELLI, R.A., M. CHEN, T-Y. CHEN *et al.* 2002. Severe low-affinity fast-channel syndrome due to a heteroallelic nonsense/missense mutation in the acetylcholine receptor ε-subunit [abstract]. Neurology **58**(suppl. 3)**:** A228.
98. SIEB, J.P., S. KRANER, M. RAUCH & O.K. STEINLEIN. 2000. Immature end-plates and utrophin deficiency in congenital myasthenic syndrome caused by epsilon-AChR subunit truncating mutations. Hum. Genet. **107:** 160–464.
99. OHNO, K., T. FUKUDOME, S. NAKANO *et al.* 1996. Mutational analysis in a congenital myasthenic syndrome reveals a novel acetylcholine receptor epsilon subunit mutation. Soc. Neurosci. Abstr. **22:** 234–234.
100. BRENGMAN, J.M., K. OHNO, X-M. SHEN & A.G. ENGEL. 1998. Congenital myasthenic syndrome due to two novel mutations in the acetylcholine receptor ε subunit gene [abstract]. Muscle Nerve **21**(suppl. 7)**:** S120.
101. HERCEGFALVI, A., A. ABICHT, V. KARCAGI & H. LOCHMÜLLER. 2000. Case report: congenital myasthenic syndrome in a Gipsy family showing pseudodominant pattern of inheritance. Acta Myol. **19:** 49–51.
102. SIEB, J.P., S. KRANER, B. SCHRANK *et al.* 2000. Severe congenital myasthenic syndrome due to homozygosity of the 1293insG epsilon-acetylcholine receptor subunit mutation. Ann. Neurol. **48:** 379–383.
103. DEYMEER, F., P. SERDAROGLU, Y. GÜLSEN-PARMAN *et al.* 2000. Clinical characteristics of a group of Turkish patients having a benign CMS phenotype with ptosis and marked ophthalmoparesis and mutations in the acetylcholine receptor epsilon subunit gene. Acta Myol. **19:** 29–32.
104. OHNO, K., A. TSUJINO, B. ANLAR & A.G. ENGEL. 2001. A 16-bp duplication of splice-acceptor site results in silencing of the downstream copy of the splice acceptor site: how are duplicated splice-acceptor sites selected in pre-mRNA splicing? Am. J. Hum. Genet. (Suppl.) **69:** 368 [abstract].
105. TSUJINO, A., C. MAERTENS, K. OHNO *et al.* 2003. Myasthenic syndrome caused by mutation of the *SCN4A* sodium channel. Proc. Natl. Acad. Sci. USA **100:** 7377–7382.

Autoimmune Diseases as the Loss of Active "Self-Control"

JEAN-FRANÇOIS BACH

Hôpital Necker, INSERM U580, 75015 Paris, France

ABSTRACT: Converging experimental evidence indicates that the clinical expression of autoimmunity is under the control of T cell–mediated immunoregulatory circuits. Several types of suppressor T cells have been described. Some of them are closely dependent upon cytokines such as TH2 cells and Tr1 cells. Others appear to rely more on cell-cell contact (such as CD25+ CD62L+ T cells), although some cytokines, notably TGF-β, may be involved in their growth or their mode of action. It is tempting to separate suppressor cells that appear spontaneously, such as CD25+ T cells and NKT cells (innate immunoregulation), from those that are only observed after antigen administration, such as TH2 cells and Tr1 cells (adaptive immunoregulation). The role of these diverse cell types in the control of the onset or the progression of autoimmune diseases is likely, but still a matter of debate. A central question is to determine whether immune dysregulation precedes the burst of pathogenic autoimmunity.

KEYWORDS: immunoregulation; CD25+ T cells; NKT cells; autoimmune diseases

INTRODUCTION

Autoimmune diseases (AIDs) result from the breakdown of self-tolerance that protects healthy individuals from the potential harmful effects of autoreactive B and T cells. Such autoreactive cells are found in any normal subject. In fact, a large spectrum of autoreactive cells escapes the deletion that takes place in the thymus and, to a lesser extent, in the periphery. These autoreactive B and T cells usually have low avidity receptors for autoantigens, but this avidity may increase during antigen-driven differentiation of the effector cells. This has been known for many years for autoreactive B cells. It has recently been well documented for CD8 T cells in the nonobese diabetic (NOD) mouse.[1] It is remarkable, though, that in the absence of T cell activation, autoreactive T cells do not aggress their target cell or organ. This apparent paradox, named "ignorance" by Zinkernagel, is illustrated by the fact that double transgenic mice that express large amounts of a lymphochoriomeningitis virus (LCMV) glycoprotein in the β cells of the islets of Langerhans, and also express an LCMV glycoprotein-specific T cell receptor, do not develop diabetes. Diabetes appears, however, when the mice are infected by LCMV, which activates glycoprotein-specific T cells.[2] The question, then, is to determine which are the factors that activate

Address for correspondence: Prof. Jean-François Bach, Hôpital Necker, INSERM U580, 161, rue de Sèvres, 75015 Paris, France. Voice: +331-44-49-53-71; fax: +331-43-06-23-88. bach@necker.fr

Ann. N.Y. Acad. Sci. 998: 161–177 (2003). © 2003 New York Academy of Sciences.
doi: 10.1196/annals.1254.017

the T cells at the origin of autoimmune diseases, either as effector cells or as CD4+ helper cells, as well as the mechanisms by which T cell tolerance is bypassed (antigen mimicry, local inflammation, superantigens).

Another major question is to determine what the regulatory mechanisms are that control the intensity and duration of the pathogenic autoimmune process. This central question is directly related to the difficult and controversial notion of suppressor T cells commonly assumed to play the major role in this regulation. The aim of this short review is to discuss the evidence supporting the role of immunoregulation in the control of AIDs and its molecular basis. The potential usage of suppressor cells as new targets for immunointervention will also be discussed.

ROLE OF T CELL–MEDIATED IMMUNOREGULATION IN THE CONTROL OF AIDs

Experimental data involving both spontaneous and experimentally induced AIDs provide evidence for the role of regulatory T cells in the prevention or control of the progression of AIDs.

Induction of Autoimmune Diseases by Thymectomy

Neonatal thymectomy (Tx) prevents the onset of most experimentally induced AIDs as it prevents other T cell–dependent immune responses. Tx must be performed in the mouse within 24 h after birth to prevent T cell differentiation, even if it may still affect some T cell functions when performed at a later age.

Tx at 3–5 days of age in nonautoimmune-prone strains such as BALB/c mice induces a polyautoimmune syndrome including gastritis, thyroiditis, and oophoritis.[3] The effect of thymectomy is corrected by the administration of CD4 T cells or, even better, of the minor subset of CD4+ CD25+ T cells.[4] It is likely that diabetes and thyroiditis, which appear in adult thymectomized rats subjected to sublethal irradiation,[5] have a similar mechanism. As in the mouse day-3 Tx model, the onset of AIDs is prevented by administration of CD4+ T cells. Note that Tx accelerates diabetes onset in NOD mice, but that, at variance with the day-3 Tx model, the acceleration is still observed when Tx is performed at 3 weeks of age.[6] Collectively, these converging Tx experiments may be interpreted as triggering the onset of AIDs resulting from the depletion of selected regulatory T cell subsets that physiologically mature and leave the thymus at a later age than that at which Tx was performed. Alternatively, these T cells might be short-lived and thus rapidly disappear after Tx. It should be noted that there is no suggestion whatsoever of any evidence in these experiments of patent immunosuppression that could notably favor the development of a viral infection that, by itself, could trigger autoimmunity.

Other Models of T Cell Depletion

Depletion of selected T cell subsets has been shown to induce AIDs in other models. Thus, restoration of nude or SCID mice by CD4+ CD25– T cells that are depleted of CD25+ T cells induces a polyautoimmune syndrome similar to that just described for day-3 Tx.[4] Restoration of SCID mice with CD4+ T cells depleted of CD45 RB^{low} T cells gives rise to colitis.[7] Administration of cyclophosphamide or low-dose irradiation accelerates diabetes onset in BB rats or NOD mice.[8] In all these models, AIDs are prevented by administration of total T cells or the relevant T cell subset, arguing in the case of cyclophosphamide treatment or sublethal irradiation against a toxic effect on the target cell.

AIDs Induced by Invalidation of Genes Implicated in T Cell Function

NOD mice genetically deficient in CD28[9] or B7.1[10] develop fulminant diabetes, which is prevented by administration of wild-type CD4+ CD25+ T cells whose number is decreased in $B7.1^{-/-}$ mice.[10] MRL/l/l lupus-prone mice lacking γ/δ T cells after disruption of the Cg gene show accelerated and exacerbated lupus.[11] $Rag^{-/-}$ and SCID NOD mice transgenically expressing a T cell receptor (TCR) derived from a diabetogenic T cell clone present fulminant diabetes onset, whereas nondeficient transgenic mice show delayed appearance of the disease.[12] Similarly, transgenic mice expressing a TCR specific for myelin basic protein only show spontaneous experimental allergic encephalomyelitis (EAE) in the absence of T cells capable of generating endogenous rearrangements, as is the case after backcrossing the $C\alpha^{-/-}$ or $Rag^{-/-}$ gene in transgenic mice.[13]

Disruption of the IL-2 receptor α gene (CD25)[14] or of the IL-2 gene[15] induces the appearance of colitis and lymphoproliferation. Similarly, $IL\text{-}10^{-/-}$ mice develop severe colitis.[16] Interestingly, $IL\text{-}4^{-/-}$ mice do not develop colitis nor autoimmune disease.[17] Note lastly that $CTLA\text{-}4^{-/-}$ mice develop major lymphoproliferation and die at an early age before any putative development of autoimmune disease.[18]

Autoimmune Disease Protection Can Be Transferred in Vivo

Protection from diabetes in NOD mice by CD4+ T cells has been demonstrated in cotransfer experiments in which T cells from prediabetic mice were coadministered in irradiated or SCID syngeneic mice with diabetogenic T cells derived from a diabetic mouse.[19] Protector cells were found in the thymus and the spleen as early as 4 weeks of age. They were also found in transgenic NOD mice expressing non-NOD MHC class II that do not develop diabetes,[20] as well as in diabetic NOD mice treated with CD3 antibody (L. Chatenoud, submitted).

Similar protection has been observed in a variety of experimentally induced AIDs, including EAE, experimental allergic thyroiditis (EAT), and experimental allergic myasthenia gravis (EAMG). More limited data are available with T cell clones.

Resistance to Disease Transfer or Induction

T cell–mediated AIDs can be transferred by T cells derived from animals with established disease in syngeneic nonaffected animals. It has been observed in NOD mice that such transfer could only be obtained if the recipient does not harbor immunocompetent T cells. The transfer is obtained in neonate recipients (less than

3 weeks of age),[21] irradiated or SCID recipients, but not in normal adult mice.[22] The role of CD4+ T cells in this resistance is indicated by the sensitivity to diabetes transfer induced in adult NOD mice by adult Tx followed by treatment with a depleting anti-CD4 antibody.[23] In the case of experimentally induced AIDs, once the acute disease is cured, the animal presents a refractory state (the disease is not reinduced by antigen administration with the same protocol as that used for initial disease induction). This refractoriness can be transferred by T cells from the refractory animals to naïve animals. Low doses of cyclophosphamide administered at 2 days before the encephalitogenic challenge abrogate the unresponsiveness of disease-resistant strains and reverse the refractory state in unsensitive strains.[24]

Multiplicity of Autoimmune Manifestations in AIDs

In the hypothesis of a purely autoantigen-driven mechanism for AIDs, one would expect that the autoimmune manifestations exclusively involve the initial target organ (whether or not one postulates the existence of a secondary antigen spreading). This is not the case in many animal or human AIDs. Insulin-dependent diabetes mellitus is frequently associated with extrapancreatic autoimmune manifestations.[22] In the mouse, NOD mice concomitantly present IDDM, thyroiditis, sialitis, autoimmune hemolytic anemia, and antinuclear antibodies. These observations suggest the concept of an underlying nonantigen-specific common defect.

Interestingly, NOD mice develop chronic EAT.[25] The common defect in question is not necessarily related to immunoregulation, but it is fair to believe that immunoregulation is the most plausible mechanism.

Interpretation

Taken together, these experiments bring strong support in favor of a role for a control of autoimmunity by regulatory T cells. It should be realized, however, that all the evidence presented may be differently interpreted and that one should wait for direct results using cell clones or characterized genes or molecules. The emergence of AIDs could relate in some cases to insufficient T cell homeostasis[26a,26b] or promotion of viral infections known to trigger a variety of AIDs. The reality of CD4+ T cell–mediated immunoregulation is clearly apparent, but the autonomy (the specialization) of regulatory cells and, even more, their precise phenotype(s) and mode of action are still ill defined. Additionally, although emphasis is presently put on CD4+ T cells, there is still room for other regulatory cells, including CD8+ T cells or NK cells.

THE NATURE OF REGULATORY T CELLS AND THEIR MODE OF ACTION

A number of regulatory T cell subsets have been described over the last three decades. Not much is left of the CD8+ Ig-restricted T cells described in the 1970s. Although a very significant number of experiments performed at that time was probably correct, errors in interpretation discredited the field for many years. Now that the notion of immunoregulation-suppression T cells is back, it would certainly be interesting to have a new look at these initial experiments. It was the introduction of the THl/TH2 paradigm by Mosmann and Coffman[27] that put regulatory cells back on the map. This is why I will first discuss TH1 and TH2 cells. I shall then mention the other regulatory T cells recently described, with particular emphasis on the CD4+ CD25+ cells already mentioned in the day-3 Tx model.

TH1/TH2 Cells

Interferon γ (IFNγ) downregulates TH2 cells, and IL-10 downregulates TH1 cells. More generally, there is a reciprocal counterregulation of TH1 and TH2 cells. Logically, major efforts have been dedicated to identify a regulatory control of immune disorders by TH1 or TH2 cells depending on the cytokine dependency of each disease. Effector mechanisms of AIDs are, for the most part, dependent on TH1 cytokines, with the possible exception of some cases of systemic lupus erythematosus and of drug-induced autoimmunity. I shall thus concentrate here on the TH2 cell–mediated regulation of TH1 AIDs.

Interestingly enough, disruption of TH2 cytokine genes does not induce autoimmunity.[16,17] IL-10$^{-/-}$ mice do develop colitis,[16] but this is not strictly speaking an AID.[28] IL-4$^{-/-}$[29] and IL-10$^{-/-}$[30,31] NOD mice show normal incidence of diabetes, and similar observations have been made for lupus mice[32] for IL-4.[33] This is not, however, a definitive argument against the role of TH2 cells because IFNγ$^{-/-}$ NOD mice also show normal onset of diabetes,[31] whereas diabetes onset is prevented by anti-IFNγ mAb treatment,[34] indicating the possibility of cytokine gene redundancy. The data just discussed are not necessarily contradictory to the observation that STAT6$^{-/-}$ NOD mice, which are not able to transduce IL-4 and IL-10 signals, show accelerated diabetes.[35] Wild NOD mice showed a low incidence of diabetes in these experiments, suggesting their contamination by some infectious agents that might stimulate TH2 cells.

Systemic administration of the TH2 cytokines inhibits AIDs progression as is well demonstrated in NOD mice for IL-4, IL-10, and IL-13, in EAMG for IL-4 and IL-10, and in collagen-induced arthritis (CIA) for IL-4 and IL-10 (TABLE 1). The cases of EAE and lupus are more complex.

TABLE 1. IL-4, IL-10, and IL-13 in experimental AIDs

	NOD	EAE	EAMG	CIA
Systemic administration				
IL-4	Protection[96,97]	Protection[98]		Protection[99–101]
IL-10	Protection[102,103]	Protection[104–106] No effect or worsening[107]	Worsening[108]	Protection[109–111]
IL-13	Protection[112]	Protection[113]		Protection[101,114]
Gene disruption				
IL-4$^{-/-}$	No effect[29]	No effect[43,44] Worsening[40]	No effect[42] Worsening[39]	Worsening[41]
IL-10$^{-/-}$	No effect[30,31]	Worsening[45,115]	Protection[116]	Worsening[117]

In fact, the most convincing data derive from autoantigen-induced disease prevention experiments. The administration of various β cell autoantigens [e.g., insulin, glutamic acid decarboxylase (GAD), or heat shock protein 60 (hsp60)] induces tolerance to β cells and diabetes prevention through involvement of TH2 cells.[36] The protection is no longer observed in IL-4$^{-/-}$ NOD mice[37] and is associated with a TH2 polarization of autoimmune response.[36] Similar data have been observed in experimentally induced diseases for soluble antigens, peptides, or altered peptide ligands (APL), the action of which is blocked by anti-IL-4 mAb.[38] Interestingly, IL-4$^{-/-}$ mice show enhanced induction of EAMG,[39] EAE,[40] and CIA,[41] but these results have not always been confirmed either for EAMG[42] or EAE.[43,44] It should also be noted that IL-10$^{-/-}$ mice show exacerbated EAE.[45]

As a whole, these data would suggest that TH2 cytokines are not involved in the physiological control of autoimmunity, and thus the onset of spontaneous disease does not represent the breakdown of the control afforded by TH2 cells. In contrast, one may assume that they play a major role after triggering by exogenously introduced antigen, as in the case of tolerance induced by soluble autoantigens and that of experimental AIDs induced by autoantigens incorporated in adjuvant.

A crucial question is to determine the differences between autoantigen presentation leading to the differentiation of effector TH1 cells and regulatory TH2 cells. What are the conditions leading to TH2 cell triggering after administration of soluble autoantigens that are not found in the natural conditions where essentially non-TH2 cells are involved? A number of studies have addressed the experimental conditions leading preferentially to TH1 or TH2 stimulation. TCR low affinity for antigens has been reported to favor TH2 polarization.[46]

CD25+ T Cells (T Regs)

When Nishizuka reported in 1969 that day-3 thymectomy in BALB/c mice induced ovaritis,[3] the observation did not appear as very striking in the midst of all the reports converging in the same direction. The model was a matter of renewed interest when Sakaguchi showed, in collaboration with Nishizuka, that the thymectomy-induced autoimmune syndrome could be prevented by administration of CD25+ CD4+ T cells.[4] It was later shown by the same group,[47] and confirmed by Shevach,[48] that CD25+ T cells that are "anergic" inhibit the proliferation of CD3 antibody-stimulated CD25– T cells *in vitro*. Importantly, it was shown that the inhibition required cell-cell contact between CD25+ and CD25– T cells and that CD25+ T cells could be derived from IL-4$^{-/-}$ or IL-10$^{-/-}$ BALB/c mice.[49] It was thus apparent that CD25+ T cells did not use TH2 cytokines. The involvement of transforming growth factor β (TGF-β) was suggested by Strober in the coculture model just described.[50] The inhibition of CD25+ T cell suppressor activity by anti-TGF-β antibody and the observation of membrane expression of TGF-β on CD25+ T cells were very suggestive of a role of TGF-β in the mode of action of CD25+ T cells. The data merit validation because they have not always been confirmed. We ourselves have recently shown that diabetes protection in the cotransfer model described above is afforded, for the most part, by CD25+ T cells and is abrogated by TGF-β antibodies in a model where anti-IL-4 and anti-IL-10 antibodies are not inhibitory (L. Chatenoud, submitted).

It is tempting to attribute to the CD25+ T cells the CD4+ T cells afforded protection in the rat thymectomy-irradiation model described by Mason[5] because such cells are CD25+ T cells (at least in the thymus),[51] are depleted by thymectomy, and depend on TGF-β.[52] An important difference, however, is the blockade of their suppressor function by anti-IL-4 antibody.[52]

In fact, the phenotype of regulatory T cells is still uncertain. CD25 is an important, but not an absolute, marker. Regulatory function is still found in CD25− T cells, at least in the spleen, at a level disproportionate to the level of contamination by CD25+ T cells[51] (L. Chatenoud, submitted). Additionally, there are no data relating CD25 to the suppressor function except perhaps through the unlikely mechanism of IL-2 absorption (CD122 is expressed at a low level in regulatory CD25+ T cells).

Another interesting marker is CD62L (L-selectin), which was found to be present in regulatory T cells.[53,54] It is as yet difficult to determine to what extent this marker overlaps with CD25. We have found regulatory CD62L+ CD25− T cells, but probably only a minority of CD62L+ T cells, which represent a large proportion of CD4+ T cells, have a regulatory function. One may hope that new markers will be derived from the systematic study of the gene transcripts selectively expressed by regulatory T cells. Two studies have recently been published using this approach.[55,56] It is interesting that a glucocorticoid-induced TNF receptor (GITR), a member of the TNF receptor superfamily, was found in the two studies (whereas other identified molecules differed). It is also interesting that an antiserum selectively developed against CD25+ T cells recognized GITR.[57a] More recently, it has been reported that Foxp3, a transcription factor whose gene is mutated in a severe polyautoimmune disease named IPEX,[57b] is selectively expressed in CD25+ regulatory T cells.[57c]

The antigen specificity of T regs is also a matter of debate. Pioneering experiments by McCullagh and Mason that show organ-specific deletion of T regs after thyroid ablation or destruction in sheep and in the rat argue in favor of such specificity,[58,59] as well as Taguchi's experiments[60,61] that indicate a gender-dependent level of regulatory CD25+ T cells controlling prostatitis or oophoritis following day-3 Tx. Protective cells were found at a higher number in mice presenting the target organ than in mice not carrying this organ, either due to gender difference or to castration.

Another question is that of the molecular mode of action of T regs. TGF-β represents a strong candidate, but further experiments are needed to confirm its involvement. CTLA-4 had been proposed on the basis of the induction of gastritis in normal BALB/c mice following administration of an anti-CTLA-4 antibody and blockade of CD25+ T cell–mediated diabetes protection in NOD mice by anti-CTLA-4 antibody (L. Chatenoud, submitted). Additionally, CTLA-4 is overexpressed in T regs. The interpretation of these data is complex. One cannot exclude that the anti-CTLA-4 antibody acts by stimulating effector T cells through an agonistic effect.

IL-10-Dependent Non-TH2 Regulatory T Cells

Two sets of data have implicated non-TH2 IL-10-dependent regulatory T cells. It was first shown by Mason and Powrie in the rat,[62] and ultimately by Powrie in the mouse,[7] that immunoincompetent rats or mice restored with CD45 RB^{high} CD4 T cells developed colitis. The onset of the disease was blocked by anti-IL-10 and anti-TGF-β antibodies.[63,64]

On the other hand, antigen-specific T cells grown in the presence of IL-10 present regulatory properties that use IL-10, which are blocked by anti-IL-10 antibodies. The suppressor effect can be demonstrated *in vitro* (in coculture experiments) and *in vivo.*[65] When SCID mice are concomitantly intraperitoneally reconstituted with CD45 RB^{high} T cells and an ovalbumin-specific IL-10-dependent T cell clone, oral administration of ovalbumin prevents the onset of colitis. These regulatory T cells have been named Tr1.

It is not yet clear whether CD45 RB^{low} and Tr1 cells represent the same cell lineage. The fact that both of them use IL-10 and TGF-β, but not IL-4, is in favor of their identity. There is no evidence, however, that these cells are implicated in the control of autoreactivity. Depletion of $CD45RB^{low}$ cells does not give rise to major gastritis, as does depletion of CD25+ T cells.

NKT Cells

NKT cells represent a discrete T cell subset sharing a number of properties with NK cells.[66] They have a unique TCR, with a constant usage of the Vα14Jα18 chain and a less restricted usage of the Vβ chain. Ligands are glycolipids, the recognition of which is MHC class I–restricted or, more precisely, CD1d-restricted. Several experimental pieces of evidence indicate that NKT cells regulate immune responses. Transgenic mice overexpressing Vα14Jα18 that have a high number of functional NKT cells show high IgE levels.[67] Conversely, $\beta 2m^{-/-}$ mice that lack NKT cells do not produce normal levels of IgE in response to polyclonal B cell activation by anti-IgD antibodies.[68] However, TH2 cell differentiation still takes place in $\beta 2m^{-/-}$ or $CD1d^{-/-}$ mice.[69] The implication of NKT cells in the physiological control of autoimmunity is indicated by the acceleration of diabetes observed in $CD1d^{-/-}$[70,71] NOD mice, as well as by the prevention of diabetes in Vα14Jα18 NOD transgenic mice.[72] NKT cell number and function are deficient in young NOD mice,[73,74] and treatment of young NOD mice with a galactosyl ceramide, an NKT cell ligand derived from a sea sponge, prevents the onset of diabetes.[75,76] Similarly, data have been collected in other models of AIDs. SJL mice, which are prone to develop severe and relapsing EAE, are NKT cell–deficient like NOD mice.[68] EAE is enhanced after treatment with an antibody directed against NK1.1 (an NK and NKT cell marker).[77,78] Autoimmune uveitis onset is controlled by NKT cells in an IL-10-dependent fashion.[79] Thus, NKT cells might contribute to the T cell–mediated control of autoimmunity. They might act directly through production of IL-4 or IL-10 (pure NKT cell populations derived from Vα14Jα18 transgenic NOD mice confer diabetes protection).[72] They might also promote the differentiation or the survival of other regulatory subsets, including TH2 cells or T regs.

Other Types of Immunoregulatory Cells

Immunoregulatory cells might not be limited to the cell types mentioned above. There are experimental data suggesting a role for several other types of T cells and non-T cells.

γ/δ T Cells

$C\gamma^{-/-}$ MRL/l/l mice show accelerated lupus onset. Insulin, administered as nasal aerosol, protects from diabetes. The protection is mediated by CD8+ γ/δ+ T cells.[80]

CD8 T Cells

Independent of the initial and probably spurious reports on the role of CD8 T cells in the regulation of immune responses, CD8 T cells might indeed contribute to immunoregulation. Treatment of nonautoimune mice by a depleting CD8 antibody enhances EAE,[81] and $CD8^{-/-}$ mice show exacerbated disease.[82] CD8 T cell clones specific for CD4 T cell idiotypes have been suggested as being involved in this regulation.[81]

NK Cells

Independent of NKT cells discussed above, NK cells have been reported to down-regulate some autoimmune responses. This has notably been well documented in the case of experimental cardiomyositis.[83]

B Cells

Antibodies may have an immunoregulatory role through a number of mechanisms, some of which may involve autoimmune responses, notably anti-idiotypic antibodies.

Nonspecific Immunosuppressors

Last, one should mention soluble immunosuppressors, molecules that appear in certain conditions such as pregnancy (α fetoprotein).[84] It is difficult to assess the reality of the regulatory role of these molecules *in vivo* and even more so in AIDs. One may also mention the modulation of AIDs observed after acute or chronic stress and in sex hormone–treated animals and humans.

Interpretation

The description of more than 10 categories of regulatory cells is troublesome. Are some of these cell types connected or affiliated? Do at least some of them represent different states of activation of the same cell lineage? Are different cells involved in different immune or autoimmune responses? What is the antigen specificity of the triggering and the effector phases?

TABLE 2. Classification of regulatory cells

Innate[a]/Natural	Adaptive
CD25+ T cells	TH2 cells
NKT cells	TH3 cells
NK cells	Tr1 cells
γ/δ+ T cells (?)	$CD45RB^{low}$ cells (?)
	CD8 T cells

[a]Innate refers to the spontaneous appearance of regulatory cells, independent of TCR usage.

Phenotypic studies are extremely valuable. CD25 or CD62L have proven to be very useful in separating regulatory from effector cells. These markers, however, still do not have absolute value. As mentioned above, T regs are found among peripheral CD25– T cells. One should not repeat the error of the 1970s when suppressor cells were assigned to a single phenotype (CD8+ Ig+), which happened to be wrong. It is more than likely that different regulatory cells operate in different experimental settings. This is well illustrated by the different pattern of AIDs observed when restoring immunoincompetent mice with CD25– or CD45 RB^{high} CD4+ T cells (gastritis[4] and colitis,[7] respectively).

At the risk of oversimplification, a dichotomy may be proposed between natural and adaptive immune regulation (TABLE 2). In the first category, one would place NKT cells, NK cells, and also T regs because T reg depletion, as induced by day-3 thymectomy, gives rise to AIDs. In contrast, adaptive immunoregulation would involve TH2 cells and Tr1 cells, which share the property of being generated following antigen sensitization.

Another important issue is that of the molecular basis of effector mechanisms. Again, one is tempted to separate regulatory cells depending on IL-4 (TH2 or NKT cells), IL-10 (Tr1 or TH2 cells), or TGF-β (T regs and Tr1). Other molecules such as GITR or CTLA-4 could be involved. It will be very important to determine whether the distinction made between cytokine-mediated and cell-cell contact mechanisms holds true.

IS THERE AN INTRINSIC DEFECT OF IMMUNOREGULATION IN AUTOIMMUNE-PRONE INDIVIDUALS?

Data discussed above bring strong support to the capacity of various T cell subsets to downregulate the development of spontaneous or experimentally induced AIDs. It is not clear, however, whether there is, in some AIDs, an intrinsic deficiency of regulatory cells that confers susceptibility of developing intensive and chronic autoimmune responses, or whether the autoantigen-driven differentiation of effector cells overrides regulatory cells that are not intrinsically abnormal. One may tentatively propose that these two mechanisms exist, both submitted to a genetic control. There are situations where an intrinsic defect of immunoregulation can be invoked. This is the case in the NOD mouse where the multiplicity of autoimmune manifestations and the observation of an early loss of *in vitro* regulation of suppressor function (L. Chatenoud, submitted) and of NKT cell number and function[73,74] have been noted. In humans, one may also suspect that some of the genetically controlled polyautoimmune diseases, such as autoimmune poly-endocrinopathy candidiasis–ectodermal dystrophy (APECED),[85] or autoimmune enteropathy with diabetes and thyroiditis (IPEX),[86] are directly related to an intrinsic defect in immunoregulation. This hypothesis has recently been confirmed for IPEX, in which the implicated gene codes for the transcription factor Foxp3 selectively expressed in CD25+ regulatory T cells.[57b,57c]

On the other hand, one may assume that AIDs triggered by autoantigen mimicry, as in the case of rheumatic fever, leads to the overriding of regulation by the burst of antigen-driven effector cells, although one cannot exclude the fact that rheumatic fever preferentially develops in subjects with deficient immunoregulation.

ENVIRONMENTAL PROMOTION OF IMMUNOREGULATORY CELLS BY INFECTIONS

Discordance in AID onset in monozygotic twins is explained by different exposure to the environment. Does the environment act by triggering the disease in the affected twin or by preventing it in the unaffected one? A large body of evidence supports the latter hypothesis.

Infections have been shown to inhibit the development of AIDs in a wide spectrum of experimental models.[87a] Thus, mycobacteria can prevent the onset of diabetes in NOD mice or of EAE in nonautoimmune-prone mice. Similarly, LCMV or lactodehydrogenase virus (LDV) prevents the onset of diabetes in NOD mice, and LDV prevents the onset of lupus in MRL/l/l mice. The protective role of infections is also indicated by the higher rate of diabetes observed in germ-free NOD mice, and in humans by the increase in disease rate in subjects migrating from countries of low incidence to those of high incidence.[87b] The mechanisms of the protection are still ill defined and probably multifactorial.

Several experimental data suggest that they might involve regulatory T cells. Thus, in mycobacteria-induced diabetes protection in NOD mice, the protection can be transferred to naïve mice by CD4+ T cells.[88] The nature of the regulatory cells implicated is not clear. Since the protection has been reported to be abrogated by anti-IL-4 and anti-IL-10 antibodies,[89] it was initially thought that TH2 cells were implicated. However, protection is still observed in IL-$4^{-/-}$ or IL-$10^{-/-}$ mice.[31] The role of T regs, NKT cells, and Toll-like receptor-mediated regulation is under investigation. The infection-mediated protection represents an interesting example of bystander suppression, where the suppressive phenomena exert their effect towards immune (or autoimmune) responses directed against antigens other than the initial triggering antigen(s).[90]

THERAPEUTIC PERSPECTIVES

Today, the treatment of AIDs essentially relies on nonantigen–specific immunosuppression, with all its associated potential hazards (infections and tumors). An attractive alternative strategy consists of inducing immunoregulation, at best in an antigen-specific fashion. Without discussing the details of the several approaches that have been considered, it is worth mentioning that various products have been shown to trigger the different categories of regulatory T cells mentioned above.

Soluble autoantigens have been shown to stimulate TH2 cells and prevent diabetes in NOD mice[36] and EAE.[91] Several clinical trials are in progress, with the native protein, a constitutive peptide, or an APL. Interestingly, because of the phenomenon of bystander suppression, one does not have to determine the nature of the primary target autoantigen.

T regs have been shown to be selectively triggered by nonactivating CD3 antibodies. Administration of a nonmitogenic anti-CD3 antibody to NOD mice with recently diagnosed diabetes induces remission of the disease.[92] The protection can be transferred to non-anti-CD3-treated animals by CD25+, CD62L+, CD4+ T cells and is dependent on TGF-β and CTLA-4 (L. Chatenoud, submitted). Two clinical trials are also in progress. One of these has already confirmed in humans the effects observed in NOD mice.[93]

NKT cells can be triggered by one of their selective ligands, a galactosyl ceramide (αGalCer). Administration of αGalCer to NOD mice protects them from diabetes.[75,76] One may also mention the possibility of substituting vaccinotherapy for the immunostimulation formerly brought by infections. This has been achieved by using bacterial extract as demonstrated in the NOD mouse (unpublished data). The proof of concept of this strategy has been obtained in human atopy. Administration of lactobacilli[94] or mycobacterial extracts[95] to newborns at risk of developing atopic dermatitis, or those having started the disease, shows a clear therapeutic effect.

CONCLUSIONS

The concept of immunoregulation has been a matter of considerable renewed interest during the last decade. Major questions are still unresolved and direct proof of the implication of regulatory T cells is often lacking. Nevertheless, even if much more remains to be learned about the phenotype and the mode of action of regulatory cells, there is presently little doubt that autoimmune responses and the potential pathological consequences of AIDs are submitted to immunoregulation in which T cells play a pivotal role. The concept is important at the basic level for the understanding of the immune system. It may also prove to be a unique source of new therapeutic approaches.

REFERENCES

1. Amrani, A., J. Verdaguer, P. Serra *et al.* 2000. Progression of autoimmune diabetes driven by avidity maturation of a T-cell population. Nature **406:** 739–742.
2. Ohashi, P.S., S. Oehen, K. Buerki *et al.* 1991. Ablation of "tolerance" and induction of diabetes by virus infection in viral antigen transgenic mice. Cell **65:** 305–317.
3. Nishizuka, Y. & T. Sakakura. 1969. Thymus and reproduction: sex-linked dysgenesia of the gonad after neonatal thymectomy in mice. Science **166:** 753–755.
4. Asano, M., M. Toda, N. Sakaguchi *et al.* 1996. Autoimmune disease as a consequence of developmental abnormality of a T cell subpopulation. J. Exp. Med. **184:** 387–396.
5. Fowell, D. & D. Mason. 1993. Evidence that the T cell repertoire of normal rats contains cells with the potential to cause diabetes: characterization of the CD4+ T cell subset that inhibits this autoimmune potential. J. Exp. Med. **177:** 627–636.
6. Dardenne, M., F. Lepault, A. Bendelac *et al.* 1989. Acceleration of the onset of diabetes in NOD mice by thymectomy at weaning. Eur. J. Immunol. **19:** 889–895.
7. Powrie, F., M.W. Leach, S. Mauze *et al.* 1993. Phenotypically distinct subsets of CD4+ T cells induce or protect from chronic intestinal inflammation in C.B-17 scid mice. Int. Immunol. **5:** 1461–1471.
8. Yasunami, R. & J.F. Bach. 1988. Anti-suppressor effect of cyclophosphamide on the development of spontaneous diabetes in NOD mice. Eur. J. Immunol. **18:** 481–484.
9. Lenschow, D.J., K.C. Herold, L. Rhee *et al.* 1996. CD28/B7 regulation of Th1 and Th2 subsets in the development of autoimmune diabetes. Immunity **5:** 285–293.
10. Salomon, B., D.J. Lenschow, L. Rhee *et al.* 2000. B7/CD28 costimulation is essential for the homeostasis of the CD4+CD25+ immunoregulatory T cells that control autoimmune diabetes. Immunity **12:** 431–440.
11. Peng, S.L. & J. Craft. 1996. T cells in murine lupus: propagation and regulation of disease. Mol. Biol. Rep. **23:** 247–251.
12. Katz, J.D., B. Wang, K. Haskins *et al.* 1993. Following a diabetogenic T cell from genesis through pathogenesis. Cell **74:** 1089–1100.

13. Lafaille, J.J., K. Nagashima, M. Katsuki *et al.* 1994. High incidence of spontaneous autoimmune encephalomyelitis in immunodeficient anti-myelin basic protein T cell receptor transgenic mice. Cell **78:** 399–408.
14. Almeida, A.R., N. Legrand, M. Papiernik *et al.* 2002. Homeostasis of peripheral CD4+ T cells: IL-2R alpha and IL-2 shape a population of regulatory cells that controls CD4+ T cell numbers. J. Immunol. **169:** 4850–4860.
15. Sadlack, B., H. Merz, H. Schorle *et al.* 1993. Ulcerative colitis-like disease in mice with a disrupted interleukin-2 gene. Cell **75:** 253–261.
16. Madsen, K.L. 2001. Inflammatory bowel disease: lessons from the IL-10 gene-deficient mouse. Clin. Invest. Med. **24:** 250–257.
17. Kuhn, R., K. Rajewsky & W. Muller. 1991. Generation and analysis of interleukin-4 deficient mice. Science **254:** 707–710.
18. Waterhouse, P., J.M. Penninger, E. Timms *et al.* 1995. Lymphoproliferative disorders with early lethality in mice deficient in Ctla-4. Science **270:** 985–988.
19. Boitard, C., R. Yasunami, M. Dardenne *et al.* 1989. T cell–mediated inhibition of the transfer of autoimmune diabetes in NOD mice. J. Exp. Med. **169:** 1669–1680.
20. Singer, S.M., R. Tisch, X.D. Yang *et al.* 1993. An Abd transgene prevents diabetes in nonobese diabetic mice by inducing regulatory T cells. Proc. Natl. Acad. Sci. USA **90:** 9566–9570.
21. Bendelac, A., C. Carnaud, C. Boitard *et al.* 1987. Syngeneic transfer of autoimmune diabetes from diabetic NOD mice to healthy neonates: requirement for both L3T4+ and Lyt-2+ T cells. J. Exp. Med. **166:** 823–832.
22. Bach, J.F. 1994. Insulin-dependent diabetes mellitus as an autoimmune disease. Endocr. Rev. **15:** 516–542.
23. Sempe, P., M.F. Richard, J.F. Bach *et al.* 1994. Evidence of CD4+ regulatory T cells in the non-obese diabetic male mouse. Diabetologia **37:** 337–343.
24. Lando, Z., D. Teitelbaum & R. Arnon. 1979. Effect of cyclophosphamide on suppressor cell activity in mice unresponsive to EAE. J. Immunol. **123:** 2156–2160.
25. Damotte, D., E. Colomb, C. Cailleau *et al.* 1997. Analysis of susceptibility of NOD mice to spontaneous and experimentally induced thyroiditis. Eur. J. Immunol. **27:** 2854–2862.
26. (a) Theofilopoulos, A.N., W. Dummer & D.H. Kono. 2001. T cell homeostasis and systemic autoimmunity. J. Clin. Invest. **108:** 335–340; (b) Barthlott, T., G. Kassiotis & B. Stockinger. 2003. T cell regulation as a side effect of homeostasis and competition. J. Exp. Med. **197:** 451–460.
27. Mosmann, T.R., H. Cherwinski, M.W. Bond *et al.* 1986. Two types of murine helper T cell clone. I. Definition according to profiles of lymphokine activities and secreted proteins. J. Immunol. **136:** 2348–2357.
28. Hibi, T., H. Ogata & A. Sakuraba. 2002. Animal models of inflammatory bowel disease. J. Gastroenterol. **37:** 409–417.
29. Wang, B., A. Gonzalez, P. Hoglund *et al.* 1998. Interleukin-4 deficiency does not exacerbate disease in NOD mice. Diabetes **47:** 1207–1211.
30. Balasa, B., K. Van Gunst, N. Jung *et al.* 2000. IL-10 deficiency does not inhibit insulitis and accelerates cyclophosphamide-induced diabetes in the nonobese diabetic mouse. Cell. Immunol. **202:** 97–102.
31. Serreze, D.V., H.D. Chapman, C.M. Post *et al.* 2001. Th1 to Th2 cytokine shifts in nonobese diabetic mice: sometimes an outcome, rather than the cause, of diabetes resistance elicited by immunostimulation. J. Immunol. **166:** 1352–1359.
32. Kono, D.H., D. Balomenos, M.S. Park *et al.* 2000. Development of lupus in BXSB mice is independent of IL-4. J. Immunol. **164:** 38–42.
33. Peng, S.L., J. Moslehi & J. Craft. 1997. Roles of interferon-gamma and interleukin-4 in murine lupus. J. Clin. Invest. **99:** 1936–1946.
34. Debray-Sachs, M., C. Carnaud, C. Boitard *et al.* 1991. Prevention of diabetes in NOD mice treated with antibody to murine IFN gamma. J. Autoimmun. **4:** 237–248.
35. Chatenoud, L., B. Salomon & J.A. Bluestone. 2001. Suppressor T cells—they're back and critical for regulation of autoimmunity! Immunol. Rev. **182:** 149–163.
36. Bach, J.F. & L. Chatenoud. 2001. Tolerance to islet autoantigens and type I diabetes. Annu. Rev. Immunol. **19:** 131–161.

37. Tisch, R., B. Wang & D.V. Serreze. 1999. Induction of glutamic acid decarboxylase 65-specific Th2 cells and suppression of autoimmune diabetes at late stages of disease is epitope dependent. J. Immunol. **163:** 1178–1187.
38. Brocke, S., K. Gijbels *et al.* 1996. Treatment of experimental encephalomyelitis with a peptide analogue of myelin basic protein. Nature **379:** 343–346.
39. Karachunski, P.I., N.S. Ostlie, D.K. Okita *et al.* 1999. Interleukin-4 deficiency facilitates development of experimental myasthenia gravis and precludes its prevention by nasal administration of CD4+ epitope sequences of the acetylcholine receptor. J. Neuroimmunol. **95:** 73–84.
40. Falcone, M., A.J. Rajan, B.R. Bloom *et al.* 1998. A critical role for IL-4 in regulating disease severity in experimental allergic encephalomyelitis as demonstrated in IL-4-deficient C57BL/6 mice and BALB/c mice. J. Immunol. **160:** 4822–4830.
41. Myers, L.K., B. Tang, J.M. Stuart *et al.* 2002. The role of IL-4 in regulation of murine collagen-induced arthritis. Clin. Immunol. **102:** 185–191.
42. Balasa, B., C. Deng, J. Lee *et al.* 1998. The Th2 cytokine IL-4 is not required for the progression of antibody-dependent autoimmune myasthenia gravis. J. Immunol. **161:** 2856–2862.
43. Liblau, R., L. Steinman & S. Brocke. 1997. Experimental autoimmune encephalomyelitis in IL-4-deficient mice. Int. Immunol. **9:** 799–803.
44. Zhao, M.L. & R.B. Fritz. 1998. Acute and relapsing experimental autoimmune encephalomyelitis in IL-4- and alpha/beta T cell–deficient C57BL/6 mice. J. Neuroimmunol. **87:** 171–178.
45. Bettelli, E., M.P. Das, E.D. Howard *et al.* 1998. IL-10 is critical in the regulation of autoimmune encephalomyelitis as demonstrated by studies of IL-10- and IL-4-deficient and transgenic mice. J. Immunol. **161:** 3299–3306.
46. Constant, S.L. & K. Bottomly. 1997. Induction of Thl and Th2 CD4+ T cell responses: the alternative approaches. Annu. Rev. Immunol. **15:** 297–322.
47. Takahashi, T., Y. Kuniyasu, M. Toda *et al.* 1998. Immunologic self-tolerance maintained by CD25+CD4+ naturally anergic and suppressive T cells: induction of autoimmune disease by breaking their anergic/suppressive state. Int. Immunol. **10:** 1969–1980.
48. Thornton, A.M. & E.M. Shevach. 2000. Suppressor effector function of CD4+CD25+ immunoregulatory T cells is antigen nonspecific. J. Immunol. **164:** 183–190.
49. Shevach, E.M. 2000. Regulatory T cells in autoimmmunity. Annu. Rev. Immunol. **18:** 423–449.
50. Nakamura, K., A. Kitani & W. Strober. 2001. Cell contact–dependent immunosuppression by CD4(+)CD25(+) regulatory T cells is mediated by cell surface–bound transforming growth factor beta. J. Exp. Med. **194:** 629–644.
51. Stephens, L.A. & D. Mason. 2000. CD25 is a marker for CD4+ thymocytes that prevent autoimmune diabetes in rats, but peripheral T cells with this function are found in both CD25+ and CD25– subpopulations. J. Immunol. **165:** 3105–3110.
52. Seddon, B. & D. Mason. 1999. Regulatory T cells in the control of autoimmunity: the essential role of transforming growth factor beta and interleukin 4 in the prevention of autoimmune thyroiditis in rats by peripheral CD4(+)CD45RC– cells and CD4(+)CD8(–) thymocytes. J. Exp. Med. **189:** 279–288.
53. Herbelin, A., J.M. Gombert, F. Lepault *et al.* 1998. Mature mainstream TCR alpha beta(+)CD4(+) thymocytes expressing L-selectin mediate "active tolerance" in the nonobese diabetic mouse. J. Immunol. **161:** 2620–2628.
54. Lepault, F. & M.C. Gagnerault. 2000. Characterization of peripheral regulatory CD4(+) T cells that prevent diabetes onset in nonobese diabetic mice. J. Immunol. **164:** 240–247.
55. Zelenika, D., E. Adams, S. Humm *et al.* 2002. Regulatory T cells overexpress a subset of Th2 gene transcripts. J. Immunol. **168:** 1069–1079.
56. McHugh, R.S., M.J. Whitters, C.A. Piccirillo *et al.* 2002. CD4(+)CD25(+) immunoregulatory T cells: gene expression analysis reveals a functional role for the glucocorticoid-induced TNF receptor. Immunity **16:** 311–323.
57. (a) Shimizu, J., S. Yamazaki, T. Takahashi *et al.* 2002. Stimulation of CD25(+) CD4(+) regulatory T cells through GITR breaks immunological self-tolerance. Nat.

Immunol. **3:** 135–142; (b) BENNETT, C.L., J. CHRISTIE, F. RAMSDELL *et al.* 2001. The immune dysregulation, polyendocrinopathy, enteropathy, X-linked syndrome (IPEX) is caused by mutations of FOXP3. Nat. Genet. **27:** 20–21; (c) HORI, S., T. NOMURA & S. SAKAGUCHI. 2003. Control of regulatory T cell development by the transcription factor Foxp3. Science **299:** 1057–1061.
58. MCCULLAGH, P. 1996. The significance of immune suppression in normal self tolerance. Immunol. Rev. **149:** 127–153.
59. SEDDON, B. & D. MASON. 1999. Peripheral autoantigen induces regulatory T cells that prevent autoimmunity. J. Exp. Med. **189:** 877–882.
60. TAGUCHI, O., A. KOJIMA & Y. NISHIZUKA. 1985. Experimental autoimmune prostatitis after neonatal thymectomy in the mouse. Clin. Exp. Immunol. **60:** 123–129.
61. TAGUCHI, O. & Y. NISHIZUKA. 1980. Autoimmune oophoritis in thymectomized mice: T cell requirement in adoptive cell transfer. Clin. Exp. Immunol. **42:** 324–331.
62. POWRIE, F. & D. MASON. 1990. OX-22^{high} CD4+ T cells induce wasting disease with multiple organ pathology: prevention by the OX-22^{low} subset. J. Exp. Med. **172:** 1701–1708.
63. ASSEMAN, C., S. MAUZE, M.W. LEACH *et al.* 1999. An essential role for interleukin 10 in the function of regulatory T cells that inhibit intestinal inflammation. J. Exp. Med. **190:** 995–1004.
64. POWRIE, F., J. CARLINO, M.W. LEACH *et al.* 1996. A critical role for transforming growth factor-beta but not interleukin 4 in the suppression of T helper type 1–mediated colitis by CD45RB(low) CD4+ T cells. J. Exp. Med. **183:** 2669–2674.
65. GROUX, H., A. O'GARRA, M. BIGLER *et al.* 1997. A CD4+ T-cell subset inhibits antigen-specific T-cell responses and prevents colitis. Nature **389:** 737–742.
66. BENDELAC, A., M.N. RIVERA, S.H. PARK *et al.* 1997. Mouse CD1-specific NK1 T cells: development, specificity, and function. Annu. Rev. Immunol. **15:** 535–562.
67. BENDELAC, A., R.D. HUNZIKER & O. LANTZ. 1996. Increased interleukin 4 and immunoglobulin E production in transgenic mice overexpressing NK1 T cells. J. Exp. Med. **184:** 1285–1293.
68. YOSHIMOTO, T., A. BENDELAC, J. HU-LI *et al.* 1995. Defective IgE production by SJL mice is linked to the absence of CD4+, NK1.1+ T cells that promptly produce interleukin 4. Proc. Natl. Acad. Sci. USA **92:** 11931–11934.
69. MORRIS, S.C., R.L. COFFMAN & F.D. FINKELMAN. 1998. *In vivo* IL-4 responses to anti-IgD antibody are MHC class II dependent and beta2-microglobulin independent and develop normally in the absence of IL-4 priming of T cells. J. Immunol. **160:** 3299–3304.
70. WANG, B., Y.B. GENG & C.R. WANG. 2001. CD1-restricted NK T cells protect nonobese diabetic mice from developing diabetes. J. Exp. Med. **194:** 313–320.
71. SHI, F.D., M. FLODSTROM, B. BALASA *et al.* 2001. Germ line deletion of the CD1 locus exacerbates diabetes in the NOD mouse. Proc. Natl. Acad. Sci. USA **98:** 6777–6782.
72. LEHUEN, A., O. LANTZ, L. BEAUDOIN *et al.* 1998. Overexpression of natural killer T cells protects V alpha 14–J alpha 281 transgenic nonobese diabetic mice against diabetes. J. Exp. Med. **188:** 1831–1839.
73. GOMBERT, J.M., A. HERBELIN, E. TANCREDE-BOHIN *et al.* 1996. Early quantitative and functional deficiency of NK1(+)-like thymocytes in the NOD mouse. Eur. J. Immunol. **26:** 2989–2998.
74. CARNAUD, C., J.M. GOMBERT, O. DONNARS *et al.* 2001. Protection against diabetes and improved NW/NKT cell performance in NOD.NK1.1 mice congenic at the NK complex. J. Immunol. **166:** 2404–2411.
75. SHARIF, S., G.A. ARRAEZA, P. ZUCKER *et al.* 2001. Activation of natural killer T cells by alpha-galactosylceramide treatment prevents the onset and recurrence of autoimmune type 1 diabetes. Nat. Med. **7:** 1057–1062.
76. HONG, S., M.T. WILSON, I. SERIZAWA *et al.* 2001. The natural killer T-cell ligand alpha-galactosylceramide prevents autoimmune diabetes in non-obese diabetic mice. Nat. Med. **7:** 1052–1056.
77. ZHANG, B., T. YAMAMURA, T. KONDO *et al.* 1997. Regulation of experimental autoimmune encephalomyelitis by natural killer (NK) cells. J. Exp. Med. **186:** 1677–1687.
78. FRITZ, R.B. & M.L. ZHAO. 2001. Regulation of experimental autoimmune encephalomyelitis in the C57BL/6J mouse by NK1.1+, DX5+, alpha beta+ T cells. J. Immunol. **166:** 4209–4215.

79. SONODA, K.H., D.E. FAUNCE, M. TANIGUCHI *et al.* 2001. NK T cell–derived IL-10 is essential for the differentiation of antigen-specific T regulatory cells in systemic tolerance. J. Immunol. **166:** 42–50.
80. HARRISON, L.C., M. DEMPSEY-COLLIER, D.R. KRAMER *et al.* 1996. Aerosol insulin induces regulatory CD8 gamma delta T cells that prevent murine insulin-dependent diabetes. J. Exp. Med. **184:** 2167–2174.
81. KUMAR, V., E. COULSELL, B. OBER *et al.* 1997. Recombinant T cell receptor molecules can prevent and reverse experimental autoimmune encephalomyelitis: dose effects and involvement of both CD4 and CD8 T cells. J. Immunol. **159:** 5150–5156.
82. KOH, D.R., W.P. FUNG-LEUNG, A. HO *et al.* 1992. Less mortality but more relapses in experimental allergic encephalomyelitis in CD8–/– mice. Science **256:** 1210–1213.
83. FAIRWEATHER, D., Z. KAYA, G.R. SHELLAM *et al.* 2001. From infection to autoimmunity. J. Autoimmun. **16:** 175–186.
84. CHAKRABORTY, M. & C. MANDAL. 1993. Immuno-suppressive effect of human alpha-fetoprotein: a cross species study. Immunol. Invest. **22:** 329–339.
85. PETERSON, P., K. NAGAMINE *et al.* 1998. APECED: a monogenic autoimmune disease providing new clues to self-tolerance. Immunol. Today **19:** 384–386.
86. WILDIN, R.S., F. RAMSDELL, J. PEAKE *et al.* 2001. X-linked neonatal diabetes mellitus, enteropathy, and endocrinopathy syndrome is the human equivalent of mouse scurfy. Nat. Genet. **27:** 18–20.
87. (a) BACH, J.F. 2001. Protective role of infections and vaccinations on autoimmune diseases. J. Autoimmun. **16:** 347–353; (b) BACH, J.F. 2002. The effect of infections on susceptibility to autoimmune and allergic diseases. N. Engl. J. Med. **347:** 911–920.
88. QIN, H.Y., M.W. SADELAIN, C. HITCHON *et al.* 1993. Complete Freund's adjuvant–induced T cells prevent the development and adoptive transfer of diabetes in nonobese diabetic mice. J. Immunol. **150:** 2072–2080.
89. CALCINARO, F., G. GAMBELUNGHE & K.J. LAFFERTY. 1997. Protection from autoimmune diabetes by adjuvant therapy in the non-obese diabetic mouse: the role of interleukin-4 and interleukin-10. Immunol. Cell Biol. **75:** 467–471.
90. WEINER, H.L., A. FRIEDMAN, A. MILLER *et al.* 1994. Oral tolerance: immunologic mechanisms and treatment of animal and human organ-specific autoimmune diseases by oral administration of autoantigens. Annu. Rev. Immunol. **12:** 809–837.
91. HIGGINS, P.J. & H.L. WEINER. 1988. Suppression of experimental autoimmune encephalomyelitis by oral administration of myelin basic protein and its fragments. J. Immunol. **140:** 440–445.
92. CHATENOUD, L., E. THERVET, J. PRIMO *et al.* 1994. Anti-CD3 antibody induces long-term remission of overt autoimmunity in nonobese diabetic mice. Proc. Natl. Acad. Sci. USA **91:** 123–127.
93. HEROLD, K.C., W. HAGOPIAN, J.A. AUGER *et al.* 2002. Anti-CD3 monoclonal antibody in new-onset type 1 diabetes mellitus. N. Engl. J. Med. **346:** 1692–1698.
94. KALLIOMAKI, M., S. SALMINEN *et al.* 2001. Probiotics in primary prevention of atopic disease: a randomised placebo-controlled trial. Lancet **357:** 1076–1079.
95. ARKWRIGHT, P.D. & T.J. DAVID. 2001. Intradermal administration of a killed Mycobacterium vaccae suspension (SRL 172) is associated with improvement in atopic dermatitis in children with moderate-to-severe disease. J. Allergy Clin. Immunol. **107:** 531–534.
96. RAPOPORT, M.J., A. JARAMILLO, D. ZIPRIS *et al.* 1993. Interleukin 4 reverses T cell proliferative unresponsiveness and prevents the onset of diabetes in nonobese diabetic mice. J. Exp. Med. **178:** 87–99.
97. CAMERON, M.J., G.A. ARREAZA, P. ZUCKER *et al.* 1997. IL-4 prevents insulitis and insulin-dependent diabetes mellitus in nonobese diabetic mice by potentiation of regulatory T helper-2 cell function. J. Immunol. **159:** 4686–4692.
98. INOBE, J.I., Y. CHEN & H.L. WEINER. 1996. *In vivo* administration of IL-4 induces TGF-beta-producing cells and protects animals from experimental autoimmune encephalomyelitis. Ann. N.Y. Acad. Sci. **778:** 390–392.
99. JOOSTEN, L.A., E. LUBBERTS, M.M. HELSEN *et al.* 1999. Protection against cartilage and bone destruction by systemic interleukin-4 treatment in established murine type II collagen-induced arthritis. Arthritis Res. **1:** 81–91.

100. HORSFALL, A.C., D.M. BUTLER, L. MARINOVA *et al.* 1997. Suppression of collagen-induced arthritis by continuous administration of IL-4. J. Immunol. **159:** 5687–5696.
101. BESSIS, N., J. HONIGER, D. DAMOTTE *et al.* 1999. Encapsulation in hollow fibres of xenogeneic cells engineered to secrete IL-4 or IL-13 ameliorates murine collagen-induced arthritis (CIA). Clin. Exp. Immunol. **117:** 376–382.
102. PENNLINE, K.J., E. ROQUE-GAFFNEY & M. MONAHAN. 1994. Recombinant human IL-10 prevents the onset of diabetes in the nonobese diabetic mouse. Clin. Immunol. Immunopathol. **71:** 169–175.
103. RABINOVITCH, A., W.L. SUAREZ-PINZON, O. SORENSEN *et al.* 1995. Combined therapy with interleukin-4 and interleukin-10 inhibits autoimmune diabetes recurrence in syngeneic islet-transplanted nonobese diabetic mice: analysis of cytokine mRNA expression in the graft. Transplantation **60:** 368–374.
104. ROTT, O., B. FLEISCHER & E. CASH. 1994. Interleukin-10 prevents experimental allergic encephalomyelitis in rats. Eur. J. Immunol. **24:** 1434-1440.
105. XIAO, B.G., X.F. BAI, G.X. ZHANG *et al.* 1998. Suppression of acute and protracted-relapsing experimental allergic encephalomyelitis by nasal administration of low-dose IL-10 in rats. J. Neuroimmunol. **84:** 230–237.
106. NAGELKERKEN, L., B. BLAUW & M. TIELEMANS. 1997. IL-4 abrogates the inhibitory effect of IL-10 on the development of experimental allergic encephalomyelitis in SJL mice. Int. Immunol. **9:** 1243–1251.
107. CANNELLA, B., Y.L. GAO, C. BROSNAN *et al.* 1996. IL-10 fails to abrogate experimental autoimmune encephalomyelitis. J. Neurosci. Res. **45:** 735–746.
108. ZHANG, G.X., B.G. XIAO, L.Y. YU *et al.* 2001. Interleukin 10 aggravates experimental autoimmune myasthenia gravis through inducing Th2 and B cell responses to AChR. J. Neuroimmunol. **113:** 10–18.
109. PERSSON, S., A. MIKULOWSKA, S. NARULA *et al.* 1996. Interleukin-10 suppresses the development of collagen type II–induced arthritis and ameliorates sustained arthritis in rats. Scand. J. Immunol. **44:** 607–614.
110. TANAKA, Y., T. OTSUKA, T. HOTOKEBUCHI *et al.* 1996. Effect of IL-10 on collagen-induced arthritis in mice. Inflamm. Res. **45:** 283–288.
111. WALMSLEY, M., P.D. KATSIKIS, E. ABNEY *et al.* 1996. Interleukin-10 inhibition of the progression of established collagen-induced arthritis. Arthritis Rheum. **39:** 495–503.
112. ZACCONE, P., J. PHILLIPS, I. CONGET *et al.* 1999. Interleukin-13 prevents autoimmune diabetes in NOD mice. Diabetes **48:** 1522–1528.
113. CASH, E., A. MINTY, P. FERRARA *et al.* 1994. Macrophage-inactivating IL-13 suppresses experimental autoimmune encephalomyelitis in rats. J. Immunol. **153:** 4258–4267.
114. BESSIS, N., M.C. BOISSIER, P. FERRARA *et al.* 1996. Attenuation of collagen-induced arthritis in mice by treatment with vector cells engineered to secrete interleukin-13. Eur. J. Immunol. **26:** 2399–2403.
115. SAMOILOVA, E.B., J.L. HORTON & Y. CHEN. 1998. Acceleration of experimental autoimmune encephalomyelitis in interleukin-10-deficient mice: roles of interleukin-10 in disease progression and recovery. Cell. Immunol. **188:** 118–124.
116. POUSSIN, M.A., E. GOLUSZKO, T.K. HUGHES *et al.* 2000. Suppression of experimental autoimmune myasthenia gravis in IL-10 gene-disrupted mice is associated with reduced B cells and serum cytotoxicity on mouse cell line expressing AChR. J. Neuroimmunol. **111:** 152–160.
117. JOHANSSON, A.C., A.S. HANSSON, K.S. NANDAKUMAR *et al.* 2001. IL-10-deficient B10.Q mice develop more severe collagen-induced arthritis, but are protected from arthritis induced with anti–type II collagen antibodies. J. Immunol. **167:** 3505–3512.

Immunology of Paraneoplastic Syndromes

Overview

JEROME B. POSNER

Memorial Sloan-Kettering Cancer Center, New York, New York 10021, USA

ABSTRACT: Cancers that cause disturbances of organs or tissues remote from the site of the tumor or its metastases are called paraneoplastic syndromes. The nervous system can be affected at virtually any site, including the neuromuscular junction (e.g., Lambert-Eaton myasthenic syndrome, myasthenia gravis). Paraneoplastic syndromes affecting the central nervous system are characterized by (1) high titers of antibodies that react with both the cancer and the affected portion of the nervous system, (2) specifically reacting T cells in the blood and cerebrospinal fluid, and (3) autopsy evidence of neuronal destruction, inflammatory infiltrates, and antibody penetration. Clinically, paraneoplastic syndromes affecting the central nervous system are usually subacute in onset, rapid in evolution, and cause severe damage, but generally stabilize after several months with or without treatment. Immune suppression does not appear to be particularly effective in treating these disorders. Treatment of the underlying cancer sometimes ameliorates symptoms.

KEYWORDS: paraneoplastic; autoantibodies; cancer; autoimmunity

INTRODUCTION

Cancer can affect not only the organ in which it grows, but also organs or tissues remote from the site of the primary tumor or its metastases.[1] Because such organ or tissue dysfunction is not caused by invasion of the neoplasm (i.e., not neoplastic), but is caused by the cancer, it is generally referred to as "paraneoplastic". Paraneoplastic syndromes can affect any organ or tissue and may cause either systemic or organ-specific effects. An example of a paraneoplastic syndrome widely recognized by oncologists is the inexplicable weight loss (paraneoplastic cachexia) that occurs in some patients with small cancers despite the fact that the patient feels well and eats with a hearty appetite. Other examples include the syndrome of inappropriate ADH secretion, hypercalcemia, and a variety of skin disorders including pemphigus[2] that affect some patients with cancer.

Of interest to neurologists and neurobiologists is the fact that paraneoplastic syndromes can affect the nervous system, causing a variety of central and peripheral nervous system syndromes that often are far more devastating than the cancer that

Address for correspondence: Jerome B. Posner, M.D., Memorial Sloan-Kettering Cancer Center, 1275 York Avenue, New York, NY 10021. Voice: 212-639-7047; fax: 212-717-3551. posnerj@mskcc.org

Ann. N.Y. Acad. Sci. 998: 178–186 (2003). © 2003 New York Academy of Sciences.
doi: 10.1196/annals.1254.018

TABLE 1. Some paraneoplastic syndromes affecting the nervous system

Involved area	Examples
Cerebral hemisphere	Dementia, limbic encephalopathy
Cerebellum	Cerebellar degeneration
Cranial nerves	Carcinoma-associated retinopathy
Spinal cord	Amyotrophic lateral sclerosis
Dorsal root ganglion	Sensory neuronopathy
Peripheral nerve	Sensorimotor polyneuropathy
Neuromuscular junction	Myasthenia gravis, LEMS
Muscle	Dermatomyositis
Multiple areas	Encephalomyelitis

triggered them.[3] TABLE 1 illustrates some of the neurologic disorders that occur as paraneoplastic syndromes.

Any cancer has the potential to cause a paraneoplastic syndrome that will affect the nervous system. Certain cancers such as small-cell carcinoma of the lung are more likely to cause paraneoplastic syndromes than are others such as non-small-cell lung cancer. Furthermore, certain cancers are associated with particular paraneoplastic syndromes. For example, ovarian and breast cancer are likely to cause paraneoplastic cerebellar degeneration,[4] whereas small-cell lung cancer, although it can cause paraneoplastic cerebellar degeneration, is more likely to cause the Lambert-Eaton myasthenic syndrome (LEMS).[5] However, many cancers are associated with several different paraneoplastic syndromes that can affect the nervous system (TABLE 2).[6]

TABLE 2. Some nervous system paraneoplastic syndromes associated with thymoma

Clinical syndrome	Reference
Limbic encephalitis	23
Cortical encephalitis	24
Stiff-person syndrome	25
Myositis	26
Neuromyotonia	27, 28
"Rippling muscles"	29
Myokymia	30
Brain stem encephalitis	31
Intestinal pseudo-obstruction	32
Chorea	33
Polyneuritis	34

TABLE 3. Estimated likelihood that a neurologic disorder is a paraneoplastic syndrome

Syndrome	Percent paraneoplastic
Lambert-Eaton myasthenic syndrome	60
Subacute cerebellar degeneration	50
Subacute sensory neuronopathy	20
Opsoclonus/myoclonus (children)	<5
Opsoclonus/myoclonus	20
Sensorimotor peripheral neuropathy	<10
Dermatomyositis	10
Myasthenia gravis	10

Of particular interest to this symposium are nervous system paraneoplastic syndromes associated with thymoma. Although the relationship between thymoma and myasthenia gravis is well known, several other central and peripheral nervous system syndromes have been associated with that tumor. Thymoma is strongly associated with myasthenia gravis (about 10% of patients with myasthenia gravis will be discovered to have a thymoma and about 30% of patients with thymoma will develop myasthenia gravis). In addition, thymoma has been associated with systemic disorders such as disseminated lupus erythematosus, dermatomyositis, Graves' disease, and Sjogren's syndrome, all of which can affect the central nervous system (CNS).[6]

INCIDENCE

With the exception of myasthenia gravis, paraneoplastic syndromes of the nervous system are uncommon. Even LEMS, a disorder that second to myasthenia gravis probably represents the most common paraneoplastic syndrome, affects no more than 3% of patients with small-cell lung cancer, a cancer that in turn represents only about 20% of all lung cancers. Thus, an oncologist with a busy clinical practice may go many years without seeing or at least recognizing a patient with a paraneoplastic syndrome.

A different situation faces the clinical neurologist. Although very few people with small-cell lung cancer suffer from LEMS, most patients with LEMS suffer from small-cell lung cancer. As TABLE 3 indicates, neurologic disorders other than myasthenia and LEMS, such as paraneoplastic cerebellar degeneration, subacutely developing sensory neuropathy, or limbic encephalopathy, should lead the neurologist to suspect a paraneoplastic syndrome and initiate a search for cancer.

CLINICAL FINDINGS

Most patients with paraneoplastic syndromes affecting the nervous system develop nervous system symptoms before they are known to have cancer. The causal cancer

TABLE 4. Clinical findings suggesting a paraneoplastic syndrome

- Symptoms begin abruptly and evolve rapidly
- Symptoms often stabilize in weeks to months
- Symptoms often cause severe disability
- For CNS syndromes, a CSF pleocytosis and elevated IgG are common
- Paraneoplastic antibodies are found in serum
- Specific disorders suggest paraneoplastic syndromes (see TABLE 3)

either may be apparent on the original examination or, despite an intensive search, may not be found for several months to a couple of years after the initial search. Certain clues should lead the clinical neurologist to suspect that a patient with a neurologic disorder may be suffering from a paraneoplastic syndrome (TABLE 4), although none is unequivocal. Most patients with paraneoplastic syndromes develop symptoms rapidly over days, weeks, or months rather than years, as with most degenerative diseases of the nervous system. The nervous system disability is usually severe, in some instances causing the patient to become bedridden over a short period of time. Certain particular symptom complexes such as the LEMS and paraneoplastic cerebellar degeneration strongly suggest the presence of an underlying cancer. When the CNS is involved, the spinal fluid often contains an excess of white cells and immunoglobulins. When present, paraneoplastic antibodies (see below) are usually at a higher titer in spinal fluid than in serum. Although nervous system disability may evolve rapidly, the tumor is more likely to be small, grow slowly, and be difficult to detect.

These clues should lead the physician to search for cancer using the most sensitive technology available, including magnetic resonance imaging (MRI) and a fluorodeoxyglucose body positron emission tomography (PET) scan.[7]

PATHOGENESIS

A question that has intrigued neurologists since paraneoplastic syndromes were first described is the mechanism by which a small cancer, sequestered in an ovary (or other organs) and not detectable by most routine imaging techniques, can cause the destruction of every Purkinje cell within the cerebellum.[8] At the time of autopsy, the patient may have other evidence of CNS damage, including inflammatory infiltrates, or the CNS may appear otherwise normal. Several hypotheses have been advanced to explain this phenomenon. Although this symposium is on autoimmunity, other hypotheses have been advanced to explain the paraneoplastic syndrome (also see TABLE 5). Oppenheim, who is generally given credit for describing paraneoplastic syndromes (although what he actually described is unclear), postulated that the tumor secreted the toxin that poisoned the nervous system.[9] Denny-Brown, a towering figure in twentieth century neurology, made an important contribution to the field of paraneoplastic syndromes when, in 1948, he described what we now call subacute sensory neuronopathy associated with small-cell lung cancer. He postulated that the cancer and the dorsal root ganglion neurons (the site of pathology) competed for an

TABLE 5. The autoimmune hypothesis of paraneoplastic syndromes

- Antigens normally restricted to the nervous system (occasionally testis) are ectopically expressed in a cancer
- The immune system recognizes the antigen in the cancer as foreign
- An immune response is generated
- Tumor growth is suppressed
- Nervous system structures expressing the antigen are damaged

essential substrate that he believed was probably pantothenic acid.[10] Based on inflammatory infiltrates found in the CNS of any patient with paraneoplastic syndromes, Henson and others postulated a viral infection,[11] which was supported upon discovery that progressive multifocal leukoencephalopathy, originally classified as one of the paraneoplastic syndromes, was due to an opportunistic virus infecting the nervous system. However, Dorothy Russell pointed out that the inflammatory infiltrates could be immune in origin as well as infectious. She is probably responsible for initiating the current view that most, if not all, paraneoplastic syndromes affecting the nervous system are immune-mediated.

AUTOIMMUNE HYPOTHESIS

TABLE 5 outlines the autoimmune hypothesis as it affects paraneoplastic syndromes. Certain protein antigens are normally expressed only in the CNS or, in some instances, in the CNS and the testis (also an immune-privileged site).[12] These antigens, which are normally not expressed elsewhere in the body, are sometimes expressed in a cancer. When the antigen is expressed in a cancer, it may or may not generate an immune response. If a sufficient immune response is generated, that immune response may damage portions of the nervous system expressing the paraneoplastic antigen and may also retard the growth of the causal tumor.

Other papers in this volume present evidence for immune mediation of disorders involving the neuromuscular junction and the peripheral nervous system. In the CNS, the evidence is less clear, but several pieces of evidence suggest an immune-mediated disorder (TABLE 6). In most, but not all, of the CNS, disorders of high titer antibodies that react with both the tumor and portions of the nervous system are found in the serum.[13] Several of these antibodies have been identified and characterized and will be discussed over the course of this symposium. It is important to

TABLE 6. Evidence for autoimmunity in CNS paraneoplastic syndromes

- High titer antibodies that react only with tumor(s) and the nervous system are present
- The antibodies are synthesized within the CNS
- Antigen-specific T cells are found in blood, CSF, and brain
- Intraneuronal deposits of antibody have been described
- The tumor often grows more slowly

recognize that not all paraneoplastic syndromes with a putative immune-mediated basis have had paraneoplastic antibodies identified.[14] New ones are being identified each year.[15]

When a paraneoplastic antibody is identified in the serum of a patient with a paraneoplastic syndrome affecting the CNS, the antibody can also be found in the spinal fluid at a higher titer than that found in the serum, suggesting intrathecal synthesis of the antibody.[16] Parenthetically, the standard five plasma exchanges, although substantially decreasing the amount of antibody in the serum, have little effect on the antibody in the spinal fluid.[16] Antigen-specific T cells are found in the blood, CSF, and brain of patients with paraneoplastic syndromes affecting the nervous system. Darnell and his colleagues have identified CDR-2-specific cytotoxic T lymphocytes in the blood of all patients with paraneoplastic cerebellar degeneration having antibodies against CDR-2.[17] Voltz and colleagues identified antigen-specific T cells in the tumor and brain of patients with paraneoplastic encephalomyelitis associated with small-cell lung cancer.[18] Thus, it is likely that cytotoxic T cells play an important role in the pathogenesis of paraneoplastic syndromes affecting the CNS.

More controversial is the identification of intraneuronal deposits of antibody from the brain of patients with paraneoplastic encephalomyelitis.[19] That the antibody can enter living cells is now generally accepted for certain cells. However, the presence of antibodies within neurons of the CNS in patients with paraneoplastic disorders remains controversial. The clear identification of such antibodies would suggest that antibodies play an important role in the pathogenesis of the disorder.

Finally, there is evidence that the immune response against a paraneoplastic antigen in the tumor slows the growth of the tumor. There is now both clinical[20] and experimental[21] evidence to support this assertion. Clinical neurologists have always believed that patients with paraneoplastic syndromes had a more indolent tumor than patients with a similar cancer, but without the paraneoplastic disorder. However, because most patients with paraneoplastic syndromes develop their neurological symptomatology first, the tumor is usually identified at an earlier stage and thus might be expected to be smaller than otherwise. However, some evidence supports the better prognosis in at least some paraneoplastic syndromes. Madison and others compared the survival of patients with LEMS associated with small-cell lung cancer with those with small-cell lung cancer without LEMS. This study could not rule out the phenomenon of lead-time bias. Graus and colleagues took advantage of the fact that approximately 20% of patients with small-cell lung cancer, who do not have neurologic abnormalities, harbor in their serum low titers of the paraneoplastic anti-Hu antibody, an antibody that at high titer is associated with encephalomyelitis and sensory neuronopathy. Because these patients had the antibody, but did not have a paraneoplastic syndrome, there was no lead-time bias caused by a paraneoplastic syndrome. Patients with the anti-Hu antibody in their serum were significantly more likely to have limited, rather than extensive, small-cell lung cancer, to respond with a complete response to standard chemotherapy, and to live longer (TABLE 7). This study has been replicated at Memorial Sloan-Kettering Cancer Center (unpublished).

Not all cancers associated with paraneoplastic syndromes may be so responsive. Graus and colleagues have reported that patients with anti-Yo positive paraneoplastic cerebellar degeneration associated with ovarian cancer do not live longer than those with similar ovarian cancers, but without the paraneoplastic syndrome.[22]

TABLE 7. Clinical characteristics of 170 small-cell lung cancer patients

Clinical state (n = 170)	Anti-Hu positive (n = 27)	Anti-Hu negative (n = 143)	p value
Age (years)	60.4 ± 10.2	61.6 ± 9.6	0.572
Sex (male)	26 (96%)	128 (90%)	1.000
Performance status (ECOG = 0–2)	25 (93%)	128 (90%)	1.000
Weight ↓ <5%	20 (74%)	91 (65%)	0.361
Stage = limit	16 (59%)	54 (39%)	0.046
Complete response	15 (56%)	28 (20%)	<0.001
Survival	14.9 months	10.2 months	0.018
Survival > 36 months	26%	6%	
Anti-P53 positive	2 (7.4%)	25 (17.4%)	

NOTE: Adjusted for age, sex, and hospital. Data from ref. 20.

TREATMENT

The best treatment of a paraneoplastic syndrome is to identify the underlying tumor when it is still small and to treat it effectively. Although this does not guarantee reversal of the paraneoplastic syndrome, the disorder will usually stop progressing once effective treatment has been undertaken. In some instances, effective treatment will lead to resolution of the syndrome, as is common in LEMS. Because these disorders are immune-mediated, immune suppression of various types has been tried in many of the disorders. Immune suppression, including plasma exchange and intravenous immunoglobulin, has proved effective in the treatment of some paraneoplastic syndromes such as LEMS and, of course, myasthenia gravis. It has proved ineffective in those syndromes involving the CNS, such as paraneoplastic cerebellar degeneration and encephalomyelitis. Perhaps the early destruction of neurons in the CNS syndrome make even effective immunotherapy unlikely to reverse the clinical findings.

REFERENCES

1. POSNER, J.B. 1995. Neurologic Complications of Cancer. Davis. Philadelphia.
2. LEYN, J. & H. DEGREEF. 2001. Paraneoplastic pemphigus in a patient with a thymoma. Dermatology **202:** 151–154.
3. POSNER, J.B. & J.O. DALMAU. 2000. Paraneoplastic syndromes of the nervous system. Clin. Chem. Lab. Med. **38:** 117–122.
4. PETERSON, K., M.K. ROSENBLUM, H. KOTANIDES & J.B. POSNER. 1992. Paraneoplastic cerebellar degeneration. I. A clinical analysis of 55 anti-Yo antibody positive patients. Neurology **42:** 1931–1937.
5. MASON, W.P., F. GRAUS, B. LANG *et al.* 1997. Small-cell lung cancer, paraneoplastic cerebellar degeneration, and the Lambert-Eaton myasthenic syndrome. Brain **120:** 1279–1300.

6. LEVY, Y., A. AFEK, Y. SHERER *et al.* 1998. Malignant thymoma associated with autoimmune diseases: a retrospective study and review of the literature. Semin. Arthritis Rheum. **28:** 73–79.
7. REES, J.H., S.F. HAIN, M.R. JOHNSON *et al.* 2001. The role of [(18)F]fluoro-2-deoxy-glucose-PET scanning in the diagnosis of paraneoplastic neurological disorders. Brain **124:** 2223–2231.
8. VERSCHUUREN, J., L. CHUANG, M.K. ROSENBLUM *et al.* 1996. Inflammatory infiltrates and complete absence of Purkinje cells in anti-Yo associated paraneoplastic cerebellar degeneration. Acta Neuropathol. **91:** 519–525.
9. OPPENHEIM, H. 1888. Uber Hirnsymptome bei Carcinomatose ohne nachweisbare. Veranderungen im Gehirn. Charite-Ann. (Berlin) **13:** 335–344.
10. DENNY-BROWN, D. 1948. Primary sensory neuropathy with muscular changes associated with carcinoma. J. Neurol. Neurosurg. Psychiatry **11:** 73–87.
11. HENSON, R.A., H.L. HOFFMAN & H. URICH. 1965. Encephalomyelitis with carcinoma. Brain **88:** 449–464.
12. VOLTZ, R., S.H. GULTEKIN, M.R. ROSENFELD *et al.* 1999. A serologic marker of paraneoplastic limbic and brain-stem encephalitis in patients with testicular cancer. N. Engl. J. Med. **340:** 1788–1795.
13. GULTEKIN, S.H., M.R. ROSENFELD, R. VOLTZ *et al.* 2000. Paraneoplastic limbic encephalitis: neurological symptoms, immunological findings, and tumour association in 50 patients. Brain **123:** 1481–1494.
14. ANTUNES, N.L., Y. KHAKOO. K.K. MATTHAY *et al.* 2000. Antineuronal antibodies in patients with neuroblastoma and paraneoplastic opsoclonus-myoclonus. J. Pediatr. Hematol. Oncol. **22:** 315–320.
15. YU, Z.Y., T.J. KRYZER, G.E. GRIESMANN *et al.* 2001. CRMP-5 neuronal autoantibody: marker of lung cancer and thymoma-related autoimmunity. Ann. Neurol. **49:** 146–154.
16. FURNEAUX, H.M., L. REICH & J.B. POSNER. 1990. Autoantibody synthesis in the central nervous system of patients with paraneoplastic syndromes. Neurology **40:** 1085–1091.
17. DARNELL, R.B. & M.L. ALBERT. 2000. Cdr2-specific CTLs are detected in the blood of all patients with paraneoplastic cerebellar degeneration analyzed. Ann. Neurol. **48:** 270.
18. VOLTZ, R., J. DALMAU, J.B. POSNER & M.R. ROSENFELD. 1998. T-cell receptor analysis in anti-Hu associated paraneoplastic encephalomyelitis. Neurology **51:** 1146–1150.
19. DALMAU, J., H.M. FURNEAUX, M.K. ROSENBLUM *et al.* 1991. Detection of the anti-Hu antibody in specific regions of the nervous system and tumor from patients with paraneoplastic encephalomyelitis/sensory neuronopathy. Neurology **41:** 1757–1764.
20. GRAUS, F., J. DALMAU, R. REÑÉ *et al.* 1997. Anti-Hu antibodies in patients with small-cell lung cancer: association with complete response to therapy and improved survival. J. Clin. Oncol. **15:** 2866–2872.
21. CARPENTIER, A.F., M.R. ROSENFELD, J-Y. DELATTRE *et al.* 1998. DNA vaccination with HuD inhibits growth of a neuroblastoma in mice. Clin. Cancer Res. **4:** 2819–2824.
22. ROJAS, I., F. GRAUS, F. KEIME-GUIBERT *et al.* 2000. Long-term clinical outcome of paraneoplastic cerebellar degeneration and anti-Yo antibodies. Neurology **55:** 713–715.
23. JOHNSTON, I., D.L. GILDAY & E.B. HENDRICK. 1975. Experimental effects of steroids and steroid withdrawal on cerebrospinal fluid absorption. J. Neurosurg. **42:** 690–695.
24. RICKMAN, O.B., J.E. PARISI, Z.Y. YU *et al.* 2000. Fulminant autoimmune cortical encephalitis associated with thymoma treated with plasma exchange. Mayo Clin. Proc. **75:** 1321–1326.
25. HAGIWARA, H., S. ENOMOTO-NAKATANI, K. SAKAI *et al.* 2001. Stiff-person syndrome associated with invasive thymoma: a case report. J. Neurol. Sci. **193:** 59–62.
26. HERRMANN, D.N., M. BLAIVAS, J.J. WALD & E.E. FELDMAN. 2000. Granulomatous myositis, primary biliary cirrhosis, pancytopenia, and thymoma. Muscle Nerve **23:** 1133–1136.
27. GHEZZI, P.M., P.F. BASSO & R. MONTANINI. 1994. Association of neuromyotonia with peripheral neuropathy, myasthenia gravis, and thymoma: a case report. Ital. J. Neurol. Sci. **15:** 307–310.
28. MYGLAND, Å., A. VINCENT, J. NEWSOM-DAVIS *et al.* 2000. Autoantibodies in thymoma-associated myasthenia gravis with myositis or neuromyotonia. Arch. Neurol. **57:** 527–531.

29. Ansevin, C.F. & P. Agamanolis. 1996. Rippling muscles and myasthenia gravis with rippling muscles. Arch. Neurol. **53:** 197–199.
30. Ho, W.K.W. & J.D. Wilson. 1993. Hypothermia, hyperhidrosis, myokymia, and increased urinary excretion of catecholamines associated with a thymoma. Med. J. Aust. **158:** 787–788.
31. Kastrup, O., S. Meyring & H.C. Diener. 2001. Atypical paraneoplastic brainstem encephalitis associated with anti-Ri-antibodies due to thymic carcinoma with possible clinical response to immunoglobulins. Eur. Neurol. **45:** 285–287.
32. Kulling, D., C.E. Reed, G.N. Verne *et al.* 1997. Intestinal pseudo-obstruction as a paraneoplastic manifestation of malignant thymoma. Am. J. Gastroenterol. **92:** 1564–1566.
33. Lee, E.K., R.A. Maselli, W.G. Ellis & M.A. Agius. 1998. Morvan's fibrillary chorea: a paraneoplastic manifestation of thymoma. J. Neurol. Neurosurg. Psychiatry **65:** 857–862.
34. Ohtake, T., M. Nishimura & M. Oda. 1999. Multifocal polyradiculoneuropathy and carcinoma of the thymus. J. Neurol. Sci. **168:** 62–67.

Pathogenic Autoantibodies in the Lambert-Eaton Myasthenic Syndrome

BETHAN LANG, ASHWIN PINTO, FEDERICA GIOVANNINI, JOHN NEWSOM-DAVIS, AND ANGELA VINCENT

Neurosciences Group and Department of Clinical Neurology, Oxford University, Oxford, United Kingdom

ABSTRACT: Lambert-Eaton myasthenic syndrome (LEMS) is an autoimmune disorder of neuromuscular transmission in which antibodies are directed against voltage-gated calcium channels (VGCCs). We studied the action of LEMS immunoglobulin G (IgG) on cloned human VGCCs stably transfected into human embryonic kidney cells (HEK293). All LEMS IgGs tested bound to the surface of the P/Q-type VGCC cell line and caused a significant reduction in whole-cell calcium currents in these cells. By contrast, only 2 out of 6 IgGs bound extracellularly to the N-type VGCC cell line, and none of the LEMS IgGs tested was able to reduce whole-cell calcium currents in these cells. We used this apparent specificity of LEMS IgG for the P/Q-type VGCC to investigate the action of these IgGs on model systems where a number of different VGCC populations exist in equilibrium. LEMS IgG caused a significant down-regulation in the ω-agatoxin IVA–sensitive P/Q-type VGCCs of cultured rat cerebellar neurons, but this was accompanied by a concomitant rise in the "resistant" R-type VGCCs. By using the passive transfer model of LEMS, similar results were observed at the mouse neuromuscular junction, where a significant reduction in P/Q-type VGCCs was paralleled by an increase in L- and R-type VGCCs. These results demonstrate an unexpected plasticity in the expression of VGCCs in mammalian neurons and may represent a mechanism by which the pathogenic effects of LEMS IgG are reduced.

KEYWORDS: Lambert-Eaton myasthenic syndrome (LEMS); voltage-gated calcium channels (VGCCs); P/Q-type VGCC; passive transfer; Purkinje cell neurons

INTRODUCTION

The Lambert-Eaton myasthenic syndrome (LEMS) is an autoimmune disorder in which autoantibodies are directed against voltage-gated calcium channels (VGCCs) present on the presynaptic nerve terminal. Binding of antibodies to the VGCC results in a decrease in nerve-evoked calcium ion entry and a reduction in neurotransmitter release, leading to the characteristic muscle weakness and to the autonomic features such as dry mouth, constipation, and impotence.[1–3]

Address for correspondence: Bethan Lang, Neurosciences Group, Weatherall Institute of Molecular Medicine, John Radcliffe Hospital, Oxford OX3 9DS, United Kingdom. Voice: +044-(0)1-865-222311; fax: +044-(0)1-865-222402.
blang@hammer.imm.ox.ac.uk

Ann. N.Y. Acad. Sci. 998: 187–195 (2003). © 2003 New York Academy of Sciences.
doi: 10.1196/annals.1254.019

Small-cell lung carcinoma (SCLC), a tumor that is strongly associated with smoking, can be detected in approximately 60% of LEMS patients.[4] The SCLC is a tumor of neuroendocrine origin that shows many of the features of neurons including the expression of functional VGCCs on the cell surface.[5] It is thought that the immune response against these channels may be responsible for triggering the disease in the paraneoplastic form of LEMS. The etiology of the disease in the other 40% of patients who do not have an underlying tumor is unknown.

AUTOIMMUNE BACKGROUND

An autoimmune etiology has long been suspected in LEMS. First, there is a preponderance of females in non-SCLC LEMS patients. Second, around 25% of all LEMS patients have a past history of organ-specific autoimmune diseases such as thyroiditis, vitiligo, and celiac disease.[4,6] There is also a strong association with HLA class I marker HLA-B8.[7,8] Verschuuren *et al.* have shown that there is a significantly raised frequency (62%) of HLA-B8 in two independent cohorts of clinically defined LEMS patients compared to age- and sex-matched controls (27%). In patients with SCLC-LEMS, only 12% were HLA-B8.[9] Finally, LEMS can be successfully treated by immunomodulatory therapy, and IgG purified from patients with LEMS can passively transfer many symptoms of the disease to mice.[2,4]

VOLTAGE-GATED CALCIUM CHANNELS AS THE AUTOANTIGENIC TARGET

Antibodies purified from patients with LEMS have been shown to functionally inhibit VGCCs at the neuromuscular junction and in SCLC cell lines, with the degree of inhibition tending to correlate with disease severity.[2,10,11] In addition, abnormalities in the density and arrangement of presynaptic nerve terminal active zone particles, which are thought to be the morphological representation of VGCC, have been observed.[12]

Voltage-gated calcium channels are a family of multimeric proteins comprising α_1, β, and $\alpha_2\delta$ subunits. The classification into the different subtypes of VGCCs is partially dependent on the gene that encodes the α_1 pore-forming subunit. Neuronal VGCCs have been classified into five main subtypes (N, L, R, P, and Q).[13] The first three have been assigned to the α_{1B}, $\alpha_{1C/D}$, and α_{1E} genes, respectively; however, the P- and Q-type VGCCs appear to be splice variants of the same α_{1A} gene. The different VGCCs can also be classified according to their electrophysiological and pharmacological characteristics. The P/Q-type VGCCs were first described in the cerebellum, but now have been shown to be present both at the mammalian neuromuscular junction and on SCLC. P-type calcium channels, first described in the Purkinje cells, are highly sensitive to low concentrations of ω-agatoxin IVA (ω-AgaTx IVA), while the Q-type VGCCs, which make up the major component of the cerebellar granule cells, are less sensitive to ω-AgaTx IVA.[14] Both channels bind ω-conotoxin MVIIC (ω-CmTx MVIIC), a toxin purified from the venom of the piscivorous snail *Conus magus*. The N-type VGCCs are fast-inactivating channels that are extremely sensitive to ω-conotoxin GVIA (ω-CgTx GVIA). The L-type VGCCs can be labeled using ^{3}H-labeled derivatives of the dihydropyridines such as nifedipine or PN200. The specificity of these toxins and drugs for the different types of VGCCs has been utilized in the development of immunoprecipitation assays to detect anti-VGCC antibodies in the sera of patients with LEMS.

Antibodies that immunoprecipitate ^{125}I-CmTx MVIIC have been detected in the sera of 90% of LEMS patients. In comparison, less than 40% of patients have antibodies against N-type (^{125}I-CgTx GVIA–labeled) VGCC, and approximately 25% have antibodies to L-type (^{3}H-PN200-labeled) VGCC.[15–17] Antibodies against intracellular epitopes of the VGCCs have also been detected. Approximately a quarter of patients have antibodies against the β subunit.[18] There are four different β subunits (β_{1-4}) that may associate with any of the α_1 subunits. It is feasible that, in an immunoprecipitation assay, anti-β subunit antibodies may account for the apparent cross-reaction between the P/Q-, N-, and L-type VGCCs.

In this study, we have investigated the effect of LEMS antibodies on the function of the different subtypes of VGCC, both native and cloned, and investigated how downregulation of one channel may dynamically affect the functional expression of the other subtypes.

EFFECT OF LEMS ON CLONED VGCC

Human embryonic kidney (HEK293) cell lines were transfected with different VGCC subunits as previously described. Cell lines encoding the P/Q-type (10–13, $\alpha_{1A\text{-}2}$, β_{4a}, $\alpha_{2b}\delta$) and N-type (C2D7, $\alpha_{1B\text{-}1}$, β_{1b}, $\alpha_{2b}\delta$[boosted]) VGCCs were a gift of K. Stauderman (SIBIA Neurosciences, La Jolla, CA) and were grown as previously described.[19] We have studied the functional effect of LEMS IgGs on calcium influx into HEK293 cell lines stably transfected with different VGCC subunits by measuring K^+-stimulated changes in intracellular free calcium concentration using the Ca^{2+}-sensitive dye, fluo-3AM.[19] LEMS IgGs specifically reduced calcium influx in the cell line expressing P/Q-type VGCCs, but not in those expressing N- , L- , or R-type VGCCs.[19] However, using ^{125}I-labeled toxins, we were able to show that LEMS sera containing anti-P/Q-type and anti-N-type VGCC antibodies were able to bind to the surface of both P/Q-type and N-type VGCCs (FIG. 1). LEMS IgG was able to immunoprecipitate surface ^{125}I-CmTx MVIIC–labeled (P/Q-type) VGCC from the 10–13 cell line (FIG. 1A). In a comparable experiment (FIG. 1B), IgGs prepared from patients with positive anti-N-type VGCC antibodies were also able to bind extracellularly to surface ^{125}I-CgTx GVIA–labeled (N-type) VGCC from the C2D7 cell line.[20] It should be noted that none of the other four LEMS IgGs was able to immunoprecipitate ^{125}I-CgTx GVIA–labeled (N-type) VGCC from solubilized frontal cortex in the standard radioimmunoassay.[15]

In the present study, we have investigated further the specificity of LEMS IgGs for cloned human neuronal VGCC by measuring their effects on whole-cell calcium currents.[20] Cells were grown overnight in the presence or absence of 2 mg/mL IgG (LEMS and control) or medium alone. Incubation in LEMS IgG significantly reduced whole-cell calcium currents in the P/Q-type cell line (37.7 ± 3 pA/pF) as compared to cells incubated either in control IgGs (78.0 ± 6 pA/pF, $p < 0.0001$) or in medium alone (65.1 ± 5 pA/pF, $p < 0.0001$) (FIG. 2A). In contrast, incubation with LEMS IgGs (including a single patient with high titers of anti-N-type VGCC anti-

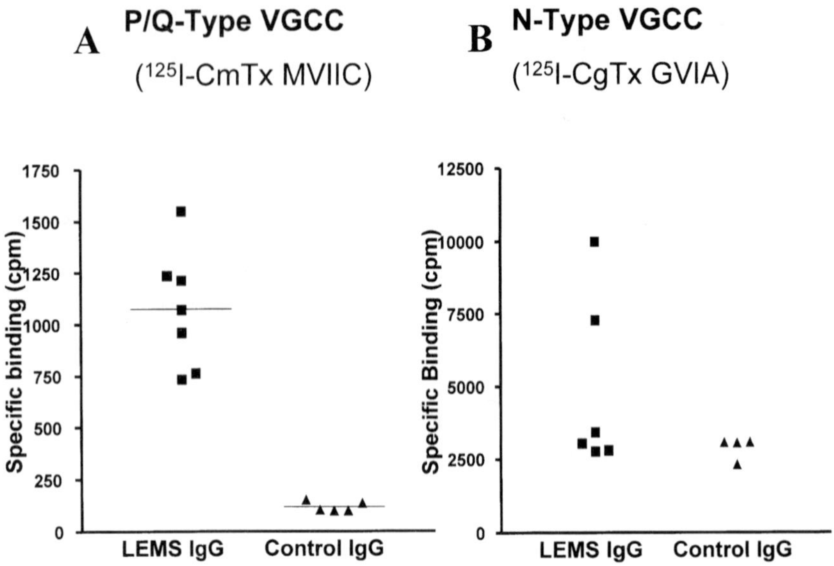

FIGURE 1. Immunoprecipitation of surface-labeled VGCCs in clonal cell lines by LEMS IgG. (**A**) Immunoprecipitation of P/Q-type VGCCs from cell line 10–13 surface-labeled with ^{125}I-CmTx MVIIC. Cells were grown at 30°C until confluent and incubated in ^{125}I-CmTx MVIIC (25–50 pM) for 1 h at 30°C. Nonspecific binding was estimated by preincubation in excess unlabeled toxin (1 µM, 30 min). LEMS (■) or control (▲) IgG (1 mg/mL) was added for an additional 2 h. After washing, the cells were extracted in digitonin (4%), and the IgG-(^{125}I-CmTx MVIIC)–labeled VGCCs were immunoprecipitated by the addition of antihuman IgG. The resulting pellet was washed and counted. Mean values for each group are shown by the horizontal bars, which are significantly different ($p < 0.0001$). **(B)** Immunoprecipitation of N-type VGCCs from cell line C2D7 surface-labeled with ^{125}I-CgTx GVIA. The experiment was carried out as above, except that the cells were grown at 37°C until confluent and that ^{125}I-CgTx GVIA (25–50 pM) was used to label the N-type VGCCs. Only two out of the six LEMS IgGs (■) showed significant binding to the N-type VGCCs as compared to controls (▲). These two patients had elevated anti-N-type VGCC antibody titers (169 and 1731 pM), while the other four LEMS patients were negative (<18 pM).

bodies) had no significant effect on whole-cell calcium currents in the N-type cell line (242 ± 17 pA/pF) as compared to cells incubated either in control IgGs (257 ± 25 pA/pF, $p = 0.60$) or in medium alone (263 ± 25 pA/pF, $p = 0.48$) (FIG. 2B).

Although these results indicate that antibodies directed against extracellular portions of the N-type VGCCs do exist in a minority of LEMS patients, it appears that they are unable to produce a pathogenic effect in the relevant cell line, as demonstrated by their lack of effect both on K^+-stimulated Ca^{2+} influx and on whole-cell calcium currents.[19,20] Using cell lines, we have shown that LEMS IgG is able to produce pathogenic effects on cell lines containing single-cloned VGCC. This model, however, is far removed from the *in vivo* situation in which several different types of VGCC coexist, presumably in dynamic equilibrium. To study this problem, we investigated two different models in which the expression of different VGCCs in the presence of LEMS IgG can be addressed.

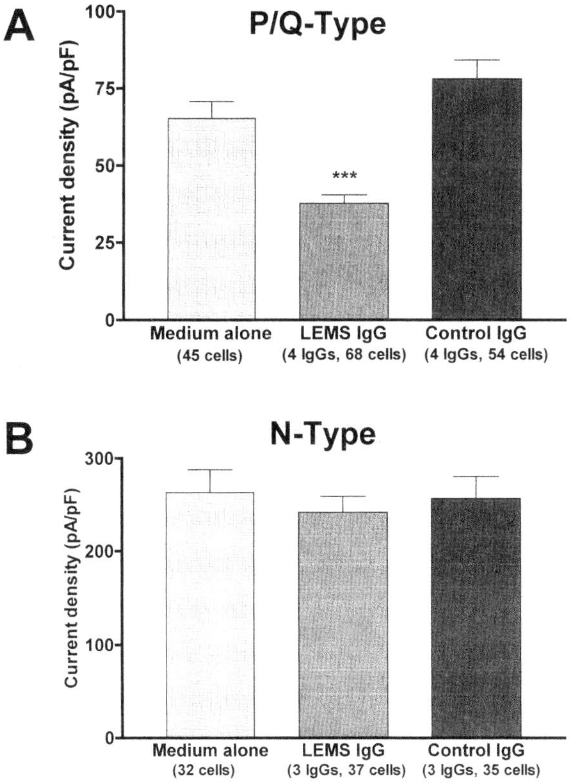

FIGURE 2. Effect of LEMS and control IgGs on whole-cell calcium currents in VGCC-transfected HEK293 cells. Results are shown for P/Q-type (10–13) and N-type (C2D7) cell lines. Cells were incubated in LEMS IgG, control IgG, or medium alone (2 mg/mL) for 18 h at either 30°C (P/Q-type cell line) or 37°C (N-type cell line), and peak current density was calculated from whole-cell calcium current recordings. **(A)** LEMS IgGs cause a significant reduction in the peak current density in the P/Q-type VGCC line as compared to cells incubated in control IgGs or medium alone ($p < 0.0001$ for both). **(B)** Treatment with LEMS IgG does not cause a significant reduction in peak current density in the N-type VGCC line compared to either cells treated with control IgGs or cells incubated in medium alone.

MODULATION OF VGCC IN PURKINJE CELL NEURONS

Cultured rat cerebellar Purkinje cells were incubated overnight in IgG (LEMS or control, 2 mg/mL) and the whole-cell current measured using standard patch-clamp techniques.[19] Incubation in IgG, prepared from two LEMS patients with high titers of anti-P/Q-type VGCC antibodies, but negative for N- and L-type VGCCs, did not significantly alter the current density as compared to that in cells incubated in healthy control IgG. However, pharmacological analysis demonstrated a large reduction in the ω-AgaTx IVA–sensitive component of the current in LEMS IgG-treated cells (11 ± 4% and 19 ± 5%) as compared to cells treated with control IgG (60 ± 6%)

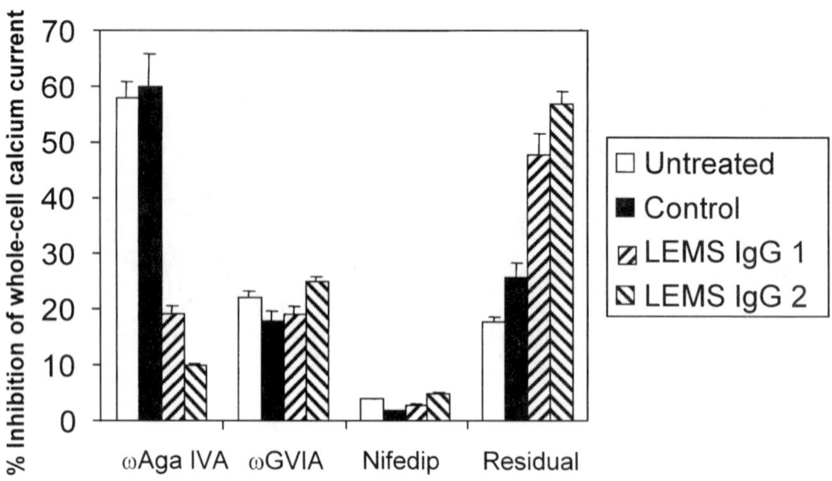

FIGURE 3. Effect of IgG (LEMS and control) on whole-cell currents in cultured rat Purkinje cells. Rat cerebellar Purkinje cells were cultured for 9–13 days *in vitro* as previously described. The cells were incubated in IgG (LEMS or control) at a concentration of 2 mg/mL for 15–22 h. The whole-cell patch-clamp technique was used to record transmembrane calcium currents in single Purkinje cells. In brief, each cell was voltage-clamped at a holding potential of −90 mV and was depolarized to a test potential of +10 mV for a duration of 50 ms every 30 s. After control currents had been recorded, the cells were superfused with ω-AgaTx IVA (50 nM) and then ω-CgTx GVIA (1 μM) and nifedipine (5 μM). Inhibition of the whole-cell currents was expressed as a percentage of the control current and the population expressed as a mean ± SEM.

and untreated cells (58 ± 4%). In parallel, there was a concomitant rise in the residual current, defined as the current that persists after the application of ω-AgaTx IVA, ω-CgTx GVIA, and nifedipine (see FIG. 3). Similar results were seen on rat cerebellar granule cells.[19] These results taken together indicate that overnight incubation in LEMS IgG causes a significant reduction in the ω-AgaTx IVA–sensitive (P/Q-type) VGCC, but leads to an increase in the magnitude of the "resistant" current. The mechanism of this interaction is unclear, but indicates that, under pathological conditions in which the P/Q-type VGCCs are downregulated, the cultured neurons are able to show plasticity by upregulation of other types of VGCC, namely R-type.

PASSIVE TRANSFER EXPERIMENTS

In order to investigate whether this phenomenon of plasticity occurs in the whole animal, passive transfer experiments were carried out. Mice were injected intraperitoneally (i.p.) daily with IgG (10 mg) purified from the plasma of patients undergoing therapeutic plasma exchange and compared to mice treated with control IgG. After 10 days, the mice were sacrificed; the phrenic nerve hemidiaphragm preparations were excised, and the nerve-evoked EPPs and MEPPs were recorded intra-

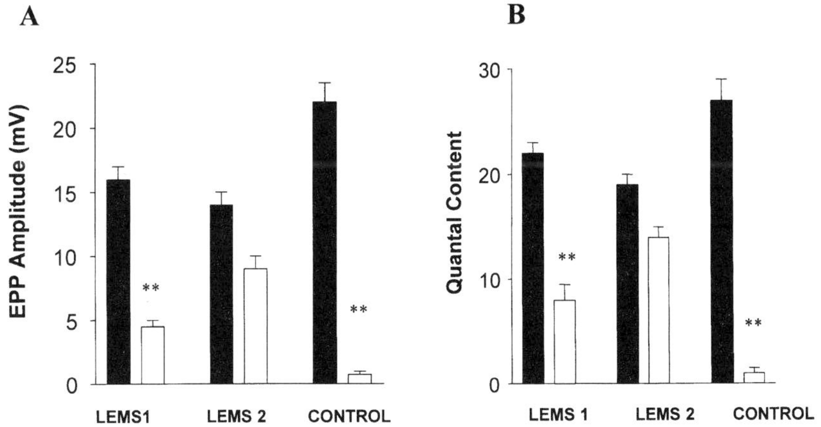

FIGURE 4. Effect of ω-AgaTx IVA on EPPs and quantal content of neuromuscular junctions of mice treated with LEMS and control IgG. Mice were injected daily with 10 mg IgG (LEMS 1, 2, and control) for 9 days, and the phrenic nerve/hemidiaphragm preparations were excised. The bar graph shows the effect of preincubation in the presence or absence of ω-AgaTx IVA (500 nM) for 1 h on EPP amplitude **(A)** and quantal content **(B)**. All experiments were carried out in the presence of 2.5 mM Ca^{2+} Krebs solution alone (*black bars*; diaphragm preparations, $n = 7$) or with ω-AgaTx IVA (*open bars*; $n = 3$). Results show the mean ± SE (**$p < 0.01$).

cellularly using standard electrophysiological techniques. The mean quantal content was calculated by the direct method.[21]

The results showed, in confirmation of others, that the EPP amplitude was reduced in mouse muscles treated with LEMS IgG (1 and 2) compared to those treated with control IgG (35% and 23%, respectively; FIG. 4A).[21–23] Similar results were obtained for the quantal content (FIG. 4B). Interestingly, ω-AgaTx IVA (500 nM), a specific P/Q-type VGCC blocker, virtually abolished both the EPP amplitude and quantal content in control-treated mice (FIGS. 4A and 4B). However, in mice treated with LEMS IgG, the same preparation of ω-AgaTx IVA only partially inhibited EPP amplitude (28% and 71%, respectively). Again, these results indicate that non P/Q-type VGCCs are recruited or unmasked on the motor nerve terminals at the neuromuscular junction in the LEMS-treated mice.

The sensitivity of these "novel" ω-AgaTx IVA–insensitive channels was investigated further by the application of other VGCC-specific blockers. L-type specific VGCC antagonists, nifedipine (5 μM) and calciseptine (1 μM), caused no significant inhibition of EPP amplitude. However simultaneous application of ω-AgaTx IVA (500 nM) and calciseptine (1 μM) to these LEMS-treated preparations caused a much larger reduction in EPP amplitude (64 ± 1%) as compared to ω-AgaTx IVA alone. The results with calciseptine indicate recruitment or "unmasking" of L-type VGCC. However, there remain VGCC channels that are insensitive to ω-AgaTx IVA and calciseptine, implying the presence of R-type channels in neuromuscular transmission in LEMS-treated mice.

CONCLUSIONS

In LEMS, in some patients at least, antibodies exist against most types of VGCCs (P/Q-, N-, and L-type). It was unclear whether these antibodies are directed either partially or completely against the pore-forming α_1 proteins or whether they cross-react through shared β subunits. Using cloned VGCCs expressed in HEK cells, we have shown that LEMS antibodies can bind extracellularly to both P/Q- and N-type VGCCs, but that the LEMS IgG exerted pathogenic effects only in the P/Q-type VGCC cell line.

In two model systems in which different VGCC subtypes exist, we have demonstrated that LEMS IgG-specific downregulation of P/Q-type VGCCs results in an upregulation of L- and R-type VGCCs. Since under normal conditions the calcium influx through P/Q-type VGCCs makes up >95% of the current evoked at the mammalian neuromuscular junction, this dynamic regulation may explain why LEMS patients are not more severely affected than in fact they are.

REFERENCES

1. Elmqvist, D. & E.H. Lambert. 1968. Detailed analysis of neuromuscular transmission in a patient with the myasthenic syndrome sometimes associated with bronchogenic carcinoma. Mayo Clin. Proc. **43:** 689–713.
2. Lang, B., J. Newsom-Davis, C. Prior & D. Wray. 1983. Antibodies to motor nerve terminals: an electrophysiological study of a human myasthenic syndrome transferred to mouse. J. Physiol. Lond. **344:** 335–345.
3. Waterman, S.A., B. Lang & J. Newsom-Davis. 1997. Effect of Lambert-Eaton syndrome immunoglobulins on autonomic neurons in the mouse. Ann. Neurol. **40:** 130–150.
4. O'Neill, J.H., N.M. Murray & J. Newsom-Davis. 1988. The Lambert-Eaton myasthenic syndrome: a review of 50 cases. Brain **111:** 577–596.
5. Benatar, M., F. Blaes, I. Johnston *et al.* 2001. Presynaptic neuronal antigens expressed by a small cell lung carcinoma cell line. J. Neuroimmunol. **113:** 153–162.
6. Guttman, L., T.W. Crosby, M. Takamori & J.D. Martin. 1972. The Eaton-Lambert syndrome and autoimmune disorders. Am. J. Med. **53:** 354–356.
7. Willcox, N., A.G. Demaine, J. Newsom-Davis *et al.* 1985. Increased frequency of IgG heavy chain Glm(2) and of HLA-B8 in the Lambert-Eaton myasthenic syndrome with and without associated lung carcinoma. Hum. Immunol. **14:** 29–36.
8. Wirtz, P.W., B.O. Roep, G.M. Schreuder *et al.* 2001. HLA I and II in Lambert-Eaton myasthenic syndrome without associated tumor. Hum. Immunol. **62:** 809–813.
9. Wirtz, P.W., N. Willcox, B.O. Roep *et al.* 2003. HLA-B8 in patients with the Lambert-Eaton myasthenic syndrome reduces likelihood of associated small cell lung carcinoma. This volume.
10. Meriney, S.D., S.C. Hulsizer, V.A. Lennon & A.D. Grinnell. 1996. Lambert-Eaton myasthenic syndrome immunoglobulins react with multiple types of calcium channels in small-cell lung carcinoma. Ann. Neurol. **40:** 739–749.
11. Lang, B., A. Vincent, N.M. Murray & J. Newsom-Davis. 1989. Lambert-Eaton myasthenic syndrome: immunoglobulin G inhibition of Ca^{2+} flux in tumor cells correlates with disease severity. Ann. Neurol. **25:** 265–271.
12. Fukuoka, T., A.G. Engel, B. Lang *et al.* 1987. Lambert-Eaton myasthenic syndrome: II. Immunoelectron microscopy localization of IgG at the mouse motor end-plate. Ann. Neurol. **22:** 200–211.
13. Birnbaumer, L., K.P. Campbell, W.A. Catterall *et al.* 1994. The naming of voltage-gated calcium channels. Neuron **13:** 505–506.
14. Mintz, I.M., V.J. Venema, K.M. Swiderek *et al.* 1992. P-type calcium channels blocked by the spider toxin omega-Aga-IVA. Nature **355:** 827–829.

15. MOTOMURA, M., B. LANG, I. JOHNSTON *et al.* 1997. Incidence of serum anti-P/Q-type and anti-N-type calcium channel autoantibodies in the Lambert-Eaton myasthenic syndrome. J. Neurol. Sci. **147:** 35–42.
16. LENNON, V.A., T.J. KRYZER, G.E. GREISMANN *et al.* 1995. Calcium channel antibodies in the Lambert-Eaton myasthenic syndrome and other paraneoplastic syndromes. N. Engl. J. Med. **332:** 1467–1474.
17. EL FAR, O., B. MARQUEZE, C. LEVEQUE *et al.* 1995. Antigens associated with N- and L-type calcium channels in Lambert-Eaton myasthenic syndrome. J. Neurochem. **64:** 1696–1702.
18. VERSCHUUREN, J.J., J. DALMAU, R. TUNKEL *et al.* 1998. Antibodies against the calcium channel beta-subunit in Lambert-Eaton myasthenic syndrome. Neurology **50:** 475–479.
19. PINTO, A., S. GILLARD, F. MOSS *et al.* 1998. Human autoantibodies specific for the alpha-1A calcium channel subunit reduce both P-type and Q-type calcium currents in cerebellar neurons. Proc. Natl. Acad. Sci. USA **95:** 8328–8333.
20. PINTO, A., K. IWASA, C. NEWLAND *et al.* 2002. The action of Lambert-Eaton myasthenic syndrome immunoglobulin G on cloned human voltage-gated calcium channels. Muscle Nerve **25:** 715–724.
21. GIOVANNINI, F., E. SHER, R. WEBSTER *et al.* 2002. Calcium channel subtypes contributing to acetylcholine release from normal, 4-aminopyridine-treated, and myasthenic syndrome auto-antibodies–affected neuromuscular junctions. Br. J. Pharmacol. In press.
22. PROTTI, D.A., R. REISIN, T.A. MACKINLEY & O.D. UCHITEL. 1996. Calcium channel blockers and transmitter release at the normal human neuromuscular junction. Neurology **46:** 1391–1396.
23. XU, Y.F., S.J. HEWETT & W.D. ATCHISON. 1998. Passive transfer of Lambert-Eaton myasthenic syndrome induces dihydropyridine sensitivity of I_{Ca} in mouse motor nerve terminals. J. Neurophysiol. **80:** 1056–1069.

LEMS IgG Binds to Extracellular Determinants on N-Type Voltage-Gated Calcium Channels, but Does Not Reduce VGCC Expression

KAZUO IWASA,[a,b] ASHWIN PINTO,[b] ANGELA VINCENT,[b]
AND BETHAN LANG[b]

[a]*Department of Neurology, Kanazawa University School of Medicine, Kanazawa 920-8641, Japan*

[b]*Neurosciences Group, Institute of Molecular Medicine, University of Oxford, Oxford OX3 9DU, United Kingdom*

KEYWORDS: LEMS; VGCC; N-type; P/Q-type; IgG; expression

Neuromuscular transmission at the mammalian neuromuscular junction is dependent on P/Q-type voltage-gated calcium channels (VGCCs). Lambert-Eaton myasthenic syndrome (LEMS) is a neurological disorder in which autoantibodies are directed against these VGCCs. Binding of the antibodies to these channels results in their subsequent downregulation and reduction in acetylcholine release, resulting in muscle weakness.[1,2]

Neurotoxins can be used to label specifically different subtypes of VGCC for radioimmunoassays. Antibodies against the P/Q-type VGCC have been detected in about 90% of LEMS patients, whereas only 30–40% have anti-N-type VGCC antibodies. It has been suggested that immunoprecipitation of N-type VGCCs may be through cross-reaction with a common intracellular β subunit. These antibodies would not be pathogenic. By contrast, if antibodies cross-react with common epitopes on the extracellular surface of the α_1 subunit of the P/Q- and N-type VGCCs, these antibodies would be expected to be pathogenic.

In this study, we used human embryonic kidney cells (HEK293) transfected with the genes encoding the N-type VGCC and studied the effects of antibody binding on surface VGCC expression.

Address for correspondence: Kazuo Iwasa, Department of Neurology, Kanazawa University School of Medicine, 13-1 Takara-machi, Kanazawa 920-8641, Japan. Voice: +81-76-265-2292; fax: +81-76-234-4253.
neuiwasa@med.kanazawa-u.ac.jp

Ann. N.Y. Acad. Sci. 998: 196–199 (2003). © 2003 New York Academy of Sciences.
doi: 10.1196/annals.1254.020

METHODS

Human embryonic kidney (HEK293) cell line (C2D7) transfected with the subunits encoding an N-type VGCC (α_{1B-1}, β_{1b}, $\alpha_{2b}\delta$ boosted) was a gift of K. Stauderman (SIBIA Neurosciences, La Jolla, CA) and was grown as previously described.[1,2]

We studied 11 patients with LEMS, 2 individual healthy controls, 1 control pool (n = 30 patients), and 3 disease controls (1 SCLC without LEMS, 2 Guillain-Barré syndrome). IgG was prepared from patients by the ethacridine lactate–ammonium sulfate method.[1]

Using standard radioimmunoassay techniques, the preparations were assayed for antibodies to P/Q-type (^{125}I-CmTx-MVIIC-labeled) VGCC and for N-type (^{125}I-CgTx-GVIA-labeled) VGCC. To assay for surface IgG binding, cells were labeled with ^{125}I-ω-CgTx-GVIA (5 fmol, 1 h, 20°C), and nonspecific binding was estimated by preincubating the cells in excess unlabeled toxin (1 μM, 30 min). Patient or control IgG (100 μL, 1 mg/mL, 90 min) was then added. The cells were washed twice and extracted in digitonin (4%). The supernatant containing the solubilized channels was harvested, and antihuman IgG (125 μL, 1:6 dilution) was added in order to form a precipitate.[1] This was then washed and the radioactivity counted.

The effect of LEMS IgG on the surface expression of N-type VGCC was studied as follows: C2D7 (2×10^5 cells/well) was incubated with IgG (1 mg/mL, patient or control) for 24 h at 37°C. After washing, the cells were incubated in ^{125}I-ω-CgTx-GVIA (5 fmol, 30 min, 20°C), washed again, and the radioactivity counted. Nonspecific ^{125}I-ω-CgTx-GVIA binding was evaluated by parallel incubation in unlabeled toxin (1 μM). The results were compared to cells grown in medium alone and to those grown in the presence of various inhibitors of protein expression. All experiments were carried out in triplicate.

RESULTS

None of the controls had VGCC antibodies above 45 pM, whereas 10 of 11 LEMS patients had P/Q-type VGCC and 4 of 11 had antibodies to N-type VGCC. The IgG preparations from these patients had P/Q-type VGCC antibody titers of 12–153 fmol/mg IgG and N-type VGCC antibody titers of 2.3–100.1 fmol/mg IgG. Two additional patients had detectable N-type VGCC antibodies using this assay system. Values for control IgG were <4.4 and <2.2 fmol/mg IgG, respectively.

To test for antibodies binding to the extracellular domains of the N-type VGCC, we exposed the VGCC expressing cells to the IgG and ^{125}I-CgTx-GVIA conotoxin, followed by washing and extraction of the VGCCs. Then, we used immunoprecipitation to quantify how many of the VGCCs had antibody attached. Four of 11 LEMS patients had antibodies that bound to the extracellular regions of N-type VGCCs, all of whom had significant N-type VGCC antibodies (TABLE 1). One patient with antibodies to solubilized N-type VGCC (6.9 fmol/mg) did not bind appreciably to the C2D7 cell line. None of the controls bound significantly to the C2D7 cell line.

Surface expression of N-type VGCCs incubated in IgG derived from patients with only P/Q-type VGCC antibodies was not significantly different to cells incubated in either control IgG or medium alone (data not shown). By contrast, incubation in IgG purified from the 2 patients with the highest N-type VGCC antibodies induced

TABLE 1. Antibodies to N-type VGCC in LEMS patients and binding to extracellular domains

	N-type antibody titer solubilized VGCC (fmol/mg IgG)[a]	Antibodies to extracellular domains (fmol)[b]
LEMS 1	100.1*	0.506**
LEMS 2	19.4*	0.769**
LEMS 3	6.9*	0.170
LEMS 4	3.4*	0.304**
LEMS 5	2.7*	0.328**
LEMS 6	2.3*	0.160
LEMS 7	0.01	0.161
LEMS 8	0.01	0.178
LEMS 9	0.01	0.174
LEMS 10	0.1	0.206
LEMS 11	0.01	0.178

[a]Anti-N-type VGCC antibody titer (fmol/mg IgG). *Results are considered positive if greater than 2.2 fmol/mg IgG (mean of controls ± 2SD, $n = 6$).

[b]Surface-(^{125}I-ω-CgTx-GVIA)-labeled N-type VGCC precipitated by IgG (fmol) compared to total ^{125}I-ω-CgTx-GVIA-surface-labeled N-type VGCC (fmol). **Results are considered positive if greater than 0.278 fmol/fmol, obtained with control IgG ($n = 6$).

increases in the level of surface expression of N-type VGCC as measured by ^{125}I-ω-CgTx-GVIA binding (FIG. 1). This upregulation was unaffected by preincubation in brefeldin A (BFA, 3 μM), which disrupts the translocation of proteins from endoplasmic reticulum to the Golgi apparatus, but abolished by incubation in nocodazole (10 μM), an inhibitor of microtubule-based vesicular transport (data not shown).[3]

DISCUSSION

Antibodies against extracellular portions of the N-type VGCC were detected in 4 out of 11 LEMS patients. Two further patients had antibodies that were probably directed against intracellular determinants as they did not bind to the extracellular surface of the VGCC. The titer of the antibodies against extracellular domains did not correlate with the titer to solubilized VGCC (TABLE 1). Preincubation in IgG from 9 patients had no apparent effect on the surface expression of N-type VGCC, consistent with results obtained using electrophysiological and calcium fluorescence techniques.[1,2] However, 2 LEMS patients with the highest anti-N-type VGCC antibody titer induced an upregulation in cell surface expression of N-type VGCC as measured by the binding of ^{125}I-ω-CgTx-GVIA (FIG. 1). Within the time course of this experiment (24 h), this upregulation was unaffected by BFA, but abolished by nocodazole, indicating that the upregulation requires the presence of a functional microtubule transport system, but does not require functional Golgi apparatus. Thus, rather than downregulating VGCCs as found in similar experiments with P/Q-type VGCCs, the N-type VGCC antibodies appear to cause upregulation of their target.

Upregulation of channels in the presence of specific anti-N-type VGCC antibodies is an unexpected result; however, similar results have been shown in a neuro-

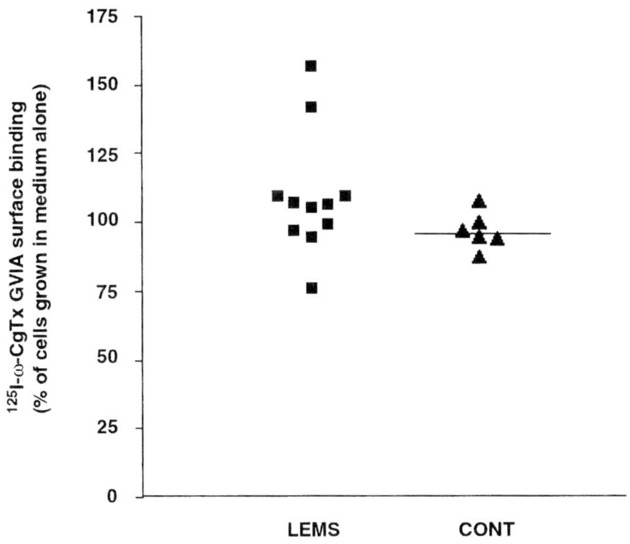

FIGURE 1. Binding of ^{125}I-ω-CgTx-GVIA to surface N-type VGCC following IgG incubation.

blastoma cell line, where administration of ω-CgTx-GVIA or cadmium ions stimulated the recruitment of novel N-type VGCCs.[4] Together, these results suggest that antibodies to N-type VGCCs do bind to the extracellular surface and initially, at least, may result in an upregulation of VGCC number. Further studies need to be carried out to establish whether these findings are representative of pathological events occurring at the neuromuscular junction in affected patients.

ACKNOWLEDGMENTS

Kazuo Iwasa was supported by the Toyobo Biotechnology Foundation.

REFERENCES

1. PINTO, A., K. IWASA, C. NEWLAND *et al.* 2002. The action of Lambert-Eaton myasthenic syndrome immunoglobulin G on cloned human voltage-gated calcium channels. Muscle Nerve **25:** 715–724.
2. PINTO, A., S. GILLARD, F. MOSS *et al.* 1998. Human autoantibodies specific for the alpha-1A calcium channel subunit reduce both P-type and Q-type calcium currents in cerebellar neurons. Proc. Natl. Acad. Sci. USA **95:** 8328–8333.
3. CID-ARREGI, A., R.G. PARTON *et al.* 1995. Nocodazole-dependent transport, and brefeldin A–sensitive processing and sorting, of newly synthesized membrane proteins in cultured neurons. J. Neurosci. **15:** 4259–4269.
4. PASSAFARO, M., F. CLEMENTI *et al.* 1994. ω-Conotoxin and Cd^{2+} stimulate the recruitment to the plasma membane of an intracellular pool of voltage operated Ca^{2+} channels. Neuron **12:** 317–326.

HLA-B8 in Patients with the Lambert-Eaton Myasthenic Syndrome Reduces Likelihood of Associated Small Cell Lung Carcinoma

PAUL W. WIRTZ,[a] NICK WILLCOX,[b] BART O. ROEP,[c] BETHAN LANG,[b] AXEL R. WINTZEN,[a] JOHN NEWSOM-DAVIS,[b] AND JAN J. VERSCHUUREN[a]

[a]*Department of Neurology, Leiden University Medical Center, Leiden, the Netherlands*

[b]*Department of Neurosciences, Weatherall Institute of Molecular Medicine, Oxford University, United Kingdom*

[c]*Department of Immunohematology, Leiden University Medical Center, Leiden, the Netherlands*

KEYWORDS: HLA-B8; Lambert-Eaton myasthenic syndrome; small cell lung carcinoma

INTRODUCTION

The Lambert-Eaton myasthenic syndrome (LEMS) is a rare autoimmune disorder of the neuromuscular junction, in which autoantibodies are directed against voltage-gated calcium channels. LEMS is associated with small cell lung carcinoma (SCLC) in about half of the patients, with its onset usually preceding detection of the SCLC.[1] Smoking is the only known predictor for the presence of SCLC in LEMS patients.[1] LEMS cases without SCLC showed an increased frequency of HLA-B8.[2,3] The aim of this study was to compare the frequency of this allele between patients with and without SCLC.

METHODS

HLA typing was done in 77 unselected Dutch and British Caucasian patients with EMG-confirmed LEMS. Diagnosis of SCLC was made by cytology or histology. Patients without SCLC were followed for at least three years. Patients with tumors other than SCLC were excluded. HLA typing was performed using the standard microcytotoxicity technique or by DNA typing. HLA-B8 frequencies in patients with and without SCLC were compared using Haldane's modification of Woolf's method. A Fisher test was used when appropriate. Odds ratios with their 95% confi-

Address for correspondence: P. W. Wirtz, M.D., Department of Neurology, Leiden University Medical Center, P. O. Box 9600, 2300 RC Leiden, the Netherlands. Voice: +31-71-5262118; fax: +31-71-5248253.

pwwirtz@lumc.nl

Ann. N.Y. Acad. Sci. 998: 200–201 (2003). © 2003 New York Academy of Sciences.
doi: 10.1196/annals.1254.021

TABLE 1. HLA-B8 in patients with the Lambert-Eaton myasthenic syndrome

	No tumor		SCLC				Odds	
	n	HLA-B8+	*n*	HLA-B8+	χ^2	*p*	ratio	95% CI
British	31	21 (68%)	17	1 (6%)	14.0	0.0002	0.030	0.003–0.257
Dutch	21	14 (67%)	8	2 (25%)	3.9	0.054	0.167	0.027–1.049
Total	52	35 (67%)	25	3 (12%)	17.5	0.00003	0.066	0.017–0.252

NOTE: The statistical comparisons are made between LEMS patients with SCLC and those without a tumor.

dence intervals were calculated. Sensitivity, specificity, and predictive values of HLA-B8 were calculated.

RESULTS

We detected SCLC in 8 of 29 (28%) Dutch LEMS patients. Two (25%) of these 8 were HLA-B8 positive, whereas HLA-B8 was found in 14 (67%) of the 21 Dutch patients without SCLC (TABLE 1). In the 48 British patients with LEMS, 17 (35%) had SCLC. Only 1 (6%) of these 17 was HLA-B8 positive, in contrast with 21 (68%) of the 31 patients without SCLC. In total, 67% of 52 LEMS patients without SCLC were HLA-B8 positive, against 12% of 25 LEMS patients with SCLC. The presence of HLA-B8 predicted the absence of SCLC with a sensitivity of 67% and a specificity of 88%. The positive predictive value of HLA-B8 for the absence of SCLC was 92%; the negative predictive value was 56%. The test had a likelihood ratio of 5.6.

CONCLUSIONS

The presence of HLA-B8 in patients with LEMS is inversely correlated with that of SCLC. In patients with LEMS associated with SCLC, the frequency of HLA-B8 was not different from that in the general population. Thus, it is unlikely that HLA-B8 protects against the development of SCLC. On the other hand, HLA-B8 was found in 67% of the patients with LEMS without tumor.[2,3] These findings emphasize the distinct genetic predisposition and immunological routes to the similar clinical presentation of LEMS with or without SCLC.

REFERENCES

1. O'NEILL, J.H., N.M. MURRAY & J. NEWSOM-DAVIS. 1988. The Lambert-Eaton myasthenic syndrome: a review of 50 cases. Brain **111:** 577–597.
2. WILLCOX, N., A.G. DEMAINE, J. NEWSOM-DAVIS *et al.* 1985. Increased frequency of IgG heavy chain Glm(2) and of HLA-B8 in Lambert-Eaton myasthenic syndrome with and without associated lung carcinoma. Hum. Immunol. **14:** 29–36.
3. WIRTZ, P.W., B.O. ROEP, G.M. SCHREUDER *et al.* 2001. HLA class I and II in Lambert-Eaton myasthenic syndrome without associated tumor. Hum. Immunol. **62:** 809–813.

Autoimmune Disorders of Neuronal Potassium Channels

JOHN NEWSOM-DAVIS,[a] CAMILLA BUCKLEY,[a] LINDA CLOVER,[a] IAN HART,[a,b] PAUL MADDISON,[a] ERDEM TÜZÜM,[a] AND ANGELA VINCENT[a]

[a]*Weatherall Institute of Molecular Medicine and Department of Clinical Neurology, University of Oxford, Oxford, United Kingdom*

[b]*Department of Neurology, Walton Hospital, Liverpool, United Kingdom*

ABSTRACT: Antibodies to voltage-gated potassium channels (VGKCs) appear likely to be the effector mechanisms in many patients with acquired peripheral nerve hyperexcitability (APNH) syndromes, a group of disorders that include neuromyotonia, cramp-fasciculation syndrome, and Isaacs' syndrome. They may contribute to the associated autonomic changes. Through a central action, they may also be the effector mechanism in those with Morvan's syndrome and in some patients with limbic encephalitis. Evidence supporting this hypothesis includes the increased association of APNH with autoimmune diseases (in particular, myasthenia gravis and thymoma), the response to plasmapheresis, passive transfer of APNH to experimental animals by patients' plasma or immunoglobulins, the action of their serum on VGKC currents studied *in vitro*, and the presence in many patients of IgG antibodies to VGKCs.

KEYWORDS: neuromyotonia; myokymia; cramp-fasciculation syndrome; peripheral nerve hyperexcitability; limbic encephalitis; Morvan's syndrome; potassium channel antibodies

INTRODUCTION

The discovery of the autoimmune nature of myasthenia gravis (MG) more than 25 years ago was seminal because it introduced the concept of antibody-mediated ion channelopathies. Moreover, the clinical observations and experimental studies that revealed the nature of MG proved invaluable in the search for other antibody-mediated disorders of the neuromuscular junction. Those early studies highlighted the clinical clues to a disorder being autoimmune, notably the association with other autoimmune diseases.[1] These studies also demonstrated the vulnerability to antibody-mediated attack of ion channels at the neuromuscular junction, which lacks the protection of the blood-nerve barrier.[2] Importantly, they also established experimental paradigms for investigating antibody-mediated effector mechanisms, notably passive transfer of the disorder to experimental animals by patients' immunoglobulins,[3]

Address for correspondence: John Newsom-Davis, Department of Clinical Neurology, University of Oxford, Oxford OX2 6HE, United Kingdom. Voice: +44 (0)1865 224940; fax: +44 (0)1865 224273.

john.newsomdavis@btinternet.com

Ann. N.Y. Acad. Sci. 998: 202–210 (2003). © 2003 New York Academy of Sciences.
doi: 10.1196/annals.1254.022

immunoprecipitation assays using target-specific neurotoxins,[4] and the clinical response to plasmapheresis.[5] Thus, prompted by the discoveries in MG, studies between 1980 and 1990 established the antibody-mediated nature of the Lambert-Eaton myasthenic syndrome (LEMS). An early clinical clue was its association in nonparaneoplastic cases with other autoimmune disorders and the response to plasmapheresis in both the paraneoplastic and nonparaneoplastic forms of the disorder.[6,7] Passive immunization of mice transferred the pathophysiological and morphological changes of the human disease,[6,8,9] and immunoprecipitation assays using the radiolabeled Cone Snail toxin MVIIC confirmed the presence of antibodies to P/Q-type voltage-gated calcium channels (VGCCs),[10,11] but our studies in LEMS raised an important new possibility, namely that the antibodies to neuronal VGCCs at the nerve terminal may also have a central action in causing the cerebellar syndrome that occurs occasionally in LEMS patients.[12]

By a similar process, evidence has been accumulating since 1990 that neuronal voltage-gated potassium channels (VGKCs) can be targeted by IgG autoantibodies, leading not only to peripheral nerve hyperexcitability syndromes, such as neuromyotonia (NMT), but probably also to central nervous system (CNS) disorders. This evidence is the focus of the present review.

VOLTAGE-GATED POTASSIUM CHANNELS

The primary VGKC structure comprises four transmembrane α-subunits and four intracellular β-subunits, arranged round a central ion pore. The α-subunit genes determine the VGKC subtype and comprise the *Shaker*-related VGKC family, which has at least six members in humans (Kv1.1–Kv1.6), as shown in TABLE 1. These combine to form homomeric or heteromeric tetramers. 4-Aminopyridine blocks all members of the family and some are blocked by specific neurotoxins such as α-dendrotoxin, a component of the venom of the green mamba snake.

VGKCs are widespread in the peripheral, autonomic, and central nervous systems and play a key role in controlling neuronal excitability. For example, compounds that block VGKCs, such as 4-aminopyridine, increase nerve excitability and may lead to repetitive peripheral nerve discharges or to seizures. Families with different point mutations in Kv1.1 can present with differing combinations of episodic ataxia, neuromyotonia, and seizures.[13] Kv1.1 knockout mice develop recurrent spontaneous seizures early in postnatal development.[14] Thus, interference with VGKC function is one potential cause of acquired neuronal hyperexcitability disorders.

ACQUIRED PERIPHERAL NERVE HYPEREXCITABILITY SYNDROMES

Several different syndromes have been described, including undulating myokymia;[15] Isaacs' syndrome,[16] in which there is severe muscle stiffness and continuous muscle fiber activity; neuromyotonia,[17] in which "pseudomyotonia" occurs (failure to relax following voluntary muscle contraction); and cramp-fasciculation syndrome.[18] A recognized cause of acquired peripheral nerve hyperexcitability (APNH) is timber rattlesnake envenomation,[19] and it may also be seen rarely in the Guillain-Barré syndrome as well as in association with other acquired neuropathies in which

TABLE 1. *Shaker*-related human VGKCs

	Kv1.1	Kv1.2	Kv1.3	Kv1.4	Kv1.5	Kv1.6
Chromosome	12	1	13	11	11	12
Channel blocker						
4-aminopyridine	+	+	+	+	+	+
α-dendrotoxin	+	+	–	–	–	+

there are abnormalities of nerve conduction. However, in the majority of patients previously reported with these disorders, the condition appeared to be idiopathic.

Patients usually first notice muscle twitching or muscle cramps.[20] Occasionally the myokymia is focal, as for example in the face.[21] Other complaints may include muscle stiffness or weakness, increased sweating, pseudomyotonia, and sensory symptoms. In addition, CNS symptoms occur in about 25% of patients. Mood change, increased irritability, and insomnia are the most common, but hallucinations or a delusional state may occur rarely (Morvan's syndrome[22]), and recently the features of limbic encephalitis have been observed (Buckley and Palace, personal communication). TABLE 1 summarizes the clinical and electromyographic findings in the three main subgroups of APNH syndromes.

Examination usually reveals muscle twitching (myokymia) either under resting conditions or following muscle contraction. However, myokymia is sometimes only revealed by electromyography. Some patients have pronounced muscle hypertrophy. Pseudomyotonia may be present, affecting handgrip or even tongue protrusion. Chvostek's sign may be elicited.

The electromyographic hallmark, first identified by Denny-Brown and Foley,[15] is the occurrence of irregular bursts of motor unit discharges with high intraburst frequencies (e.g., 40–150 Hz), referred to as "myokymic discharges". In other cases, prolonged "neuromyotonic" discharges or "after-discharges" (following voluntary muscle activation) may occur. Fasciculation or fibrillation potentials may also be present.

The peripheral nerve origin of these spontaneous discharges was demonstrated by Isaacs.[16] In many patients, the discharges were unchanged following distal peripheral nerve block, but were abolished by curare, implying that they were arising "from the terminal arborisations of motor nerves". Later studies, however, showed that peripheral nerve block sometimes substantially reduced the discharges, indicating that the impulse generators can be in proximal portions of the motor nerve,[20] perhaps even in the motoneuron itself because the electromyographic features of APNH can occasionally occur in motoneuron disease.

CLINICAL CLUES TO AN AUTOIMMUNE ETIOLOGY

There are several clinical pointers to a likely autoimmune etiology for APNH syndromes.[20] First, these disorders occur with other autoimmune disorders more frequently than would be expected by chance, in particular with MG.[23] Second, many patients have a thymoma,[20,24–28] a tumor known to associate with other autoimmune disorders in addition to MG, and to be present in about 20% of patients. Third, neuromyotonia can be provoked by penicillamine treatment,[29] as in the case of MG. Fourth, oligoclonal bands are sometimes present in the cerebrospinal fluid.[20] Finally, there appears to be an increased likelihood of these disorders occurring as paraneoplastic conditions with lung cancer or lymphoma.[30,31]

CLINICAL STUDIES

Plasma exchange (plasmapheresis) can induce a substantial and significant reduction in the quantified spontaneous motor unit discharges in patients with APNH disorders,[20,32] although not in all patients. Nevertheless, the clear-cut clinical and electromyographic improvement in some patients strongly suggests an antibody-mediated disorder. Later studies showed that patients sometimes improve after intravenous immunoglobulin infusion or following immunosuppressive treatment with prednisolone and azathioprine, further supporting an autoimmune pathogenesis.

WHAT IS THE LIKELY TARGET ANTIGEN?

The nerve action potential depends on the opening of voltage-gated sodium channels. One possible underlying mechanism might be prolonged inactivation of these channels by antibody binding, which could lead to increased nerve excitability. However, because anti-ion-channel antibodies in both MG and LEMS usually exert their actions through a process of channel loss, it seemed more likely that APNH was due to loss of functional VGKCs responsible for repolarization of the nerve membrane.

EXPERIMENTAL ELECTROPHYSIOLOGICAL STUDIES

Passive transfer of patients' immunoglobulins to experimental animals proved to be as valuable in demonstrating the antibody-mediated nature of APNH in some patients as it had been in elucidating the disease mechanisms in MG and in LEMS. Sinha and colleagues[32] showed that resistance to curare was significantly increased in mice injected with APNH plasma or immunoglobulins. Such an increase would be predicted if the patients' antibodies were reducing the number of functioning VGKCs because, like 4-aminopyridine, this would prolong the action potential at the nerve terminal, thereby increasing the quantal content of the endplate potential, that is, the number of ACh packets released, requiring a larger concentration of curare to block transmission.

In further *in vitro* studies in passively immunized mice, direct measurement of the amplitudes of the miniature endplate potentials and of the endplate potential using microelectrodes allowed the quantal content to be calculated. In sets of mice injected with six different APNH IgGs, the mean quantal content was increased by 21% relative to control values ($p < 0.005$),[33] consistent with a reduction in the number of VGKCs. In addition, rat dorsal root ganglion cells incubated for 24 h *in vitro* in IgG at 2 mg/mL, and then studied in whole cell patch mode, showed a marked increase in repetitive firing in the presence of APNH IgG, compared with controls.

Similar repetitive firing was produced by the application of 3,4-diaminopyridine, which blocks VGKCs.[33] Thus, APNH IgGs appeared to contain antibodies to VGKCs that can induce hyperexcitability changes in motor and sensory nerves.

Patch-clamp studies of a human neuroblastoma cell line NB-1, which expresses Kv1.1 and 1.2, and of CHO cells transfected with either Kv1.1 or 1.6 provided direct evidence that APNH IgGs (from NMT and from idiopathic myokymia patients) can downregulate VGKCs of these subtypes.[34] It was necessary to incubate cells for 3 days rather than 1 day for the suppression of K^+ currents to be observed, implying that the action was exerted through an intracellular processing mechanism rather than by direct pharmacological block. These findings confirmed earlier studies in the rat PC-12 cell line.[35] Studies on the neuroblastoma cell line NB-1 also showed that the APNH IgGs tested did not block voltage-gated sodium channels, helping to resolve the issue of whether or not the effects of APNH antibodies might be exerted through the prolonged activation of these channels.[34]

The APNH IgGs did not affect the time course of activation or inactivation of the outward K^+ currents, indicating that the observed effects were due to a reduction in the number of functional VGKCs rather than to an action on channel kinetics.[34]

DETECTION OF ANTIBODIES TO VGKCs

Antibodies specific to VGKCs were first detected in NMT patients by an immunoprecipitation assay using human frontal cortex as the source of antigen.[33,36] Membranes were extracted in 1% digitonin and labeled with ^{125}I-α-dendrotoxin (DnTx), which is known to block Kv1.1, 1.2, and 1.6 (TABLE 1). Raised serum titers were found in about 50% of patients, but not in MG, LEMS, or healthy controls. Positive titers were found more frequently in those with thymoma (FIG. 1).

A molecular-histochemical method in which the cRNA for an individual VGKC α-subunit was injected into *Xenopus* oocytes proved to be much more sensitive,

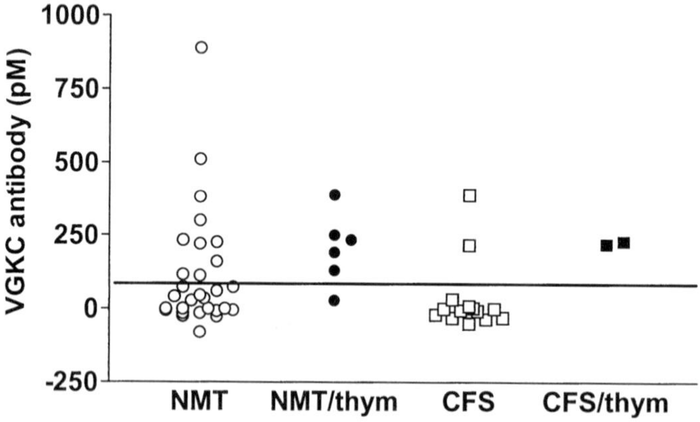

FIGURE 1. Scatter plot of serum VGKC antibody titers in patients with neuromyotonia (NMT) or cramp-fasciculation syndrome (CFS) alone or with thymoma (thym). Titers were regarded as positive if greater than the mean + 3 SDs of control sera (100 pM).

although not suitable for routine use. Antibodies were detected to the relevant VGKC expressed in the oocyte cytoplasm by immunohistochemistry on frozen sections.[36] By this means, antibodies to Kv1.1, 1.2, or 1.6 were detected to one or more of these VGKC subtypes in more than 17 of 19 NMT patients studied.[23] This finding, together with the clinical autoimmune associations and the experimental pathophysiological studies described above, strongly implicate VGKC autoantibodies in the pathogenesis of APNH.

DO APNH SYNDROMES HAVE A COMMON PATHOGENESIS?

The three main subtypes of APNH outlined in TABLE 2 have distinct clinical and electromyographic features. To investigate whether cramp-fasciculation syndrome (C-F) and neuromyotonia (NMT) have a common pathogenesis, we analyzed the clinical, autoimmune, and electrophysiological features of 60 patients presenting with features of peripheral nerve hyperexcitability.[23] Patients with APNH were grouped according to an electromyographic criterion: the presence (group A) or absence (group B) of myokymic EMG discharges (spontaneous bursts of doublet, triplet, or multiplet motor unit discharges with 40–300 Hz intraburst frequency). Group A ($N = 42$) broadly accorded with the NMT subtype, while group B ($N = 18$) broadly accorded with the C-F syndrome. The analysis showed that the two groups had a similar average age of onset (45 and 48 years, respectively), an increased frequency of associated autoimmune disorders, and association with thymoma and acetylcholine receptor antibodies or with lung cancer. Moreover, serum VGKC autoantibodies were detected in 38% of group A and 28% of group B using the ^{125}I-α-DnTx immunoprecipitation assay. Thus, autoimmunity and specifically antibodies to VGKCs are strongly implicated in the pathogenesis of both groups, the EMG features reflecting quantitative rather than qualitative differences. Creatine kinase was raised in about half the patients in each group. VGKC antibodies may also be detected in patients with focal NMT.[21]

Interestingly, mild CNS symptoms also occurred in both groups (mood change and insomnia). In a recent study, Liguori and colleagues[37] reported raised serum antibodies in an elderly man with Morvan's syndrome, who presented with NMT, dysautonomia, impaired slow-wave sleep, and abnormal REM sleep. He also had oligoclonal bands in his cerebrospinal fluid. Symptoms improved after plasmapheresis, suggesting that his disorder was antibody-mediated. Thus, it seems likely that antibodies to VGKCs are implicated in Morvan's syndrome, as in C-F syndrome and NMT.

The increased sweating experienced by some APNH patients, although possibly accounted for by the increased muscle activity, might also represent antibody-mediated hyperactivity within the autonomic nervous system. VGKC antibodies may also have a pathogenetic role in some patients with acquired gut dysmotility.[38]

From the present findings, it cannot be argued that all patients with APNH have an antibody-mediated disorder. In the study by Hart and colleagues,[23] 25% of group A patients had an associated disorder of nerve conduction that was usually axonal in type and could have contributed to the NMT. Moreover, we have observed typical features of NMT in two patients who had amyotrophic lateral sclerosis.

TABLE 2. Typical clinical features of APNH syndromes

Disorder	Clinical features	EMG findings
Cramp-fasciculation syndrome (C-F)	Muscle cramps, stiffness fasciculations	Spontaneous single MU discharges, fasciculations, after-discharges
Neuromyotonia (NMT)	As for C-F plus: myokymia, pseudomyotonia, muscle hypertrophy, increased sweating	As for C-F plus: spontaneous continuous MU discharges and myokymic discharges
Morvan's syndrome	As for NMT plus: hallucinations, insomnia, mood change	As for NMT

LIMBIC ENCEPHALITIS AND VGKC ANTIBODIES

Limbic encephalitis is characterized by the subacute onset of agitation, disorientation, loss of recent memory, and sometimes hallucinations and temporal lobe seizures. It may occur in isolation or as a paraneoplastic condition. Associated tumors include thymoma,[39] small cell lung cancer, and testicular tumors. The clinical similarity between limbic encephalitis and the CNS features of Morvan's syndrome led Buckley and colleagues[40] to investigate the presence of serum VGKC antibodies in two patients with limbic encephalitis, one of whom had MG and a recurrent thymoma. The serum VGKC antibody titer in this patient rose sharply from normal values at the time of thymoma recurrence, having been undetectable in stored serial serum samples taken during the first 10 years of her illness. After a course of plasmapheresis, both her MG and the manifestations of encephalitis subsided, and were accompanied by a decline in the AChR and VGKC antibody titers. The second patient with limbic encephalitis, which included tonic-clonic seizures and developed in isolation, had very high titers of VGKC antibodies. An MR T2-weighted brain scan showed an area of increased signal in the left hippocampus. Her disorder improved spontaneously, associating with a decline in VGKC antibodies. Immunohistochemistry showed staining of the middle third of the molecular layer of the dentate gyrus by serum taken during the acute phase of her illness, but not by her convalescent serum. It was concluded that the encephalitis was likely to be antibody-mediated in view of the temporal relationships between VGKC antibody titers and her psychological state. The above patients had no evident myokymia on examination, but electromyographic studies were not done. However, recently in another similar patient with limbic encephalitis and no myokymia on clinical examination, electromyography clearly showed the changes of NMT (Buckley and Palace, personal communication). Thus, the serum of patients with limbic encephalitis should be tested for VGKC antibodies and for the presence of subclinical myokymia by electromyography.

REFERENCES

1. SIMPSON, J.A. 1966. Myasthenia gravis as an autoimmune disease: clinical aspects. Ann. N.Y. Acad. Sci. **135:** 506–516.
2. PATRICK, J. & J. LINDSTROM. 1973. Autoimmune response to acetylcholine receptor. Science **180:** 871–872.
3. TOYKA, K.V., D.B. DRACHMAN, A. PESTRONK & I. KAO. 1975. Myasthenia gravis: passive transfer from man to mouse. Science **190:** 397–399.
4. LINDSTROM, J.M., M.E. SEYBOLD, V.A. LENNON *et al.* 1976. Antibody to acetylcholine receptor in myasthenia gravis: prevalence, clinical correlates, and diagnostic value. Neurology **26:** 1054–1059.
5. PINCHING, A.J., D.K. PETERS & J. NEWSOM-DAVIS. 1976. Remission of myasthenia gravis following plasma-exchange. Lancet **2:** 1373–1376.
6. LANG, B., J. NEWSOM-DAVIS, D. WRAY *et al.* 1981. Autoimmune aetiology for myasthenic (Eaton-Lambert) syndrome. Lancet **2:** 224–226.
7. NEWSOM-DAVIS, J. & N.M. MURRAY. 1984. Plasma exchange and immunosuppressive drug treatment in the Lambert-Eaton myasthenic syndrome. Neurology **34:** 480–485.
8. LANG, B., J. NEWSOM-DAVIS, C. PRIOR & D. WRAY. 1983. Antibodies to motor nerve terminals: an electrophysiological study of a human myasthenic syndrome transferred to mouse. J. Physiol. **344:** 335–345.
9. FUKUNAGA, H., A.G. ENGEL, B. LANG *et al.* 1983. Passive transfer of Lambert-Eaton myasthenic syndrome with IgG from man to mouse depletes the presynaptic membrane active zones. Proc. Natl. Acad. Sci. USA **80:** 7636–7640.
10. MOTOMURA, M., I. JOHNSTON, B. LANG *et al.* 1995. An improved diagnostic assay for Lambert-Eaton myasthenic syndrome. J. Neurol. Neurosurg. Psychiatry **58:** 85–87.
11. LENNON, V.A., T.J. KRYZER, G.E. GRIESMANN *et al.* 1995. Calcium-channel antibodies in the Lambert-Eaton syndrome and other paraneoplastic syndromes. N. Engl. J. Med. **332:** 1467–1474.
12. PINTO, A., S. GILLARD, F. MOSS *et al.* 1998. Human autoantibodies specific for the alpha1A calcium channel subunit reduce both P-type and Q-type calcium currents in cerebellar neurons. Proc. Natl. Acad. Sci. USA **95:** 8328–8333.
13. ZUBERI, S.M., L.H. EUNSON, A. SPAUSCHUS *et al.* 1999. A novel mutation in the human voltage-gated potassium channel gene (Kv1.1) associates with episodic ataxia type 1 and sometimes with partial epilepsy. Brain **122**(part 5)**:** 817–825.
14. RHO, J.M., P. SZOT, B.L. TEMPEL *et al.* 1999. Developmental seizure susceptibility of kv1.1 potassium channel knockout mice. Dev. Neurosci. **21:** 320–327.
15. DENNY-BROWN, D. & J.M. FOLEY. 1948. Myokymia and the benign fasciculation of muscular cramps. Trans. Assoc. Am. Physicians **61:** 88–96.
16. ISAACS, H.A. 1961. Syndrome of continuous muscle fibre activity. J. Neurol. Neurosurg. Psychiatry **24:** 319–325.
17. MERTENS, H-G. & S. ZSCHOCKE. 1965. Neuromyotonie. Klin. Wochensschr. **43:** 917–925.
18. TAHMOUSH, A.J., R.J. ALONSO, G.P. TAHMOUSH & T.D. HEIMAN-PATTERSON. 1991. Cramp-fasciculation syndrome: a treatable hyperexcitable peripheral nerve disorder. Neurology **41:** 1021–1024.
19. GUTMANN, L. & L. GUTMANN. 1996. Axonal channelopathies: an evolving concept in the pathogenesis of peripheral nerve disorders. Neurology **47:** 18–21.
20. NEWSOM-DAVIS, J. & K.R. MILLS. 1993. Immunological associations of acquired neuromyotonia (Isaacs' syndrome): report of five cases and literature review. Brain **116**(part 2)**:** 453–469.
21. GUTMANN, L., J.G. TELLERS & S. VERNINO. 2001. Persistent facial myokymia associated with K(+) channel antibodies. Neurology **57:** 1707–1708.
22. MORVAN, A. 1890. De la choree fibrillaire. Gaz. Hebdomad. Med. Chirurg. **27:** 173–200.
23. HART, I.K., P. MADDISON, J. NEWSOM-DAVIS *et al.* 2002. Phenotypic variants of autoimmune peripheral nerve hyperexcitability. Brain **125:** 1887–1895.
24. LEE, E.K., R.A. MASELLI, W.G. ELLIS & M.A. AGIUS. 1998. Morvan's fibrillary chorea: a paraneoplastic manifestation of thymoma. J. Neurol. Neurosurg. Psychiatry **65:** 857–862.

25. HEIDENREICH, F. & A. VINCENT. 1998. Antibodies to ion-channel proteins in thymoma with myasthenia, neuromyotonia, and peripheral neuropathy. Neurology **50:** 1483–1485.
26. VERNINO, S., R.G. AUGER, A.M. EMSLIE-SMITH *et al.* 1999. Myasthenia, thymoma, presynaptic antibodies, and a continuum of neuromuscular hyperexcitability. Neurology **53:** 1233–1239.
27. EVOLI, A., M.M. LO, R. MARRA *et al.* 1999. Multiple paraneoplastic diseases associated with thymoma. Neuromuscul. Disord. **9:** 601–603.
28. MYGLAND, A., A. VINCENT, J. NEWSOM-DAVIS *et al.* 2000. Autoantibodies in thymoma-associated myasthenia gravis with myositis or neuromyotonia. Arch. Neurol. **57:** 527–531.
29. REEBACK, J., S. BENTON, M. SWASH & M.S. SCHWARTZ. 1979. Penicillamine-induced neuromyotonia. Br. Med. J. **1**(6176)**:** 1464–1465.
30. WALSH, J.C. 1976. Neuromyotonia: an unusual presentation of intrathoracic malignancy. J. Neurol. Neurosurg. Psychiatry **39:** 1086–1091.
31. CARESS, J.B., W.K. ABEND, D.C. PRESTON & E.L. LOGIGIAN. 1997. A case of Hodgkin's lymphoma producing neuromyotonia. Neurology **49:** 258–259.
32. SINHA, S., J. NEWSOM-DAVIS, K. MILLS *et al.* 1991. Autoimmune aetiology for acquired neuromyotonia (Isaacs' syndrome). Lancet **338:** 75–77.
33. SHILLITO, P., P.C. MOLENAAR, A. VINCENT *et al.* 1995. Acquired neuromyotonia: evidence for autoantibodies directed against K^+ channels of peripheral nerves. Ann. Neurol. **38:** 714–722.
34. NAGADO, T., K. ARIMURA, Y. SONODA *et al.* 1999. Potassium current suppression in patients with peripheral nerve hyperexcitability. Brain **122:** 2057–2066.
35. SONODA, Y., K. ARIMURA, A. KURONO *et al.* 1996. Serum of Isaacs' syndrome suppresses potassium channels in PC-12 cell lines. Muscle Nerve **19:** 1439–1446.
36. HART, I.K., C. WATERS, A. VINCENT *et al.* 1997. Autoantibodies detected to expressed K^+ channels are implicated in neuromyotonia. Ann. Neurol. **41:** 238–246.
37. LIGUORI, R., A. VINCENT, L. CLOVER *et al.* 2001. Morvan's syndrome: peripheral and central nervous system and cardiac involvement with antibodies to voltage-gated potassium channels. Brain **124:** 2417–2426.
38. KNOWLES, C.H., B. LANG, L. CLOVER *et al.* 2002. A role for autoantibodies in some cases of acquired non-paraneoplastic gut dysmotility. Scand. J. Gastroenterol. **37:** 166–170.
39. FUJII, N., A. FURUTA, H. YAMAGUCHI *et al.* 2001. Limbic encephalitis associated with recurrent thymoma: a postmortem study. Neurology **57:** 344–347.
40. BUCKLEY, C., J. OGER, L. CLOVER *et al.* 2001. Potassium channel antibodies in two patients with reversible limbic encephalitis. Ann. Neurol. **50:** 73–78.

Neuronal Ganglionic Acetylcholine Receptor Autoimmunity

STEVEN VERNINO[a] AND VANDA A. LENNON[a,b,c]

Departments of [a]Neurology, [b]Immunology, and [c]Laboratory Medicine and Pathology, Mayo Clinic, Rochester, Minnesota 55905, USA

ABSTRACT: We have developed and validated an assay to detect serum antibodies specific for the ganglionic AChR. The assay uses ganglionic AChR solubilized from membranes of the human neuroblastoma cell line (IMR-32) as antigen. The ganglionic AChR is radiolabeled by complexing with ^{125}I-epibatidine. Among patients with acquired dysautonomia, seropositivity is highly associated with the diagnosis of idiopathic or paraneoplastic autonomic neuropathy and can distinguish these disorders from other forms of autonomic dysfunction. Ganglionic AChR binding antibodies are detectable in 50% of patients with subacute autoimmune autonomic neuropathy (AAN). These patients often have a high antibody value (>0.2 nmol/L). Lower values (0.05–0.20 nmol/L) are found in ~10% of patients with limited AAN.

KEYWORDS: autonomic neuropathy; thymoma; gastrointestinal dysmotility; orthostatic hypotension

In patients with myasthenia gravis (MG), antibodies specific for the muscle nicotinic acetylcholine receptor (AChR) interfere with neuromuscular junction transmission.[1] Structurally similar neuronal AChRs are found throughout the central nervous system. Neuronal nicotinic AChRs are also expressed in the peripheral nervous system where they mediate fast synaptic transmission through autonomic ganglia in both the sympathetic and parasympathetic nervous systems. The ganglionic AChR contains the α3 neuronal AChR subunit, most commonly associated with the β4 subunit. Transgenic mice that are homozygous for null mutations in the α3 gene lack ganglionic AChR and have profound autonomic dysfunction.[2] By analogy with MG, autoantibodies specific for neuronal ganglionic AChR could disrupt cholinergic synaptic transmission in autonomic ganglia and lead to autonomic failure.

The syndrome now recognized as autoimmune autonomic neuropathy (AAN) is also known as idiopathic autonomic neuropathy, subacute autonomic neuropathy, or acute pandysautonomia. In its usual presentation, AAN presents as severe panautonomic failure that reaches peak deficit within 3 months and often within a few days or weeks.[3–5] The course is generally monophasic, with slow and incomplete recovery. Less commonly, patients have a chronic progressive course.[5] Sympathetic failure is

Address for correspondence: Steven Vernino, Department of Neurology, Mayo Clinic, 200 First Street SW, Rochester, MN 59905. Voice: 507-284-8726; fax: 507-284-1814.
verns@mayo.edu

Ann. N.Y. Acad. Sci. 998: 211–214 (2003). © 2003 New York Academy of Sciences.
doi: 10.1196/annals.1254.023

manifested as orthostatic hypotension and anhidrosis, and parasympathetic failure as dry mouth and eyes, sexual dysfunction, urinary retention, impaired pupillary light response, and fixed heart rate. Gastrointestinal dysmotility is common and may present as anorexia, early satiety, postprandial abdominal pain and vomiting, diarrhea, constipation, or intestinal pseudo-obstruction. Motor and sensory nerve abnormalities are minimal or absent. An identical presentation can occur in a paraneoplastic context with small-cell lung cancer or thymoma, but there are often accompanying elements of a subacute encephalomyeloneuropathy.[6]

The concept that AAN is an autoimmune disease was initially based on several observations: (1) clinical associations with lung cancer, Lambert-Eaton myasthenic syndrome, myasthenia gravis, and thymoma;[7,8] (2) clinical similarity to the acute autonomic disturbances that accompany Guillain-Barré syndrome;[8] (3) the high frequency of organ-specific autoantibodies (thyroid, gastric parietal cell, and glutamic acid decarboxylase antibodies) in patients with subacute autonomic neuropathy; (4) commonly associated antecedent symptoms of a viral illness; (5) elevated spinal fluid protein; and (6) individual case reports of benefit from intravenous immune globulin therapy.[9,10]

We have developed and validated an assay to detect serum antibodies specific for the ganglionic AChR.[11] The assay uses ganglionic AChR solubilized from membranes of the human neuroblastoma cell line (IMR-32) as antigen, and this is radiolabeled by complexing with ^{125}I-epibatidine. Serum IgG and IgM antibodies that bind to this complex are precipitated by adding goat anti-human IgG/IgM.

Ganglionic AChR autoantibodies are not found in heathy control subjects. Among patients with acquired dysautonomia, seropositivity is highly associated with the diagnosis of idiopathic or paraneoplastic autonomic neuropathy and can distinguish these disorders from other forms of autonomic dysfunction (TABLE 1).[6] Ganglionic AChR binding antibodies are detectable in 50% of patients with subacute AAN. These patients often have a high antibody value (>0.2 nmol/L). Lower values

TABLE 1. Ganglionic receptor antibody frequency in patients with dysautonomia and other disorders

Diagnostic group	No. of patients tested	% seropositive
Autonomic disorders		
Subacute AAN	28	50
Paraneoplastic AAN	18	28
Postural tachycardia syndrome	20	10
Idiopathic gastrointestinal dysmotility	34	9
Diabetic autonomic neuropathy	18	11
Multiple system atrophy	10	0
Other disorders		
Lambert-Eaton syndrome	113	6
Myasthenia gravis without thymoma	62	0
Paraneoplastic disorders with thymoma	36	19
Paraneoplastic disorders with SCLC	69	3

NOTE: None of 150 healthy control subjects were seropositive for ganglionic AChR antibodies.

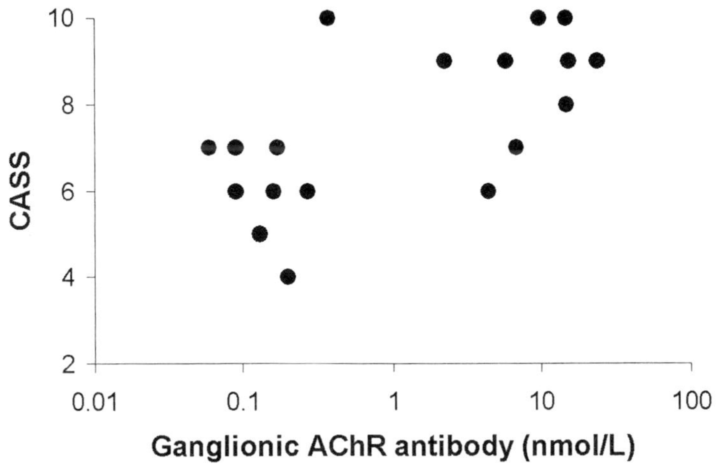

FIGURE 1. Serum ganglionic AChR antibody levels correlate with severity of dysautonomia.[5] Antibody values for individual patients are plotted on a logarithmic scale. The composite autonomic severity score (CASS)[15] is significantly correlated with antibody level ($p < 0.01$, Spearman).

(0.05–0.20 nmol/L) are found in ~10% of patients with limited AAN, including those with isolated gastrointestinal dysmotility, diabetic autonomic neuropathy, or postural tachycardia syndrome.

Serum levels of ganglionic AChR binding antibody are significantly correlated with severity of autonomic dysfunction (FIG. 1) and, on follow-up testing, the ganglionic AChR antibody level correlates with changes in clinical and laboratory indices of autonomic dysfunction.[6] Improvement in autonomic function is usually associated with a decline in antibody levels. These findings suggest that ganglionic AChR antibodies are direct pathophysiologic effectors of autonomic dysfunction.

Ganglionic AChR antibodies are found (usually at lower levels) in 5–10% of patients with other paraneoplastic neurological disorders related to thymoma and small-cell lung cancer (including Lambert-Eaton syndrome) (TABLE 1). These antibodies are also found in patients with acquired disorders of neuromuscular hyperexcitability such as Isaacs' syndrome (acquired neuromyotonia).[12] About 50% of patients with neuromyotonia have antibodies specific for α-dendrotoxin-sensitive voltage-gated potassium channels. A subset of those without detectable potassium channel antibodies are seropositive for ganglionic AChR antibodies (TABLE 2). It is possible that ganglionic AChR antibodies are also pathophysiologically important in neuromuscular hyperexcitability. Presynaptic neuronal nicotinic AChRs found at the motor nerve terminal have been reported to be α3-immunoreactive.[13] These receptors may modulate neuromuscular function through both positive and negative feedback regulation of ACh release.[14] Antibody-induced loss of inhibitory presynaptic regulation could give rise to an inappropriate increase in action potential–induced motor nerve terminal activity.

TABLE 2. Autoantibodies in patients with neuromuscular hyperexcitability[12]

Diagnosis	No. of patients	No. (%) of antibody positive		
		VGKC antibody	Ganglionic AChR antibody	Either antibody
Neuromyotonia	35	19 (54%)	5 (14%)	22 (63%)
Cramp-fasciculation syndrome	32	5 (16%)	2 (6%)	7 (22%)
Acquired rippling muscle syndrome	5	1 (20%)	1 (20%)	2 (40%)

ACKNOWLEDGMENTS

This work was supported by K08NS02247 and the Mayo Clinic Cancer Center.

REFERENCES

1. DRACHMAN, D. 1994. Myasthenia gravis. N. Engl. J. Med. **330:** 1797–1810.
2. XU, W. *et al.* 1999. Megacystis, mydriasis, and ion channel defect in mice lacking the alpha3 neuronal nicotinic acetylcholine receptor. Proc. Natl. Acad. Sci. USA **96:** 5746–5751.
3. YOUNG, R.R. *et al.* 1975. Pure pan-dysautonomia with recovery. Brain **98:** 613–636.
4. SUAREZ, G.A. *et al.* 1994. Idiopathic autonomic neuropathy: clinical, neurophysiologic, and follow-up studies on 27 patients. Neurology **44:** 1675–1682.
5. KLEIN, C.M. *et al.* 2003. The spectrum of autoimmune autonomic neuropathies. Ann. Neurol. **53:** 752–758.
6. VERNINO, S. *et al.* 2000. Autoantibodies to ganglionic acetylcholine receptors in autoimmune autonomic neuropathies. N. Engl. J. Med. **343:** 847–855.
7. VERNINO, S., W.P. CHESHIRE & V.A. LENNON. 2001. Myasthenia gravis with autoimmune autonomic neuropathy. Autonom. Neurosci. **88:** 187–192.
8. LOW, P.A. & J.G. MCLEOD. 1997. The autonomic neuropathies. *In* Clinical Autonomic Disorders, pp. 397–401. Little, Brown. Boston.
9. SMIT, A. *et al.* 1997. Unusual recovery from acute panautonomic neuropathy after immunoglobulin therapy. Mayo Clin. Proc. **72:** 333–335.
10. VENKATARAMAN, S., M. ALEXANDER & C. GNANAMUTHU. 1998. Postinfectious pandysautonomia with complete recovery after intravenous immunoglobulin therapy. Neurology **51:** 1764–1765.
11. VERNINO, S., T. KRYZER & V. LENNON. 2002. Autoantibodies in autoimmune autonomic neuropathies and neuromuscular hyperexcitability disorders. *In* Manual of Clinical Laboratory Immunology, pp. 1013–1017. ASM Press. Washington, D.C.
12. VERNINO, S. & V.A. LENNON. 2002. Ion channel and striational antibodies define a continuum of autoimmune neuromuscular hyperexcitability. Muscle Nerve **26:** 702–707.
13. TSUNEKI, H., I. KIMURA & K. DEZAKI. 1995. Immunohistochemical localization of neuronal nicotinic receptor subtypes at the pre- and postjunctional sites in mouse diaphragm muscle. Neurosci. Lett. **196:** 13–16.
14. FU, W-M. & J-J. LIU. 1997. Regulation of acetylcholine release by presynaptic nicotinic receptors at developing neuromuscular synapses. Mol. Pharmacol. **51:** 390–398.
15. LOW, P.A. 1993. Composite autonomic scoring scale for the laboratory quantification of generalized autonomic failure. Mayo Clin. Proc. **68:** 748–752.

Humoral and Cellular Autoimmune Responses in Stiff Person Syndrome

TOBIAS LOHMANN,[a] MARCO LONDEI,[b] MOHAMMED HAWA,[c] AND R. DAVID G. LESLIE[c]

[a]*Department of Medicine I, University of Erlangen, 91054 Erlangen, Germany*

[b]*Kennedy Institute of Rheumatology, London W6 8LW, United Kingdom*

[c]*St. Bartholomew's Hospital, London EC1A 7BE, United Kingdom*

ABSTRACT: Stiff person syndrome (SPS) is a chronic autoimmune disease associated with humoral and cellular immune responses to glutamic acid decarboxylase (GAD) 65. Another chronic autoimmune disease, type 1 diabetes (T1D), is also associated with autoimmune responses to this antigen, but T1D patients develop SPS only extremely rarely and only a third of SPS patients develop T1D (mostly mild manifestations in adulthood). In a previous study, we described important differences between T1D and SPS in the autoimmune response to GAD 65: (1) T cells of SPS patients recognize epitopes in the middle of GAD 65 (amino residues 81–171 and 313–403), whereas patients with T1D preferentially recognize another middle (161–243) and a C-terminal region (473–555); and (2) GAD antibodies (Abs) were nearly exclusively of the Th1-associated IgG1 type in T1D, whereas SPS patients had both Th1- and Th2-associated IgG4 and IgE GAD Abs. These differences were not simply related to different HLA alleles. Fine epitope mapping revealed further distinct T cell epitopes in both diseases despite similar HLA background. Therefore, a single autoantigen can elicit different immune responses causing distinct chronic autoimmune diseases possibly related to a Th1 or Th2 bias of the disease.

KEYWORDS: stiff person syndrome; autoimmune disease; type 1 diabetes; glutamic acid decarboxylase 65

INTRODUCTION

The synthesizing enzyme for the inhibitory neurotransmitter γ-amino butyric acid (GABA), glutamic acid decarboxylase (GAD), exists in two major isoforms, GAD 65 and 67.[1,2] Both proteins are encoded by two nonallelic genes and share homology that differs remarkably in different parts of the molecules. Both isoforms are expressed in human neurons, pancreatic beta cells, and other neuroendocrine tissues, but GAD 65 seems to be the major isoform expressed in human pancreatic beta cells.[3] Autoantibodies to GAD 65 and GAD 67 have been detected in the sera of

Address for correspondence: Tobias Lohmann, Department of Medicine I, University of Erlangen, Ulmenweg 18, 91054 Erlangen, Germany. Voice: +49-9131-85-35229; fax: +49-9131-85-35231.

tobias.lohmann@med1.imed.uni-erlangen.de

Ann. N.Y. Acad. Sci. 998: 215–222 (2003). **© 2003 New York Academy of Sciences.**
doi: 10.1196/annals.1254.024

patients with type 1 diabetes (T1D) and a rare neurological disorder, stiff man or stiff person syndrome (SPS).[2,4] SPS is diagnosed in less than one in one million of the general population and is clinically characterized by stiffness of axial muscles and painful muscular spasms.[5] T1D develops in about 30% of the patients with SPS,[6,7] mainly as mild manifestations in adulthood. GAD is implicated as an important autoantigen in T1D.[8] SPS is caused by an impairment of GABA-ergic neurotransmission in the central nervous system, possibly caused directly by the anti-GAD immune attack.[9,10]

Islet cell antibodies (ICA) are a feature of T1D, occurring in the sera of approximately 80% of newly diagnosed cases. ICA recognize a number of different antigens including GAD, insulin, and protein tyrosine phosphatases. ICA are polyclonal and, in general, are restricted to IgG1 isotype belonging to the IgG subclass.[11] The isotype profile of antigen-specific antibodies has been shown to reflect T cell (Th1 or Th2) effector functions in animal models.[12] Interferon-γ-dependent antibody isotypes in mice are mainly IgG2a and IgG3 (human homologues probably IgG1 and IgG3), which reflects a Th1 response, while a Th2 response is predominantly IgE or IgG1 (human homologues probably IgE and IgG4). Restriction of ICA to IgG1 in IDDM in humans may thus represent a Th1 dominant immune response. ICA are also a feature of SPS; in these patients, the antibodies are predominantly attributable to GAD antibodies. The isotype profile of antigen-specific antibodies, including GAD antibodies, in T1D and SPS has not been characterized. However, monoclonal antibodies isolated from T1D patients are usually of the IgG1 isotype.[13] We therefore established assays for the isotypes of GAD antibodies and estimated them in SPS and T1D patients.

Furthermore, distinct dominant epitopes of GAD have been described for GAD specific autoantibodies in T1D and SPS.[6,7,14–16] It was hypothesized that the different recognition of GAD by the immune system may explain the low penetration of T1D in SPS.[7] Our group[17] and others[18] have described dominant T cell epitopes of GAD in T1D, but nothing was known about the T cell epitopes to GAD in SPS. In this study, we investigated 8 patients with SPS (3 of them were diabetic) for their reactivity to overlapping synthetic peptides covering completely GAD 65 and 67 and compared the results to our described data on T cell reactivity to GAD peptides in T1D and healthy controls.[17]

METHODS

Fourteen patients with clinical and neurological features of SPS (7 of them had T1D) were selected for this study. The diagnosis was confirmed independently by a neurologist and included typical clinical symptoms, electromyogram findings, clinical improvement by diazepam, and mostly GAD antibodies. Mean age was 45 years (range 23–67; 4 men and 10 women). All patients had no other diseases beside SPS or T1D. GAD-antibody responses of these SPS patients were compared to 17 T1D patients (mean age: 23 years; range: 3–45 years). Their duration of diabetes was similar to that of the 7 SPS patients with diabetes (3–7 years). Eight of the SPS patients were compared for T cell responses to GAD with the T1D patients (<5 years from diagnosis) and 10 healthy controls described elsewhere.[17] Two SPS patients with T cell responses to region 81–171 and 1 patient for region 313–403 were studied again for responses to single peptides of these regions.

Antibody Assays

In vitro transcribed and translated GAD labeled with ^{35}S-methionine was used as the antigen, prepared as previously described.[19] The isotype-specific GAD antibody assay is described in detail elsewhere.[20]

To establish a cutoff for positivity, the results were calculated in 37 control subjects of similar age and sex ratio: (1) as the mean cpm for each antibody isotype and (2) as the mean cpm for all antibody isotypes. Positive results in patients were defined as a cpm value greater than 3 standard deviations (SD) above the mean of the control levels using both methods.

T Cell Assays

All 15-mers overlapping by 11 residues covering both GAD 65 and 67 completely were synthesized by the multipin method.[21] Peptides were cleaved in 0.05 mol/L HEPES, pH 7.6–7.8, in 40% acetonitrile (HPLC grade) in water; the purity of peptides was confirmed by HPLC to be >80%. The peptides were used pooled (20 per pool) or as single peptides in a final concentration of 2 μg/mL in proliferation assays. Negative control wells contained the same dilution of buffer without peptide. Both toxic and mitogenic effects of the peptide pools were excluded. Again, T cell proliferation assays are described in detail elsewhere.[17]

The number of positive wells for each antigen was calculated;[21] positive wells exceeded the mean cpm plus 3 SD (pools) or plus 2 SD (single peptides) of 32 negative control wells. Frequencies of positive responses significant at the $p < 0.0025$ level are reported.[21] The pool with the most positive wells was regarded as the "dominant" pool for each individual. Fisher's exact test was used to analyze differences between SPS, T1D, and control patients ($p < 0.05$ was considered significant). Analysis was only done when a dominant pool was found in 2 or more SPS patients and in 3 or more T1D patients.

HLA typing of SPS patients was performed using antibodies provided by the Xth HLA-Tissue Typing Workshop. Furthermore, HLA-DQ subtyping was performed by the single-step allele-specific polymerase chain reaction as described elsewhere.[22]

RESULTS

Antibodies to GAD were detected in 11 of 17 T1D patients and 11 of 14 SPS patients. Only GAD antibody–positive patients are analyzed for isotype responses (11 T1D and 11 SPS patients). GAD IgG1 was the most prevalent isotype both in T1D and SPS patients. GAD isotypes other than IgG1 were detected in 0 of 11 T1D patients, but in 8 of 11 SPS patients; thus, these antibodies were more prevalent in SPS than in the T1D patients (Fisher's exact $p = 0.003$). IgG4 or IgE isotypes were found in 5 of 11 SPS compared to none of 11 T1D patients ($p = 0.012$). Of the 7 SPS patients with diabetes, 5 had an antibody profile similar to that found in T1D (i.e., IgG1, but no IgG4 or IgE), but the other 2 patients had IgG4 and IgE GAD antibodies similar to the profile in 3 of 7 patients without diabetes. GAD 65 isotypes were not related to disease duration or HLA type in SPS and T1D patients.

T cell responses to pools of overlapping peptides of GAD 65 in SPS patients were compared to groups of T1D patients and healthy controls described previously.[17] The experimental design (including media or plastics used) and evaluation were absolutely identical to our previous work to get optimal comparibility of the data. Six of 8 SPS patients, 12 of 17 T1D patients, and 9 of 10 controls had significant T cell responses to GAD 65 peptide pools; only these probands with T cell responses were analyzed for the comparison of epitope specificity of the T cell response. In contrast to T1D patients or healthy controls, the T cell response to GAD 65 peptides in SPS patients was mainly restricted to two regions of GAD 65, that is, 81–171 and 313–403, in the middle of the molecule. Region 81–171 was dominantly recognized in 3 of 6 SPS patients compared to 0 of 12 T1D patients ($p < 0.025$) or 1 of 9 healthy controls ($p > 0.1$). It should be stated that region 81–171 was also recognized in 4 of 20 long-term T1D patients (>5 years after diagnosis; unpublished data). Region 313–403 was dominantly recognized in 3 of 6 SPS patients compared to 1 of 12 T1D patients ($p < 0.05$) or 1 of 9 healthy controls ($p > 0.1$).

In our previous report,[17] we have described the region 473–555 of GAD 65 as immunodominant in T1D since the T cells of 6 of 12 T1D patients responded dominantly to this region. In our present study, none of the 6 SPS patients showed a T cell response to this region ($p < 0.05$). Furthermore, the T cells of 5 of 9 healthy controls recognized region 161–243 in a dominant manner[17] and, again, no significant T cell reactivity to this region was observed in SPS patients ($p < 0.05$).

In the same study,[17] 8 of 15 T1D patients and 3 of 10 healthy controls recognized dominantly region 153–243 of GAD 67, but no significant differences between healthy controls and T1D patients were found for T cell reactivity to GAD 67 pools. In this study, T cells of 6 of 8 SPS patients recognized GAD 65 and of 3 of 8 SPS patients GAD 67 peptide pools. Therefore, the T cell response in SPS can be directed to both GAD 65 and GAD 67, but also for GAD 67 the recognized epitopes in SPS patients differed from those in T1D patients and healthy controls (e.g., 73–163 or 465–555 in SPS patients and 153–243 in T1D patients and controls).

For 2 SPS patients, we were able to decode the GAD T cell response to single epitopes of the region 81–171. Remarkably, 2 peptides (101–115 and 145–159) were recognized by T cells of both patients, despite completely different HLA types. The latter epitope (145–159) overlaps a GAD 65 epitope recognized by a T cell line from a recent onset T1D patient, which was restricted by DR2.[23] The dominant T cell epitope in SPS patients, however, seems to be located in the middle of this region (113–127 for patient 1; 117–135 for patient 2). Peptides 113–127 and 117–135 mainly overlap a peptide (115–127) described as immunogenic in a DR401 transgenic mouse model[24] and, indeed, 1 patient had the DR401 haplotype. Furthermore, peptide 88–99 has been described as an immunodominant DRB1*0101 restricted epitope in a T1D patient.[25] This peptide was found in our study as a subdominant epitope for 1 patient who also had the haplotype DRB1*0101. One patient was tested again for responses to single peptides of region 313–403 and her T cells responded to an array of peptides in this region (337–351, 349–363, 369–383, 385–403), including the binding site of pyridoxal phosphate (390–402) and an epitope (339–352) described by others for SPS T cells[26] and showing cross-reactivity to a peptide of cytomegalovirus.[27]

DISCUSSION

Our observations on GAD antibody isotypes suggest a bias in T1D patients towards a Th1-type immune response, which was not evident in the SPS patients. In contrast, SPS patients showed evidence for spreading of the immune response to IgG isotypes other than IgG1, including IgG4 and IgE, associated with a Th2 response. Such a Th2 response has been associated with at least preliminary protection from islet cell destruction,[28] while a bias to Th1 immunity in the cytokine network of T1D has been described already by others.[29] Possibly, such a Th2 bias of islet cell autoimmunity is correlated to the phase of "benign autoimmunity" in NOD mice, in contrast to the Th1-biased "malignant autoimmunity" causing islet cell destruction and full blown diabetes.[30] The reason for the Th1/Th2 bias in autoimmune disease may have several possible explanations. It might be due to the nature of the antigen, abnormalities in immunoregulation, or genetic factors that influence class switching.

The differences in epitope recognition between SPS patients and T1D patients or controls may simply reflect differences in HLA types rather than disease specificity. However, 2 SPS patients had the T1D-related HLA haplotype DR4/DQ0302 highly correlated with T cell responses to GAD 473–555 in T1D in our previous study,[17] but the T cells of these SPS patients still responded preferentially to GAD 81–171. In this region 81–171, we found responses to peptides of GAD 65 described as immunogenic in the HLA transgenic mice, supporting the feasibility of our approach for epitope decoding. Some epitopes detected in region 81–171 had been described as epitopes of T cell lines of T1D patients of the same HLA haplotype, but were rather subdominant epitopes in our SPS patients. However, we cannot completely exclude HLA dependence of T cell epitope specificity because it is impossible to match SPS and T1D patients for HLA since the HLA linkage differs between these diseases.[31]

Region 313–403 of GAD 65 was recognized by 3 of 8 of our SPS patients and contains 2 linear epitopes of GAD antibodies (residues 354–368 and 390–402) described by others.[7] Moreover, region 390–402 contains the binding site of the GAD cofactor, pyridoxal 5′-phosphate, and an immune attack against this region has been proposed as a possible pathogenetic mechanism in SPS.[6] Remarkably, the 3 SPS patients with dominant T cell responses to region 313–403 elicited very high GAD antibody titers and a broad antibody response with isotypes other than IgG1. Larger studies about T cell responses to GAD epitopes are necessary to define a possible link between T and B cell epitopes in SMS since the existence of linear GAD antibody epitopes in SPS,[6,7] in contrast to the preferentially conformational GAD antibody epitopes in T1D,[14] may offer such a direct link.

The comparison of immune responses to GAD between SPS and T1D patients or healthy controls is hampered by the small number of SPS patients available (SPS is diagnosed in $<1/10^6$ of the general population).[7] Nevertheless, regions 81–171 and 313–403 of GAD 65 seem to be recognized by T cells of a remarkable fraction of SPS patients, while the region 473–555 of GAD 65 was never recognized in SPS patients in contrast to T1D patients, although 3 of 8 SPS patients had developed T1D. There may be different explanations for the absence of T1D in most of the SPS patients: (1) T1D is progressing very slowly in these patients such that the future development of T1D in these individuals cannot be excluded; (2) differences in HLA types as proposed by Pugliese[31] are responsible for T1D development; or (3) a Th2-like immune response protects SPS patients from development of T1D. Supporting

TABLE 1. T cell autoimmunity against a single autoantigen, GAD65, in two distinct diseases, SPS and T1D

	Type 1 diabetes (T1D)	Stiff person syndrome (SPS)
Dominant T cell	477–555	88–171
Epitopes	161–243	313–403
GAD-Ab isotypes	IgG1 (IgG3)	IgG1 + IgG4 + IgE
Th1/Th2 bias	pure Th1	mixed Th1/Th2
Islet outcome	"Malignant" islet cell destruction	"Benign" islet inflammation

the second possibility, some SPS patients not developing T1D had HLA DQ6 subtypes that were proposed as protective against T1D in SPS patients.[31] In support of the third outcome, all 3 patients with GAD antibody isotypes suggestive for a Th2-type immune response were free of diabetes. This is in line with numerous reports on a defective Th2 immune response in T1D.[29,32–34]

In summary, the isotype profile of the GAD antibody response and the dominant T cell epitopes of GAD 65 and GAD 67 differed between SPS and T1D. Therefore, the immune response to a single autoantigen may be qualitatively and/or quantitatively different, resulting in distinct or only partially overlapping autoimmune disease entities (TABLE 1). These differences may explain the low penetration of T1D in SPS and, more importantly, the Th1- or Th2-like preference of the immune attack in both diseases.[35] Since the switch of a Th1- to a Th2-like immune response was proposed as a therapeutic approach in T1D,[36] the differences in epitope recognition between SPS and T1D may give clues about the conditions that prime the different immune reactions to GAD 65 and may possibly be exploited in therapeutic interventions. On the other hand, the development of SPS has to be considered as a possible hazard in such interventions.

ACKNOWLEDGMENTS

This work was supported by grants of the Deutsche Forschungsgemeinschaft (Lo 532) and the Deutsche Diabetesgesellschaft (to T. Lohmann), Diabetes UK, Diabetic Twin Research Trust, Action Research and the Joint Research Board of St. Bartholomew's Hospital (to R. D. G. Leslie), and the Eli Lilly Award (to M. Hawa).

REFERENCES

1. BU, D-F., M.G. ERLANDER, B.C. HITZ *et al.* 1989. Two human glutamate decarboxylases, 65-kD and 67-kD GAD, are each encoded by a single gene. Proc. Natl. Acad. Sci. USA **89:** 2115–2119.
2. BAEKKESKOV, S., H-J. AANSTOOT, S. CHRISTGAU *et al.* 1990. Identification of the 64 K autoantigen in insulin-dependent diabetes mellitus as the GABA-synthesizing enzyme glutamic acid decarboxylase. Nature **347:** 151–156.
3. HAGOPIAN, W.A., B. MICHELSEN, A.E. KARLSEN *et al.* 1993. Autoantibodies in IDDM primarily recognize the 65,000-M_r rather than the 67,000-M_r isoform of glutamic acid decarboxylase. Diabetes **42:** 631–636.

4. SOLIMENA, M., F. FOLLI, S. DENIS-DONINI *et al.* 1988. Autoantibodies to glutamic acid decarboxylase in a patient with stiff-man syndrome, epilepsy, and type-1 diabetes. N. Engl. J. Med. **318:** 1012–1020.
5. MOERSCH, F.P. & H.W. WOLTMAN. 1957. Progressive fluctuating muscular rigidity and spasm ("stiff-man" syndrome): report of a case and some observations in 13 other cases. Mayo Clin. Proc. **31:** 421–427.
6. LI, L., W.A. HAGOPIAN, H.R. BRASHEAR *et al.* 1994. Identification of autoantibody epitopes of glutamic acid decarboxylase in stiff-man syndrome patients. J. Immunol. **152:** 930–934.
7. KIM, J., M. NAMCHUK, T. BUGAWAN *et al.* 1994. Higher autoantibody levels and recognition of a linear NH_2-terminal epitope in the autoantigen GAD_{65} distinguish stiff-man syndrome from insulin-dependent diabetes mellitus. J. Exp. Med. **180:** 595–606.
8. YOON, J.W., C.S. YOON, H.W. LIM *et al.* 1999. Control of autoimmune diabetes in NOD mice by GAD expression or suppression in beta cells. Science **284:** 1183–1187.
9. SOLIMENA, M., F. FOLLI, R. APARISI *et al.* 1990. Autoantibodies to GABA-ergic neurons and pancreatic beta cells in stiff-man syndrome. N. Engl. J. Med. **322:** 1555–1560.
10. DINKEL, K., H.M. MEINCK, K.M. JURY *et al.* 1998. Inhibition of gamma-aminobutyric acid synthesis by glutamic acid decarboxylase autoantibodies in stiff-man syndrome. Ann. Neurol. **44:** 194–201.
11. MILLWARD, B.A., M.J. HUSSAIN, M. PEAKMAN *et al.* 1988. Characterisation of islet cell antibody in insulin dependent diabetes: evidence for IgG1 subclass restriction and polyclonality. Clin. Exp. Immunol. **71:** 353–366.
12. ABBAS, A.K., K.M. MURPHY & A. SHER. 1996. Functional diversity of helper T lymphocytes. Nature **383:** 787–793.
13. MADEC, A-M., F. ROUSSET, S. HO *et al.* 1996. Four IgG anti-islet human monoclonal antibodies isolated from a type 1 diabetes patient recognize distinct epitopes of glutamic acid decarboxylase. J. Immunol. **156:** 3541–3549.
14. RICHTER, W., Y. SHI & S. BAEKKESKOV. 1993. Autoreactive epitopes defined by diabetes-associated human monoclonal antibodies are localized in the middle and C-terminal domains of the smaller form of glutamate decarboxylase. Proc. Natl. Acad. Sci. USA **90:** 2832–2836.
15. BUTLER, M.H., M. SOLIMENA, R. DIRKX *et al.* 1993. Identification of a dominant epitope of glutamic acid decarboxylase (GAD-65) recognized by autoantibodies in stiff-man syndrome. J. Exp. Med. **178:** 2097–2106.
16. BJÖRK, E., L.A. VELLOSO, O. KÄMPE & F.A. KARLSSON. 1993. GAD autoantibodies in IDDM, stiff-man syndrome, and autoimmune polyendocrine syndrome type I recognize different epitopes. Diabetes **43:** 161–165.
17. LOHMANN, T., R.D.G. LESLIE, M. HAWA *et al.* 1994. Immunodominant epitopes of glutamic acid decarboxylase 65 and 67 in insulin-dependent diabetes mellitus. Lancet **343:** 1607–1608.
18. ATKINSON, M.A., M.A. BOWMAN, L. CAMPBELL *et al.* 1994. Cellular immunity to a determinant common to glutamate decarboxylase and Coxsackie virus in insulin-dependent diabetes. J. Clin. Invest. **94:** 2125–2129.
19. HAWA, M., R. ROWE, M.S. LAN *et al.* 1997. Value of antibodies to islet protein tyrosine phosphatase–like molecule in predicting type 1 diabetes. Diabetes **46:** 1270–1275.
20. HAWA, M.I., D. FAVA, F. MEDICI *et al.* 2000. Antibodies to IA2 and GAD65 in type 1 and type 2; isotype restriction and polyclonality. Diab. Care **23:** 228–233.
21. REECE, J.C., H.M. GEYSEN & S.J. RODDA. 1993. Mapping the major human T helper epitopes of tetanus toxin. J. Immunol. **151:** 6175–6184.
22. PICARD, J. 1993. Single-step allele-specific polymerase chain reaction HLA-DQ subtyping using ARMS primers. Hum. Immunol. **38:** 115–122.
23. ENDL, J., H. OTTO, G. JUNG *et al.* 1997. Identification of naturally processed T cell epitopes from glutamic acid decarboxylase presented in the context of HLA-DR alleles by T lymphocytes of recent onset IDDM patients. J. Clin. Invest. **99:** 2405–2415.
24. WICKER, L.S., S.L. CHEN, G.T. NEPOM *et al.* 1996. Naturally processed T cell epitopes from human glutamic acid decarboxylase identified using mice transgenic for the type 1 diabetes–associated human MHC class II allele, DRB1*0401. J. Clin. Invest. **98:** 2597–2603.

25. BACH, J-M., H. OTTO, G.T. NEPOM *et al.* 1997. High affinity presentation of an autoantigenic peptide in type 1 diabetes by an HLA class II protein encoded in a haplotype protecting from disease. J. Autoimmun. **10:** 375–386.
26. SCHLOOT, N.C., M.C. BATSTRA, G. DUINKERKEN *et al.* 1999. GAD65-reactive T cells in a non-diabetic stiff-man syndrome patient. J. Autoimmun. **12:** 289–296.
27. HIEMSTRA, H.S., N.C. SCHLOOT, P.A. VAN VEELEN *et al.* 2001. Cytomegalovirus in autoimmunity: T cell crossreactivity to viral antigen and autoantigen glutamic acid decarboxylase. Proc. Natl. Acad. Sci. USA **98:** 3988–3991.
28. TIAN, J. & D.L. KAUFMAN. 1998. Attenuation of inducible Th2 immunity with autoimmune disease progression. J. Immun. **161:** 5399–5403.
29. KALLMANN, B.A., M. HUTHER, M. TUBES *et al.* 1997. Systemic bias of cytokine production toward cell-mediated immune regulation in IDDM and toward humoral immunity in Graves' disease. Diabetes **46:** 237–243.
30. DILTS, S.M. & K.J. LAFFERTY. 1999. Autoimmune diabetes: the involvement of benign and malignant autoimmunity. J. Autoimmun. **12:** 229–232.
31. PUGLIESE, A., R. GIANANI, G.S. EISENBARTH *et al.* 1994. Genetics of susceptibility and resistance to insulin-dependent diabetes in stiff-man syndrome. Lancet **344:** 1027–1028.
32. KUKREJA, A., G. COST, J. MARKER *et al.* 2002. Multiple immuno-regulatory defects in type-1 diabetes. J. Clin. Invest. **109:** 131–140.
33. RABINOVITCH, A. 1994. Immunoregulatory and cytokine imbalances in the pathogenesis of IDDM: therapeutic intervention by immunostimulation? Diabetes **44:** 859–862.
34. LOHMANN, T., S. LAUE, U. NIETZSCHMANN *et al.* 2002. Reduced expression of Th1 associated chemokine receptors on peripheral blood lymphocytes at diagnosis of type 1 diabetes. Diabetes **51:** in press.
35. ELLIS, T.M. & M.A. ATKINSON. 1996. The clinical significance of an autoimmune response against glutamic acid decarboxylase. Nat. Med. **2:** 148–153.
36. LIBLAU, R.S., S.M. SINGER & H.O. MCDEVITT. 1995. TH1 and TH2 CD4+ T cells in the pathogenesis of organ-specific autoimmune diseases. Immunol. Today **16:** 34–38.

The Role of Thymomas in the Development of Myasthenia Gravis

ALEXANDER MARX, HANS KONRAD MÜLLER-HERMELINK,
AND PHILIPP STRÖBEL

Institute of Pathology, University of Würzburg, D-97080 Würzburg, Germany

ABSTRACT: Thymic pathology occurs in 80–90% of myasthenia gravis patients. Significant associations between different thymic alterations and clinical findings are discussed. To highlight peculiarities in thymoma-associated myasthenia gravis, we briefly review myasthenia gravis associated with thymic lymphofollicular hyperplasia (TFH) and thymic atrophy.

KEYWORDS: thymoma; paraneoplastic myasthenia gravis; thymic atrophy; thymic lymphofollicular hyperplasia

INTRODUCTION

Seropositive myasthenia gravis (MG) is an autoimmune disease associated with autoantibodies to the nicotinic acetylcholine receptor (AChR) at the neuromuscular junction.[1,2] Thymoma-associated MG (paraneoplastic MG) is a seropositive subtype. Thymic pathology occurs in 80–90% of MG patients and is at its most subtle in seronegative MG.[3,4] There are significant associations between different thymic alterations and clinical findings[5–7] (TABLE 1). To highlight peculiarities in thymoma-associated MG, we briefly review MG associated with thymic lymphofollicular hyperplasia (TFH) and thymic atrophy.

HISTOPATHOLOGY OF THE THYMUS IN MG

TFH

TFH occurs in 70% of MG patients.[8] It is characterized by lymphoid follicles with or without germinal centers extending into perivascular spaces (PVSs). The basal membrane around PVSs is disrupted by lymphoid follicle development,[9] resulting in a fusion of the medulla (i.e., a part of the thymus parenchyma) and PVSs (thought to belong to the peripheral immune system).[10,11] Myoid cells are noninnervated myoblast- or myotube-like muscle cells that occur in the thymic medulla and most probably express both fetal and adult-type AChR[10,12–14] in the normal thymus

Address for correspondence: Alexander Marx, Institute of Pathology, University of Würzburg, Josef-Schneider-Strasse 2, D-97080 Würzburg, Germany. Voice: +49-931-201-47421; fax: +49-931-201-47505.
path031@mail.uni-wuerzburg.de *or* path036@mail.uni-wuerzburg.de

**Ann. N.Y. Acad. Sci. 998: 223–236 (2003). © 2003 New York Academy of Sciences.
doi: 10.1196/annals.1254.025**

TABLE 1. MG subtypes according to thymus pathology: correlation with clinical, epidemiological, and genetic findings[6,9,57–59,70,73,87]

	Hyperplasia[a]	Thymoma	Atrophy
Onset of symptoms: age (years)	10–39	15–80	>40
Sex (m:f)	1:3	1:1	2:1
HLA association	B8; DR3	(DR2, A24)	B7; DR2
CTLA-4 polymorphism (allele 104)	Normal	Increased	Normal
TNFA*T1/B*2 homozygosity	Rare	Very frequent	Frequent
TNFA*T2, TNFB1, TNFB*1, C4A*QO, C4B*1, DRB1*03	Frequent	Rare	Rare
Autoantibodies against:			
AChR	80%	>95%	90%
Striated muscle	10–20%	>90%	30–60%
Titin	<10%	>90%	30–40%
Ryanodine receptor	<5%	50–60%	20%
IL-12, IFN-α[b]	Infrequent	63–88%	Infrequent

[a]Early-onset MG.

[b]Cumulative percentage for nonthymoma MG patients was reported as 12%; the percentage in non-MG thymoma patients was reported as 30%.[56]

and in TFH. For unknown reasons, myoid cells in TFH are frequently located in intimate apposition to dendritic cells.[10] Such contacts are rare in the normal thymus. The thymic cortex in TFH shows the normal age-dependent morphology.

Thymomas in Paraneoplastic MG

Thymoma occurs in about 10% of MG patients. Thymomas are epithelial tumors of the thymus. Criteria for their histological diagnosis have recently been defined by the World Health Organization (WHO),[15,16] distinguishing type A (medullary), AB (mixed), B1 (organoid), B2 (cortical), B3 ("well differentiated thymic carcinoma"), and C (nonorganoid thymic carcinomas, e.g., with squamous cell differentiation resembling carcinomas in other parts of the body). Of note, only type A, AB, and B1–3 thymomas exhibit "thymus-like features", that is, they have the capacity to promote intratumorous T cell development (see below) and only these thymoma subtypes are associated with MG.[15,17] The genetic basis of thymoma oncogenesis is currently being elucidated.[18–20]

Thymus Atrophy in MG

Thymic atrophy is encountered in 10–20% of MG patients.[21] It is probably not the end-stage of TFH and, except from a slight increase in medullary B cells and dendritic cells,[22] the thymuses in these patients are equivalent to age-matched controls, including a normal number of myoid cells per thymic tissue area.[10,23]

PATHOGENIC CONCEPTS IN SEROPOSITIVE MG

Pathogenesis of MG in TFH

It is now generally accepted that TFH-associated MG results from an intrathymic pathogenesis with acetylcholine receptors (AChR) on thymic myoid cells being primarily involved as (triggering) autoantigen.[24] This concept is supported by the fact that a substantial percentage of autoantibodies in TFH/MG patients recognize the fetal AChR.[25] Fetal AChR (i.e., AChR with a γ- instead of an ε-subunit) is expressed only on thymic myoid cells and a few extraocular muscle fibers.[14,26–28] Extrathymic immunization with AChR can induce experimental autoimmune MG (EAMG), but does not elicit TFH.[29] By contrast, transplantation of TFH-affected thymus into SCID mice results in prolonged production of anti-AChR autoantibodies, showing that TFH contains all constituents of a self-sustaining autoimmune reaction.[30–32] Since myoid cells remain largely negative for MHC class II in MG, they are probably unable to prime AChR-reactive CD4+ T cells.[33] Therefore, dendritic cells may take up AChR from myoid cells and present AChR peptides to potentially AChR-reactive T cells (which occur as nontolerized T cells in the normal T cell repertoire[34–36]) and are increased in TFH.[37,38] If activated, such autoreactive T cells may provide help to B cells for autoantibody production both inside and outside the thymus.[39,40]

TFH occurs frequently in MG[41] and commonly in other autoimmune diseases,[21] but rarely in healthy persons.[42] Its actual trigger is not known, but a genetic contribution to the etiology of TFH-associated MG has been demonstrated for several polymorphic genes, such as MHC class I and II,[43,44] IL-1β,[45] TNFα,[46–48] IL-10,[49] and the AChR α-subunit.[50–52]

Pathogenesis of Thymoma-Associated MG

Distinct Autoantigens, Autoantibodies, Genetics, and Associated Autoimmune Paraneoplastic Syndromes in Thymoma Patients

There is a large body of evidence showing that the pathogenesis of thymoma-associated MG differs from LFH-associated MG.[7,17,53] There is a broad spectrum of paraneoplastic autoimmune diseases that occur either in isolation or associated with MG in thymoma (TABLE 2). In some of these paraneoplastic syndromes, the autoantigens and autoantibodies and their pathogenic relevance have been characterized. Some authors found no increase of nonmuscle autoimmune diseases in MG+ thymoma patients.[54,55] Antibodies to IL-12 and IFN-α might be involved in the pathogenesis of paraneoplastic MG and are sensitive markers to detect thymoma recurrences.[56] Titers of anti-ryanodine receptor antibodies significantly correlate with clinical MG severity,[57,58] while anti-titin autoantibodies as markers for disease severity are not unequivocally established.[58,59]

A major morphological difference between thymoma and TFH is the presence of AChR-expressing myoid cells in LFH, but their absence in thymomas. A striking functional difference is the absence (with few exceptions[60]) of autoantibody production inside thymomas.[61]

TABLE 2. Paraneoplastic diseases of presumed autoimmune pathogenesis reported to be associated with thymoma

Addison's disease	Panhypopituitarism
Agranulocytosis	Pernicious anemia
Alopecia areata	Polymyositis
Aplastic anemia	Pure red cell aplasia
Autoimmune colitis (GvHD-like)	Rheumatoid arthritis
Cushing's syndrome	Rippling muscle disease
Hemolytic anemia	Sarcoidosis
Hypogammaglobulinemia	Scleroderma
Intestinal pseudo-obstruction	Sensory motor neuropathy
Limbic encephalitis	Stiff-person syndrome
Myasthenia gravis	Systemic lupus erythematosus
Myocarditis	Thyroiditis
Neuromyotonia	

NOTE: In the majority of these diseases, the immunopathogenesis has not been resolved.

Shared Features among MG-Associated Thymomas

The pathogenesis of paraneoplastic MG might be heterogeneous in terms of various morphological and functional findings.[17] However, MG-associated thymomas share common features:

(1) All MG-associated thymomas are either type A, AB, or B1–3 thymomas according to the WHO classification and share morphological and functional features with the normal thymus. In particular, they provide signals for the homing of immature hematopoietic precursors and promote their differentiation to apparently mature T cells.[62–64] It is not yet clear whether a few type A thymomas might be an exception to this rule since they generate at most very few T cells. Anyway, thymic carcinomas (type C thymomas), thymic neuroendocrine tumors, or thymic lymphomas do not exhibit intratumorous thymopoiesis and are unassociated with MG.[17]

(2) MG-associated thymomas are enriched for autoreactive T cells with specificity for the AChR α-subunit and the ε-subunit.[64–68] There is strong evidence that they are, in part, generated by intratumorous, nontolerogenic thymopoiesis.[67,68]

(3) All MG-associated thymomas export naïve mature T cells[69,70] and it was hypothesized that export of autoreactive CD4+ T cells is of pathogenic relevance. This hypothesis was directly proven by Buckley and colleagues[71] using the quantification of T cell receptor excision circles (TRECs) in blood T cells, showing that both naïve CD4+ and CD8+ T cells are increased in thymoma patients with MG. Very recently, we found that MG-positive and MG-negative thymomas differ with respect to their capacity to complete intratumorous maturation of the CD4 T cell lineage, that is, to generate CD4+CD45RA+ naïve T cells.[70] Terminal CD4 T cell maturation is aborted in MG(–) thymomas, and MG(–) patients exhibit decreased naïve CD4 T cell levels in the peripheral blood (FIG. 1).

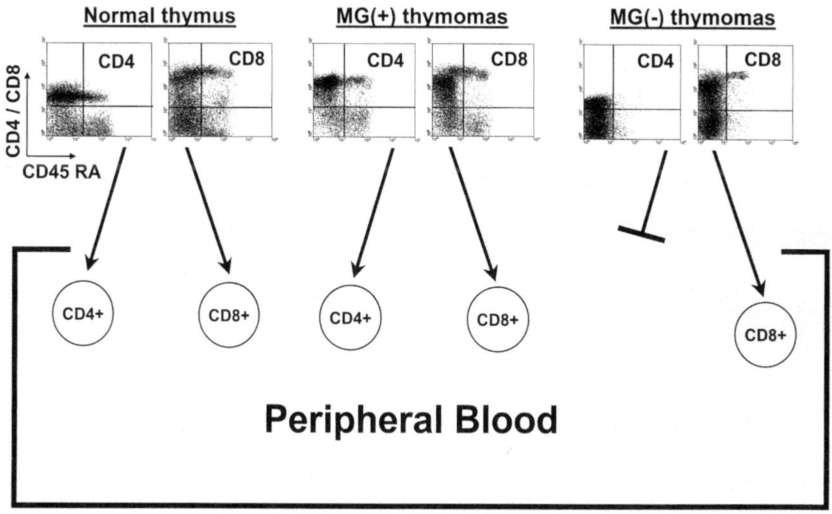

FIGURE 1. T cell export from thymus and thymomas to the blood in either MG(+) or MG(−) patients. Recent data suggest that the presence of MG is highly correlated with the capacity of a thymoma to complete intratumorous CD4 T cell maturation and to export the mature naïve T cells into the peripheral blood.

(4) Almost all MG-associated thymomas exhibit reduced expression of major histocompatibility complex (MHC) class II molecules on neoplastic epithelial cells.[72] In parallel, thymopoiesis in thymomas is quantitatively less efficient.[62,72] In addition, reduced MHC class II levels might be one reason why thymopoiesis in thymomas is not tolerogenic, that is, qualitatively abnormal (see below).[73]

(5) Concurrent autoimmunity against four apparently unrelated types of autoantigens is highly characteristic of paraneoplastic MG. These autoantigens are the AChR;[74] striational muscle antigens, including titin;[75] neuronal antigens;[76] and cytokines (IL-12, IFN-α).[56] Autoimmunity to the ryanodine receptor is also highly characteristic, but less frequent.[57,77] A common theme shared by MG-associated thymomas is the occurrence of mRNA coding for the autoantigens mentioned.[78–80] Except for the cytokines, however, there appears to be an apparent lack of the respective proteins,[77,81–84] although it is not excluded that translation into very small amounts of autoantigenic protein occurs, with potential implications for autoimmunization.[85–88]

Diverse Features among MG-Associated Thymomas

Apart from shared features among MG-associated thymomas, there are also features that are clearly diverse. One such feature is the abnormal (hyper)expression of proteins unrelated to the autoantigens, but expressing AChR-, titin- or ryanodine receptor-like epitopes[68,77,81,84] in neoplastic epithelial cells. These antigens occur in a subset of thymomas only. While the role of such "cross-reacting" proteins as specific immunogens has been seriously questioned recently,[68,89] it appears likely that abnormally expressed proteins might disturb the normal pool of endogenous peptides for presentation by MHC II proteins on thymoma epithelial cells.[73] Since quality and quantity of thymic endogenous epithelial cell peptides have a major impact on T cell selection and tolerance induction,[90–93] altered expression of endogeneous proteins in thymoma might be an indirect mechanism resulting in nontolerogenic intratumorous T cell development (see below).[17] Loss of heterozygosity (LOH) for the MHC locus in neoplastic epithelium mainly of MG-associated thymomas appears to be particularly frequent among MG(+) thymomas, although more cases have to be evaluated. This LOH may result in a MHC chimerism between the hemizygous thymoma epithelium (presumed to perform T cell selection) and the heterozygous intratumorous dendritic cells and the peripheral immune system. MHC chimerism might be one among other mechanisms of nontolerogenic T cell selection in a subset of thymomas.[17,19]

Finally, there is diversity as to the occurrence of activated mature T cells in thymomas. Some type A (medullary) thymomas, which are rarely associated with MG, have been found to harbor increased numbers of activated CD25+CD4+ mature T cells compared to the normal thymus.[63] By contrast, almost all type AB, B2, and B3 thymomas (that collectively are frequently MG-associated) were devoid of activated CD4+ T cells.[64,94] These findings argue for a different pathogenesis of paraneoplastic MG in type A versus type AB and B thymomas (see below).

PATHOGENETIC MODEL OF PARANEOPLASTIC MG

Taken together, the following findings await explanation by an appropriate pathogenic model:

(1) Paraneoplastic MG occurs in thymomas that contain immature T cells and promote their maturation.[17,73]

(2) Thymomas express reduced levels of MHC class II antigens[72,95–97] and loss of one MHC locus on chromosome 6p21 in many thymomas may result in a qualitatively altered MHC/peptide repertoire on thymoma epithelial cells.[19] Physiological MHC levels are particularly important for negative selection (tolerization) of the thymic T cell repertoire.[98,99]

(3) Thymoma epithelial cells often exhibit hyperexpression of endogenous proteins.

(4) MG-associated thymomas are enriched in autoreactive T cells,[38] which are probably generated in the thymoma, and are restricted to the minority HLA isotypes DP14 and DR52α, which are infrequent in MG patients without thymoma.[67] Furthermore, intratumorous and blood T cells exhibit unusual autoantigen specificities.[68]

(5) Thymomas export CD4[71] and CD8 T cells[69] and paraneoplastic MG is associated with export of CD4 T cells.[70,71] MG(−) thymomas fail to complete terminal intratumorous CD4+ T cell maturation[70] (FIG. 1).

(6) Intratumorous activation of mature T cells is restricted to rare type A thymomas.[94]

(7) Intratumorous autoantibody production is exceptionally rare.[60,61]

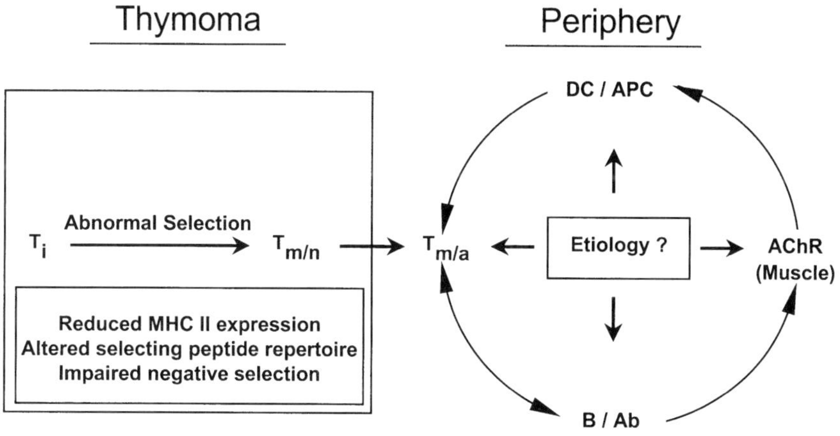

FIGURE 2. Hypothetical pathogenic model for paraneoplastic MG in WHO type AB and B thymomas. MG-associated thymomas promote T cell maturation from immature precursors (T_i) to fully mature, naïve CD4 T cells ($T_{m/n}$). Thymocyte maturation might be accompanied by abnormal positive and nontolerogenic negative T cell selection. After export to the "periphery" (i.e., residual thymus, lymph nodes, bone marrow, and eventually muscle), naïve T cells are primed by antigen-presenting dendritic cells (DC/APC) to become mature, activated CD4 T cells ($T_{m/a}$) that provide help to autoantibody (Ab)–producing B cells. Whether the AChR in skeletal muscle or thymic myoid cells is the primary (triggering) autoantigen or becomes secondarily involved is unknown. Likewise, the events initiating the autoimmune cascade (etiology) have not been identified. The pathogenesis of MG in WHO type A thymomas, which are virtually nonthymopoietic, has not been resolved.

Taken together, we favor the hypothesis that type AB and type B thymomas [90–95% of MG(+) thymoma cases] contribute to autoimmunization by nontolerogenic thymopoiesis and export of naïve but potentially autoreactive mature T cells to the periphery.[69] Export of naïve T cells might gradually replace the normally tolerant, thymus-derived T cell repertoire by a chimeric autoimmunity-prone T cell repertoire derived from both the thymoma and the thymus. To become pathogenically relevant, nonactivated but potentially autoantigen-reactive T cells have to become activated (by whatever etiological mechanism, see below) in order to provide help for autoantibody-producing B cells outside the thymoma (FIG. 2).[94] At this stage of pathogenesis, a role for a "CTLA-4 low" phenotype[100] and for anti-IL-12 or anti-IFN-α autoantibodies[56] can be envisaged facilitating the CD4 T cell–dependent production of anti-AChR autoantibodies.

ETIOLOGY OF PARANEOPLASTIC MG

The mechanisms that activate the autoimmunity-prone T cell repertoire, that is, the etiologies triggering the MG-provoking autoimmune cascade, have yet to be defined. We have observed paraneoplastic MG following unspecific infectious or

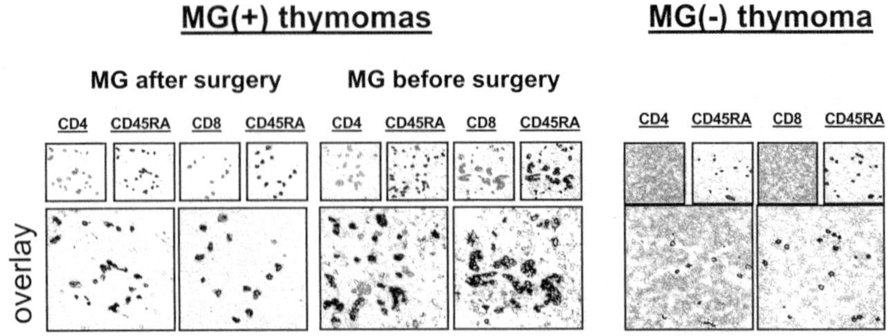

FIGURE 3. Confocal laser microscope immunofluorescence staining of a thymoma with MG at the time of surgery and of a patient who developed MG months after surgical removal of the tumor with abundant mature naïve (CD4+CD45RA+) T cells in both the MG+ thymomas. By contrast, this T cell subset is highly reduced in MG(–) thymomas, while the CD8+ subset appears to be preserved. Detection of intratumorous mature naïve CD4 T cells in the thymoma of patients without autoimmune phenomena at the time of surgery may indicate an increased risk to develop postsurgery MG.

traumatic "stimuli", but in most cases no major event can be spotted.[17] Whether CD8+ T cells[101] and genetic susceptibility[102,103] contribute to the etiological events has yet to be proven. The "periphery" (outside the thymoma), where emigrant T cells become activated, can clearly be the residual thymus,[104] which we found enriched in autoreactive T cells in many thymoma cases (unpublished). However, other lymphoid organs and probably the bone marrow also play a role in this process,[7] given that even complete surgical removal of thymoma plus residual thymus is often not followed by a decline of autoantibody titers.[105]

POSTSURGERY MG

MG can occur weeks or even years after thymectomy in a small minority of thymoma patients.[106] In accordance with the pathogenic model shown in FIGURE 2, postsurgery MG has been taken as circumstantial evidence for a scenario in which thymomas start to alter the peripheral T cell repertoire during the nonmyasthenic phase of thymoma growth.[101] Furthermore, the model suggests the testable prediction that postsurgery MG thymomas may generate and export mature naïve CD4+ T cells, like MG+ thymomas, but unlike "true" MG(–) thymomas. Recently, this prediction could be verified in a single postsurgery MG thymoma (FIG. 3) that harbored fully mature naïve CD4+CD45RA+ T cells, while such cells were virtually absent from all other investigated thymomas that were MG(–) at the time of surgery ($N = 14$). These findings suggest a low risk for developing postsurgery MG for patients that are nonmyasthenic at the time of surgery. However, detection of naïve CD4 T cells in a "nonmyasthenic" thymoma may predict that the risk for postsurgery MG is increased. More cases need to be studied to verify this hypothesis.

MAJOR UNRESOLVED QUESTIONS IN PARANEOPLASTIC MG

It has remained enigmatic why nontolerogenic thymopoiesis in type AB and B thymomas results in only a quite narrow spectrum of autoimmune phenomena and an even narrower spectrum of autoimmune diseases, with MG outnumbering cytopenias or central nervous system alterations by far.[17,67] It is tempting to speculate that the lack of myoid cells in thymomas might play a role in this respect.

Another enigma has been the pathogenesis of paraneoplastic MG in type A thymomas (5% of MG-associated thymomas). In this thymoma subtype, the frequency of paraneoplastic MG is the lowest, while the frequency of cytopenias, particularly pure red cell aplasia, is the highest among all potentially MG-associated thymoma subtypes (A, AB, B1–3). Type A thymomas usually exhibit minimal or virtually absent intratumorous thymopoiesis (in terms of both immature CD4+CD8+ and naïve CD4+ T cells).[63,69] Considering the central role of intratumorous thymopoiesis for the pathogenic model given in FIGURE 2 for type AB and B thymomas, we believe that MG in type A thymomas might have another pathogenesis, which may be based on CD8+ T cells that appear to be produced by type A thymomas[69] or on CD25+ T cells that are increased in type A, but reduced in all other thymoma subtypes.[94]

Finally, it has not been elucidated which autoantigens maintain the prolonged autoantibody response after thymoma surgery, but the AChR itself is an obvious candidate. The destruction of skeletal muscle endplates by autoantibodies or cytotoxic T cells could release AChR and striational antigens, which may be processed and presented to autoreactive T cells by the intramuscular inflammatory infiltrate[107] or by antigen-presenting cells in regional lymph nodes.[7,73]

FINAL QUESTIONS

Pathogenic models based on experimental data have not been suggested for thymic atrophy–associated MG. Heterogeneity of autoantibodies to striational antigens,[4] and particularly titin,[108,109] suggest heterogeneity among MG patients with thymic atrophy. Given that thymoma-associated MG and thymic atrophy–associated MG share striational autoantibodies (TABLE 1) and more protracted effects of thymectomy on MG,[4] we speculate that atrophic thymuses might resemble thymomas as to the pathogenesis of MG. Specifically, atrophic thymuses might contribute new, but less efficiently tolerized T cells to the T cell repertoire because of age-associated thymic insufficiencies.[23,110,111] As in thymomas, the recently exported, but autoimmunity-prone T cells may gradually replace the more tolerant "historic" T cell repertoire from the pre-atrophic era. Individual genetic or environmental susceptibility factors may then determine whether and when tolerance breakdown occurs in the periphery.[16] According to this model, activation of autoreactive T cells should occur outside the atrophic thymus, in agreement with a recent histological study.[108]

REFERENCES

1. LINDSTROM, J.M. *et al.* 1998. Antibody to acetylcholine receptor in myasthenia gravis: prevalence, clinical correlates, and diagnostic value. Neurology **51:** 933–939.

2. TSARTOS, S.J. *et al.* 1998. Anatomy of the antigenic structure of a large membrane autoantigen, the muscle-type nicotinic acetylcholine receptor. Immunol. Rev. **163:** 89–120.
3. WILLCOX, N. *et al.* 1991. The thymus in seronegative myasthenia gravis patients. J. Neurol. **238:** 256–261.
4. WILLIAMS, C.L. *et al.* 1992. Paraneoplastic IgG striational autoantibodies produced by clonal thymic B cells and in serum of patients with myasthenia gravis and thymoma react with titin. Lab. Invest. **66:** 331–336.
5. WILLCOX, N. 1993. Myasthenia gravis. Curr. Opin. Immunol. **5:** 910–917.
6. DRACHMAN, D.B. 1994. Myasthenia gravis. N. Engl. J. Med. **330:** 1797–1810.
7. MARX, A. *et al.* 1997. Pathogenesis of myasthenia gravis. Virch. Arch. **430:** 355–364.
8. MÜLLER-HERMELINK, H.K. & A. MARX. 1999. Pathological aspects of malignant and benign thymic disorders. Ann. Med. **31**(suppl. 2): 5–14.
9. ROXANIS, I., K. MICKLEM & N. WILLCOX. 2001. True epithelial hyperplasia in the thymus of early-onset myasthenia gravis patients: implications for immunopathogenesis. J. Neuroimmunol. **112:** 163–173.
10. KIRCHNER, T. *et al.* 1986. Immunohistological patterns of non-neoplastic changes in the thymus in myasthenia gravis. Virch. Arch. B Cell. Pathol. **52:** 237–257.
11. FLORES, K.G. *et al.* 1999. Analysis of the human thymic perivascular space during aging. J. Clin. Invest. **104:** 1031–1039.
12. NAVANEETHAM, D. *et al.* 2001. Human thymuses express incomplete sets of muscle acetylcholine receptor subunit transcripts that seldom include the delta subunit. Muscle Nerve **24:** 203–210.
13. GEUDER, K.I. *et al.* 1992. Pathogenetic significance of fetal-type acetylcholine receptors on thymic myoid cells in myasthenia gravis. Dev. Immunol. **2:** 69–75.
14. SCHLUEP, M. *et al.* 1987. Acetylcholine receptors in human thymic myoid cells *in situ*: an immunohistological study. Ann. Neurol. **22:** 212–222.
15. ROSAI, J. 1999. Histological Typing of Tumours of the Thymus. Springer-Verlag. Berlin/New York.
16. MARX, A. & H.K. MÜLLER-HERMELINK. 1999. From basic immunobiology to the upcoming WHO-classification of tumors of the thymus. Pathol. Res. Pract. **195:** 515–533.
17. MULLER-HERMELINK, H.K. & A. MARX. 2000. Thymoma. Curr. Opin. Oncol. **12:** 426–433.
18. PARRENS, M. *et al.* 1998. Expression of NGF receptors in normal and pathological human thymus. J. Neuroimmunol. **85:** 11–21.
19. ZETTL, A. *et al.* 2000. Recurrent genetic aberrations in thymoma and thymic carcinoma. Am. J. Pathol. **157:** 257–266.
20. ZHOU, R. *et al.* 2001. Thymic epithelial tumors can develop along two different pathogenetic pathways. Am. J. Pathol. **159:** 1853–1860.
21. MÜLLER-HERMELINK, H.K. & A. MARX. 1996. Thymus. *In* Anderson's Pathology. Tenth edition, pp. 1218–1243. Mosby. St. Louis.
22. KIRCHNER, T. *et al.* 1988. Pathogenesis of myasthenia gravis: acetylcholine receptor–related antigenic determinants in tumor-free thymuses and thymic epithelial tumors. Am. J. Pathol. **130:** 268–280.
23. SEMPOWSKI, G.D. *et al.* 2000. Leukemia inhibitory factor, oncostatin M, IL-6, and stem cell factor mRNA expression in human thymus increases with age and is associated with thymic atrophy. J. Immunol. **164:** 2180–2187.
24. WEKERLE, H. & U.P. KETELSEN. 1977. Intrathymic pathogenesis and dual genetic control of myasthenia gravis. Lancet **1:** 678–680.
25. WEINBERG, C.B. & Z.W. HALL. 1979. Antibodies from patients with myasthenia gravis recognize determinants unique to extrajunctional acetylcholine receptors. Proc. Natl. Acad. Sci. USA **76:** 504–508.
26. GEUDER, K.I. *et al.* 1992. Genomic organization and lack of transcription of the nicotinic acetylcholine receptor subunit genes in myasthenia gravis–associated thymoma. Lab. Invest. **66:** 452–458.
27. KAMINSKI, H.J., L.L. KUSNER & C.H. BLOCK. 1996. Expression of acetylcholine receptor isoforms at extraocular muscle endplates. Invest. Ophthalmol. Vis. Sci. **37:** 345–351 [published erratum: 1996. Invest. Ophthalmol. Vis. Sci. **37**(8): 6A].

28. MacLennan, C. *et al.* 1997. Acetylcholine receptor expression in human extraocular muscles and their susceptibility to myasthenia gravis [see comments]. Ann. Neurol. **41:** 423–431.
29. Meinl, E., W.E. Klinkert & H. Wekerle. 1991. The thymus in myasthenia gravis: changes typical for the human disease are absent in experimental autoimmune myasthenia gravis of the Lewis rat. Am. J. Pathol. **139:** 995–1008.
30. Schonbeck, S. *et al.* 1993. Transplantation of myasthenia gravis thymus to SCID mice. Ann. N.Y. Acad. Sci. **681:** 66–73.
31. Spuler, S. *et al.* 1994. Myogenesis in thymic transplants in the severe combined immunodeficient mouse model of myasthenia gravis: differentiation of thymic myoid cells into striated muscle cells. Am. J. Pathol. **145:** 766–770.
32. Spuler, S. *et al.* 1996. Thymoma-associated myasthenia gravis: transplantation of thymoma and extrathymomal thymic tissue into SCID mice. Am. J. Pathol. **148:** 1359–1365.
33. Baggi, F. *et al.* 1993. Presentation of endogenous acetylcholine receptor epitope by an MHC class II–transfected human muscle cell line to a specific CD4+ T cell clone from a myasthenia gravis patient. J. Neuroimmunol. **46:** 57–65.
34. Melms, A. *et al.* 1992. T cells from normal and myasthenic individuals recognize the human acetylcholine receptor: heterogeneity of antigenic sites on the alpha-subunit. Ann. Neurol. **31:** 311–318.
35. Jermy, A., D. Beeson & A. Vincent. 1993. Pathogenic autoimmunity to affinity-purified mouse acetylcholine receptor induced without adjuvant in BALB/c mice. Eur. J. Immunol. **23:** 973–976.
36. Salmon, A.M. *et al.* 1998. An acetylcholine receptor alpha subunit promoter confers intrathymic expression in transgenic mice: implications for tolerance of a transgenic self-antigen and for autoreactivity in myasthenia gravis. J. Clin. Invest. **101:** 2340–2350.
37. Melms, A. *et al.* 1988. Thymus in myasthenia gravis: isolation of T-lymphocyte lines specific for the nicotinic acetylcholine receptor from thymuses of myasthenic patients. J. Clin. Invest. **81:** 902–908.
38. Sommer, N. *et al.* 1990. Myasthenic thymus and thymoma are selectively enriched in acetylcholine receptor–reactive T cells. Ann. Neurol. **28:** 312–319.
39. Hohlfeld, R. & H. Wekerle. 1999. The immunopathogenesis of myasthenia gravis. *In* Myasthenia Gravis and Myasthenic Disorders, pp. 87–110. Oxford University Press. Oxford.
40. Sims, G.P. *et al.* 2001. Somatic hypermutation and selection of β cells in thymic germinal centers responding to acetylcholine receptor in myasthenia gravis. J. Immunol. **167:** 1935–1944.
41. Vincent, A. 1994. Aetiological factors in development of myasthenia gravis. Adv. Neuroimmunol. **4:** 355–371.
42. Middleton, G. & E.M. Schoch. 2000. The prevalence of human thymic lymphoid follicles is lower in suicides. Virch. Arch. **436:** 127–130.
43. Compston, D.A. *et al.* 1980. Clinical, pathological, HLA antigen, and immunological evidence for disease heterogeneity in myasthenia gravis. Brain **103:** 579–601.
44. Degli-Esposti, M.A. *et al.* 1992. An approach to the localization of the susceptibility genes for generalized myasthenia gravis by mapping recombinant ancestral haplotypes. Immunogenetics **35:** 355–364.
45. Huang, D. *et al.* 2001. Disruption of the IL-1beta gene diminishes acetylcholine receptor–induced immune responses in a murine model of myasthenia gravis. Eur. J. Immunol. **31:** 225–232.
46. Skeie, G.O. *et al.* 1999. TNFA and TNFB polymorphisms in myasthenia gravis. Arch. Neurol. **56:** 457–461.
47. Huang, D.R. *et al.* 1999. Tumour necrosis factor-alpha polymorphism and secretion in myasthenia gravis. J. Neuroimmunol. **94:** 165–171.
48. Franciotta, D. *et al.* 2001. Polymorphic markers in MHC class II/III region: a study on Italian patients with myasthenia gravis. J. Neurol. Sci. **190:** 11–16.
49. Huang, D.R. *et al.* 1999. Markers in the promoter region of interleukin-10 (IL-10) gene in myasthenia gravis: implications of diverse effects of IL-10 in the pathogenesis of the disease. J. Neuroimmunol. **94:** 82–87.

50. Garchon, H.J. *et al.* 1994. Involvement of human muscle acetylcholine receptor alpha-subunit gene (CHRNA) in susceptibility to myasthenia gravis. Proc. Natl. Acad. Sci. USA **91:** 4668–4672.
51. Djabiri, F. *et al.* 1997. No evidence for an association of AChR beta-subunit gene (CHRNB1) with myasthenia gravis. J. Neuroimmunol. **78:** 86–89.
52. Giraud, M. *et al.* 2001. Linkage of HLA to myasthenia gravis and genetic heterogeneity depending on anti-titin antibodies. Neurology **57:** 1555–1560.
53. Vincent, A. *et al.* 1998. Determinant spreading and immune responses to acetylcholine receptors in myasthenia gravis. Immunol. Rev. **164:** 157–168.
54. Aarli, J.A. *et al.* 1992. Myasthenia gravis with thymoma is not associated with an increased incidence of non-muscle autoimmune disorders. Autoimmunity **11:** 159–162.
55. Christensen, P.B. *et al.* 1995. Associated autoimmune diseases in myasthenia gravis: a population-based study [see comments]. Acta Neurol. Scand. **91:** 192–195.
56. Meager, A. *et al.* 1997. Spontaneous neutralising antibodies to interferon-alpha and interleukin-12 in thymoma-associated autoimmune disease [letter]. Lancet **350:** 1596–1597.
57. Mygland, A. *et al.* 1994. Ryanodine receptor antibodies related to severity of thymoma associated myasthenia gravis. J. Neurol. Neurosurg. Psychiatry **57:** 843–846.
58. Romi, F. *et al.* 2000. The severity of myasthenia gravis correlates with the serum concentration of titin and ryanodine receptor antibodies. Arch. Neurol. **57:** 1596–1600.
59. Yamamoto, A.M. *et al.* 2001. Anti-titin antibodies in myasthenia gravis: tight association with thymoma and heterogeneity of nonthymoma patients. Arch. Neurol. **58:** 885–890.
60. Fujii, Y. *et al.* 1984. Antibody to acetylcholine receptor in myasthenia gravis: production by lymphocytes from thymus or thymoma. Neurology **34:** 1182–1186.
61. Newsom-Davis, J. *et al.* 1987. Immunological heterogeneity and cellular mechanisms in myasthenia gravis. Ann. N.Y. Acad. Sci. **505:** 12–26.
62. Takeuchi, Y. *et al.* 1995. Accumulation of immature CD3–CD4+CD8– single-positive cells that lack CD69 in epithelial cell tumors of the human thymus. Cell. Immunol. **161:** 181–187.
63. Nenninger, R. *et al.* 1997. Abnormal T lymphocyte development in myasthenia gravis–associated thymomas. *In* Epithelial Tumors of the Thymus, pp. 165–177. Plenum. New York.
64. Nenninger, R. *et al.* 1998. Abnormal thymocyte development and generation of autoreactive T cells in mixed and cortical thymomas. Lab. Invest. **78:** 743–753.
65. Sommer, N. *et al.* 1991. Acetylcholine receptor–reactive T lymphocytes from healthy subjects and myasthenia gravis patients. Neurology **41:** 1270–1276.
66. Conti-Fine, B.M. *et al.* 1998. T cell recognition of the acetylcholine receptor in myasthenia gravis. Ann. N.Y. Acad. Sci. **841:** 283–308.
67. Nagvekar, N. *et al.* 1998. A pathogenetic role for the thymoma in myasthenia gravis: autosensitization of IL-4-producing T cell clones recognizing extracellular acetylcholine receptor epitopes presented by minority class II isotypes. J. Clin. Invest. **101:** 2268–2277.
68. Schultz, A. *et al.* 1999. Neurofilament is an autoantigenic determinant in myasthenia gravis. Ann. Neurol. **46:** 167–175.
69. Hoffacker, V. *et al.* 2000. Thymomas alter the T-cell subset composition in the blood: a potential mechanism for thymoma-associated autoimmune disease. Blood **96:** 3872–3879.
70. Ströbel, P. *et al.* 2002. Paraneoplastic myasthenia gravis correlates with generation of mature naive T cells in thymomas. Blood **100:** in press.
71. Buckley, C. *et al.* 2001. Mature, long-lived CD4+ and CD8+ T cells are generated by the thymoma in myasthenia gravis. Ann. Neurol. **50:** 64–72.
72. Ströbel, P. *et al.* 2001. Evidence for distinct mechanisms in the shaping of the CD4 T cell repertoire in histologically distinct myasthenia gravis–associated thymomas. Dev. Immunol. **8:** 279–290.
73. Müller-Hermelink, H.K. *et al.* 1997. Characterization of the human thymic microenvironment: lymphoepithelial interaction in normal thymus and thymoma. Arch. Histol. Cytol. **60:** 9–28.

74. VINCENT, A. 1999. Antibodies to ion channels in paraneoplastic disorders. Brain Pathol. **9:** 285–291.
75. AARLI, J.A. *et al.* 1998. Muscle striation antibodies in myasthenia gravis: diagnostic and functional significance. Ann. N.Y. Acad. Sci. **841:** 505–515.
76. MARX, A. *et al.* 1992. Neurofilament epitopes in thymoma and antiaxonal autoantibodies in myasthenia gravis. Lancet **339:** 707–708.
77. MYGLAND, A. *et al.* 1995. Thymomas express epitopes shared by the ryanodine receptor. J. Neuroimmunol. **62:** 79–83.
78. HARA, Y. *et al.* 1991. Neoplastic epithelial cells express alpha-subunit of muscle nicotinic acetylcholine receptor in thymomas from patients with myasthenia gravis. FEBS Lett. **279:** 137–140.
79. SKEIE, G.O. *et al.* 1998. Titin transcripts in thymomas. Ann. N.Y. Acad. Sci. **841:** 422–426.
80. KUSNER, L.L., A. MYGLAND & H.J. KAMINSKI. 1998. Ryanodine receptor gene expression thymomas. Muscle Nerve **21:** 1299–1303.
81. MARX, A. *et al.* 1990. Characterization of a protein with an acetylcholine receptor epitope from myasthenia gravis–associated thymomas [see comments]. Lab. Invest. **62:** 279–286.
82. SIARA, J., R. RUDEL & A. MARX. 1991. Absence of acetylcholine-induced current in epithelial cells from thymus glands and thymomas of myasthenia gravis patients. Neurology **41:** 128–131.
83. MARX, A. *et al.* 1992. A striational muscle antigen and myasthenia gravis–associated thymomas share an acetylcholine-receptor epitope. Dev. Immunol. **2:** 77–84.
84. MARX, A. *et al.* 1996. Expression of neurofilaments and of a titin epitope in thymic epithelial tumors: implications for the pathogenesis of myasthenia gravis. Am. J. Pathol. **148:** 1839–1850.
85. WAKKACH, A. *et al.* 1996. Expression of acetylcholine receptor genes in human thymic epithelial cells: implications for myasthenia gravis. J. Immunol. **157:** 3752–3760.
86. WILISCH, A. *et al.* 1999. Association of acetylcholine receptor alpha-subunit gene expression in mixed thymoma with myasthenia gravis. Neurology **52:** 1460–1466.
87. KLEIN, L., B. ROETTINGER & B. KYEWSKI. 2001. Sampling of complementing self-antigen pools by thymic stromal cells maximizes the scope of central T cell tolerance. Eur. J. Immunol. **31:** 2476–2486.
88. DERBINSKI, J. *et al.* 2001. Promiscuous gene expression in medullary thymic epithelial cells mirrors the peripheral self. Nat. Immunol. **2:** 1032–1039.
89. NAGVEKAR, N. *et al.* 1998. Epitopes expressed in myasthenia gravis (MG) thymomas are not recognized by patients' T cells or autoantibodies. Clin. Exp. Immunol. **112:** 17–20.
90. FUKUI, Y. *et al.* 1997. Positive and negative CD4+ thymocyte selection by a single MHC class II/peptide ligand affected by its expression level in the thymus. Immunity **6:** 401–410.
91. BARTON, G.M. & A.Y. RUDENSKY. 1999. Requirement for diverse, low-abundance peptides in positive selection of T cells. Science **283:** 67–70.
92. DONGRE, A.R. *et al.* 2001. *In vivo* MHC class II presentation of cytosolic proteins revealed by rapid automated tandem mass spectrometry and functional analyses. Eur. J. Immunol. **31:** 1485–1494.
93. WONG, P. *et al.* 2001. Dynamic tuning of T cell reactivity by self-peptide–major histocompatibility complex ligands. J. Exp. Med. **193:** 1179–1187.
94. MARX, A. *et al.* 1998. Paraneoplastic autoimmunity in thymus tumors. Dev. Immunol. **6:** 129–140.
95. WILLCOX, N. *et al.* 1987. Myasthenic and nonmyasthenic thymoma: an expansion of a minor cortical epithelial cell subset? Am. J. Pathol. **127:** 447–460.
96. INOUE, M. *et al.* 1999. Impaired expression of MHC class II molecules in response to interferon-gamma (IFN-gamma) on human thymoma neoplastic epithelial cells. Clin. Exp. Immunol. **117:** 1–7.
97. KADOTA, Y. *et al.* 2000. Altered T cell development in human thymoma is related to impairment of MHC class II transactivator expression induced by interferon-gamma (IFN-gamma). Clin. Exp. Immunol. **121:** 59–68.

98. LAUFER, T.M., L. FAN & L.H. GLIMCHER. 1999. Self-reactive T cells selected on thymic cortical epithelium are polyclonal and are pathogenic *in vivo*. J. Immunol. **162:** 5078–5084.
99. VAN MEERWIJK, J.P. & H.R. MACDONALD. 1999. *In vivo* T-lymphocyte tolerance in the absence of thymic clonal deletion mediated by hematopoietic cells. Blood **93:** 3856–3862.
100. HUANG, D. *et al.* 2000. Dinucleotide repeat expansion in the CTLA-4 gene leads to T cell hyper-reactivity via the CD28 pathway in myasthenia gravis. J. Neuroimmunol. **105:** 69–77.
101. VINCENT, A. & N. WILLCOX. 1999. The role of T-cells in the initiation of autoantibody responses in thymoma patients. Pathol. Res. Pract. **195:** 535–540.
102. HUANG, D. *et al.* 1998. Genetic association of Ctla-4 to myasthenia gravis with thymoma. J. Neuroimmunol. **88:** 192–198.
103. MACHENS, A. *et al.* 1999. Correlation of thymic pathology with HLA in myasthenia gravis. Clin. Immunol. **91:** 296–301.
104. CONTI-TRONCONI, B.M. *et al.* 1994. The nicotinic acetylcholine receptor: structure and autoimmune pathology. Crit. Rev. Biochem. Mol. Biol. **29:** 69–123.
105. SOMNIER, F.E. 1994. Exacerbation of myasthenia gravis after removal of thymomas [see comments]. Acta Neurol. Scand. **90:** 56–66.
106. NAMBA, T., N.G. BRUNNER & D. GROB. 1978. Myasthenia gravis in patients with thymoma, with particular reference to onset after thymectomy. Medicine (Baltimore) **57:** 411–433.
107. MASELLI, R.A., D.P. RICHMAN & R.L. WOLLMANN. 1991. Inflammation at the neuromuscular junction in myasthenia gravis. Neurology **41:** 1497–1504.
108. MYKING, A.O. *et al.* 1998. The histomorphology of the thymus in late onset, non-thymoma myasthenia gravis. Eur. J. Neurol. **5:** 401–405.
109. LUBKE, E. *et al.* 1998. Striational autoantibodies in myasthenia gravis patients recognize I-band titin epitopes. J. Neuroimmunol. **81:** 98–108.
110. HAYNES, B.F. *et al.* 2000. The role of the thymus in immune reconstitution in aging, bone marrow transplantation, and HIV-1 infection. Annu. Rev. Immunol. **18:** 529–560.
111. FAGNONI, F.F. *et al.* 2000. Shortage of circulating naive CD8(+) T cells provides new insights on immunodeficiency in aging. Blood **95:** 2860–2868.

Scenarios for Autoimmunization of T and B Cells in Myasthenia Gravis

H. SHIONO,[a] I. ROXANIS,[a] W. ZHANG,[a] G. P. SIMS,[b] A. MEAGER,[c] L. W. JACOBSON,[a] J-L. LIU,[a] I. MATTHEWS,[a] Y-L. WONG,[a] M. BONIFATI,[a] K. MICKLEM,[d] D. I. STOTT,[b] J. A. TODD,[e] D. BEESON,[a] A. VINCENT,[a] AND N. WILLCOX[a]

[a]*Neuroscience Group, Weatherall Institute for Molecular Medicine, University of Oxford, Oxford OX3 9DS, United Kingdom*

[b]*Department of Immunology and Bacteriology, Western Infirmary, University of Glasgow, Glasgow G11 6NT, United Kingdom*

[c]*Department of Immunobiology, National Institute of Biological Standards and Control, Potter's Bar EN6 3QG, United Kingdom*

[d]*Department of Cellular Science, John Radcliffe Hospital, University of Oxford, Oxford OX3 9DU, United Kingdom*

[e]*Department of Medical Genetics, Addenbrooke's Hospital, University of Cambridge, Cambridge CB2 2XY, United Kingdom*

ABSTRACT: We have studied responses in thymoma patients to interferon-α and to the acetylcholine receptor (AChR) in early-onset myasthenia gravis (EOMG), seeking clues to autoimmunizing mechanisms. Our new evidence implicates a two-step process: (step 1) professional antigen-presenting cells and thymic epithelial cells prime AChR-specific T cells; then (step 2) thymic myoid cells subsequently provoke germinal center formation in EOMG. Our unifying hypothesis proposes that AChR epitopes expressed by neoplastic or hyperplastic thymic epithelial cells aberrantly prime helper T cells, whether generated locally or infiltrating from the circulation. These helper T cells then induce antibody responses against linear epitopes that cross-react with whole AChR and attack myoid cells in the EOMG thymus. The resulting antigen-antibody complexes and the recruitment of professional antigen-presenting cells increase the exposure of thymic cells to the infiltrates and provoke local germinal center formation and determinant spreading. Both these and the consequently enhanced heterogeneity and pathogenicity of the autoantibodies should be minimized by early thymectomy.

KEYWORDS: acetylcholine receptor (AChR); autoantibodies; autoimmunization; germinal center; interferon-α; interleukin-12; myasthenia gravis; thymic hyperplasia; thymoma

Address for correspondence: Nick Willcox, Neuroscience Group, Weatherall Institute for Molecular Medicine, Headington, Oxford OX3 9DS, United Kingdom. Voice: +44-1865-222325; fax: +44-1865-222402.

nick.willcox@imm.ox.ac.uk

Ann. N.Y. Acad. Sci. 998: 237–256 (2003). © 2003 New York Academy of Sciences.
doi: 10.1196/annals.1254.026

INTRODUCTION

In humans, very little is known about mechanisms of autoimmunization in general. In myasthenia gravis (MG), in particular, there are two challenging puzzles. The pathogenic autoantibodies to the acetylcholine receptor (AChR) are clearly dependent on helper T cells (Th),[1,2] but how can these Th be first primed when the AChR is not normally coexpressed with HLA-class II? Once activated (presumably against linear AChR epitopes), how do these Th then come to induce responses in the pathogenic B cells, whose antibodies are almost exclusively specific for the (extracellular) native AChR conformation,[3] and how do these B cells first come to process/present native AChR? Interestingly, this second step clearly can follow α138–199 peptide immunization, which eventually evokes AChR conformation-specific autoantibodies in rabbits.[4] Resolving these issues might suggest new approaches to prevention or therapy.

Most unusually, in MG, there are several invaluable clues, notably in the distinct patient subgroups, in the associated thymomas found in ~10% of patients (who show distinctive serology) and in the thymic infiltrates ("hyperplasia") in nearly every case with early-onset myasthenia gravis (EOMG) (onset < age 40).[1,2,5] These include lymph node–type high endothelial venules, T cell areas, and germinal centers (GC). They compress the residual parenchyma into characteristic medullary epithelial bands (MEB)[5] and may be originally attracted there by the rare medullary myoid cells[6] that express the complete AChR, especially of the fetal isoform[7] so often preferred by these patients' autoantibodies.[3] The myoid cells may also help to stimulate the typical spontaneous anti-AChR autoantibody production by EOMG thymic cells;[1,5,8] these terminally differentiated plasma cell responses have clearly been selectively activated *in situ*, unlike the many other B cells specific for extraneous antigens, such as influenza virus.[8]

AUTOIMMUNIZATION IN THYMOMAS

Responses against IL-12 and IFN-α

Thymomas are epithelial tumors; in MG, they usually resemble disorganized cortex, containing abundant developing thymocytes and exporting many of their progeny to the periphery.[1,9] In addition to their anti-AChR, these patients almost always have other autoantibodies recognizing various striational muscle antigens, notably titin.[10] At least some of its epitopes are expressed in thymomas[11] and may be selecting or even autoimmunizing some of the nearby T cells.

At diagnosis, we found that patients with thymoma and MG had, quite unexpectedly, autoantibodies to IFN-α (in >70%) and to IL-12 (in >50%), often at high titers,[12] but not against the many other cytokines tested, except rarely GM-CSF. We found similar antibodies to IFN-α and IL-12 in ~30% of late-onset MG (LOMG) patients without thymomas (FIG. 1B) and against titin in ~80%, but they were all very uncommon in EOMG.[13] Both antibodies neutralize their respective cytokines in bioassays.[12] Titers against IFN-α and IL-12 correlate so poorly that they must be independent specificities.[12] They also show no obvious correlation with thymoma histology ($N \approx 70$) or HLA type ($N \approx 90$). Both increase sharply in the unusual cases whose thymomas recur[13] (FIG. 1C), perhaps a valuable early warning. Evidently, these antibodies are more directly associated with the thymomas than are the anti-AChR and the anti-titin, which tend to remain stable.[13]

To pursue such associations, we measured specific autoantibody production in culture by cells from thymomas, from the adjacent thymic remnant (when available),

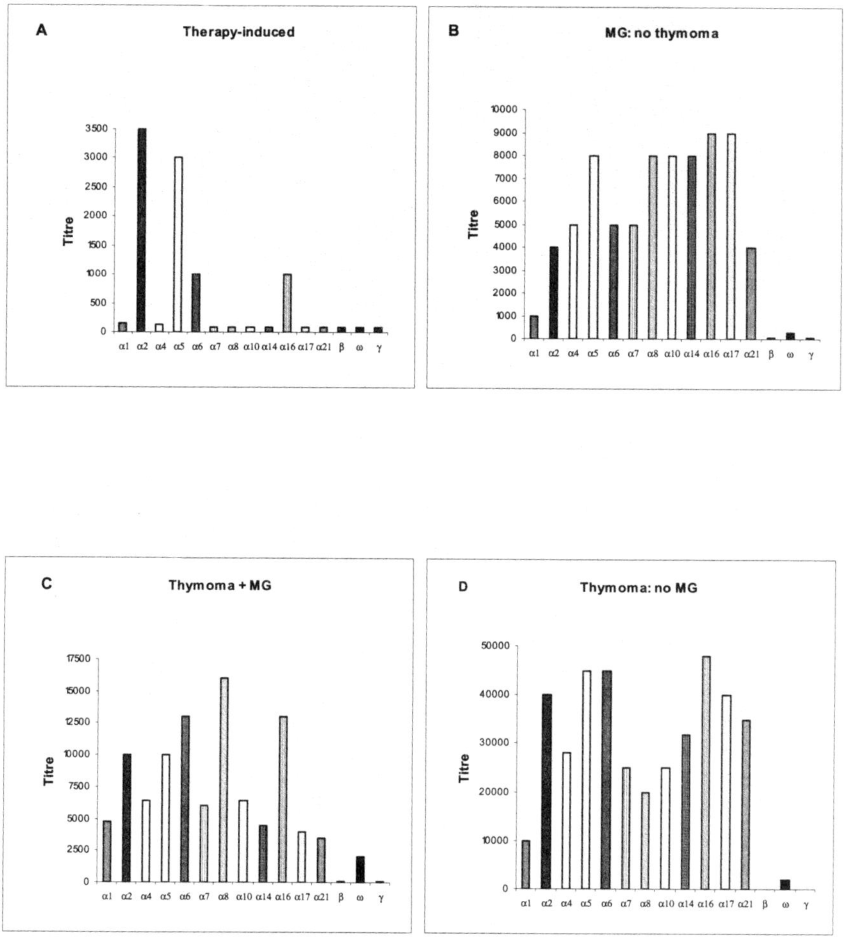

FIGURE 1. Cross-neutralization of IFN-α subtypes by sera from 4 patients. **(A)** A carcinoma patient previously treated with IFN-α2. **(B)** A late-onset MG patient followed for >7 years without evidence of thymoma (anti-AChR titer, 10 nM). **(C)** An MG-thymoma patient negative for these antibodies at thymomectomy in 1990. By 1997, when in hospital for ~5 months with persistent sinus/lung infections with *Haemophilus influenzae*, she was strongly positive for antibodies to IL-12 as well as IFN-α (shown in panel C). A thymoma recurrence was noted in 2002. **(D)** A thymoma patient without MG, but with anti-AChR titer of 15.1 nM. We assayed neutralization of antiviral effects.[12] IFN-ω is more closely related to IFN-α than is IFN-β.

TABLE 1. Autoantibody production in culture by cells from thymoma, thymic remnant, and PBL

	Thymoma		Thymic remnant		PBL	
	PWM−	PWM+	PWM−	PWM+	PWM−	PWM+
Anti-AChR	**6.4**	50.0	17.1	23.2	–	–
	2/19	5/19	5/15	4/15	0/11	0/11
Anti-IFN-α	**28.2**	14.0	15.7	15.2	–	33.0
	7/17	2/17	8/13	3/13	0/7	3/7
Anti-IL-12	**37.4**	3.1	12.4	11.3	–	53.1
	2/15	1/15	3/10	2/10	0/7	1/7
Anti-titin	–	10.8	–	5.1	nd	nd
	0/12	3/12	0/9	2/10		

NOTE: The top values are the mean percent of the maximal cpm precipitated by the positive samples after background subtraction for each RIA (using 75 μL of culture supernatant); the fractions are the number of positive cultures/total number of seropositive cases tested. The pokeweed mitogen (PWM) responses (i.e., those where the value was at least doubled) are shown as the mean increment above the levels in the unstimulated cultures. nd = not done.

and from blood, with or without the T cell–dependent B cell stimulant pokeweed mitogen (PWM; TABLE 1). As noted,[14] spontaneous anti-AChR production was much more often seen in the remnant, which includes myoid cells, than in the thymoma where intact AChR has never been detected.[15] Even though several thymomas contained PWM-responsive B cells, these showed almost no sign of prior activation against AChR (TABLE 1). Likewise, with titin, we found only rare/weak PWM-stimulated responses in occasional thymomas (Shiono *et al.*, 2003. *Int. Immunol.* **15:** 903–913).

There was a striking contrast with IFN-α and IL-12; cells from the thymomas produced either autoantibody spontaneously at least as frequently/vigorously as those from the remnants (TABLE 1), clearly indicating specific prestimulation by the native cytokines *in situ*. To us, these results strongly imply that some cell type(s) in thymomas expresses native IFN-α and/or IL-12 that is recognizable by both T and B cells, but only linear AChR epitopes that cannot drive a conformation-specific antibody response there. Identifying the cell type(s) responsible should be easier for these smaller and simpler cytokine molecules than for the sparser and less stable AChR.

Autoimmunizing Cell Type(s)

Further clues come from the specificities of the serum anticytokine autoantibodies. In many patients, the anti-IL-12 antibodies recognize its inducible p40 subunit, as well as the native p70 heterodimer, on Western blots (Meager and colleagues, in preparation). The anti-IFN antibodies are even more interesting. They very rarely recognize the distantly related IFN-κ (produced by keratinocytes) or IFN-β (from fibroblasts), despite its immunogenicity during therapy (e.g., for multiple sclerosis), and never (detectably) the unrelated type II IFN-γ (from T and NK cells) (FIG. 1). In patients treated with IFN-α (e.g., for renal carcinoma or hepatitis C), antibodies are also common, but they cross-neutralize a narrow range of the 12 different IFN-α subtypes (FIG. 1A). In stark contrast, even the earliest positive MG sera tested to date cross-neutralize a very wide spectrum of subtypes (FIG. 1C), and the pattern varies little in serial samples after thymomectomy. Very interestingly, the 30% of positive LOMG sera show similarly broad reactivity (FIG. 1B).

The coincident recognition of native IL-12 and almost the full gamut of IFN-α subtypes, but not other type I or II IFNs, implicates dendritic cells (DC) as the auto-immunizing cell type, which collectively are the producers par excellence of both cytokines.[16] Interestingly, they can be generated from a common pre-T/pre-NK progenitor in the thymus.[17] Since thymopoiesis is often grossly excessive in thymomas, aberrant DC production/behavior seem plausible too. Moreover, DC seem a likely connecting thread not only among thymomas of widely varying histology and HLA type, but also in some LOMG cases, whose very similar serology[13] must hold precious clues (Meager *et al.*, 2003. *Clin. Exp. Immunol.* **132:** 128–136).

Potential Effects in Patients

In humans, both IFN-α and especially IL-12 are proinflammatory cytokines that strongly favor Th1 (IFN-γ)–producing Th. Therefore, one might expect their neutral-

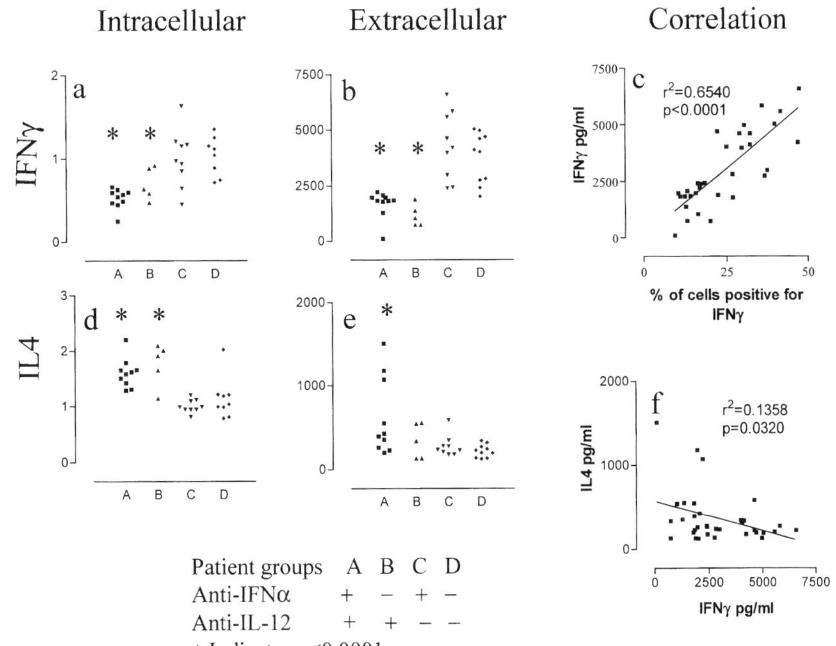

FIGURE 2. Effects of MG-thymoma sera on IFN-γ and IL-4 responses of PBL from a healthy donor to autologous LPS-matured DC. For **(a)** and **(d)**, we show the percentage of the responder blasts labeled for the cytokines after permeabilization; for **(b)** and **(e)**, their levels in the supernatants, assayed by ELISA. **(c, f)** There was a much stronger inverse correlation between the IFN-γ^{+} and IL-4^{+} cells ($r^2 = 0.78$; $p < 0.0001$) than for the secreted cytokines (see **f**). Sera were tested at 1/100. The asterisked groups differed from group D, $p < 0.0001$.

ization in the patients to predispose to infections (though IFN-β might compensate). Surprisingly, infections are uncommon, even though most MG-thymoma patients need immunosuppressive therapy. However, chronic mucocutaneous candidiasis is well described in thymoma patients; we have also noted occasional cases with prolonged infections (e.g., FIG. 1C; including *Herpes zoster*), and deaths from an "AIDS-like" syndrome or cryptococcal meningitis.[12]

We therefore looked for effects of our patients' sera on Th1/Th2 polarization. To maximize comparability, we tested responses of $CD4^+$ T cells from healthy donors to autologous DC matured with LPS, which produce high levels of IL-12, but little IFN-α.[18] Sera containing anti-IL-12 antibodies consistently reduced IFN-γ responses 3- to 5-fold (FIG. 2), as did mAbs to IL-12 (not shown). So far, effects have not been consistent with sera containing anti-IFN-α alone (FIG. 2, group C), but they might be more obvious with more potent IFN-α-producing stimulator cells. Some sera with both antibodies enhanced IL-4 responses (FIGS. 2d and 2e).

Since many established memory responses are already Th1- or Th2-committed,[19] responses to previously encountered pathogens are probably not affected by these antibodies in our (mostly middle-aged) seropositive cases. We propose that their occasional intractable infections are to "newcomer organisms" and might respond to cautious use of IFN-γ, against which we never find antibodies (FIG. 1).[12]

AUTOSENSITIZATION OF TH: A ROLE FOR MEDULLARY THYMIC EPITHELIAL CELLS?

The medullary thymic epithelial cells (TEC) show clear evidence of true hyperplasia in EOMG, analogous to regenerating epithelia elsewhere.[20] In the "palisades" at the edges of the MEB, they are more densely packed, with fewer processes. Especially where the laminin borders of the MEB break down, clusters of TEC appear to migrate into the infiltrates (FIG. 5d). Near these "epicenters", they express several integrins, notably αvβ5, plus the EGFR, and do so more uniformly than in the normal medulla.[20] However, while all are clearly HLA-class I^+, only a minority express class II (weakly); even in these epicenters, they also have an unpromising costimulatory phenotype, unlike the adjacent professional antigen-presenting cells (APC).[20] Furthermore, while TEC cultured from thymomas presented peptides well to our AChR-specific Th clones, they processed longer polypeptides much less efficiently than the APC from blood.[21]

Expression of Autoepitopes by TEC

Insulin and Thyroid Peroxidase

There is much evidence for the expression of "peripheral tissue-specific" autoantigens such as insulin[22] and gastric Na^+/H^+ ATPase in the normal thymus,[23] as well as for thymic selection of regulatory T cells (Treg) that help to prevent autoimmunity.[24–26] However, the selecting cell type(s) has rarely been identified in the human thymus.

We therefore studied (pro-)insulin expression as a positive control. In EOMG and control samples, the two mAbs with the highest affinities[27] (3B1 and A6) consistently labeled foci of cells in the subcapsular region and scattered cells in the medulla, most

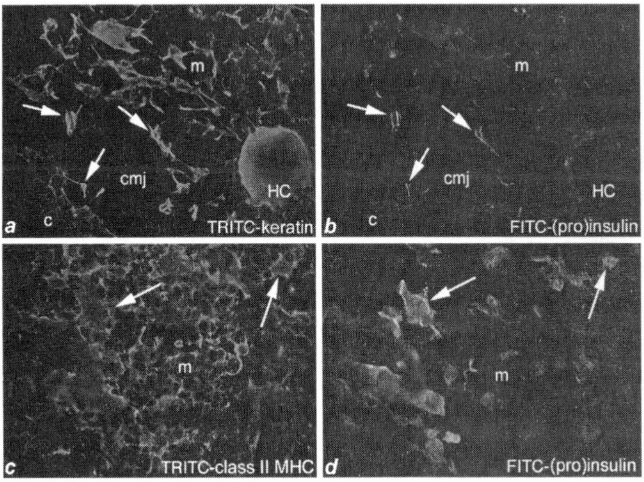

FIGURE 3. Two-color immunofluorescence labeling for (pro-)insulin **(b, d)** (with the high-affinity mAb 3B1) in thymus from a 12-year-old control. In **(a, b)**, the medullary (pro-)insulin$^+$ cells are clearly keratin$^+$ (*arrow*); in **(c, d)**, some are evidently also HLA-class II$^+$ (*arrow*), with the (pro-)insulin labeling clearly internal to the class II. Results were negative with the two lower affinity anti-insulin mAbs[27] (1E2 and ANT-1). Note that the Hassall's corpuscle (HC) is negative for (pro-)insulin **(b)**. Terms: c, cortex; m, medulla; cmj, cortico-medullary junction.

of which proved to be TEC (FIGS. 3a–3d). We saw no labeling in the cortex (TABLE 2). All the (pro-)insulin$^+$ cells were HLA class I$^+$. However, in much of the medulla, class II staining normally appears confluent, and we could only be sure of its expression on about 10% of the (pro-)insulin$^+$ cells there (FIGS. 3c and 3d). In addition, we saw a similar picture with an mAb to thyroid peroxidase (TPO),[28] another important autoantigenic target.

AChR Subunits

Many groups have detected thymic expression of AChR subunit mRNAs (apart from the δ) using very sensitive RT-PCR assays.[15,29–31] The ε gave the strongest signals in thymomas in one study with less sensitive RNase protection assays.[32] When tested, expression was apparently by the TEC[15,30] and by myoid cells,[15] as expected. At the protein level, the intact AChR is clearly present in myoid cells,[7] but has never been detected in thymomas.[15] However, since nearly all the available mAbs recognize conformational epitopes exclusively, isolated subunits are hard to detect and rarely sought. We thus used sera from rabbits immunized with synthetic peptides (20–40 amino acids long) from the human α, β, γ, and ε sequences to stain sections of normal and EOMG thymus (TABLE 2). For the α, these were pooled into four subgroups. We also tested individual sera, for example, against the P3A insert.[33] In addition, we included single antisera against β44–68, γ69–93, and ε329–365, as well as an anti-fibulin as a negative control. All of these sera specifically recognized the

TABLE 2. Reactivity of rabbit anti-AChR antisera and an anti-(pro-)insulin mAb in thymic compartments and thymomas

	Control or EOMG			EOMG	Thymoma + MG (no. of positive samples)		
Antisera/mAb	Sub-capsular	Cortex	Medulla	MEB	A ($N = 1$)	B_2 ($N = 4$)	B_3 ($N = 7$)
Anti-(α1–56)	–	–	+	+	1	1 + 1[a]	6
Anti-(α62–129)	–	–	–	–	0	1 + 1	1 + 4
Anti-(α138–199)	–	+	+	+	1	3 + 1	3 + 2[b]
Anti-(α138–199): peptide blocked	–	↓	↓	↓	↓	↓	↓
Anti-P3A[c]	–	–	–	–	0 + 1	0 + 2	3 + 2
Anti-(α310–389)	–	–	–	–	nd	1	3/5
Anti-β (β44–68)	+	–	+	+	nd	nd	nd
Anti-γ (γ69–93)	+	–	+	+	nd	nd	nd
Anti-ε (ε329–365)	+	–	+	+	0	2/2	2/2
Anti-(pro-)insulin	+	–	+	+	1	2/2	1/2
Anti-fibulin	–	–	–	–	0	0	0

NOTE: We studied thymus from 8 EOMG cases (aged 13 to 34 years with MG durations of 9 to 49 months and anti-AChR titers ranging from 13 to 46 nM) and 3 pediatric cardiac surgery controls. One case with a WHO type B_2 thymoma, and all of those with type A or B_3, had been pretreated with corticosteroids. The indirect immunoperoxidase labeling was for 30 min for each step. ↓ indicates substantially reduced staining intensity after overnight preblocking with homologous peptides. The anti-(pro-)insulin was mAb26 ("3B1"); the others were rabbit antisera raised against synthetic peptides; those against the AChR-α were pools of 2–4 antisera, apart from the single anti-P3A. nd = not done.

[a]One case with clearly positive cells and one with weaker positivity.

[b]These weakly positive cells were mainly macrophages in perivascular spaces.

[c]Anti-α51–58:P3A insert [25 amino acids]:59–65.

homologous peptides in dot blots (at 0.01 μg/mL); only the anti-α138–199 pool[4] and the anti-α309–368 bound intact human AChR, and did so weakly. We tested them at 1/1000–1/200 by immunoperoxidase and at 1/500–1/100 by indirect immunofluorescence. In general, we saw clear staining for β, γ, and ε, but for only two of the four α subunit regions (TABLE 2); with all of these, it was evident at 1/1000–1/200 dilutions (without special amplification), but it was not significant with several other sera—even at 1/10—despite their strong dot blot signals.

Myoid cells provided a convenient internal positive control and showed surprisingly strong staining for the α, γ, and ε regions tested (FIGS. 4e and 4f). This implies that they contain unfolded subunits/sequential epitopes, even including the ε. As expected, they also labeled for γ (confirmed with an affinity-purified antibody fraction).

In "normal" areas (whether in EOMG or control thymus), most of these sera showed similar staining patterns to those for insulin and TPO, although fewer TEC were positive, both in subcapsular foci or scattered in the medulla (TABLE 2).

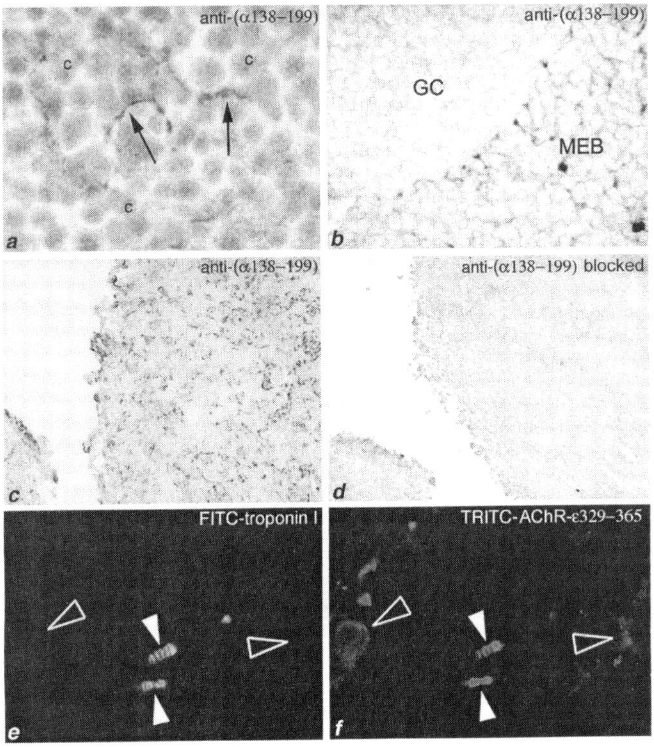

FIGURE 4. **(a–d)** Indirect immunoperoxidase labeling for AChR α138–199 in thymus from **(a)** a 2-month-old control, **(b)** an EOMG patient, and **(c, d)** a cortical thymoma (WHO B_2). **(a)** In the cortex ("c"), typical reticular TEC are weakly positive (*arrow*); in **(b)**, some labeled palisading cells in the MEB are probably epithelial too. In the thymoma **(c, d)**, the scattered TEC are no longer positive after prior overnight blocking of the pooled antisera with homologous peptides **(d)**. **(e, f)** Two-color immunofluorescence labeling for troponin I to detect myoid cells **(e)** (*solid arrowheads*; FITC) and ε329–365 **(f)** (TRITC), which is seen in some additional cells (probably medullary TEC; *open arrowheads*). Donors for **(b)** a 23-year-old EOMG female with MG duration of 16 months and anti-AChR titer > 29.5 nM); for **(c, d)**, a 50.8-year-old MG female with anti-AChR titer of 30.9 nM; for **(e, f)**, a 13.3-year-old EOMG female with a 45-month duration and anti-AChR titer of 31.3 nM.

Palisading cells were also occasionally positive at the edges of the MEB (FIG. 4b). With the α, we saw these interesting differences: subcapsular TEC stained minimally for any of its four regions; medullary TEC labeled only for α1–56 and α138–199; and the latter also weakly stained some typical reticular cortical TEC (FIG. 4a).

Prima facie evidence of specificity is the generally similar staining pattern with the anti-(pro-)insulin and TPO mAbs; the highly selective labeling of occasional TEC with only some of the antisera, despite their strong signals on blots and their minimal staining of macrophages and Hassall's corpuscles (both notorious for non-specific binding) (FIG. 3); the labeling of myoid cells; the similar results with the affinity-purified anti-γ antibodies; and the successful blocking of the anti-α138–199 with the homologous peptides (FIGS. 4c and 4d).

However, we saw no signs specifically incriminating the AChR subunit$^+$ TEC in the response in EOMG—that is, no clear differences (apart from the MEB) between EOMG and control samples, no striking change in numbers or staining intensity, and no colocalization with CD4$^+$ or CD8$^+$ T cells or APC or at sites of MEB fragmentation. Nevertheless, if such changes are early or focal, they could easily be missed.

Our limited study on thymomas included 4 cortical (WHO type B_2) and 8 mostly epithelial tumors that had been enriched by the MG donor's prior corticosteroid treatment [1 type A, 7 type B_3]. Some of each type showed clear labeling for (pro-)-insulin in scattered TEC (TABLE 2). The same anti-AChR antisera as above detected sporadic TEC, and so did others—against α62–129 and the P3A insert and even sometimes α310–389—especially in the more epithelial tumors. As expected from its labeling of normal cortical TEC, the anti-α138–199 pool stained both the cortical and the epithelial tumors consistently, peptide blocking again supporting its specificity (FIGS. 4c and 4d). Interestingly, one of the type B_3 thymomas was the source of a Vβ2$^+$ T cell clone[34] specific for α138–167, and its parenchyma labeled for this AChR region; Vβ2$^+$ T cells had been noted in the perivascular spaces,[34] where we now also saw some macrophages labeling for α138–199, as in another type B_3 thymoma.

Thus, the main differences in the thymomas were the absence of myoid cells and rarity of GC, the greater total number of positive cells (in these sometimes very bulky tumors), and some staining of CD68$^+$ macrophages in the perivascular spaces, a possible sign of antigen uptake by these cells.

Interpretation

These results require independent confirmation with further affinity-purified or monoclonal antibodies, ideally combined with *in situ* hybridization and immunochemical studies on the expressed polypeptides to exclude cross-recognition of other autoantigens, as seen with anti-α371–380 mAbs.[35] Our frequently negative results for this latter region and some others (e.g., α62–129) may reflect differences either in fine specificities and affinities of our antisera or in their sensitivities to fixation or to maturational/conformational changes.[36]

Despite all these reservations, we conclude that (1) at least some AChR transcripts are indeed translated into protein in both the normal and EOMG thymus as well as thymoma and (2) along with myoid cells, medullary TEC are the likeliest AChR subunit–autoimmunizing cell type,[15,30] as suspected for other peripheral tissue-specific antigens.

MYOID CELLS AND GERMINAL CENTERS IN EOMG

Thymic Myoid Cells and Conformation-Specific B Cell Responses

In the EOMG thymus, the TEC in the MEB are largely separated from the infiltrates by laminin$^+$ borders (FIG. 5). However, these borders are usually fenestrated near the germinal centers (GC)[5,6,20] and sometimes at other foci too (see below). That disposition could permit exposure of medullary TEC to mature peripheral-type T and B cells, something that would not occur in the normal thymus. In previous

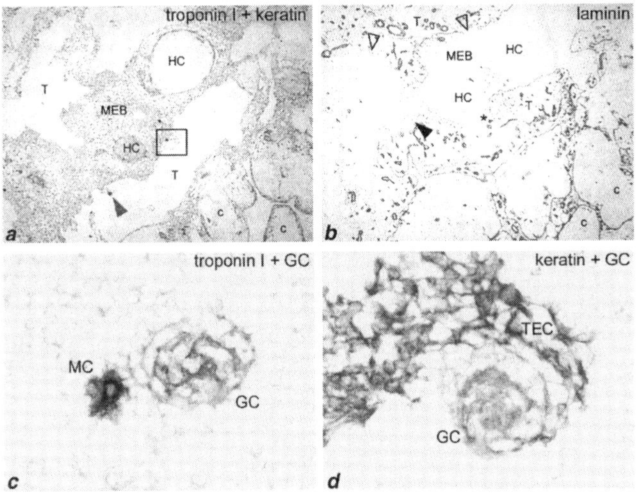

FIGURE 5. Colocalization of a myoid cell with a nascent GC at a site of laminin breakdown in an EOMG thymus.[6] A large keratin$^+$ MEB **(a)** with conspicuous Hassall's corpuscles (HC) is compressed between two large T cell areas ("T"). The intervening laminin$^+$ border is fenestrated at one focus (*boxed* in **a** and *asterisked* in **b**) where TEC break out into the infiltrate **(d)**. A single "exposed" myoid cell ("MC"; troponin I$^+$) **(c)** at this very site is contacting a small GC (labeled for B cells and FDC) **(c, d)**. Other laminin fenestrations have either an adjacent myoid cell (*solid arrowheads* in **a** and **b**) or no nearby myoid cells or GC (*open arrowheads* in **b**)]. Donor is a 22-year-old EOMG female with MG duration of 37 months and anti-AChR titer > 34.8 nM.

studies,[5] we suspected that the infiltrates might be a nonspecific effect, for example, of circulating AChR/autoantibody complexes depositing locally and initiating GC formation.[37] Although they remained plausible culprits, we had no firm evidence[5] to incriminate the long-suspected myoid cells;[2,38] regardless of their precise location, they are rarely HLA-class II$^+$, have an unpromising costimulatory phenotype, and seem unlikely to prime Th directly.[6]

To reexamine the potential of myoid cells, we next quantitated their distribution, whether in areas of relatively normal medulla (sometimes deep within MEB) or "exposed" at either focal laminin fenestrations—where they contacted both the TEC in the MEB and the infiltrates—or wholly within the latter[6] (FIG. 5). To include early cases, we also studied 4 "seroconverters", typical myasthenics who became anti-AChR seropositive only 1–32 months postthymectomy, as well as 36 widely representative EOMG samples.

As expected, myoid cell frequencies were extremely variable, being almost zero in some cases; their exposure to the infiltrates increased almost significantly with MG duration.[6] In view of their overall rarity, we were surprised to find myoid cells at 24% of the laminin fenestrations in seropositive EOMG (FIG. 5). Interestingly, this percentage was even higher (67%) in the seroconverters, whereas GC outnumbered them (63%) in established seropositive EOMG. Moreover, in both patient groups, the occurrence of a myoid cell at a fenestration significantly increased the chances

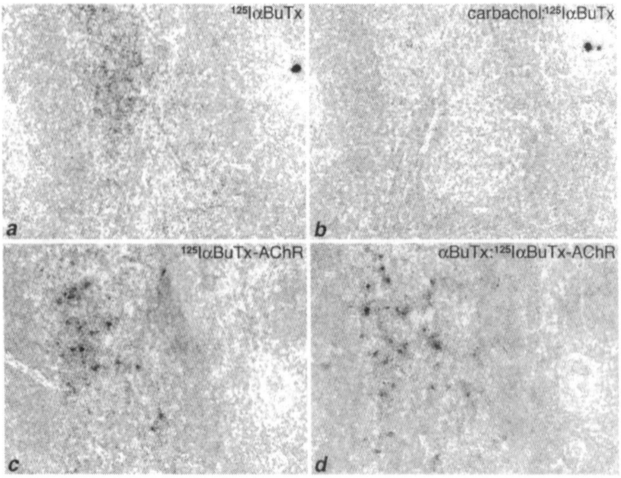

FIGURE 6. Detection of AChR **(a, b)** and AChR-specific plasma cells/plasmablasts **(c, d)** in adjacent sections of a GC in an EOMG thymus, with ^{125}I-α-BuTx **(a, b)** or AChR-^{125}I-α-BuTx **(c, d)**. For **(b)**, the section was preincubated (2 h) with 10^{-4} M carbamylcholine to prevent the ^{125}I-α-BuTx from binding to AChR, while a Hassall's corpuscle still labels non-specifically (*upper right*). In **(d)**, similar preincubation with unlabeled α-BuTx did not reduce the AChR-^{125}I-α-BuTx binding. Donor is an 11.5-year-old EOMG female with an 8-month duration and anti-AChR titer of 12.2 nM.

of finding a nearby GC[6] (FIG. 5). This unexpected co-occurrence was our most MG-specific finding;[6] it was not seen in an extremely hyperplastic thymus from an SLE patient without MG (or anti-AChR antibodies) and strongly implicates myoid cells as *agents provocateurs*.

Specific GC in EOMG Thymus

Our previous evidence suggested that spontaneous anti-AChR antibody production correlated better with the T cell areas than the GC.[5] We next located specific plasma cells/precursors definitively in autoradiographs of sections labeled with soluble human AChR-^{125}I-α-bungarotoxin (α-BuTx), which inevitably contains some free ^{125}I-α-BuTx. Interestingly, when tested alone as a control, this gave weak diffuse labeling in ~50% of the GC in EOMG thymi (FIGS. 6a and 6b), but not in tonsils. Clear blocking by 10^{-4} M carbamylcholine indicated that this binding was specific, presumably to AChR fragments in immune complexes trapped by follicular dendritic cells (FDC).[39]

With ^{125}I-α-BuTx-AChR, we saw two striking differences. In about 20% of the GC (up to 80% in one case), we saw much more strongly/more discretely labeled, and often numerous, single cells (FIGS. 6c and 6d). Their labeling was frequently so intense that it must indicate underlying plasma cells, even within GC. Further, these were also seen scattered in the adjacent T cell areas, not always close to labeled GC.[40] We are currently checking the AChR-specific GC for colocalizing myoid cells.

Because of limited sensitivity, low levels of intracellular Ig in GC centroblasts, and possible differences in fine AChR specificity, we must surely be underestimating the truly AChR-reactive B lineage cells. For example, we have noted no significant binding to any resting B cells in GC coronas. Nevertheless, these findings are clear evidence of ongoing responses to AChR in the EOMG thymus and thus fit very well with the specific *in situ* activation of terminal plasma cells already inferred from culture responses.[1,5,8]

Antibody Mutations in EOMG Thymi

It is well established that GC are the sites of antibody diversification and antigen-driven selection of high-affinity somatic mutant B cell clones.[39] Because the strongly AChR-binding cells must be a rich source of antibody transcripts, we were encouraged to isolate specific Fabs from combinatorial libraries prepared from EOMG thymic cells. From our first typical case, we obtained four distinct Fabs, two specific for the MIR and one for fetal rather than adult AChR.[41]

From the second, we microdissected cells from serial sections from four GC and sequenced a total of 263 rearranged VH genes;[40] they were biased towards the widely used VH3 genes, but also to VH5. Although GC often have oligoclonal B cell origins in animal studies,[39] we found a remarkable sequence diversity even in two GC that contained numerous AChR-binding cells, one of them with extensive ^{125}I-α-BuTx labeling too.[40] The GC contained singly represented B cells, some without mutations and others with >30 (FIG. 7). We also found numerous, small, clonally related families, sometimes spanning up to five adjacent sections. Their genealogical trees showed branching patterns with accumulating mutations.[40] In some, these included the original germline sequence ("recent clones"). In others, they stemmed from a deduced clonal progenitor that already had 5–26 mutations (FIG. 7)—clear evidence of successive rounds of diversification in this ongoing response.

We next isolated ~36 Fabs from two unusual EOMG mothers with previous arthrogryposis multiplex congenita (AMC) babies,[42] AChR-binding thymic GC (as above), and serum antibodies that greatly preferred fetal to adult AChR, selectively inhibiting its ion channel function.[42] Interestingly, this fetal AChR specificity is considerably more common in parous than nonparous patients,[43] suggesting autoimmunization by AChR from the fetus (A. Vincent and colleagues, this volume).

All but one of the Fabs showed a strong fetal AChR-binding preference, competing well with fetal AChR-specific mAbs. Disappointingly, none substantially affected ion channel function.[43] All their VH and most of their Vκ sequences were highly mutated. Even though these Fabs were derived from bulk thymus cells, we found a dominant VH clone in each case (again from the VH3 family), paired, in one, with a similarly related Vκ family (from the O2/12 group). Even more interestingly, each clonally related family stemmed from a highly mutated progenitor with 25–44 mutations from germline (similar to 15D in FIG. 7B). We inferred (1) an initial round of selection against AChR from the fetus itself (? in uterine lymph nodes) and (2) attraction of some of the resulting memory cells to the thymus by the fetal AChR of myoid cells, which (3) drives further rounds of diversification in the nearby GC.

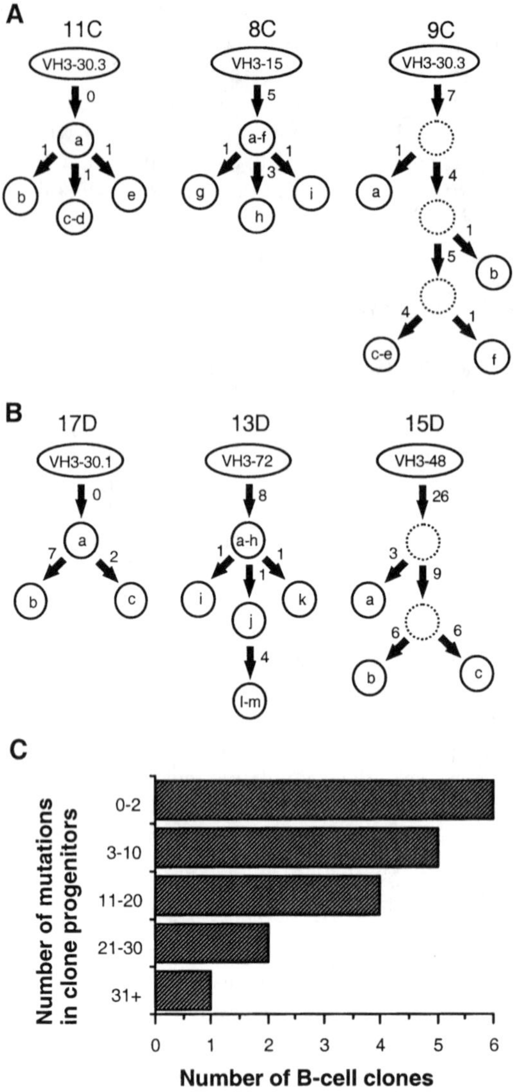

FIGURE 7. Heterogeneity of VH sequences in microdissected GC cells from an EOMG patient. Strongly ^{125}I-α-BuTx-AChR-binding cells were numerous in the GC used in **A**, but fewer in **B**; in both, the FDC labeled well with ^{125}I-α-BuTx alone.[40] Genealogical trees were constructed with maximal parsimony. The best-matching germline sequence is given in the ellipse; letters in the circles refer to individual isolated sequences, and the dotted circles to deduced intermediates. Beside the arrows are the numbers of intervening mutations. The data for **C** derive from 4 GC. Dissecting more sections would surely reveal even greater diversity. Donor is a 34.5-year-old EOMG female with 31-month MG duration and anti-AChR titer > 41 nM. (From ref. 40 with permission.)

TOWARDS A UNIFYING HYPOTHESIS: AUTOIMMUNIZATION OF TH AND B CELLS IN SUCCESSIVE STEPS

We propose that successive steps occur in the autoimmunization of Th and B cells. For the first step, medullary TEC are more plausible candidates than muscle or myoid cells for initially autosensitizing T cells against linear epitopes. For the second, we propose that these T cells induce "early autoantibodies", which subsequently help to provoke GC formation and so broaden the antibody specificities.

Step 1

The TEC are implicated partly by their hyperplasia,[20] especially at the "epicenters" in EOMG, and by their expression of class II and costimulatory molecules, as well as by their AChR subunit mRNA transcripts and even polypeptides[15,30] (FIG. 4). Even if few of the TEC are class II$^+$, they might nevertheless be highly immunogenic in this professional lymphoid microenvironment,[44] perhaps with the help of the abundant bystander professional APC. Remarkably, many EOMG patients have serum autoantibodies to subcapsular/medullary TEC,[45] independent evidence that they actually do autoimmunize in this subgroup (whereas muscle seems an unlikely culprit[46]). Complete AChR has not been detected convincingly in TEC; incomplete subunit assembly probably favors rapid degradation[36] and might generate T cell epitopes more efficiently. Interestingly, TEC express the ε subunit,[15,32] which contains an apparently immunodominant epitope presented to Th1 T cells by HLA-DR52a,[47] a candidate susceptibility allele in EOMG. We are currently developing epitope–HLA-class II multimers to characterize these Th further from patients' blood and thymus, and especially to assess their susceptibility *ex vivo* to specific tolerance induction (U. Kishore and colleagues, this volume).

Their expression of selected peripheral tissue-specific autoantigens suggests less stringent transcriptional controls in TEC than elsewhere or possibly some thymus-specific expression element in their promoters. Their scarcity may explain the evident lack of self-tolerance to AChR.[48] Instead, these TEC seem normally to select and/or prime Treg against a variety of peripheral self-antigens, a process that appears to be critically IL-2-dependent.[49,50] Possibly, a mere shift in the local cytokine balance might switch pre-Treg towards a pathogenic and/or cytotoxic behavior that eventually leads to autoantibody production. In the EOMG thymus, IL-2$^+$ cells have been noted in T cell areas.[51] Together with IL-1 and IL-6, which are produced by TEC,[52] they could contribute to GC formation.[39,53] Moreover, the 3:1 female bias in EOMG, its stronger HLA associations in females,[54] and its onset between puberty and menopause recall the known hormonal influences of prolactin[55] on TEC behavior, potentially another important predisposing factor.

Step 2

It is hard to explain how Th recognizing unfolded AChR sequences activate conformation-specific B cell responses without invoking *de novo* class II expression on muscle or myoid cells in response to unlikely second insults, such as viral infections (which have not been implicated in MG[2,8]). Determinant spreading offers a particularly neat solution. For example, rabbits immunized with α138–199 peptides eventually make conformation-specific antibodies against rabbit AChR.[4] We propose that the isolated AChR subunits (α or ε) in TEC similarly evoke "early" antibody responses that cross-react with native AChR, including its extracellular domain. The progressive involvement of thymic myoid cells in seroconversion and local GC formation[6] (FIG. 5) strongly suggests that they are the key targets for these antibodies (or those evoked by AChR from the fetus in parous mothers[43]). The ensuing damage could then readily recruit professional APC and release antigen/antibody complexes—known potent stimulators of GC formation.[37,39] Indeed, that may be a critical step; the clear antigen-driven diversification there[40,41,43] must enhance the complement activation and thus the pathogenicity of the antibodies.

This proposal not only avoids any need to postulate myoid cell infections or co-stimulation, but also neatly explains the preference of these patients' autoantibodies for the fetal AChR[1–4] that myoid cells express.[2,7] Moreover, these early antibodies would focus the response onto their AChR rather than their other muscle antigens that are rarely recognized in EOMG, despite their evident immunogenicity in MG-thymoma patients.[1–3,10,11] Although there is little evidence,[56] cytotoxic T cell responses could play an analogous damaging role, but one would then expect reactions to these other muscle antigens.

In MG-thymoma patients, we believe, like others,[1,2,15,29] that the neoplastic TEC initially prime T cells in the thymoma, possibly against other muscle antigens or against some shared motif,[14] with no dominant HLA-restriction yet identified. The apparent absence of myoid cells and native AChR[15] in thymomas correlates with the rarity of GC and spontaneous anti-AChR production there, unlike in the adjacent thymic remnant (TABLE 1), where we see similar hyperplasia/infiltration and clonal diversification in AChR- and IFN-α-specific Fabs (Shiono *et al.*, 2003. *Int. Immunol.* **15:** 903–913). Alternatively, step 2 could take place in muscle, where lymphocytic infiltrates have long been noted, although not at endplates.[46] Since thymomas often generate more single $CD8^+$ than $CD4^+$ T cells, a cytotoxic attack on myoid or muscle cells seems likely; it might account for the autoantibody responses to other (striational) muscle antigens and/or expose cryptic epitopes, potentially a key step in autoimmunization.[57]

Effects versus Causes

It remains possible that the response in EOMG is initiated in the periphery, for example, by mimetic microbes, although there is little evidence in their favor.[1–3,8] The thymus could, in theory, only become involved secondarily because it is receptive/responsive to circulating immune complexes or activated T cells.[5] However, this "dull hypothesis" makes few predictions, and our new evidence further implicating both TEC and myoid cells argues strongly against it.

A TESTABLE HYPOTHESIS

Our hypothesis makes many testable predictions: (1) the essential early changes involve T and then B cell priming by the TEC against linear AChR epitopes and may well be focal; (2) early in EOMG, there should be antibodies that cross-react between unfolded subunits and whole AChR; (3) the HLA-DR3-B8 haplotype favors

Th responses to AChRε, leading to myoid cell damage and conformation-specific antibody responses to the fetal as well as adult AChR; in certain seronegative MG patients, this "switch" may never occur, perhaps because they rarely have this haplotype (unpublished); (4) exposed myoid cells in EOMG should have bound anti-AChR antibodies and complement components, which should correlate with the numbers of GC and the proportion of fetal AChR-specific autoantibodies; (5) any GC close to exposed myoid cells in EOMG should be largely AChR-specific; and (6) variability in myoid cell numbers, involvement, or its timing, might help to explain the variable benefits of thymectomy.

Finally, analogous processes might occur in other autoimmune diseases, explaining the thymic hyperplasia and GC noted sometimes in humans and animal models.[58–60] The extent of GC formation might depend on the accessibility there of native autoantigen to antibody attack. Indeed, in human autoimmunity, an ideal test of our hypothesis would be a systematic comparison of thymic changes in diseases differing in thymic autoantigen expression and in antibody- versus T cell–mediated pathogeneses.

ACKNOWLEDGMENTS

We are extremely grateful to many colleagues for access to patients and samples, and to N. Hales, G. Janossy, P. Banga, and G. K. Dhoot for antibodies. This work was supported by the Muscular Dystrophy Campaign, the Myasthenia Gravis Association, the Sir Jules Thorn Charitable Trust, and the Medical Research Council of Great Britain. H. Shiono and I. Roxanis contributed equally to this study.

REFERENCES

1. WILLCOX, N. 1993. Myasthenia gravis. Curr. Opin. Immunol. **5:** 910–917.
2. DRACHMAN, D.B. 1994. Myasthenia gravis. N. Engl. J. Med. **330:** 179–181.
3. TZARTOS, S.J., T. BARKAS, M.T. CUNG *et al.* 1998. Anatomy of the antigenic structure of a large membrane autoantigen, the muscle-type nicotinic acetylcholine receptor. Immunol. Rev. **163:** 89–120.
4. VINCENT, A., N. WILLCOX, M. HILL *et al.* 1998. Determinant spreading and immune responses to acetylcholine receptors in myasthenia gravis. Immunol. Rev. **164:** 157–168.
5. SCHLUEP, M., N. WILLCOX, M.A. RITTER *et al.* 1988. Myasthenia gravis thymus: clinical, histological, and culture correlations. J. Autoimmun. **1:** 445–467.
6. ROXANIS, I., K. MICKLEM, N. WILLCOX *et al.* 2002. Thymic myoid cells and germinal center formation in myasthenia gravis: possible roles in pathogenesis. J. Neuroimmunol. **125:** 185–197.
7. SCHLUEP, M., N. WILLCOX, A. VINCENT *et al.* 1987. Acetylcholine receptors in human thymic myoid cells *in situ*: an immunohistological study. Ann. Neurol. **22:** 212–222.
8. WILLCOX, N. & A. VINCENT. 1988. Myasthenia gravis as an example of organ-specific autoimmune disease. *In* B Lymphocytes in Human Disease, pp. 469–506. Oxford University Press. Oxford.
9. BUCKLEY, C., D. DOUEK, J. NEWSOM-DAVIS *et al.* 2001. Mature, long-lived $CD4^+$ and $CD8^+$ T cells are generated by the thymoma in myasthenia gravis. Ann. Neurol. **50:** 64–72.
10. AARLI, J.A., K. STEFANSSON, L.S.G. MARTON & R.L. WOLLMAN. 1990. Patients with myasthenia gravis and thymoma have in their sera IgG autoantibodies against titin. Clin. Exp. Immunol. **82:** 284–288.
11. SKEIE, G.O., A. FREIBURG, B. KOLMERER *et al.* 1997. Titin transcripts in thymomas. J. Autoimmun. **10:** 551–557.

12. MEAGER, A., A. VINCENT, J. NEWSOM-DAVIS & N. WILLCOX. 1997. Spontaneous neutralising antibodies to interferon-α and interleukin-12 in thymoma-associated autoimmune disease. Lancet **350:** 1596–1597.
13. BUCKLEY, C., J. NEWSOM-DAVIS, N. WILLCOX & A. VINCENT. 2001. Do titin and cytokine antibodies in MG patients predict thymoma or thymoma recurrence? Neurology **57:** 1579–1582.
14. YOSHIKAWA, H. & V.A. LENNON. 1997. Acetylcholine receptor autoantibody secretion by thymocytes: relationship to myasthenia gravis. Neurology **49:** 562–567.
15. WILISCH, A., S. GUTSCHE, V. HOFFACKER *et al.* 1999. Association of acetylcholine receptor α subunit gene expression in mixed thymoma with myasthenia gravis. Neurology **52:** 1460–1466.
16. MOSER, M. & K.M. MURPHY. 2000. Dendritic cell regulation of Th1-Th2 development. Nat. Immunol. **1:** 199–205.
17. SPITS, H., F. COUWENBERG, A.Q. BAKKER *et al.* 2000. Id2 and Id3 inhibit development of $CD34^+$ stem cells into predendritic cell (pre-DC)2, but not into pre-DC1: evidence for a lymphoid origin of pre-DC2. J. Exp. Med. **192:** 1775–1783.
18. ZHANG, W., J-L. LIU, A. MEAGER *et al.* 2003. Autoantibodies to IL-12 in myasthenia gravis patients with thymoma: effects on the IFN-γ responses of healthy $CD4^+$ T cells. J. Neuroimmunol. **139:** 102–108.
19. WANG, X. & T. MOSSMAN. 2001. *In vivo* priming of CD4 T cells that produce interleukin (IL)-2, but not IL-4 or IFN-γ, and can subsequently differentiate into IL-4- or IFN-γ-secreting cells. J. Exp. Med. **194:** 1069–1080.
20. ROXANIS, I., K. MICKLEM & N. WILLCOX. 2001. True epithelial hyperplasia in the thymus of early-onset myasthenia gravis patients: implications for immuno-pathogenesis. J. Neuroimmunol. **112:** 163–173.
21. GILHUS, N.E., N. WILLCOX, G. HARCOURT *et al.* 1995. Antigen presentation by thymoma epithelial cells from myasthenia gravis patients to potentially pathogenic T cells. J. Neuroimmunol. **56:** 65–76.
22. SMITH, K.M., D.C. OLSON, R. HIROSE & D. HANAHAN. 1997. Pancreatic gene expression in rare cells of thymic medulla: evidence for functional contribution to T cell tolerance. Int. Immunol. **9:** 1355–1365.
23. ALDERUCCIO, F., P.A. GLEESON, S.P. BERZINS *et al.* 1997. Expression of the gastric H/K ATPase α subunit in the thymus may explain the dominant role of the β subunit in the pathogenesis of autoimmune gastritis. Autoimmunity **25:** 167–175.
24. SEDDON, B. & D. MASON. 2000. The third function of the thymus. Trends Immunol. **21:** 95–99.
25. JORDAN, M.S., A. BOESTEANU, A.J. REED *et al.* 2001. Thymic selection of $CD4^+CD25^+$ regulatory T cells induced by an agonist self peptide. Nat. Immunol. **2:** 301–306.
26. SHEVACH, E.M. 2001. Certified professionals: $CD4^+CD25^+$ suppressor T cells. J. Exp. Med. **193:** F41– F45.
27. CROWTHER, N.J., B. XIAO & C.N. HALES. 1994 Epitope analysis of human insulin and intact proinsulin. Protein Eng. **7:** 137–144.
28. EWINS, D.L., P.S. BARNETT, R.W. TOMLINSON *et al.* 1992. Mapping epitope specificities of monoclonal antibodies to thyroid peroxidase using recombinant antigen preparations. Autoimmunity **11:** 141–149.
29. HARA, H., K. HAYASHI, K. OHTA *et al.* 1993. Nicotinic acetylcholine receptor mRNAs in myasthenic thymuses: association with intrathymic pathogenesis of myasthenia gravis. Biochem. Biophys. Res. Commun. **194:** 1269.
30. WAKKACH, A., T. GUYON, C. BRUAND *et al.* 1996. Expression of acetylcholine receptor genes in human thymic epithelial cells: implications for myasthenia gravis. J. Immunol. **157:** 3753–3760.
31. WHEATLEY, L.M., D. URSO, K. TUMAS *et al.* 1992. Molecular evidence for the expression of nicotinic acetylcholine receptor α-chain in mouse thymus. J. Immunol. **148:** 3105–3109.
32. MACLENNAN, C.A., D. BEESON, N. WILLCOX *et al.* 1998. Muscle nicotinic acetylcholine receptor mRNA expression in hyperplastic and neoplastic myasthenia gravis thymus. Ann. N.Y. Acad. Sci. **841:** 407–410.

33. BEESON, D., A. MORRIS, A. VINCENT & J. NEWSOM-DAVIS. 1990. The human muscle acetylcholine receptor α-subunit exists as two isoforms: a novel exon. EMBO J. **9:** 2101–2106.
34. NAGVEKAR, N., A-M. MOODY, P. MOSS *et al.* 1998. A pathogenic role for the thymoma in myasthenia gravis; autosensitization of IL-4-producing T cell clones recognizing extracellular acetylcholine receptor epitopes presented by minority class II isotypes. J. Clin. Invest. **101:** 2268–2277.
35. MARX, A., R. O'CONNOR, K.I. GEUDER *et al.* 990. Characterization of a protein with an acetylcholine receptor epitope from myasthenia gravis–associated thymomas. Lab. Invest. **62:** 279–286.
36. CARLIN, B.E., J.C. LAWRENCE, J.M. LINDSTROM & J.P. MERLIE. 1986. An acetylcholine receptor precursor α subunit that binds α-bungarotoxin, but not *d*-tubocurarine. Proc. Natl. Acad. Sci. USA **83:** 498–502.
37. KUNKL, A. & G.G.B. KLAUS. 1981. The generation of memory cells. IV. Immunisation with antigen/antibody complexes accelerates the development of memory cells, the formation of germinal centres, and the maturation of antibody affinity in the secondary response. Immunology **43:** 371–378.
38. WEKERLE, H. & U-P. KETELSEN. 1976. Intrathymic pathogenesis and dual genetic control of myasthenia gravis. Lancet **i:** 678–680.
39. MACLENNAN, I.C.M. 1994. Germinal centers. Annu. Rev. Immunol. **12:** 117–139.
40. SIMS, G.P., H. SHIONO, N. WILLCOX & D.I. STOTT. 2001. Somatic hypermutation and selection of B cells in thymic germinal centers responding to acetylcholine receptor in myasthenia gravis. J. Immunol. **167:** 1935–1944.
41. FARRAR, J., S. PORTOLANO, N. WILLCOX *et al.* 1997. Diverse Fab specific for acetylcholine receptor epitopes from a myasthenia gravis combinatorial library. Int. Immunol. **9:** 1311–1318.
42. RIEMERSMA, S., A. VINCENT, D. BEESON *et al.* 1996. Association of arthrogryposis multiplex congenita with maternal antibodies inhibiting fetal acetylcholine receptor function. J. Clin. Invest. **98:** 2358–2363.
43. MATTHEWS, I., G.P. SIMS, S. LEDWIDGE *et al.* 2002. Antibodies to human acetylcholine receptor in parous women: evidence for immunization by fetal antigen. Lab. Invest. **82:** 1407–1417.
44. KÜNDIG, T., M.F. BACHMANN, C. DI PAOLO *et al.* 1995. Fibroblasts as efficient antigen-presenting cells in lymphoid organs. Science **268:** 1343–1347.
45. SAFAR, D., C. AIME, S. COHEN-KAMINSKY & S. BERRIH-AKNIN. 1991. Antibodies to thymic epithelial cells in myasthenia gravis. J. Neuroimmunol. **35:** 101–110.
46. NAKANO, S. & A.G. ENGEL. 1993. Myasthenia gravis: quantitative immunocytochemical analysis of inflammatory cells and detection of complement membrane attack complex at the end-plate in 30 patients. Neurology **43:** 1167–1172.
47. HILL, M., D. BEESON, P. MOSS *et al.* 1999. Early-onset myasthenia gravis: a recurring T cell epitope in the adult-specific acetylcholine receptor ε subunit presented by the susceptibility allele HLA-DR52a. Ann. Neurol. **45:** 224–231.
48. JERMY, A., D. BEESON & A. VINCENT. 1993. Pathogenic autoimmunity to affinity purified mouse acetylcholine receptor induced without adjuvant in BALB/c mice. Eur. J. Immunol. **23:** 973–976.
49. SADLACK, B., H. MERZ, H. SCHORLE *et al.* 1993. Ulcerative colitis-like disease in mice with a disrupted interleukin-2 gene. Cell **75:** 253–261.
50. ITOH, M., T. TAKAHASHI, N. SAKAGUCHI *et al.* 1999. Thymus and autoimmunity: production of $CD25^+$ $CD4^+$ naturally anergic and suppressive T cells as a key function of the thymus in maintaining self-tolerance. J. Immunol. **162:** 5317–5326.
51. EMILIE, D., M.C. CREVON, S. COHEN-KAMINSKY *et al.* 1991. *In situ* production of interleukins in hyperplastic thymus from myasthenia gravis patients. Hum. Pathol. **22:** 461–468.
52. LE, P.T., D.T. TUCK, C.A. DINARELLO *et al.* 1987. Human thymic epithelial cells produce interleukin 1. J. Immunol. **138:** 2520–2526.
53. KOSCO-VILBOIS, M.H., J-Y. BONNEFOY & Y. CHVATCHKO. 1997. The physiology of murine germinal center reactions. Immunol. Rev. **156:** 127–136.

54. JANER, M., A. COWLAND, J. PICARD *et al.* 1999. A susceptibility region extending into the HLA-class I sector telomeric to HLA-C. Hum. Immunol. **60:** 909–917.
55. DARDENNE, M. & W. SAVINO. 1994. Control of thymus physiology by peptidic hormones and neuropeptides. Immunol. Today **15:** 518–523.
56. CURNOW, S.J., N. WILLCOX & A. VINCENT. 1998. Induction of primary immune responses by allogeneic human myoblasts: dissection of the cell types required for proliferation, IFN-γ secretion, and cytotoxicity. J. Neuroimmunol. **86:** 53–62.
57. CASCIOLA-ROSEN, L., F. ANDRADE, D. ULANET *et al.* 1999. Cleavage by granzyme B is strongly predictive of autoantigen status: implications for initiation of autoimmunity. J. Exp. Med. **190:** 815–826.
58. BURNET, F.M. & I.R. MACKAY. 1962. Lymphoepithelial structures and autoimmune disease. Lancet **ii:** 1030–1033.
59. MURAKAMI, M., Y. HOSOI, T. NEGISHI *et al.* 1996. Thymic hyperplasia in patients with Graves' disease: identification of thyrotropin receptors in human thymus. J. Clin. Invest. **98:** 2228–2234.
60. EAST, J., M.A.B. DE SOUSA & D.M.V. PARROTT. 1965. Immunopathology of New Zealand black (NZB) mice. Transplantation **3:** 711–729.

A New Model Linking Intrathymic Acetylcholine Receptor Expression and the Pathogenesis of Myasthenia Gravis

ARNOLD I. LEVINSON, YI ZHENG, GLEN GAULTON, JONNI MOORE, C. HANK PLETCHER, DECHENG SONG, AND LISA M. WHEATLEY

Allergy and Immunology Section, University of Pennsylvania School of Medicine, Philadelphia, Pennsylvania 19104-6160, USA

ABSTRACT: The thymus is thought to play an important role in the pathogenesis of myasthenia gravis (MG), an autoimmune disease characterized by skeletal muscle weakness. However, its role remains a mystery. The studies described represent our efforts to determine how intrathymic expression of the neuromuscular type of acetylcholine receptors (nAChRs) is involved in the immunopathogenesis of MG. We review our work characterizing the expression of the alpha subunit of nAChR (nAChRα) in the thymus and advance a new hypothesis that examines the intrathymic expression of this autoantigen in disease pathogenesis.

KEYWORDS: thymus; myasthenia gravis; acetylcholine receptor alpha subunit

INTRODUCTION

Myasthenia gravis (MG) is an autoimmune disease caused by IgG antibodies directed at neuromuscular acetylcholine receptors (nAChRs). These autoantibodies impair neuromuscular transmission by reducing the number of receptors (reviewed in ref. 1). The events that lead to the abrogation of self-tolerance to nAChRs remain a mystery. The thymus gland has long been considered to hold the key to solving this mystery, although the nature of its involvement remains to be elucidated. Interest in a primary role for the thymus has been fueled by pathologic, clinical, and immunologic lines of evidence (reviewed in ref. 2).

INTRATHYMIC EXPRESSION OF AChR

It is now clear that nAChRs are expressed on cells in the thymus. This finding led to the hypothesis, first espoused by Wekerle,[3] that the thymus represents a potentially important focus for initiating or perpetuating the autoimmune response

Address for correspondence: Arnold I. Levinson, M.D., Chief, Allergy and Immunology Section, University of Pennsylvania School of Medicine, Room 1014 BRB II/III, 421 Curie Boulevard, Philadelphia, PA 19104-6160. Voice: 215-898-4592; fax: 215-898-0193.
frog@mail.med.upenn.edu

Ann. N.Y. Acad. Sci. 998: 257–265 (2003). © 2003 New York Academy of Sciences.
doi: 10.1196/annals.1254.027

TABLE 1. Summary of nAChRα RT-PCR studies

nAChRα mRNA expression
Normal mouse, control human, and MG thymus
Human thymic epithelial cell line (TEC)
Mouse thymic stromal lines
Dendritic cells
Cortical and medullary epithelial cell lines
Thymus nAChRα nucleotide sequences identical to counterparts at myoneural junction

in MG (in contrast to the more traditional role of the thymus in tolerance induction). We have been particularly interested in the intrathymic expression of the nAChR alpha subunit (nAChRα) since this subunit contains disease-relevant B and T cell epitopes.[4–7] Expression of the receptor α chain has been reported on a wide variety of thymic cells including epithelial cells,[8] thymocytes,[9] and myoid cells.[10–12] Until recently, myoid cells were viewed as the principal nAChR-expressing cells in thymus.[12] These cells, which share phenotypic and functional properties with skeletal muscle cells, are found in the medulla of both normal and MG thymus.

Using RT-PCR, several groups, including our own, reexamined this question. We initially reported that mRNA for the nAChRα was expressed in normal mouse, normal human, and MG thymus.[13,14] In addition, we reported that nAChRα mRNA was expressed on transformed murine thymic cortical and medullary epithelial cell lines and thymic dendritic cell lines.[13] Moreover, we provided evidence for the first time that mRNAs encoding both major isoforms of the human nAChRα, that is, $P3A^+$ and $P3A^-$, were expressed in normal and MG thymus and normal human thymic epithelial cells.[14,15] We also showed that the nucleotide sequences of these isoforms were identical to their counterparts expressed at the myoneural junction and provided evidence for the expression of a third, albeit minor, nAChRα isoform. The above results are summarized in TABLE 1. Subsequently, others reported that nAChRα protein as well as mRNA were expressed on human thymic epithelial cells.[16]

Given the potential role of nAChRs expressed on thymic epithelial cells (TEC) in the pathogenesis of MG, we expanded our work to address additional features of nAChRα expression on these cells.[15] We found that the smaller $P3A^-$ isoform was present in a 5-fold excess in both control and MG thymus and a 2.5-fold excess in a normal human thymic epithelial cell line, relative to the larger $P3A^+$ isoform. This clearly differs from the relationship of these isoforms in control and MG muscle where they are expressed to an equivalent degree.[16,17] These results, summarized in TABLE 2, indicate that the expression of the $P3A^-$ and $P3A^+$ isoforms is differentially regulated in thymus and muscle compartments.

We subsequently observed that $P3A^-$ mRNA expression was 2.5-fold greater in MG thymus than in control thymus, whereas $P3A^+$ expression was 2.8-fold greater in MG thymus than control thymus.[15] These results parallel findings in skeletal muscle where mRNA expression was found to be greater in MG muscle than in control muscle.[18] There is currently no explanation for the observed increased nAChRα

TABLE 2. Expression of nAChRα P3A⁻ and P3A⁺ isoforms

Control and MG thymus	
	P3A⁻ expression 5-fold > P3A⁺
Human TEC	
	P3A⁻ expression 2.5-fold > P3A⁺
Human skeletal muscle	
	P3A⁻ and P3A⁺ expression equivalent

TABLE 3. Cytokine regulation of P3A⁻ and P3A⁺ expression in human TEC

Cytokine	P3A⁻	P3A⁺
IL-1	No effect	No effect
IL-4	No effect	No effect
IL-6	No effect	No effect
IFN-γ	2.7×	2.8×

mRNA expression in MG thymus. However, it may reflect the antecedent action of local environmental factors including anti-ACHRα antibodies and cytokines.

The thymus in MG is characterized by increased epithelial cell production of IL-1 and IL-6.[19,20] Since there is evidence that cytokines elaborated by normal TEC have autocrine function,[21] it seemed possible that these cytokines or perhaps others produced by cells in the thymus might regulate TEC expression of nAChRα. Indeed, our recent studies indicate that neither IL-1, IL-6, nor IL-4 impacts on expression of nAChRα mRNA by a human TEC line.[15] In contrast, interferon-γ (IFN-γ) increased expression of the P3A⁻ and P3A⁺ isoforms by factors of 2.7 and 2.8, respectively (TABLE 3). It is known that IFN-γ upregulates the expression of MHC class II antigens on thymic epithelial cells.[21,22] This dual effect of IFN-γ on nAChRα and MHC antigens raises the possibility that this cytokine, and perhaps others, may alter expression of thymic nAChRα *in vivo* in a manner that leads to the development or perpetuation of MG. However, understanding how this might occur requires a brief review of the thymus' role in the development of T cell tolerance and a consideration of how the thymus could serve as a site of immune activation.

INTRATHYMIC NACHR: AN ARCHITECT OF CENTRAL TOLERANCE AND SENSITIZATION

The thymus plays a fundamental role in the generation of the peripheral T cell repertoire.[23–25] Thymocytes with low affinity receptors for self-proteins are thought to be positively selected for export to the peripheral lymphoid tissues where they comprise the T cell repertoire that recognizes exogenous antigens.[23,24] In contrast, T cell tolerance to self derives largely from the process of central deletion/inactivation, wherein developing thymocytes with high affinity receptors for self-peptide are silenced by apoptosis or anergy. Whereas there is widespread agreement that presentation of self-peptides by cortical epithelial cells is necessary for positive selection,[24–26] there is still controversy over the identity of the thymic APC (antigen presenting cell) involved in negative selection. Indeed, there is evidence supporting roles for thymic medullary epithelial cells and bone marrow–derived macrophages and dendritic cells in this process.[25,27–30] However, central deletion is not complete even though a broad array of self-peptides is expressed on medullary thymic epithelial cells.[31] Self-reactive T cells appear to escape from the thymus in small numbers, perhaps due to the fact that limiting levels of self-antigen limit the efficiency of tolerance induction.[32–34] However, such self-reactive T cells are thought to be held in check because of their anergic or ignorant status, that is, they never encounter self-antigen in the periphery in a manner that leads to immune activation, or they are suppressed by regulatory T cells.[35]

BIDIRECTIONAL TRAFFICKING OF T CELLS FROM AND TO THE THYMUS

The thymus is not generally considered to be a site of immune activation. Based on the classic studies of Gowans, traffic of lymphocytes is generally considered to be unidirectional, that is, out of the thymus into the blood and peripheral lymphoid organs.[36] However, there is evidence that peripheral immunocompetent T cells migrate back to the thymus in small numbers where they typically enter the thymic medullary compartment.[37–43] The evidence suggests that activated peripheral T cells account for the bulk of thymic immigrants,[38,39,42] although there is also evidence for the entry of resting T cells.[43] It is not known if the number of thymic immigrants would be increased nonspecifically by an inflammatory reaction in the thymus. Also, it is not known if self-reactive T cell immigrants would be activated were they to engage their specific antigen in the thymus. When self-reactive T cells encounter their antigens in other tissue compartments in the presence of requisite costimulatory signals, they can be activated to express their differentiation program.[44] One mechanism that leads to a milieu that promotes the abrogation of tolerance peripherally is infection. Local infection can lead to the upregulation of MHC antigens and costimulatory molecules on cells that express low levels of self-antigens, thereby leading to activation of autoreactive T cells.[44]

PERIPHERAL T CELL HOMING TO THE THYMUS: A NEW MODEL OF THE INTRATHYMIC PATHOGENESIS OF MG

Our ability to uncover the molecular events, particularly in the thymus, that direct the initiation of MG, has been hampered by the lack of a model system. Thymic pathology is not a feature of experimental models of MG in rodents. Although such models have provided insight into the pathogenesis of MG,[45] they have not served to elucidate the role played by the thymus. To circumvent this problem, we have developed a new model of intrathymic inflammation (FIG. 1).[46] The hypothesis to be tested is that an inflammatory reaction to an unrelated antigen within the medulla of

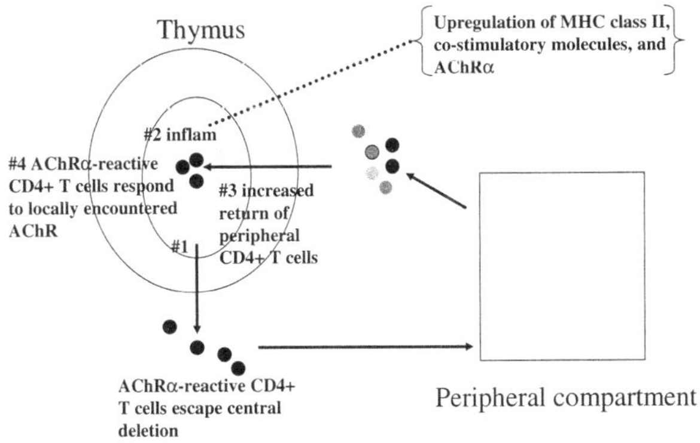

FIGURE 1. Intrathymic pathogenesis of myasthenia gravis. See text for details.

TABLE 4. Rationale for intrathymic pathogenesis hypothesis

nAChRα-reactive CD4+ T cells can be found in the blood of healthy donors as well as MG patients
nAChRα-reactive T and B cells are recovered from MG thymus, but not "control" thymus
nAChRα is constitutively expressed on thymic myoid cells and thymic epithelial cells
nAChRα mRNA and MHC class II protein expression on human thymic epithelial cells is upregulated by IFN-γ
Peripheral T cells traffic to thymus where they enter the medulla

the thymus facilitates entry of peripheral nAChRα-reactive CD4+ T cells that escaped central deletion. These cells enter the thymus in the medullary compartment, where they encounter nAChRα expressed on APCs. The concomitant intrathymic inflammatory reaction creates a milieu that favors activation of these cells, that is, upregulation of MHC class II antigens, costimulatory molecules on APCs, and perhaps upregulation of AChR expression. Presentation of nAChRα epitopes to the CD4+ thymic immigrants leads to their activation, help for locally stimulated αAChR-reactive B cells, production of anti-AChR antibodies and germinal centers, and the development of MG. The rationale for this hypothesis is outlined in TABLE 4.

To test this hypothesis, we devised an experimental protocol for inducing intrathymic inflammation targeted to the thymic medulla, the compartment entered by returning peripheral T cells. We generated molecular variants of the well-characterized thymotrophic gross murine leukemia virus (G-MLV), GD-17, which had previously been shown to exclusively infect medullary thymic epithelium following intrathymic injection in naïve mice.[47] The thymotropic MLV vectors were created by ligating a 425-bp fragment containing the U3 region of GD-17 into the LTR backbone of the well-defined M-MLV vector LXSH (FIG. 2). The parental LXSH vector includes 5′ M-MSV LTR, the Psi packaging site and 5′ Gag region, the hygromycin resistance

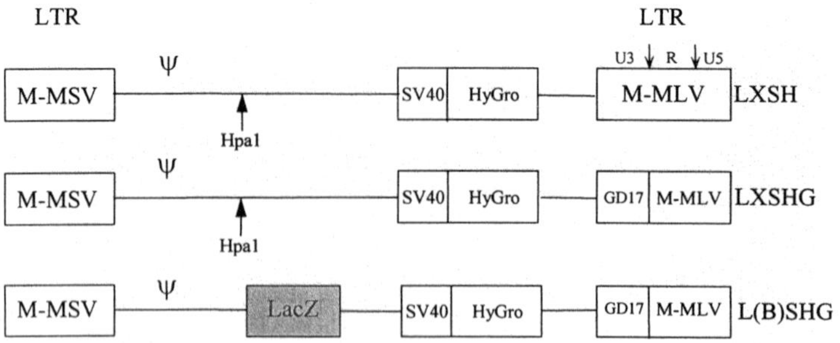

FIGURE 2. Schematic diagram of MLV-based vectors. The vectors used in these studies are presented in linear form. The parental LXSH vector includes 5′ M-MSV LTR, the Psi packaging site and 5′ Gag region, the hygromycin resistance gene under control of the SV40 promoter, and the 3′ LTR of M-MLV. Vectors are modified by insertion of either GD-17 U3 or LacZ.

gene under control of the SV40 promoter, and the 3′ LTR of M-MLV. For our experimental protocol, we modified this vector by insertion of the Lac Z gene [L(B)SHG]. We utilized L(B)SHG and LXSHG as our experimental and control vectors, respectively. As was true for GD-17, we found that these vectors target the thymic medullary epithelium for expression of virally encoded genes.

In our experimental model, Balb/c mice were immunized to β-galactosidase (β-gal) and then were injected intrathymically (i.t.) with the β-gal encoding vector L(B)SHG or the control vector LXSHG. Hematoxylin and eosin–stained sections of thymus obtained four days after i.t. injection of L(B)SHG, but not LXSHG, showed obliteration of the cortical/medullary architecture with marked cellular expansion of the medulla. To determine whether this local inflammatory reaction nonspecifically augmented the entry of peripheral T cells into the thymus, β-gal-immunized mice were injected i.v. with a population of CFSE-labeled CD4+ T cells specific for an unrelated antigen four days after i.t. injection of L(B)SHG or LXSHG. Animals that received L(B)SHG had 4.2-fold more CFSE-labeled CD4+ thymic immigrants than animals that received the control vector.

CONCLUSIONS

The studies described herein review our recent attempts to elucidate the role of the thymus in the pathogenesis of MG. A central focus of these efforts is the role played by the intrathymic expression of nAChRs. We have established a model of inflammation in the thymic medulla and report that such an inflammatory process promotes the nonspecific entry of peripheral CD4+ T cells into the thymus. Using this model, we are in the process of determining whether (1) nAChRα-reactive CD4+ T cell homing to the thymus is also augmented by a concurrent intrathymic inflammatory response to an unrelated antigen and (2) nAChRα-reactive T cell immigrants undergo activation following their engagement of autoantigen in this inflammatory milieu, provide help for the production of anti-AChR antibodies by immigrant autoreactive B cells, and thereby promote the development of a myasthenic syndrome.

ACKNOWLEDGMENTS

Studies described in this report were supported by a grant from the Muscular Dystrophy Association and National Institutes of Health (Grant No. AI 50058). We thank Cecelia Willitt for assistance with preparation of the manuscript.

REFERENCES

1. LEVINSON, A.I., B. ZWEIMAN & R.P. LISAK. 1987. Immunopathogenesis and treatment of myasthenia gravis. J. Clin. Immunol. **7:** 187–197.
2. LEVINSON, A.I. & L. WHEATLEY. 1995. The thymus and the pathogenesis of myasthenia gravis. Clin. Immunol. Immunopathol. **78:** 1–5.
3. WEKERLE, H., U.P. KETELSON, A.D. ZURN & B.W. FULPIUS. 1978. Intrathymic pathogenesis of myasthenia gravis: transient expression of acetylcholine receptors on thymus-derived myogenic cells. Eur. J. Immunol. **8:** 579–582.
4. HOHLFELD, R., K.V. TOYKA, S.J. TZARTOS *et al.* 1987. Human helper T lymphocytes in myasthenia gravis recognize the nicotinic receptor α subunit. Proc. Natl. Acad. Sci. USA **84:** 5379–5383.
5. ZHANG, Y., M. SCHLUEP, S. FRUTIGER *et al.* 1990. Immunologic heterogeneity of autoreactive T lymphocytes against the nicotinic acetylcholine receptor in myasthenic patients. Eur. J. Immunol. **20:** 2577–2583.
6. OSHIMA, M., T. ASHIZAWA, M.S. POLLACK & M.Z. ATASSI. 1990. Autoimmune T cell recognition of human acetylcholine receptor: the sites of T cell recognition in myasthenia gravis on the extracellular part of the α-subunit. Eur. J. Immunol. **20:** 2563–2569.
7. FUJI, Y. & J. LINDSTROM. 1988. Specificity of the T cell immune response to acetylcholine receptor in experimental autoimmune myasthenia gravis. J. Immunol. **140:** 1830–1837.
8. ENGEL, W., J.L. TROTTER, D.E. MACFARLIN & C.L. MCINTOSH. 1977. Thymic epithelial cells contain acetylcholine receptor. Lancet **1:** 1310–1311.
9. FUCHS, S., I. SCHMIDT-HOPFELDD & G. TRIDENTE. 1980. Thymic lymphocytes bear a surface antigen which cross-reacts with acetylcholine receptor. Nature **287:** 162–164.
10. KAO, I. & D.B. DRACHMAN. 1977. Thymic muscle cells bear acetylcholine receptors: possible relation to myasthenia gravis. Science **195:** 74–75.
11. WEKERLE, H., U.P. KETELSON, A.D. ZURN & B.W. FULPIUS. 1978. Intrathymic pathogenesis of myasthenia gravis: transient expression of acetylcholine receptors on thymus-derived myogenic cells. Eur. J. Immunol. **8:** 579–582.
12. SCHLUEP, M.N., N. WILCOX, A. VINCENT *et al.* 1987. Acetylcholine receptor in human thymic myoid cells *in situ*: an immunologic study. Ann. Neurol. **22:** 212–222.
13. WHEATLEY, L.M., D. URSO, K. TUMAS *et al.* 1992. Molecular characterization of the nicotinic acetylcholine receptor alpha chain in mouse thymus. J. Immunol. **148:** 3105–3109.
14. WHEATLEY, L.M., D. URSO, Y. ZHENG *et al.* 1993. Molecular analysis of intrathymic nicotinic acetylcholine receptor. Ann. N.Y. Acad. Sci. **681:** 74–82.
15. ZHENG, Y., L.M. WHEATLEY, T. LIU & A.I. LEVINSON. 1999. Acetylcholine receptor alpha subunit mRNA expression in human thymus: augmented expression in myasthenia gravis and upregulation by interferon-γ. Clin. Immunol. **1:** 170–177.
16. WAKKACH, A., T. GUYON, C. BRUAND *et al.* 1978. Expression of acetylcholine receptor genes in human thymic epithelial cells: implications for myasthenia gravis. J. Immunol. **157:** 3752–3760.
17. BEESON, D., A. MORRIS, A. VINCENT & J. NEWSOM-DAVIS. 1990. The human muscle nicotinic acetylcholine receptor α-subunit exists as two isoforms: a novel exon. EMBO J. **9:** 2101–2106.

18. GUYON, T., P. LEVASSEUR, F. TRUFFAULT *et al.* 1993. Nicotinic acetylcholine receptor α subunit variants in human myasthenia gravis: quantification of steady-state levels of messenger RNA in muscle biopsy using the polymerase chain reaction. J. Clin. Invest. **94:** 16.
19. COHEN-KAMINSKY, S., R. DELATTRE, O. DEVERGNE *et al.* 1991. Synergistic induction of interleukin-6 production and gene expression in human thymic epithelial cells by LPS and cytokines. Cell. Immunol. **138:** 79–93.
20. EMILIE, D., M.C. CREVEN, S. COHEN-KAMINSKY *et al.* 1991. *In situ* production of interleukins in hyperplastic thymus from myasthenia gravis patients. Hum. Pathol. **22:** 461–468.
21. GALY, A.H. & H. SPITS. 1991. IL-1, IL-4, and IFN-γ differentially regulate cytokine production and cell surface molecule expression in cultured human thymic epithelial cells. J. Immunol. **147:** 3823–3830.
22. BERRIH-AKNIN, S., F. ARENZANA-SEISDEDOS, S. COHEN *et al.* 1985. Interferon-gamma modulates HLA class II antigen expression on cultured human thymic epithelial cells. J. Immunol. **35:** 1165–1171.
23. SPRENT, J., D. LO, E.K. GAO & Y. RON. 1988. T cell selection in the thymus. Immunol. Rev. **101:** 173–190.
24. KISIELOW, P. & M.V. BOEHMER. 1990. Negative and positive selection of immature thymocytes: timing and the role of the ligand for T cell receptor. Semin. Immunol. **2:** 35–44.
25. ANDERSON, G., N.C. MOORE, J.J. OWEN & E.J. JENKINSON. 1996. Cellular interactions in thymocyte development. Annu. Rev. Immunol. **14:** 73–99.
26. ALAM, S.M., P.J. TRAVERS, J.L. WUNG *et al.* 1996. T-cell-receptor affinity and thymocyte positive selection. Nature **381:** 616–620.
27. HUGO, P., J.W. KAPPLER, D.I. GODFREY & P.C. MARRACK. 1994. Thymic epithelial cell lines that mediate positive selection can also induce thymocyte clonal deletion. J. Immunol. **152:** 1022–1031.
28. BLACKMAN, M., J. KAPPLER & P. MARRACK. 1990. The role of the TCR in positive and negative selection of developing cells. Science **248:** 1335–1341.
29. BONOMO, A. & P. MATZINGER. 1993. Thymus epithelium induces tissue-specific tolerance. J. Exp. Med. **177:** 1153–1164.
30. HOFFMAN, M.W., W.R. HEATH, D. RUSCHMEYER & J.F. MILLER. 1995. Deletion of high-avidity T cells by thymic epithelium. Proc. Natl. Acad. Sci. USA **92:** 9851–9855.
31. KLEIN, L. & B. KYEWSKI. 2000. "Promiscuous" expression of tissue antigens in the thymus: a key to T-cell tolerance and autoimmunity? J. Mol. Med. **78:** 483–494.
32. OEHEN, S.U., P.S. OHASHI, K. BURKI *et al.* 1994. Escape of thymocytes and mature T cells from clonal deletion due to limiting tolerogen expression levels. Cell. Immunol. **158:** 342–352.
33. IWABUCHI, K., K.I. NAKAYAMA, R.L. MCCOY *et al.* 1992. Cellular and peptide requirements for *in vitro* clonal deletion of immature thymocytes. Proc. Natl. Acad. Sci. USA **89:** 9000–9004.
34. ADELSTEIN, S., H. PRITCHARD-BRISCOE, T.A. ANDERSON *et al.* 1991. Induction of self-tolerance in T cells, but not β cells of transgenic mice expressing little self-antigen. Science **251:** 1223–1225.
35. SHEVACH, E. 2000. Regulatory T cells in autoimmunity. Adv. Rev. Immunol. **18:** 423–449.
36. GOWANS, J.L. & E. KNIGHT. 1964. The route of re-circulation of lymphocytes in the rat. Proc. R. Soc. London **B159:** 257–282.
37. NAPARSTEK, Y., J. HOLOSHITZ, S. EISSENSTEIN *et al.* 1982. Effector T lymphocyte line cells migrate to the thymus and persist there. Nature **300:** 262–264.
38. NAPARSTEK, Y., A. BEN-NUN, J. HOLOSHITZ *et al.* 1993. T lymphocyte lines producing or vaccinating against autoimmune encephalomyelitis (EAE): functional activation induces peanut agglutinin receptors and accumulation in the brain and thymus of line cells. Eur. J. Immunol. **13:** 418–423.
39. MICHIE, S.A., E.A. KIRKPATRICK & R.V. ROUSE. 1988. Rare peripheral T cells migrate to and persist in normal mouse thymus. J. Exp. Med. **168:** 1929–1934.
40. HIROKAWA, K., M. UTSUYAMA & T. SADO. 1989. Immunohistological analysis of immigration of thymocyte-precursors into the thymus: evidence for immigration of peripheral T cells into the thymic medulla. Cell. Immunol. **119:** 160–170.

41. GOSSMANN, J., J. LOHLER & F. LEHMANN-GRUBE. 1991. Entry of antivirally active T lymphocytes into the thymus of virus-infected mice. J. Immunol. **146:** 293–297.
42. AGUS, D., C.D. SURH & J. SPRENT. 1991. Reentry of T cells to the adult thymus is restricted to activated cells. J. Exp. Med. **173:** 1039–1046.
43. WESTERMANN, J., T. SMITH, U. PETERS *et al.* 1991. Both activated and nonactivated leukocytes from the periphery continuously enter the thymic medulla of adult rats: phenotypes, sources, and magnitude of traffic. Eur. J. Immunol. **26:** 1866–1874.
44. MONDINO, A., A. KHOURTS & M.K. JENKINS. 1996. The anatomy of T-cell activation and tolerance. Proc. Natl. Acad. Sci. USA **93:** 2245–2252.
45. CHRISTADOSS, P., M. POUSSIN & C. DENG. 2000. Animal models of myasthenia gravis. Clin. Immunol. **94:** 75–87.
46. LEVINSON, A., Y. ZHENG, S. MURPHY *et al.* 2002. Peripheral T cell homing to the inflamed thymus: relevance to myasthenia gravis. J. Allergy Clin. Immunol. **109:** S280.
47. MARSHALL, D.J. & G.N. GAULTON. 1996. The role of the immune response in MuLV-induced lymphomagenesis. Leukemia **10:** 1860–1866.

Human Myoid Cells Protect Thymocytes from Apoptosis

ROZEN LE PANSE-RUSKONÉ AND SONIA BERRIH-AKNIN

CNRS UMR 8078, IPSC, Université Paris XI, Hôpital Marie Lannelongue, 92350 Le Plessis-Robinson, France

KEYWORDS: myoid cells; apoptosis; thymocytes; thymus

INTRODUCTION

Thymus provides a complex environment essential for $CD4^+$ and $CD8^+$ T cell maturation. In addition to cortical and medullary epithelial cells, other stromal cell types can influence thymocyte development.[1] Myoid cells in the thymus correspond to a rare cellular population essentially localized in the medulla and the cortico-medullary junction.[2] They possess the antigenic characteristics of skeletal muscle cells within the thymus. Their biological role is unclear, but their involvement in myasthenia gravis has been suggested.[3] Using a human myoid cell line established in our laboratory, we investigated the effects of myoid cells on thymocyte behavior and phenotype *in vitro*.

RESULTS

Establishment of a Myoid Cell Line

In all our experiments, we used fresh thymic fragments from children undergoing corrective cardiovascular surgery at the Marie Lannelongue Hospital (Le Plessis-Robinson, France).

Thymic stromal cells were immortalized using a plasmid vector encoding the SV40T oncogene. Among the cell lines obtained, one possessed cellular characteristics and markers of skeletal muscle cells observed on normal myoid cells (TABLE 1)[4] and was designated MITC (myoid immortalized thymic cells).

Thymocyte Antiapoptotic Effects of MITC

To investigate the *in vitro* effects of MITC on thymocytes, freshly isolated thymocytes were seeded onto confluent MITC cultures or directly onto plastic

Address for correspondence: Rozen Le Panse-Ruskoné, CNRS UMR 8078, IPSC, Université Paris XI, Hôpital Marie Lannelongue, 92350 Le Plessis-Robinson, France. Voice: +33-1-40-94-55-97; fax: +33-1-46-30-45-64.
rozen.lepanse@ccml.u-psud.fr

**Ann. N.Y. Acad. Sci. 998: 266–269 (2003). © 2003 New York Academy of Sciences.
doi: 10.1196/annals.1254.028**

TABLE 1. Characterization of MITC as myoid cells, a rare cellular population in the thymus sharing characteristics with skeletal muscle cells[4]

Skeletal muscle cell–related components observed in MITC
Myogenic transcription factor (MyoD1) mRNA
α-, β-, δ-, ε-, γ-acetylcholine receptor subunit mRNA
Troponin T antigen
Desmin antigen
MITC characteristics as skeletal muscles
Differentiation and fusion of MITC with cytosine arabinose
Functional AChR in patch-clamp studies

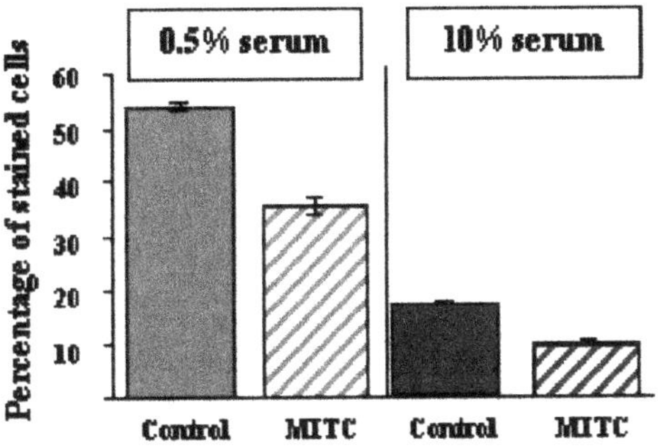

FIGURE 1. Annexin-V-FITC staining of thymocytes. Freshly isolated thymocytes were seeded onto confluent MITC or directly onto plastic culture in 6-well plates. Thymocyte culture experiments were carried out using RPMI medium complemented with 10% or 0.5% of fetal calf serum (FCS). After 24 h, thymocytes were stained with annexin-V-FITC (Boehringer Mannhein) and analyzed in the appropriate gate by a FACSCalibur analyzer. The bar chart corresponds to a representative experiment out of three, and the bars represent the SD calculated from the analysis of three different wells for each culture condition.

culture. The apoptotic state of thymocytes was analyzed 24 h later. Using flow cytometry, we determined the percentage of annexin-V-FITC-stained thymocytes in the gate corresponding to viable thymocytes.

We demonstrated that *in vitro* coculture of myoid cells and thymocytes for 24 h protected thymocytes from apoptosis by strongly decreasing the number of annexin-positive cells regardless of the percentage of serum used (FIG. 1).

We then analyzed whether this protective effect of MITC was not due to an increase in thymocyte proliferation in the coculture model with MITC. We did not observe any variation in the number of thymocytes after 24 h in culture with or without MITC (data not shown). Mitomycin C is an antiproliferative compound. The

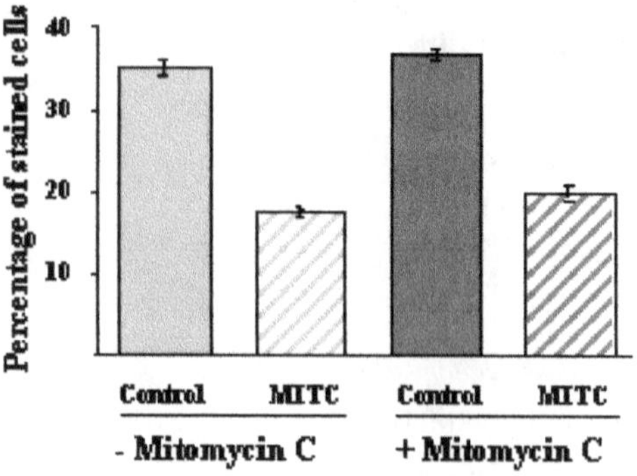

FIGURE 2. Annexin-V-FITC staining of thymocytes. Freshly isolated thymocytes were incubated 45 min at 37°C in RPMI supplemented with 2% FCS and 0.5 mg/mL mitomycin C (Sigma). Thymocytes were then washed twice in RPMI supplemented with 10% FCS and seeded onto confluent MITC or directly onto plastic culture in 6-well plates. After 24 h, thymocytes were stained with annexin-V-FITC and analyzed in the appropriate gate by a FACSCalibur analyzer. The bar chart corresponds to a representative experiment out of three, and the bars represent the SD calculated from the analysis of three different wells for each culture condition.

antiapoptotic effect of myoid cells on thymocytes was similar for mitomycin C–treated or nontreated thymocytes (FIG. 2).

CONCLUSIONS

We observed in our coculture model that myoid cells protected thymocytes from apoptosis independently of any effect on the proliferative state of thymocytes. This antiapoptotic effect could be due to the release of soluble factors by myoid cells. Kamo and colleagues observed that conditioned culture medium from rat thymic myoid cells can stimulate thymocyte proliferation.[5] Indeed, in culture, these cells produce numerous cytokines.[6] However, the myoid antiapoptotic effect observed here could also be due to direct cellular contacts between myoid cells and thymocytes. Preliminary experiments carried out in our laboratory tend to support this last hypothesis (data not shown).

Myoid cells have been especially observed in the medulla and the cortico-medullary junction[2] and consequently colocalized with mature T cells. We then investigated the effects of myoid cells on mature T cells to check if the antiapoptotic effect on thymocytes is devoted to one particular type of T cells. So far, the effects of myoid cells on thymocyte apoptosis can be observed on any subtype of thymocytes analyzed, but it seemed that this coculture model could especially favor CD4 single positive thymocyte survival (data not shown). Myoid cells could thus play an important role in the thymus by participating in thymic selection processes.

Whether this phenomenon is involved in the selection of autoreactive T cells in MG thymuses deserves further investigation.

ACKNOWLEDGMENT

This work was supported by Grant No. NS 39869 from the National Institute of Health.

REFERENCES

1. ANDERSON, G. & E.J. JENKINSON. 2001. Lymphostromal interactions in thymic development and function. Nat. Immunol. **1:** 31–39.
2. SCHLUEP, M., N. WILLCOX, A. VINCENT *et al.* 1987. Acetylcholine receptors in human thymic myoid cells *in situ*: an immunohistological study. Ann. Neurol. **22:** 212–222.
3. BAGGI, F., M. NICOLLE, A. VINCENT *et al.* 1993. Presentation of endogenous acetylcholine receptor epitope by an MHC class II–transfected human muscle cell line to a specific $CD4^+$ T cell clone from a myasthenia gravis patient. J. Neuroimmunol. **46:** 57–66.
4. WAKKACH, A., S. POEA, E. CHASTRE, *et al.* 1999. Establishment of a human thymic myoid cell line. Am. J. Pathol. **155:** 1229–1240.
5. KAMO, I., A. TADA-KIKUCHI, S. FURUKAWA *et al.* 1983. Effects of thymic myoid cell culture supernatant on cells from lymphatic tissues. Cell. Immunol. **94:** 587–597.
6. IWAKAWI, N., A. KIKUCHI, T. KUNISHITA *et al.* 1996. Analysis of the lymphoproliferative cytokines produced by thymic myoid cells. Immunology **87:** 108–112.

Analysis of SjTREC Levels in Thymus from MG Patients and Normal Children

LAURA PASSERINI,[a] PIA BERNASCONI,[a] FULVIO BAGGI,[a]
FERDINANDO CORNELIO,[b] AND RENATO MANTEGAZZA[a]

[a]*Immunology and Muscular Pathology Unit,* [b]*Department of Neuromuscular Diseases, Istituto Nazionale Neurologico "Carlo Besta", 20133 Milan, Italy*

Keywords: myasthenia gravis (MG); sjTREC; thymopoiesis; thymic output

INTRODUCTION

The sensitization to the myasthenia gravis (MG) autoantigen (AChR) and possibly the maintenance of the autoimmune attack are likely to occur within thymus: MG is often associated with abnormalities in thymic tissue (hyperplasia and thymoma), but the pathological basis of this association is still unknown.[1]

During intrathymic development, immature T cells rearrange the T cell receptor (TCR) gene to generate functional TCRs. During this process, excisional DNA products, called TCR rearrangement excision circles (TRECs), are released. The rearrangement events that occur in 70% of αβ T cells are identical, generating a unique signal-joint TREC (sjTREC) in naïve αβ T cells.[2] TRECs remain within the cell during export from the thymus and persist in one daughter cell at each cell cycle. TREC levels in peripheral blood reflect the balance between thymic export of T cells and their rate of proliferation.[3] Quantification of sjTRECs can be used as a measure of thymic function; measurement of sjTREC levels in thymocytes of adult subjects has demonstrated ongoing thymopoiesis well into adulthood.[4]

In this study, we have used sjTREC analysis to quantitate thymopoiesis in normal and MG thymus as well as in peripheral blood mononuclear cells (PBMCs) from healthy donors and MG patients, before and after thymectomy, as a marker of thymic export of T cells to the periphery.

MATERIALS AND METHODS

Patients and Peripheral Blood Samples

Specimens of thymus, removed by VATET approach from 34 MG patients, were frozen over liquid nitrogen fumes and stored in liquid nitrogen until use. There were 17 hyperplastic and 7 involuted thymuses, according to standard histopathological

Address for correspondence: Renato Mantegazza, Immunology and Muscular Pathology Unit, Istituto Nazionale Neurologico "Carlo Besta", via Celoria 11, 20133 Milan, Italy. Voice: +39-02-2394372; fax: +39-02-70633874.
rmantegazza@istituto-besta.it

Ann. N.Y. Acad. Sci. 998: 270–274 (2003). © 2003 New York Academy of Sciences.
doi: 10.1196/annals.1254.029

criteria,[1] and 10 thymomas diagnosed and classified according to WHO classification.[5] Normal thymus samples were obtained from 4 children who underwent corrective cardiovascular surgery. PBMCs were isolated from 20 MG patients (7 hyperplastic, 4 involuted thymuses, and 9 thymomas) and 10 healthy age-matched donors by Ficoll-Paque gradient centrifugation (Amersham-Pharmacia). For 6 MG patients, samples of thymic tissue were available. Twelve MG patients (6 with thymoma and 6 without thymoma) were prospectively studied before and 2–12 months after thymectomy. Cells were stored at –80°C until use.

DNA Extraction

DNA was extracted from whole thymic tissue and PBMCs according to phenol-chloroform standard procedure and stored at –20°C pending PCR amplification.

Quantification of sjTRECs

A competitor DNA identical to the region amplified by the signal-joint primers, but containing a 102-bp deletion, was constructed by amplifying DNA using the sjTREC-specific reverse primer modified at the 3′ end (5′-AGGCTGATCTTGTCT-GACATTTGCTCCGTGGAGGGCTG-3′). A 0.5-μg sample of DNA was coamplified with known concentrations of the competitor in 25 μL of PCR mixture containing 1× PCR buffer (Finnzymes), 200 μM each dNTP (PE Applied Biosystems), 1 μM sjTREC-specific primers, and 1 U DynaZyme DNA polymerase (Finnzymes). PCR conditions were 1 cycle at 95°C for 5 min, followed by 30 cycles at 90°C, 60°C, and 72°C, each for 30 s. Primer sequences, based on previously published sequences, are located ~180 bp on either side of the recombination joints.[3] PCR products were resolved on 2% agarose gel stained with ethidium bromide. Fluorescence of both competitor and target was quantitated (as absorbance) by densitometry using the Kodak Digital Science software (Eastman Kodak, distributed by Amersham-Pharmacia Biotech) and the amount of sjTREC-specific DNA was determined as previously described.[6] The results were expressed as fg of sjTREC DNA/0.5 μg of DNA.

Statistical Analysis

Data are presented as mean ± SE. Values were compared using the two-tailed Student's *t* test.

RESULTS

In order to quantitate thymopoiesis, we studied sjTREC levels within thymus from 34 MG patients and 4 normal children. Results are presented in FIGURE 1. SjTREC levels were significantly raised in the thymus of patients with thymoma (24.4 ± 5.7 fg/0.5 μg DNA) compared to MG patients with involuted thymus (4.9 ± 2 fg/0.5 μg DNA) ($p = 0.01$); they were higher, but not significantly, in hyperplastic thymus (15 ± 3.6 fg/0.5 μg DNA) compared to involuted thymus ($p = 0.15$). No statistically significant difference was observed when sjTREC levels of nonpathological young thymuses (28.2 ± 3.6 fg/0.5 μg DNA) were compared with those found in thymoma ($p = 0.7$) or hyperplasia ($p = 0.1$).

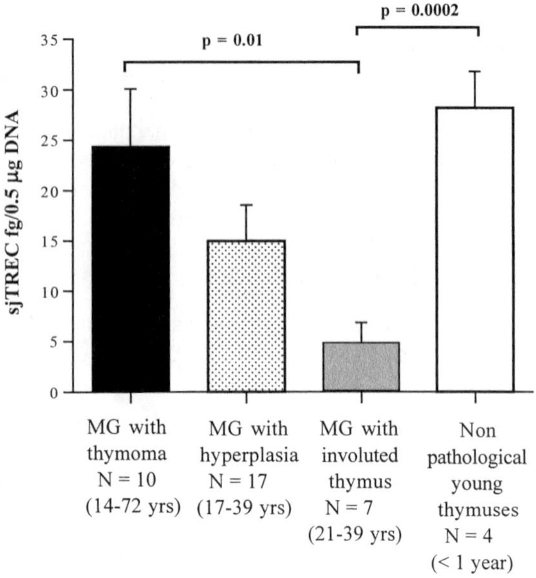

FIGURE 1. SjTREC levels in thymus from MG patients and controls. In involuted thymuses, sjTREC levels were significantly lower than in the thymus of MG patients with thymoma ($p = 0.01$) and in nonpathological young thymuses ($p = 0.0002$). No statistically significant difference was observed when thymoma sjTREC levels were compared with those found in nonpathological young thymuses ($p = 0.7$) or in patients with hyperplasia ($p = 0.15$). The levels in MG hyperplastic thymus were not significantly different from the levels measured in MG involuted thymus and in nonpathological young thymuses ($p = 0.1$). Results are presented as mean ± SE.

To evaluate thymic T cell export in MG patients and adult healthy controls, we measured sjTREC levels in peripheral blood. We found that sjTREC levels in healthy controls were low, with a relatively small variation between individuals (0.176 ± 0.05 fg/0.5 µg DNA). In MG patients with thymoma, sjTREC levels were approximately 7-fold greater than in healthy individuals (1.25 ± 0.44 fg/0.5 µg DNA, $p = 0.02$), but not significantly higher than in MG patients without thymoma (hyperplasia: 1.01 ± 0.21 fg/0.5 µg DNA, $p = 0.6$; involuted thymus: 0.87 ± 0.31 fg/0.5 µg DNA, $p = 0.6$). In these patients, sjTREC levels were significantly raised compared to healthy controls ($p = 0.0004$, hyperplastic thymus versus healthy controls; $p = 0.005$, involuted thymus versus healthy controls) (FIG. 2).

Twelve MG patients who underwent therapeutic thymectomy were subsequently studied up to 12 months after surgery. Results are presented in TABLE 1. Before thymectomy, sjTREC levels in 3 of 6 MG patients with thymoma doubled those measured in patients without thymoma (range: 1.59–3.76 fg/0.5 µg DNA and 0.20–1.73 fg/0.5 µg DNA, respectively). These levels rapidly declined and remained low at 6 to 12 months after thymectomy (range: 0.51–1.65 fg/0.5 µg DNA). In the other 3 thymoma patients, basal sjTREC levels were low (range: 0.14–0.41 fg/0.5 µg DNA) and were decreased or unchanged after thymectomy. In 4/6 (67%) patients, the clinical

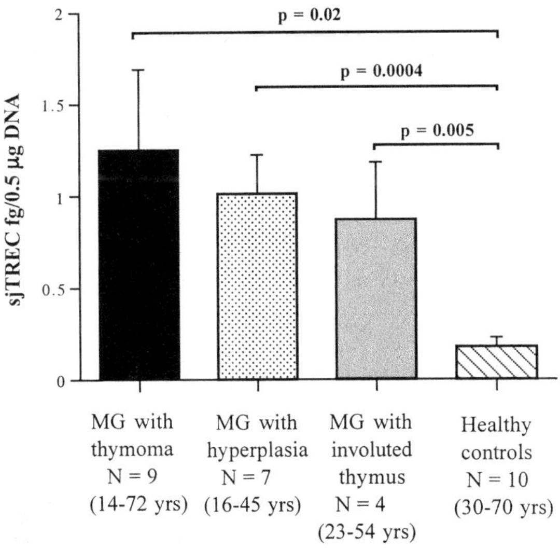

FIGURE 2. SjTREC levels in PBMCs from MG patients and controls. TREC levels in PBMCs from MG patients were significantly raised when compared to healthy donors ($p = 0.02$, 0.0004, and 0.005 for MG with thymoma, hyperplasia, and involuted thymus versus healthy controls, respectively). SjTREC levels in MG patients with thymoma were not significantly higher than in MG patients without thymoma ($p = 0.6$). Results are presented as mean ± SE.

TABLE 1. Serial sjTREC levels in PBMCs from MG patients before and after thymectomy

MG patients	Clinical course[a]						
	Pre	Post	0 months[b]	2 months[b]	6 months[b]	12 months[b]	Outcome[c]
1	G	G	1.59	0.35	1.06	0.51	U
2	B	G	3.76	0.83	1.65	na	I
3	G	PR	2.94	1.15	na	0.52	I
4	G	G	0.41	0.27	0.31	0.53	U
5	G	PR	0.14	0.20	nd	nd	I
6	G	O	0.18	0.13	na	0.42	I
7	O	R	1.73	1.15	1.41	1.19	R
8	G	G	0.20	0.53	0.91	0.14	U
9	G	PR	1.02	1.60	1.22	0.66	I
10	G	G	1.42	0.38	na	0.30	U
11	G	R	1.45	3.25	2.80	0.90	R
12	O	R	0.50	na	0.98	na	R

NOTE: MG patients 1–6: patients with thymoma; MG patients 7–12: patients without thymoma. Results are expressed as fg of sjTREC DNA/0.5 μg DNA.

[a]G, generalized; B, bulbar; O, ocular; R, remission; PR, pharmacological remission.

[b]Time after thymectomy; time 0, day of thymectomy; na, not available; nd, not detectable.

[c]U, unchanged; I, improved; R, remission.

outcome at 12 months after thymectomy correlates with the variation in sjTREC levels (TABLE 1). MG patients without thymoma showed that basal TREC levels were either unchanged or raised for the first few months after surgery, but there was a substantial decrease (average 33%) at 1 year after. As in thymoma patients, correlation between clinical outcome and sjTREC levels was observed (TABLE 1).

CONCLUSIONS

The present study revealed that sjTREC levels are significantly raised in the thymus of MG patients with thymoma compared to those with involuted thymus ($p = 0.01$). The low sjTREC levels in involuted thymus are in line with the different response to thymectomy observed among the MG patients affected by different thymic histology (see Mantegazza and colleagues, this volume). Furthermore, thymoma sjTREC levels do not differ from levels detected in hyperplasia nor in nonpathological young thymuses, suggesting that, in thymoma, thymopoiesis is as active as in infancy and confirming that thymoma generates mature T cells from immature precursors.[7] The high sjTREC levels detected in peripheral blood of thymoma patients support the hypothesis that the tumor sustains the export of self-reactive T cells to the periphery in MG, in line with results by Buckley and colleagues[8] and as reported by Hoffacker and colleagues.[9]

We found that thymectomy in MG (with or without thymoma) resulted in a substantial decrease in sjTREC$^+$ cells, in particular in those patients with high levels of sjTREC at the time of surgery (TABLE 1).

The discrepancy between sjTREC levels in thymus and peripheral blood of patients with involuted thymus (FIGS. 1 and 2) suggests that the MG thymus generates long-lasting T cells that persist in the periphery even when the thymus is no longer producing major quantities of mature T cells.

REFERENCES

1. MARX, A. *et al.* 1997. Pathogenesis of myasthenia gravis. Virch. Arch. **430:** 355–364.
2. VERSCHUREN, M.C. *et al.* 1997. Preferential rearrangements of the T cell receptor-delta-deleting elements in human T cells. J. Immunol. **158:** 1208–1216.
3. DOUEK, D.C. *et al.* 1998. Changes in thymic function with age and during the treatment of HIV infection. Nature **396:** 690–695.
4. JAMIESON, B.D. *et al.* 1999. Generation of functional thymocytes in the human adult. Immunity **10:** 569–575.
5. ROSAI, J. & G.D. LEVINE. 1999. Histological typing of tumors of the thymus. *In* World Health Organisation, International Histological Classification of Tumors, pp. 1–65. Springer. Heidelberg.
6. BERNASCONI, P. *et al.* 1995. Expression of transforming growth factor-beta 1 in dystrophic patient muscles correlates with fibrosis: pathogenetic role of a fibrogenic cytokine. J. Clin. Invest. **96:** 1137–1144.
7. STRÖBEL, P. *et al.* 2002. Paraneoplastic myasthenia gravis correlates with generation of mature naive CD4(+) T cells in thymomas. Blood **100:** 159–166.
8. BUCKLEY, C. *et al.* 2001. Mature, long-lived CD4+ and CD8+ T cells are generated by the thymoma in myasthenia gravis. Ann. Neurol. **50:** 64–72.
9. HOFFACKER, V. *et al.* 2000. Thymomas alter the T-cell subset composition in the blood: a potential mechanism for thymoma-associated autoimmune disease. Blood **96:** 3872–3879.

Analysis of $CD4^+CD25^+$ Cell Population in the Thymus from Myasthenia Gravis Patients

A. BALANDINA,[a] A. SAOUDI,[b] P. DARTEVELLE,[c] AND S. BERRIH-AKNIN[a]

[a]*CNRS UMR 8078, IPSC, Université Paris XI, Hôpital Marie Lannelongue, Le Plessis-Robinson, France*

[b]*INSERM U-28, Hôpital Purpan, Toulouse, France*

[c]*Service de Chirurgie Thoracique, Hôpital Marie Lannelongue, Le Plessis-Robinson, France*

ABSTRACT: The present study is aimed at exploring the regulatory $CD4^+CD25^+$ T cells in the thymus from myasthenia gravis (MG) patients. In early-onset MG, the thymus is hyperplastic and contains autoreactive activated T cells. Preliminary studies indicate that these $CD4^+CD25^+$ cells include activated autoreactive T cells. Studies to characterize the phenotype and suppressive capacity of these cells will be discussed.

KEYWORDS: $CD4^+CD25^+$ T cells; myasthenia gravis; thymus; thymocyte population

Myasthenia gravis (MG) is mediated by autoantibodies to the acetylcholine receptor (AChR) at the neuromuscular junction. The high titer of anti-AChR antibodies is associated with thymic abnormalities. In early-onset MG, the thymus is hyperplastic and contains autoreactive activated T cells, being the effector site of the autoimmune anti-AChR response. $CD4^+CD25^+$ T cells, which express the α-chain of the IL-2 receptor, have emerged as an important immunoregulatory T cell subset. These regulatory T cells are generated in the thymus and prevent the induction of autoimmune diseases in a number of experimental animal models.[1] Such T cells are able to suppress the proliferation of $CD4^+CD25^-$ cells and represent about 10% of $CD4^+$ cells. This subpopulation has also been described in the thymus and peripheral blood of healthy humans.[2] Induction of MG can be associated with the deficiency in immunoregulatory cells. We analyzed the number of $CD25^+$ cells and their distribution between the different thymocyte populations in the thymus from MG patients.

Address for correspondence: A. Balandina, CNRS UMR 8078, IPSC, Université Paris XI, Hôpital Marie Lannelongue, 92350 Le Plessis-Robinson, France. Voice: +33-1-40-94-55-97; fax: +33-1-46-30-45-64.

anna.balandina@ccml.u-psud.fr

Ann. N.Y. Acad. Sci. 998: 275–277 (2003). © 2003 New York Academy of Sciences.
doi: 10.1196/annals.1254.030

METHODS

Thymic tissue was obtained at thymectomy of the patients selected according to thymic histology. Patients with thymomas or those on steroid treatment were excluded from the study. Control thymuses were obtained from children aged from 11 days to 8 months who were undergoing heart surgery. Thymocytes were retrieved by gentle scraping of fresh thymic tissue, filtering, and washing them once in Hanks' balanced solution (HBSS). They were stained with mAbs to CD4, CD8, and CD25 and analyzed by flow cytometry.

RESULTS

FIGURE 1 shows an analysis of CD25 expression in one representative MG patient with positive anti-AChR antibody titer and in one healthy control. CD25 expression is limited mostly to $CD4^{hi}CD8^-$ T cells in both patients and controls; however, the percentage of $CD25^+$ cells among $CD4^+$ cells is augmented in patients, 20% compared to 10% in controls. Our data on five thymuses show that CD25 expression is increased in $CD4^+$ and $CD4^-CD8^-$ cells from patients with positive titer of anti-AChR antibodies, from 12% to 35% of $CD4^+$ cells, whereas $CD25^+$ cells comprise 10–16% of $CD4^+$ thymocytes in control subjects. The increased expression of CD25

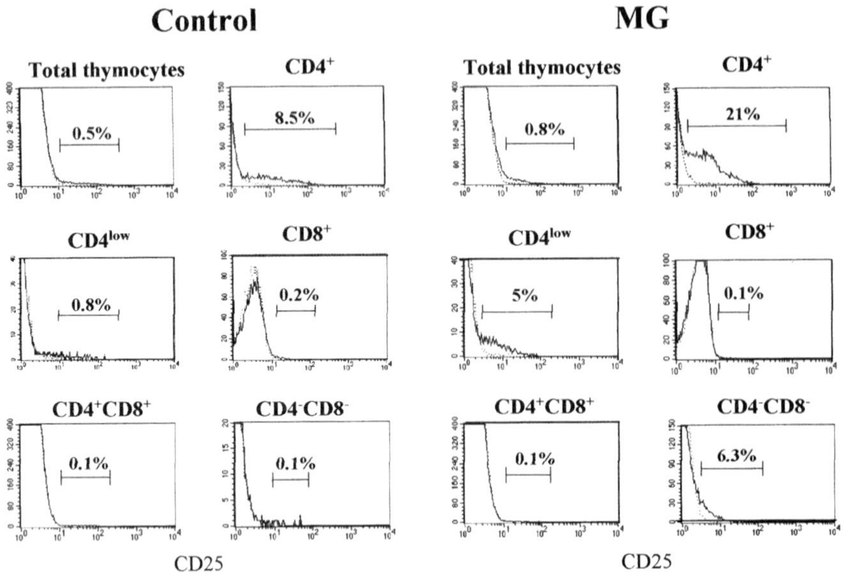

FIGURE 1. Analysis of CD25 expression in the thymus of an MG patient with anti-AChR antibody titer of 11 nmol/L and in a healthy newborn control. Freshly isolated thymocytes were stained with mAbs to CD8-FITC, CD4-PerCP, and CD25-PE and analyzed by flow cytometry. Expression of CD25 in different populations is shown with a solid line, and the staining with an isotype IgG2 control with a dotted line.

in $CD4^-CD8^-$ cells in MG patients could be related to the activated state described in the B cell population of MG thymus.[3] In contrast, there is no significant difference in the numbers of $CD4^+CD25^+$ cells between seronegative patients and controls. This finding correlates with the results that the proportion of cells with high levels of Fas expression is increased in all thymocyte populations from MG patients with high titers of anti-AChR antibodies.[4] $CD4^+Fas^{hi}$ thymocytes had been shown to be enriched in AChR-reactive activated cells. Since CD25 is transiently expressed upon activation of naïve $CD4^+$ T cells, $CD4^+CD25^+$ cells from MG thymus must contain both the activated pathogenic cells and the resting or activated regulatory cells. Even in healthy adults, the T cell population should be enriched in activated memory cells as they encounter the foreign antigens during the course of life. In conclusion, CD25 does not represent a perfect marker for regulatory human CD4 T cells. The analysis of other cell markers in combination with CD25 will be necessary to discriminate between activated and regulatory cells.

ACKNOWLEDGMENTS

This work was supported by Grant No. NS39869 from the National Institute of Health.

REFERENCES

1. SHEVACH, E.M. 2002. $CD4^+CD25^+$ suppressor T cells: more questions than answers. Nat. Rev. Immunol. **2:** 389–400.
2. STEPHENS, L.A. *et al.* 2001. Human $CD4^+CD25^+$ thymocytes and peripheral T cells have immune suppressive activity *in vitro*. Eur. J. Immunol. **31:** 1247–1254.
3. LEPRINCE, C. *et al.* 1990. Thymic B cells from myasthenia gravis patients are activated B cells: phenotypic and functional analysis. J. Immunol. **145:** 2115–2122.
4. MOULIAN, N. *et al.* 1997. Thymocyte Fas expression is dysregulated in myasthenia gravis patients with anti-acetylcholine receptor antibody. Blood **89:** 3287–3295.

Expression of Transforming Growth Factor-β1 in Thymus of Myasthenia Gravis Patients

Correlation with Pathological Abnormalities

PIA BERNASCONI,[a] LAURA PASSERINI,[a] ANDREA ANNONI,[a]
FEDERICA UBIALI,[a] CRISTIANA MARCOZZI,[a] PAOLO CONFALONIERI,[b]
FERDINANDO CORNELIO,[b] AND RENATO MANTEGAZZA[a]

[a]*Immunology and Muscular Pathology Unit,* [b]*Department of Neuromuscular Diseases, Istituto Nazionale Neurologico "Carlo Besta", 20133 Milan, Italy*

KEYWORDS: **transforming growth factor-β; thymus; myasthenia gravis**

INTRODUCTION

Several lines of evidence indicate that the thymus plays a critical role in the pathogenesis and development of myasthenia gravis (MG).[1] In the thymus, T cell maturation/differentiation is achieved via interaction with thymic epithelial cells (TECs).[2] TECs express on their surfaces MHC class II molecules and produce immunoregulatory cytokines, such as interleukins (IL)-1α, IL-1β, and IL-6, and leukemia-inhibitory factor (LIF), all of which are involved in T cell development.[3]

Transforming growth factor-β (TGF-β) is a pleiotropic cytokine present ubiquitously in tissues and produced by a variety of cell types. In humans, three different isoforms have been identified (TGF-β1, β2, and β3).[4]

In primary human TEC cultures, TGF-β1 and β3 modulate cell function by increasing gene expression and production of IL-1α, IL-1β, and IL-6.[5] In MG hyperplastic thymus, the expression of IL-1β, IL-2, and IL-6 mRNAs is increased.[6] Both Th1- and Th2-related cytokines promote the development of experimental autoimmune MG and may help autoreactive B cells to produce anti-AChR antibodies in MG.[7] Moreover, in thymectomized MG patients, there are more circulating cells expressing TGF-β1 mRNA than in nonthymectomized patients.[8]

To elucidate the involvement of TGF-β in MG, we investigated its localization and level of expression in thymus tissue from a series of MG patients with diverse thymus pathology.

Address for correspondence: Pia Bernasconi, Immunology and Muscular Pathology Unit, Istituto Nazionale Neurologico "Carlo Besta", Via Celoria 11, 20133 Milan, Italy. Voice: +39-02-2394369; fax: +39-02-70633874.

pbernasconi@istituto-besta.it

Ann. N.Y. Acad. Sci. 998: 278–283 (2003). © 2003 New York Academy of Sciences.
doi: 10.1196/annals.1254.031

MATERIALS AND METHODS

Tissue Samples

Twenty-two thymus specimens (10 hyperplastic, 6 involuted, and 6 thymomas)[1,9] were obtained from MG patients and 4 from children who underwent corrective cardiovascular surgery; the thymus specimens from the latter patients will be thereafter indicated as nonpathological young thymus. The tissues were frozen over liquid nitrogen fumes and stored in liquid nitrogen until use.

Polymerase Chain Reaction

Total RNA, prepared from 10–15 mg of frozen thymus using the RNAfast-II kit (Molecular Systems, San Diego, CA), was reverse-transcribed and subjected to PCR using primers specific for the three TGF-β isoforms. TGF-β1 transcript was also analyzed by quantitative-PCR (Q-PCR), as elsewhere described.[10]

Immunohistochemistry

Cryostat sections of thymus, fixed in acetone and blocked with 3% bovine serum albumin in PBS, were incubated with primary mouse monoclonal antibodies (anti-pan-cytokeratin, Dako, Copenhagen, Denmark; anti-CD1a, American Type Culture Collection, Rockville, MD; anti-human TGF-β1, Serotec, Oxford, United Kingdom; anti-CD22, Dako) for 2 h at the working dilution as indicated by the manufacturers. The staining was revealed using the ABC technique. Adjacent sections were stained with hematoxylin-eosin to relate antibody localization to tissue histology.

Statistical Analysis

Data are presented as means ± standard deviation (SD). Values were compared using the two-tailed Student's *t* test.

RESULTS

TGF-β2, not detectable in nonpathological young thymuses, was expressed at about the same level in all MG thymuses, while for TGF-β3 the expression was similar in all MG and nonpathological young thymuses (data not shown). In hyperplastic thymus, TGF-β1 levels (mean ± SD: 34 ± 19.3 fg/200 ng total RNA) were significantly different from those in involuted thymus (1.77 ± 1.6) and thymoma (3.55 ± 3) ($p < 0.005$), which did not differ significantly from each other ($p > 0.1$). In nonpathological young thymus, the range was 6.5 to 36 fg/200 ng total RNA (17.3 ± 12.7), significantly different from MG involuted thymus and thymoma ($p < 0.05$), but not from hyperplastic thymus ($p = 0.08$) (FIG. 1).

By immunohistochemistry, TGF-β1 protein was detected in all thymus samples. In hyperplastic thymus, it was mainly distributed in the medulla (identified by the presence of Hassall's bodies, FIG. 2B) in areas also positive for cytokeratin (FIG. 2A); no signal was detected in the cortex, positive for CD1a (not shown), or in germinal centers, characterized by the presence of $CD22^+$ cells (FIG. 2C). In thymoma, TGF-β1

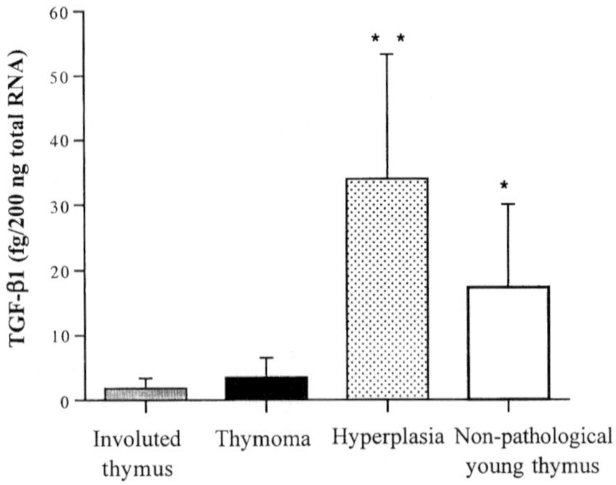

FIGURE 1. Quantitative PCR analysis of TGF-β1 mRNA in nonpathological young thymuses and MG thymuses. Values are presented as means ± SD. Statistical analysis was performed by the two-tailed Student's *t* test: **TGF-β1 mRNA levels in hyperplastic thymuses vs. involuted thymuses and thymoma, $p < 0.005$; *TGF-β1 mRNA levels in nonpathological young thymuses vs. involuted thymuses and thymoma, $p < 0.05$.

was present as clusters of positive staining (FIG. 3C), in areas diffusely positive for cytokeratin within neoplastic areas (FIG. 3D), and in the connective tissue (data not shown). In involuted thymus, TGF-β1 was present almost entirely in the connective tissue, which has replaced the majority of thymic tissue, leaving only small areas of keratin$^+$ TECs (data not shown). In nonpathological young thymuses, TGF-β1 was present in connective tissue septa, nonuniformly in CD1a$^+$ cells of the cortex and in the medulla, and not in CD22$^+$ germinal centers (data not shown).

CONCLUSIONS

The significantly higher levels of TGF-β we found in hyperplastic thymus than in thymoma or involuted thymuses, similar to those quantified in thymuses from young children, and its localization exclusively in the medulla, in association with keratin$^+$ TECs, and not within the cortex or germinal centers, suggest that TGF-β1 may be involved, together with other proinflammatory cytokines, in the medullary cell proliferation, characteristic of hyperplastic thymus, rather than in thymocyte selection, as in normal conditions.[11] It remains to be elucidated whether the action of TGF-β1 in MG is biased towards an altered immunoregulation within hyperplastic thymus.

In nonpathological young thymus, we found high levels of TGF-β1, together with its location both in the cortex and in the medulla, and this is consistent with its active involvement in the regulation of T cell development in thymus.[11]

In MG thymoma (all with benign histopathological features), TGF-β1 does not seem to play a crucial role in neoplastic development as it does in many types of tumors. Its involvement in thymoma development needs further investigation.

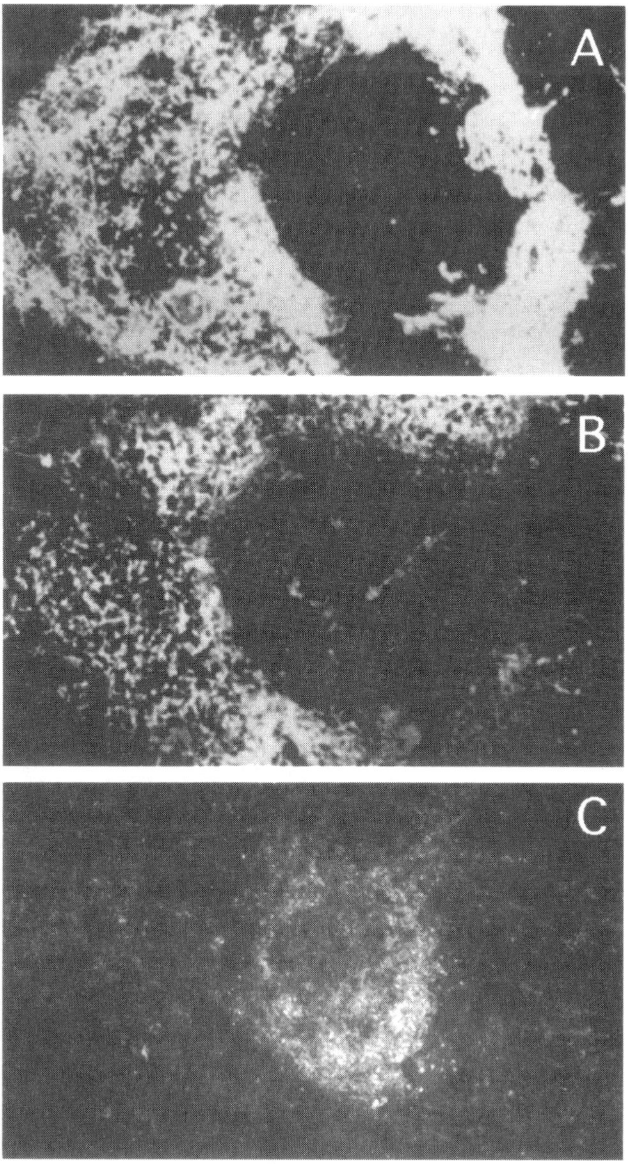

FIGURE 2. Immunofluorescence staining of TGF-β1 in hyperplastic thymus from an MG patient. Serial sections stained with **(A)** anti-pan-cytokeratin antibody and marker for TEC, **(B)** anti-TGF-β1, and **(C)** anti-CD22 (marker for germinal center). TGF-β1 is widely distributed in relation to TECs, but completely absent in germinal centers. Magnification: ×400.

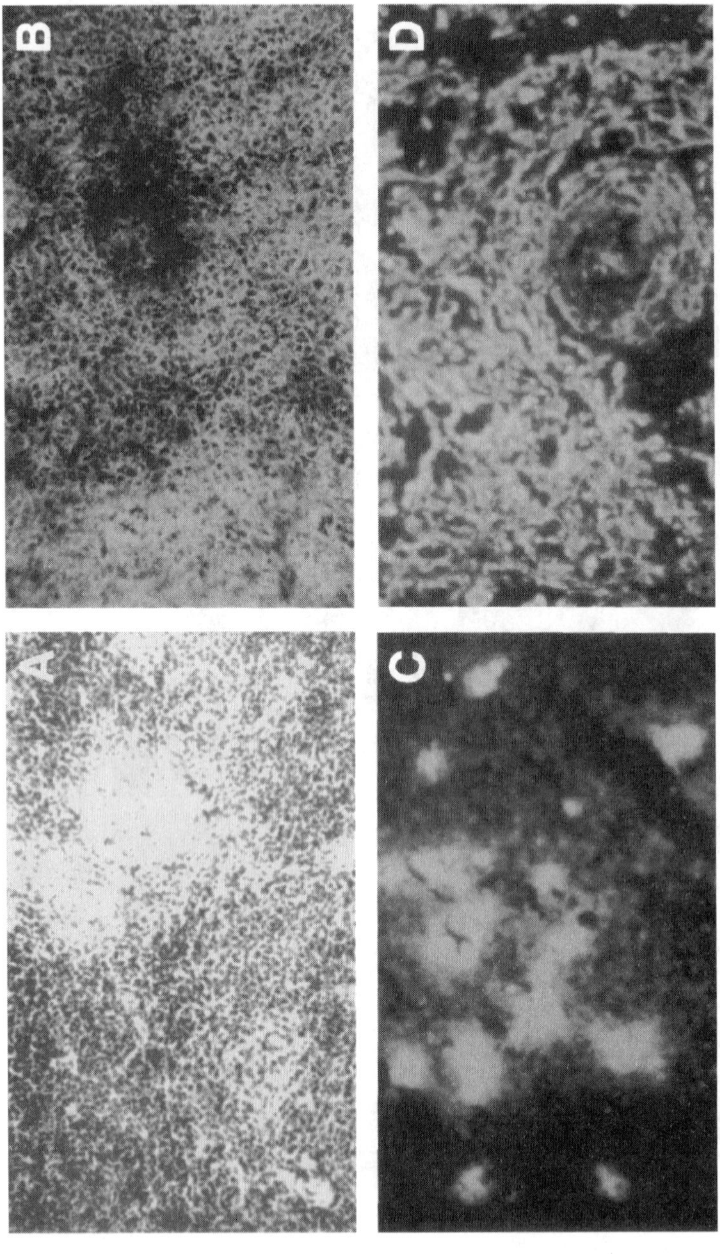

FIGURE 3. Sections showing location of TGF-β1 in corticomedullary thymoma from an MG patient. Serial sections showing gross structure of thymic tissue with **(A)** hematoxylin-eosin and **(B)** CD1a immunofluorescence staining revealing proliferation of thymic cortex. Serial sections showing that **(C)** TGF-β1 immunofluorescence staining is present in patchy areas of **(D)** keratin-positive cells. Magnification: ×400.

REFERENCES

1. MARX, A. *et al.* 1997. Pathogenesis of myasthenia gravis. Virch. Arch. **430:** 355–364.
2. SPRENT, J. *et al.* 1988. T cell selection in the thymus. Immunol. Rev. **101:** 173–190.
3. SHORTMAN, K. 1992. Cellular aspects of early T-cell development. Curr. Opin. Immunol. **4:** 140–146.
4. WAHL, S.M. 1994. Transforming growth factor beta: the good, the bad, and the ugly. J. Exp. Med. **180:** 1587–1590.
5. SCHLUNS, K.S., J.E. COOK & P.T. LE. 1997. TGF-β differentially modulates epidermal growth factor-mediated increases in leukemia-inhibitory factor, IL-6, IL-1α, and IL-1β in human thymic epithelial cells. J. Immunol. **158:** 2704–2712.
6. EMILIE, D. *et al.* 1991. *In situ* production of interleukins in hyperplastic thymus from myasthenia gravis patients. Hum. Pathol. **22:** 461–468.
7. LI, H. *et al.* 1998. Cytokine and chemokine mRNA expressing cells in muscle tissues of experimental autoimmune myasthenia gravis. J. Neurol. Sci. **161:** 40–46.
8. BATOCCHI, A.P. *et al.* 1998. Low level of TGF-β in early stages of myasthenia gravis. Ann. N.Y. Acad. Sci. **841:** 342–346.
9. ROSAI, J. & G.D. LEVINE. 1999. Histological typing of tumors of the thymus. *In* World Health Organisation, International Histological Classification of Tumors, pp. 1–65. Springer. Heidelberg.
10. BERNASCONI, P. *et al.* 1995. Expression of transforming growth factor-beta 1 in dystrophic patient muscles correlates with fibrosis: pathogenetic role of a fibrogenic cytokine. J. Clin. Invest. **96:** 1137–1144.
11. WAHL, S.M., J.M. ORENSTEIN & W. CHEN. 2000. TGF-β influences the life and death decisions of T lymphocytes. Cytokine Growth Factor Rev. **11:** 71–79.

T Cells and Cytokines in the Pathogenesis of Acquired Myasthenia Gravis

MONICA MILANI,[a] NORMA OSTLIE,[a] WEI WANG,[a]
AND BIANCA M. CONTI-FINE[a,b,c]

[a]*Department of Biochemistry, Molecular Biology, and Biophysics,*
[b]*Department of Pharmacology, University of Minnesota,*
Minneapolis, Minnesota 55455, USA

ABSTRACT: Although the symptoms of myasthenia gravis (MG) and experimental MG (EAMG) are caused by autoantibodies, CD4$^+$ T cells specific for the target antigen, the nicotinic acetylcholine receptor, and the cytokines they secrete, have an important role in these diseases. CD4$^+$ T cells have a pathogenic role, by permitting and facilitating the synthesis of high-affinity anti-AChR antibodies. Th1 CD4$^+$ cells are especially important because they drive the synthesis of anti-AChR complement-fixing IgG subclasses. Binding of those antibodies to the muscle AChR at the neuromuscular junction will trigger the complement-mediated destruction of the postsynaptic membrane. Thus, IL-12, a crucial cytokine for differentiation of Th1 cells, is necessary for development of EAMG. Th2 cells secrete different cytokines, with different effects on the pathogenesis of EAMG. Among them, IL-10, which is a potent growth and differentiation factor for B cells, facilitates the development of EAMG. In contrast, IL-4 appears to be involved in the differentiation of AChR-specific regulatory CD4$^+$ T cells, which can prevent the development of EAMG and its progression to a self-maintaining, chronic autoimmune disease. Studies on the AChR-specific CD4$^+$ cells commonly present in the blood of MG patients support a crucial role of CD4$^+$ T cells in the development of MG. Circumstantial evidence supports a pathogenic role of IL-10 also in human MG. On the other hand, there is no direct or circumstantial evidence yet indicating a role of IL-4 in the modulatory or immunosuppressive circuits in MG.

KEYWORDS: experimental myasthenia gravis; CD4$^+$ T cell; IL-10; IL-4

INTRODUCTION

Acquired myasthenia gravis (MG) and its animal model, experimental autoimmune myasthenia gravis (EAMG), are antibody (Ab)–mediated, T cell–dependent autoimmune diseases. The nicotinic acetylcholine receptor (AChR) at the neuromuscular junction (NMJ) is the target of the autoimmune attack, which results in the symptoms of MG and EAMG.

Address for correspondence: Dr. Monica Milani, Department of Biochemistry, Molecular Biology, and Biophysics, University of Minnesota, 6-155 Jackson Hall, 321 Church Street, Minneapolis, MN 55455. Voice: 612-624-3790; fax: 612-625-2163.
mmilani@cbs.umn.edu
[c]Previously known as Bianca M. Conti-Tronconi.

Ann. N.Y. Acad. Sci. 998: 284–307 (2003). **© 2003 New York Academy of Sciences.**
doi: 10.1196/annals.1254.032

Anti-AChR Abs cause AChR loss, damage of the postsynaptic membrane at the NMJ, and failure of the neuromuscular transmission.[1–4] In contrast, CD4$^+$ T helper cells are not directly involved in the damage of the NMJ. Yet several findings support their important role in the pathogenesis of MG: (1) the pathogenic anti-AChR Abs in MG patients are high-affinity IgG,[5,6] produced by B cells only after intervention of cytokines secreted by CD4$^+$ T helper cells; (2) MG patients have AChR-reactive CD4$^+$ T cells in the blood and thymus;[7,8] (3) peripheral blood mononuclear cells (PBMC) from MG patients grafted in severe combined immunodeficiency (SCID) mice induce synthesis of human anti-AChR Ab and myasthenic symptoms only if the grafted cells include the CD4$^+$ cells;[9] (4) treatment of MG patients with anti-CD4 Abs causes clinical and electrophysiologic improvements and abolishes the response of their T cells to the AChR *in vitro*.[10]

Different studies have proven that CD4$^+$ T helper cells are necessary for EAMG development. A first, pivotal study used an *in vivo* cell transfer model: sublethally irradiated, thymectomized rats grafted with a mixture of B cells and CD4$^+$ T cells from rats immunized with AChR developed anti-AChR Ab and myasthenic symptoms, whereas the graft of B cells alone did not induce these effects.[11] Other studies have verified the crucial role of CD4$^+$ T cells in rodent EAMG by showing that administration of Abs against the CD4 or the MHC class II molecules prevented EAMG[12,13] and that mice genetically deficient in CD4$^+$ cells (because of a disruption of the MHC class II genes) were resistant to EAMG.[14]

The role of CD8$^+$ cells in MG and EAMG is still debated. In MG, CD8$^+$ T cells might have a modulatory role.[15–17] In EAMG, some studies concluded that CD8$^+$ T cells have a pathogenic role, and other studies that they have a protective function.[18–20]

CD4$^+$ T cells comprise different subclasses, which secrete characteristic cytokines.[21–23] A simple classification separates Th1, Th2, and Th3 cells (FIG. 1). Th1 cells produce proinflammatory cytokines, such as IL-2, IL-18, and IFN-γ. They are involved in cell-mediated immune responses and induce production by B cells of IgG subclasses, which bind complement (e.g., IgG2a and IgG2b in the mouse). Th2 cells produce anti-inflammatory cytokines, such as IL-4 and IL-10, which may reduce the intensity of an immune response. However, Th2 cells have an important role in the induction of humoral immune responses: they drive the synthesis of IgA, IgE, and IgG subclasses that do not fix complement (e.g., IgG1 in the mouse). Th1 and Th2 cells downregulate each other. A subset of CD4$^+$ T cells with regulatory functions produce TGF-β and require IL-4 for their development: they are referred to as Th3 cells.[24] Other CD4$^+$ T cell subclasses may have immunoregulatory functions. Those include CD4$^+$ cells, which secrete IL-10 primarily, termed Tr1 cells;[25] and CD25$^+$CD4$^+$ T cells, which may exert their suppressive action by direct cell contact and perhaps also by secreting anti-inflammatory cytokines.[26]

The role (or roles) of the different CD4$^+$ T cell subsets and cytokines in the pathogenesis of autoimmune diseases is complex and still unclear. Several studies have addressed these issues in T cell–mediated experimental autoimmune disease: their sometimes conflicting conclusions underline the difficulties of identifying the specific role for immune mediators like the cytokine, which are pleiotropic, have overlapping functions, and may have different and contrasting effects on the immune responses, depending on the time and place where they exert their action.[27,28] Defining the role of the different cytokines and CD4$^+$ T cell subsets in Ab-mediated diseases like MG will be an especially formidable task since both T cells and B cells

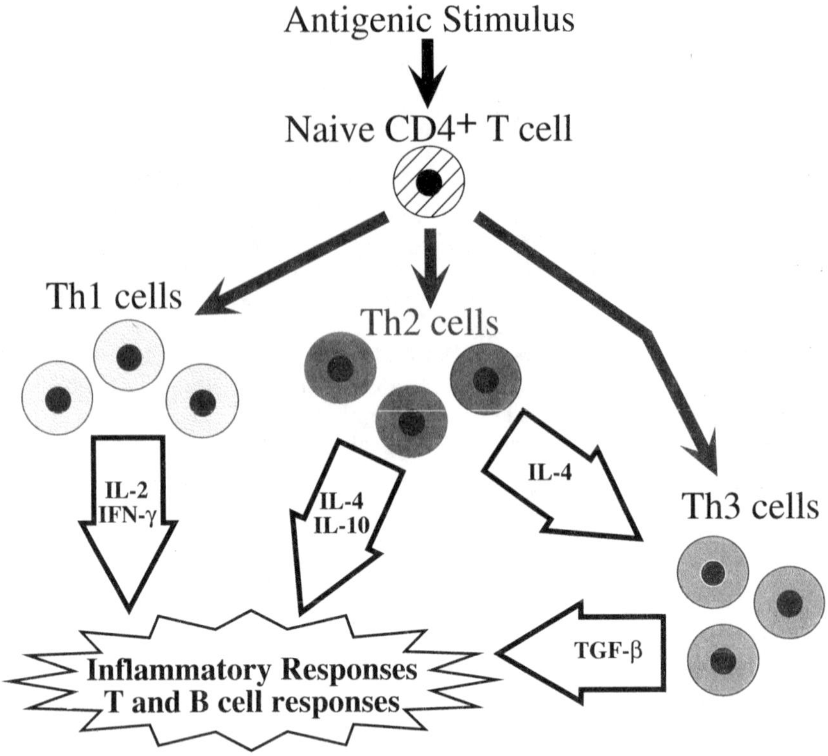

FIGURE 1. A simplified model of the Th1/Th2/Th3 cytokine network.

contribute to their immunopathogenesis, and both may be affected by the action of $CD4^+$ T cells and their cytokines, sometimes with opposite effects.

$CD4^+$ T CELLS AND CYTOKINES IN MG

Anti-AChR $CD4^+$ T Cells in Ocular and Generalized MG

MG includes two clinical subtypes: ocular MG (oMG), in which the myasthenic weakness is limited to the extraocular muscles (EOM), and generalized MG (gMG), in which the symptoms involve all striated muscles.[1–4,29] Sometimes, the disease of oMG patients progresses and their symptoms became generalized. Given the role of $CD4^+$ T cells in the pathogenesis of MG, it is of importance to understand how they recognize the AChR and how their anti-AChR response evolves over time and correlates with the progression of the symptoms.

Muscle AChR is formed by four homologous subunits and exists in two developmentally regulated isoforms. Embryonic muscle AChR contains α, β, γ, and δ subunits. After muscle innervation, the ε subunit replaces the γ subunit. However, adult

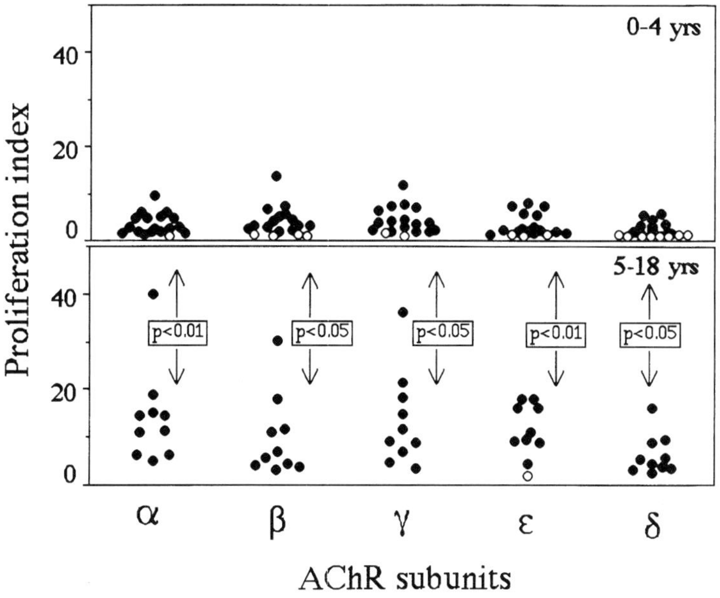

FIGURE 2. Proliferation indexes of CD4+ T cells from gMG during the course of the disease, stimulated with the AChR subunit peptide pools as indicated below the plot. The proliferation indexes are separated in two groups, according to the duration of their symptoms, as indicated in each plot. The black symbols in the plots represent significant proliferative responses, as compared to the spontaneous cell proliferation observed in the absence of any antigen. The significance of the difference in the average responses to different AChR subunits in the two groups is indicated inside the plots. Reprinted with the permission of *Neurology*.

EOM still express the γ subunit, in addition to the ε subunit. Both embryonic and adult AChRs comprise two α subunits and only one copy of the other subunits.[30]

We have studied the proliferative response of CD4+ T cells from the blood of gMG and oMG patients to the different subunits of human muscle AChR. As representative antigens, we have used pools of overlapping synthetic peptides, approximately 20 residues long, spanning the sequence of each subunit.[31–41] We have also used the individual peptides to determine the sequence regions of the different AChR subunits that formed epitopes recognized by the patients' CD4+ T cells. Some gMG patients in the early stages of their disease did not recognize all the subunits. However, when the disease had lasted for 5 years or longer, CD4+ T cell sensitization had spread to all AChR subunits, including the ε and γ subunits (FIG. 2).[40] Furthermore, the proliferative responses to the individual subunits were higher in those patients whose disease had lasted for more than 5 years than in those with a shorter history of myasthenic symptoms. These findings suggest that, in gMG, the sensitization of the autoimmune CD4+ cells spreads over time to an increasingly larger number of epitopes on each of the AChR subunits.

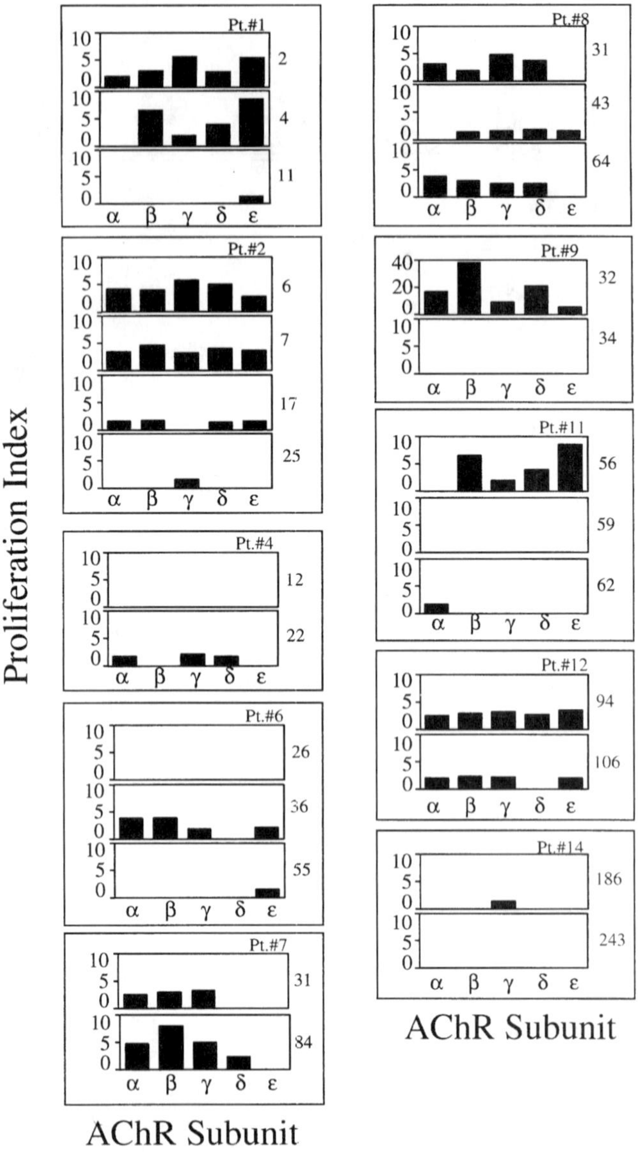

FIGURE 3. Proliferation indexes of CD4$^+$ T cells obtained from oMG stimulated with the AChR subunit peptide pools. The numbers at the right of the plots indicate the duration of the disease, in months, at the time of the experiment. Reprinted with the permission of *Journal of Neuroimmunology.*

Also, the CD4$^+$ T cells from oMG patients could recognize any of the AChR subunits, even though their responses were lower than those responses observed in gMG patients.[41] However, the CD4$^+$ T cells of the individual oMG patients frequently did not recognize all of the AChR subunit, even when their EOM weakness had been present for a number of years. Furthermore, the subunits that evoked a proliferative response of the CD4$^+$ cells of individual oMG patients changed over time: the recognition of a subunit could appear and disappear even over relative short periods of time (weeks or months) (FIG. 3). Also, the epitopes recognized by individual oMG patients changed over time.[41] This is in contrast with the stable recognition of AChR subunits and epitopes in gMG: in the individual gMG patients, once the CD4$^+$ T cells became sensitized to a subunit, or an individual epitope, their response persisted, even for periods as long as 10 years.[35,36] The minimal and unstable sensitization of anti-AChR CD4$^+$ T cells in oMG patients is in agreement with their low and inconsistent synthesis of anti-AChR Abs.[1,3] These findings suggest that residual modulatory mechanisms able to downregulate the autoimmune anti-AChR response may still survive in oMG patients.

The CD4$^+$ cells of both oMG and gMG patients recognized the δ subunit less intensely than the other subunits.[40] The lesser recognition of the δ subunit might be related to the earlier event in the anti-AChR sensitization, which likely occurs in the thymus,[1–4] because the human thymus seldom expresses the δ AChR subunit.[42]

The CD4$^+$ T cells of MG patients recognize a complex epitope repertoire on each of the AChR subunits.[43] To examine whether the CD4$^+$ epitope repertoire was different in oMG and gMG patients, we determined the sequence regions of the ε and γ subunits that elicited a proliferative response of the patients' CD4$^+$ T cells. CD4$^+$ cells from oMG and gMG patients recognized overlapping, yet different, epitope repertoires.[41]

The AChR Contains Universal CD4$^+$ Epitope Sequences

Although each MG patient recognized a unique set of sequences on each AChR subunit, we identified a few sequences recognized by most MG patients, regardless of their MHC haplotype ("universal" epitope sequences; UES). The UES are comprised within the following residues: 48–67, 101–120, 118–137, 304–322, and 403–437 of the α subunit; 181–200, 271–290, and 316–350 of the β subunit; 75–94 and 321–340 of the γ subunit; and 91–110 and 141–160 of the δ subunit. These sequences are recognized by a large number of CD4$^+$ T cells: thus, they form CD4$^+$ epitopes that are both universal and immunodominant. The UES on the α subunit were identified both by the use of CD4$^+$ T cell lines propagated from MG patients by stimulation with a pool of synthetic peptides spanning the α subunit sequence and by the use of unselected blood CD4$^+$ cells: these different approaches identified the same UES.[35–38]

Experiments that used mice transgenic for human MHC class II molecules that present AChR epitopes in MG patients supported the identification of the UES on the AChR α subunit: the CD4$^+$ T cells of transgenic mice immunized with purified human AChR in adjuvant recognized α subunit peptide sequences that included the UES described above.[44]

Experiments in SCID mice grafted with PBMC from gMG patients depleted in CD4$^+$ T cells, and "reconstituted" with UES-specific CD4$^+$ T cells from the same

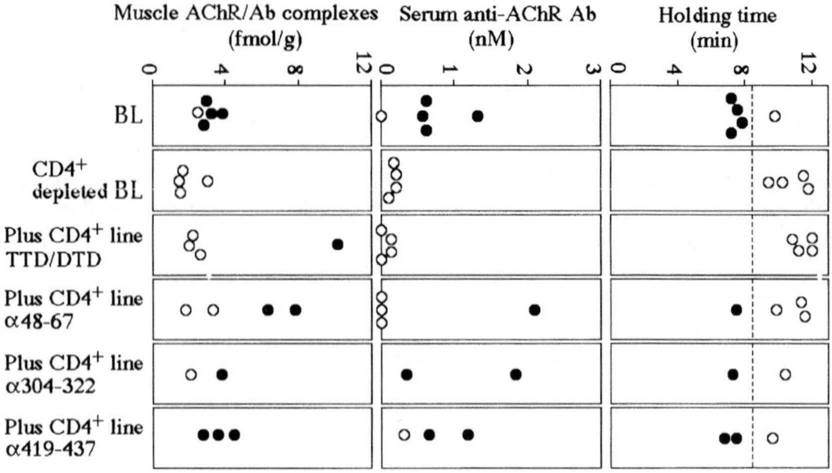

FIGURE 4. CD4+ cells specific for "universal" α subunit epitopes (UES) drive the synthesis of pathogenic anti-AChR Ab and permit transfer of MG symptoms. SCID mice were engrafted with PBMC (indicated in the figure as "blood lymphocytes", BL) or CD4+-depleted PBMC from a gMG patient, or with the patient's CD4+-depleted PBMC supplemented with CD4+ cell lines propagated from this same patient, and specific for tetanus and diphteria toxoids (TTD/DTD), or the universal CD4+ epitope sequences α48–67, α304–322, and α419–437 of the human muscle AChR, as indicated below the plots. The figure reports the average strength of the mice (measured as holding time in an inverted grid holding test described previously[56,69]), 4–10 weeks after the engraftment, and the concentration of human anti-AChR Ab in their sera, 7 weeks after the engraftment. The lowest panels report the concentration of AChR Ab complexes in the mouse muscle at the end of the observation period, 12 weeks after the engraftment. *Black symbols* represent mice with a significantly reduced holding time, or with significant concentrations of serum anti-AChR Ab and muscle AChR/Ab complexes. The *dotted line* in the top panels indicates the holding time below which we considered the mice to have a significant reduction of their strength (average holding time of SCID mice engrafted with PBMC from normal controls minus two SD). Reprinted with the permission of *Neurology*.

patients (α48–67, α304–322, and α419–437), demonstrated that the UES-specific CD4+ cells drive the synthesis of pathogenic anti-AChR Abs (FIG. 4).[9]

Cytokine Phenotype of the Anti-AChR CD4+ T Cells

Several lines of evidence suggest that, in MG patients, most of the anti-AChR CD4+ T cells have Th1 phenotype. Most CD4+ T cell lines propagated from MG patients and specific for AChR subunits or individual epitopes secreted IL-2, but not IL-4, when challenged with the relevant AChR antigen.[37,38] Moreover, studies on the frequency of IFN-γ producing CD4+ T cells (i.e., Th1 cells) specific for individual AChR subunits and epitopes in the blood of MG patients showed that all oMG and gMG patients had Th1 cells sensitized to each of the AChR subunits (FIG. 5).[40] In gMG patients, the frequency in the blood of AChR-specific Th1 cells compared with or exceeded that of Th1 cells specific for a commonly encountered exogenous antigen,

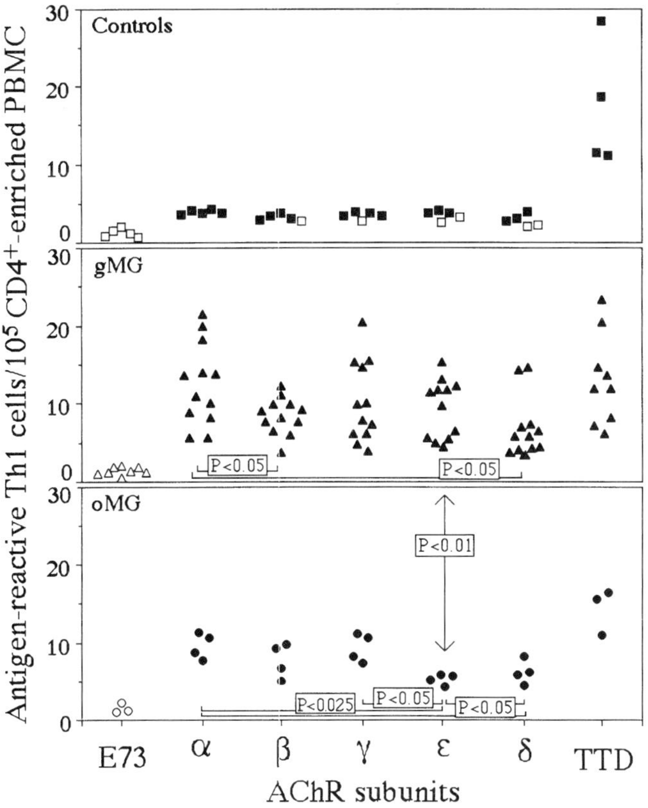

FIGURE 5. Average number of IFN-γ secreting cells in cultures of 10^5 $CD4^+$ enriched PBMC that responded specifically to the AChR subunit peptide pools, or to TTD, as indicated below the plots. The *black symbols* indicate values significantly higher than the number of T cells secreting IFN-γ spontaneously. We also report the results obtained when the cells were cultured in the presence of the control peptide E73. The significance of the difference in the responses to different AChR subunits in the three groups is indicated in boxes. Reprinted with the permission of *Neurology*.

tetanus toxoid.[40] We used individual overlapping peptides spanning the sequence of the α subunit and an IFN-γ ELISPOT assay to identify the sequence regions of the α subunit recognized by $CD4^+$ Th1 cells in a group of gMG patients. Each patient had a characteristic pattern of peptide recognition, but most of them had Th1 $CD4^+$ cells that produced IFN-γ in response to some of the AChR UES described above (FIG. 6).[39]

Anti-AChR CD4⁺ T Cells Are Necessary for the Synthesis of MG-Inducing Abs

Experiments in SCID mice grafted with immune cells from the blood of MG patients proved that synthesis of pathogenic anti-AChR Abs and the development of myasthenic symptoms requires anti-AChR $CD4^+$ T cells.[9]

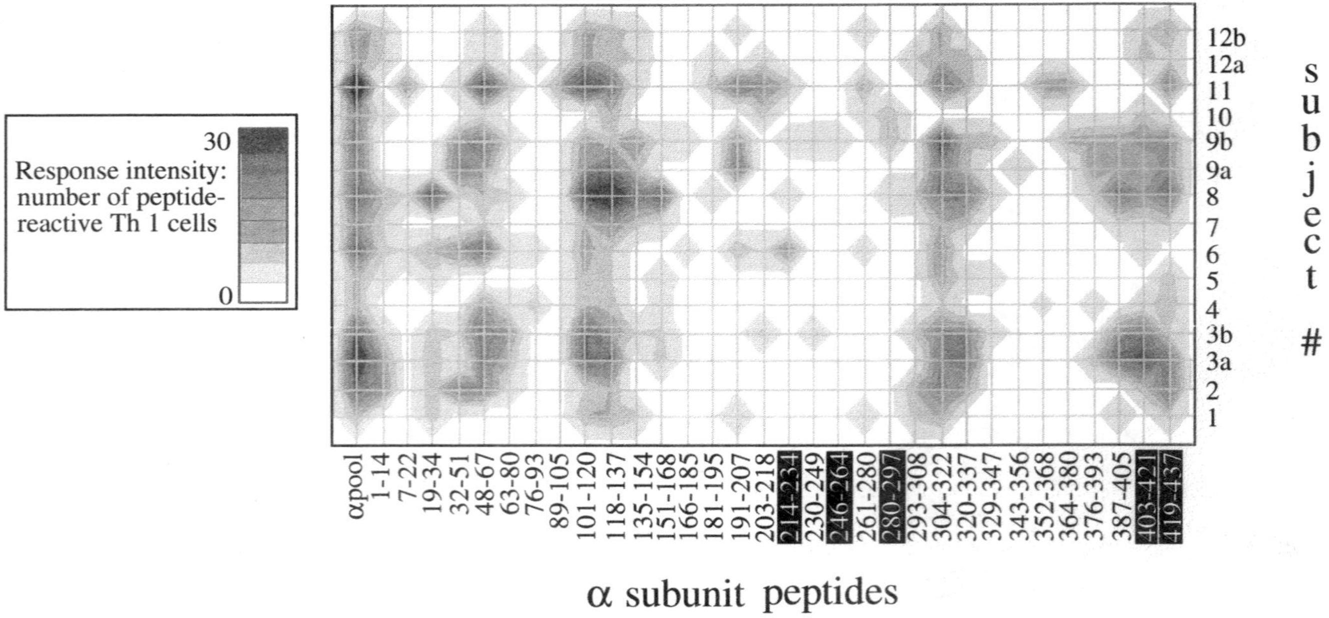

FIGURE 6. Summary representation of the frequency of $CD4^+$ T cells that secrete IFN-γ in response to the α subunit peptide pool, and to the individual peptides spanning the AChR α subunit, in 13 gMG patients. The data are represented as a contour map. Each horizontal strip represents the results obtained with the $CD4^+$-enriched PBMC of one patient in one experiment, as indicated at the right of the plot. The response to a subunit peptide pool, reported at the extreme left, is followed by that to the individual peptides (one peptide for each vertical line), starting with the amino-terminal peptide sequence. The average ($N = 3$) number of cells/culture of 10^5 $CD4^+$-enriched PBMC that significantly responded to the presence of the individual peptide antigens is indicated using the code depicted at the right. The background values, that is, the average number of cells that in a given patient and in a given experiment spontaneously secreted IFN-γ, were subtracted from the data reported here. Reprinted with the permission of *Neurology*.

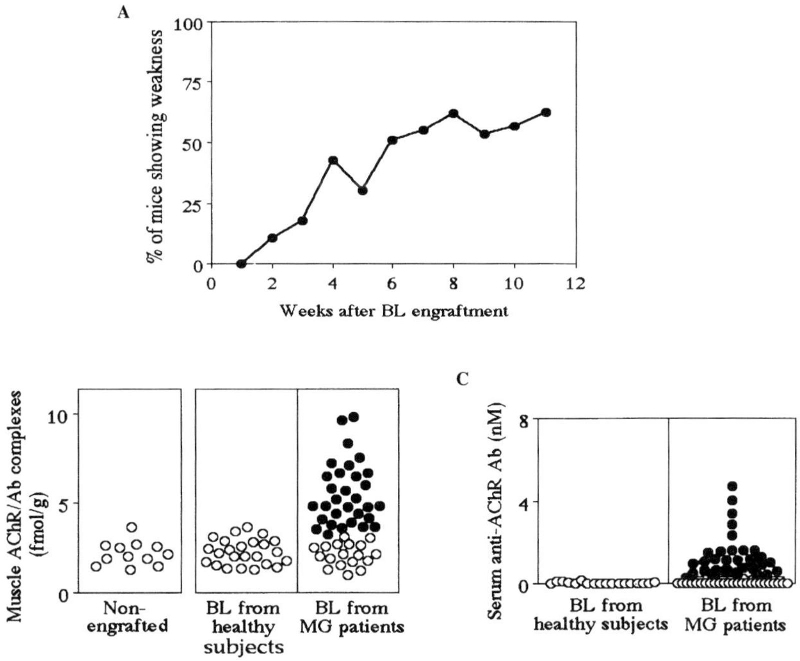

FIGURE 7. **(A)** Frequency of significant muscle weakness in mice engrafted with BL from MG patients, revealed by the hanging grid test described previously.[56,69] The frequency of the significantly affected mice increased with time. It reached a plateau from week 7 onwards after the graft, when 40 of the 62 mice (65%) engrafted with BL from MG patients had myasthenic weakness. **(B)** Human anti-AChR Ab in sera of individual SCID mice, 7–10 weeks after a graft of PBMC (indicated in the figure as BL) from 17 gMG patients or 4 healthy subjects. **(C)** AChR bound by human anti-AChR Ab in muscle of individual SCID mice, 7–18 weeks after a graft of PBMC (indicated in the figure as BL) from 17 gMG patients or 4 healthy subjects, as indicated below the plots. Negative controls were muscle samples from 12 untreated SCID mice (indicated in the plot as "non-engrafted"). In panels B and C, the *black symbols* indicate the presence of a significant concentration and the *white symbols* indicate absence of serum anti-AChR Ab or of muscle AChR/Ab complexes. Reprinted with the permission of *Neurology*.

SCID mice have an aberrant rearrangement of the genes encoding the immunoglobulin and the T cell receptor: they do not have functional mature B and T cells and they tolerate xenograft.[45,46] They are a useful tool to examine the functional interplay between anti-AChR B and T cells, and the roles of $CD4^+$ and $CD8^+$ T cells and of anti-UES T $CD4^+$ cells, in the development of myasthenic symptoms.

Intraperitoneal graft of PBMC from gMG patients, but not from healthy subjects, reproduced the clinical and immunological characteristic of MG in SCID mice. Most of the SCID mice grafted with PBMC from gMG patients developed myasthenic weakness, and had human anti-AChR Abs in the serum and bound to the AChR at the NMJ (FIG. 7). The presence of $CD4^+$ T cells was necessary to transfer the disease. SCID mice grafted with myasthenic PBMC depleted in $CD4^+$ cells did not develop muscle weakness and did not synthesize human anti-AChR Ab. In contrast, depletion of the CD8$^+$ cells did not affect the ability of PBMC from MG patients to induce myasthenic weakness and anti-AChR Ab synthesis.

The anti-AChR CD4$^+$ T cells, but not CD4$^+$ T cells specific for other antigens, can support the synthesis of anti-AChR Ab and induce development of myasthenic symptoms. This was demonstrated by the finding that CD4$^+$ depleted PBMC from MG patients reacquired the ability to transfer the myasthenic weakness and the synthesis of human anti-AChR Ab in SCID mice if they were supplemented with AChR-specific CD4$^+$ T cells from the same patients, but not with CD4$^+$ T cells specific for other antigens.[9]

ANTI-AChR CD4$^+$ T CELLS AND CYTOKINES IN MOUSE EAMG

Immunization with purified AChR in adjuvant induces EAMG in a variety of animal species.[1,47] Because of the high degree of sequence similarity of AChRs from different species, the abundant and easily purified AChR from the *Torpedo* fish (TAChR) is commonly used to induce EAMG.[1,47]

Among rodents, Lewis rats are most susceptible to EAMG.[48] Mice, because of the high "safety factor" of their neuromuscular transmission, are relatively resistant to EAMG.[47] (The term "safety factor" indicates the ability of the mouse NMJ to maintain its normal function even when a substantial fraction of the AChR molecules are missing or nonfunctioning. It is likely due to the presence, in the mouse NMJ postsynaptic membrane, of much more AChR than needed for neuromuscular transmission.) Even the most EAMG-susceptible strains, like the C57Bl/6 (B6) mice,[49,50] develop myasthenic weakness only after repeated injection of TAChR in Freund's adjuvant, and seldom in all of the immunized mice. Also, their myasthenic symptoms may be minimal or subclinical.[1,47] Still, mouse EAMG is a good model to study the immune mechanisms that induce or modulate the anti-AChR Ab response. This is because of the abundance of mutant mouse strains, usually available in the EAMG-susceptible B6 genetic background, which carry knockout mutations of gene encoding important immune receptors and modulators, or transgenes for those immune molecules expressed in defined immune cell types.

In TAChR-immunized mice, anti-TAChR Abs that cross-react with the mouse muscle AChR cause the myasthenic symptoms. In contrast, in B6 mice, the TAChR-sensitized CD4$^+$ T cells that drive the synthesis of pathogenic Abs do not cross-react with mouse AChR. The finding that the immunization with TAChR does not trigger a self-reactive response of CD4$^+$ T cells may explain why mouse EAMG is not self-maintaining like human MG: the mice that survive EAMG will recover within weeks after the end of the TAChR immunization.[1,47]

We have studied the role of several Th1 and Th2 cytokines (IL-12, IFN-γ, IL-4, and IL-10) in EAMG, using B6 mice genetically deficient in or transgenic for an individual cytokine.

Role of IL-12 and IFN-γ in EAMG

Th1 cells, which can be cytotoxic, are implicated in the pathogenesis of T cell–mediated experimental autoimmune diseases.[27,28] Because Th1 cytokines are less broadly effective on the growth and differentiation of B cells than Th2 cytokines, their role in Ab-mediated autoimmune diseases might have been overlooked. However, Th1 cells induce synthesis of complement-fixing Abs, which cause tissue damage most effectively.[21–23] Therefore, they likely have an important role in the pathogenesis of those Ab-mediated autoimmune diseases, where, like MG and EAMG, the destruction of a specific tissue or cellular structure causes the symptoms.

IL-12 and IFN-γ are important for the differentiation and effector function of Th1 cells. IL-12 is the most important stimulant of the differentiation of naïve T cells in Th1 cells and it provides a costimulus for maximal IFN-γ production by the antigen-activated Th1 cells.[51,52] Mice genetically deficient in IL-12 (IL-$12^{-/-}$) have severely reduced Th1 responses.[53] Also, they have increased secretion of IL-4 after Ag stimulation, suggesting a polarization of their immune responses toward Th2 sensitization.[53] IFN-γ, which is secreted by activated Th1 cells, promotes their further proliferation and activates macrophages.[21,23] Mice genetically deficient in IFN-γ (IFN-$\gamma^{-/-}$) have reduced function of both Th1 cells and macrophages.[54]

Genetic Absence of IL-12 or IFN-γ Has Different Effects on EAMG in B6 Mice

IL-$12^{-/-}$ mice immunized with TAChR did not develop EAMG (FIG. 8).[55,56] They developed serum anti-TAChR Ab in amounts comparable to those of wild-type B6

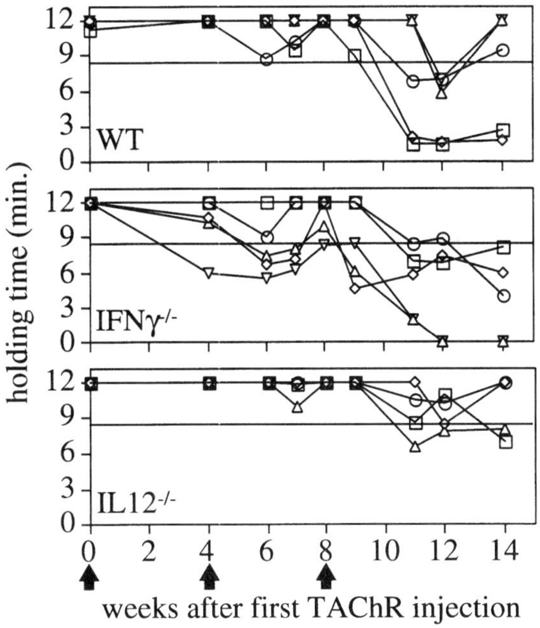

FIGURE 8. Strength of 5 WT, 5 IFN-$\gamma^{-/-}$, and 4 IL-$12^{-/-}$, as indicated inside the panels, measured as holding time.[56,69] The mice received three TAChR injections at the times indicated with *arrowheads*. The tests at 0, 4, and 8 weeks were carried out just before the TAChR immunizing injections. The horizontal line indicates the holding time below which a mouse has EAMG. Reprinted with the permission of *Journal of Immunology*.

(WT) mice, but they had a reduced synthesis of the complement-fixing anti-TAChR IgG2b and IgG2c. In contrast, we found that IFN-$\gamma^{-/-}$ mice were susceptible to EAMG to an extent comparable to that of WT mice (FIG. 8).[55] The IFN-$\gamma^{-/-}$ mice had serum anti-TAChR Ab in amounts comparable to those observed in the IL-$12^{-/-}$ and WT mice. They had a reduced serum concentration of anti-TAChR IgG2c as compared to WT mice, but a comparable concentration of the complement-fixing anti-TAChR IgG2b. WT, IL-$12^{-/-}$, and IFN-$\gamma^{-/-}$ mice had similar amounts of Ab-complexed AChR in their muscles. Thus, the EAMG resistance of the IL-$12^{-/-}$ mice was not due to inability of their anti-TAChR Ab to bind mouse muscle AChR. The different susceptibility to EAMG of these strains was related to the ability of the anti-TAChR Ab to bind to muscle and fix complement: after TAChR immunization, all mice had IgG bound to the NMJ, but only WT and IFN-$\gamma^{-/-}$ mice had complement as well.

These findings demonstrated that IL-12 has a crucial role in the immunopathogenesis of EAMG and verified the limited importance of Th2-driven anti-AChR Ab in causing myasthenic symptoms. They also suggested that IFN-γ has a disposable role in EAMG development since the complement-fixing IgG2b, whose synthesis does not require IFN-γ, suffices for the development of the disease.

The results of other studies supported a pathogenic role of IFN-γ in mouse EAMG. Two studies[57,58] investigated the effects of disrupting the genes for IFN-γ and its receptor on EAMG using mice of mixed genetic background [129/SvEv × C57Bl/6)F_2]. Because genetic factors other than the MHC alleles influence susceptibility to EAMG as well,[49,50,59] the different genetic background of the mice used in the studies on the role of IFN-γ in EAMG[57,58] complicates the comparison of their results.

One study[57] found that (129/SvEv × C57Bl/6) F_2 mice genetically deficient in IFN-γ did not synthesize anti-TAChR Ab (including Th2-driven IgG subclasses) or develop EAMG after TAChR immunization. Absence of IFN-γ reduces the effectiveness of Ag presentation: IFN-$\gamma^{-/-}$ mice have reduced macrophage function and expression of MHC class II molecules.[54] A suboptimal immunization, perhaps due to TAChR degradation by proteases that copurify with the TAChR,[60,61] might explain the lack of anti-TAChR response in that study.[57] Another study[58] found that (129/SvEv × C57Bl/6) F_2 mice genetically deficient in IFN-γ receptor developed less anti-AChR Ab than nonmutated mice and had less frequent and less severe EAMG. This indicated that IFN-γ signaling was a facilitating, albeit disposable, factor for EAMG development.

The more important facilitating effect of IFN-γ on EAMG in (129/SvEv×C57Bl/6) F_2 mice[57,58] than in B6 mice[55] may be because IFN-γ may trigger pathogenic mechanisms other than those mediated by anti-TAChR Ab: transgenic expression of IFN-γ in mouse muscle resulted in cellular infiltrates, deposition of IgG at the NMJ, and disruption of neuromuscular transmission without synthesis of anti-AChR Ab.[62] IFN-γ has complex and sometimes contrasting effects in other autoimmune responses too.[63–65]

Role of IL-10 in EAMG

IL-10 is an important effector cytokine of activated Th2 cells. However, IL-10 is secreted by a variety of other immune and nonimmune cells, including Ly-1 B cells, keratinocytes, activated macrophages, and mast cells.[21–23] IL-10 has a broad and complex range of activities.[21–23] They include anti-inflammatory activity, costimulation of thymocytes, stimulation of mast cell proliferation, stimulation of B cell differentiation, and downregulation of Th1 responses.[66] To understand the role of IL-10 in the pathogenesis of EAMG, we first examined the susceptibility to EAMG of B6 mice genetically deficient in IL-10 (IL-$10^{-/-}$) (Ostlie and Conti-Fine, unpublished observations). Those experiments suggested that TAChR immunization in adjuvant did not induce muscle weakness of a myasthenic nature in the IL-$10^{-/-}$ mice. However, the gastrointestinal pathology that commonly occurs in these mice, and the resulting losses in water and electrolytes, made it difficult to assess the muscle strength of the IL-$10^{-/-}$ mice reliably because the weakness that commonly occurs in these mice may have masked a subclinical weakness induced by the TAChR immunization. Yet, another study on the susceptibility to EAMG of IL-$10^{-/-}$ mice also concluded that genetic absence of IL-10 made the mutant mice resistant to EAMG induction.[67] To examine the role of IL-10 in EAMG in a different experimental system, we used IL-10 transgenic (TG) B6 mice, in which the T cell–specific IL-2 promoter drove the expression of the IL-10 transgene.[68] The T cells that synthesize IL-10 include activated, IL-2 secreting Th1 cells, which produce IL-10 transiently, in response to T cell activation.[68] Because of the transient expression of the transgene, the immune system of these TG mice is not significantly different from the control littermates.[68] For example, although IL-10 is a potent downregulator of Th1 cells, IFN-γ synthesis is reduced, but not eliminated in these TG mice, which have normal serum IgG levels and numbers and phenotype of T and B cells.[68]

We immunized IL-10 TG and WT mice three times with 30 or 2 μg TAChR in Freund's adjuvant.[69] The first dose is effective at inducing EAMG in WT B6 mice, whereas the second, lower dose is not. The IL-10 TG mice were much more susceptible to EAMG than WT mice. Most of them had EAMG weakness 10 weeks after the first immunization with 2 μg TAChR, whereas none of the WT mice immunized

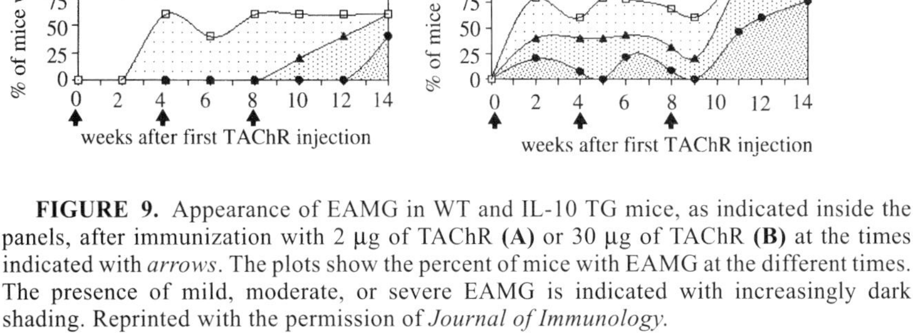

FIGURE 9. Appearance of EAMG in WT and IL-10 TG mice, as indicated inside the panels, after immunization with 2 μg of TAChR **(A)** or 30 μg of TAChR **(B)** at the times indicated with *arrows*. The plots show the percent of mice with EAMG at the different times. The presence of mild, moderate, or severe EAMG is indicated with increasingly dark shading. Reprinted with the permission of *Journal of Immunology*.

with this low dose of TAChR developed EAMG at any time (FIG. 9A). After immunization with the higher dose of TAChR, both IL-10 TG and WT mice developed EAMG, but in IL-10 TG mice the myasthenic weakness was more frequent, more severe, and longer lasting than in WT mice (FIG. 9B).

IL-10 TG mice had higher serum concentrations of anti-TAChR Abs than WT mice. The serum concentrations of anti-mouse AChR Abs were not significantly different in IL-10 TG and WT mice. However, after immunization with the high dose of TAChR, the anti-mouse AChR Abs appeared in the sera of IL-10 TG mice earlier than in WT mice; and after the low dose TAChR immunization, they were more frequent in IL-10 TG mice than WT mice. The relative amounts of anti-TAChR IgG of different subclasses were similar in all WT and IL-10 TG mice: thus, IL-10 TG mice had increased synthesis of all IgG subclasses, including those induced by Th1 cytokines. This suggests that the increased synthesis of anti-TAChR Ab in IL-10 TG mice resulted from the action of IL-10 on B cells, not by a reduced anti-TAChR Th1 response. The transgenic expression of IL-10 simultaneous with IL-2 synthesis facilitated the anti-AChR Ab response, including the synthesis of Th1-driven IgG subclasses, resulting in the increased susceptibility to EAMG. Therefore, at least when synthesized together with IL-2, the effects of IL-10 as a differentiation and proliferation stimulant for B cells, and a switch factor for a variety of Ig classes and subclasses[70–74] and possibly for all IgG isotypes,[75] overshadowed the action of IL-10 as a downregulator of Th1 cells and APC.

IL-10, especially in combination with IL-2, facilitates $CD8^+$ cytotoxic T cell responses.[76–80] The role of $CD8^+$ cells in EAMG is not clear. However, the results of some studies suggested that $CD8^+$ cells are necessary for EAMG development.[81,82] If $CD8^+$ cells facilitate rodent EAMG, their stimulation by the transgenic IL-10 may have played a role in the increased susceptibility to EAMG of the IL-10 TG mice.

Because of its ability to downregulate Th1 cells and the synthesis of a variety of cytokines, IL-10 is considered a possible therapy of undesirable immune responses.[83,84] However, the effects of IL-10 on T cell–mediated experimental autoimmune responses are complex and conflicting. Also, IL-10 has an important pathogenic role in an Ab-mediated autoimmune disease, systemic lupus erythematosus. In this disease, the Ig production is IL-10-dependent and an increased production of IL-10 by B cells and monocytes may be a critical pathogenic mechanism.[85,86] The increased susceptibility to EAMG of IL-10 TG mice, and the observation that MG patients have increased blood levels of AChR-specific cells that secrete IL-10,[87] raises concerns about the suitability of IL-10 as a treatment to curb Ab-mediated autoimmune diseases. IL-10 might be a target, rather than a tool, in the suppression of undesirable Ab responses.

Role of IL-4 in EAMG

IL-4 is another important Th2 cytokine, which is both an effector of activated Th2 cells and a stimulant of their differentiation and proliferation.[21–23] When secreted by activated Th2 cells, IL-4 further stimulates their proliferation, and facilitates the differentiation of naïve Th cells into Th2 cells, when they encounter their antigen.

IL-4 has complex effects on immune cells other than Th2 cells and therefore on the adaptive immune responses. IL-4 is a potent growth and differentiation factor for B cells and it induces synthesis of different Ig isotypes, including IgG subclasses that do not fix the complement.[21–23] However, IL-4 also has anti-inflammatory effects, that downregulate immune responses by reducing the function of activated APC and Th1 cells.[21–23] Also, it is a growth factor for Th3 cells, which downregulate the immune responses by secreting TGF-β.[24]

We have investigated the role of IL-4 in the pathogenesis and prevention of EAMG using B6 mice genetically deficient for IL-4 (IL-4$^{-/-}$). IL-4$^{-/-}$ mice have an effective Th1 response, but a severely impaired Th2 function.[88]

IL-4 Is Not Necessary for EAMG Development and Its Absence Increases the Susceptibility to EAMG

In an initial set of experiments, we immunized IL-4$^{-/-}$ and WT B6 mice with TAChR, using doses and procedures that induce EAMG in WT mice. Approximately 58% of the WT mice developed EAMG. In contrast, all of the IL-4$^{-/-}$ mice developed EAMG. The WT and IL-4$^{-/-}$ mice had similar concentrations of serum anti-TAChR Ab. However in the IL-4$^{-/-}$ mice, most of the anti-TAChR IgGs were of Th1-driven, complement-binding IgG subclasses. In contrast, in WT mice, about half of the TAChR IgGs were Th2-driven IgG1. The CD4$^+$ T cells of TAChR-immunized IL-4$^{-/-}$ mice responded vigorously to the TAChR and recognized the same immunodominant and subdominant peptides (residues 146–169, 181–200, and 360–378 of the TAChR α subunit) as the CD4$^+$ T cells from WT mice. These findings demonstrate that IL-4 is not necessary for development of EAMG.

Since IL-4$^{-/-}$ mice have fully functional Th1 cells,[88] the finding that they develop EAMG demonstrates that Th1 cells alone can drive the synthesis of pathogenic anti-AChR Ab. This conclusion agrees well with the finding that genetic absence of IL-12 makes B6 mice resistant to EAMG induction.[55,56] Another study also concluded that IL-4 has a disposable role in EAMG development.[89] These findings suggest that IL-4, and therefore Th2 cells, do not have a pathogenic role in EAMG, but rather they might modulate and curb the development of anti-AChR Ab and the resulting EAMG symptoms.

Genetic Absence of IL-4 Permits the Development of a Chronic Form of EAMG

A study on the time course of EAMG in IL-4$^{-/-}$ and WT B6 mice after a single immunization with TAChR confirmed a protective role of IL-4.[90] Its genetic absence allowed development of a self-maintaining, chronic form of EAMG, characterized by an early sensitization of T cells to the autologous mouse AChR and by a persistent production of Abs specific for the mouse muscle AChR, even at times when the anti-TAChR Abs had disappeared from the serum.[90]

After a single immunizing injection of TAChR in complete Freund's adjuvant of IL-4$^{-/-}$ and WT mice, only a few WT mice developed a short-lived myasthenic syndrome. In contrast, most IL-4$^{-/-}$ mice developed EAMG weakness, which lasted for all the observation period (30 weeks). IL-4$^{-/-}$ and WT mice developed comparable concentrations of serum anti-TAChR Abs. However, IL-4$^{-/-}$ mice had anti-mouse AChR Abs in their serum much more frequently and in much higher concentrations than WT mice. Also, the anti-mouse AChR Abs persisted in the IL-4$^{-/-}$ mouse sera for the whole duration of the observation period, even when the Abs to the immunizing TAChR were not detectable anymore.

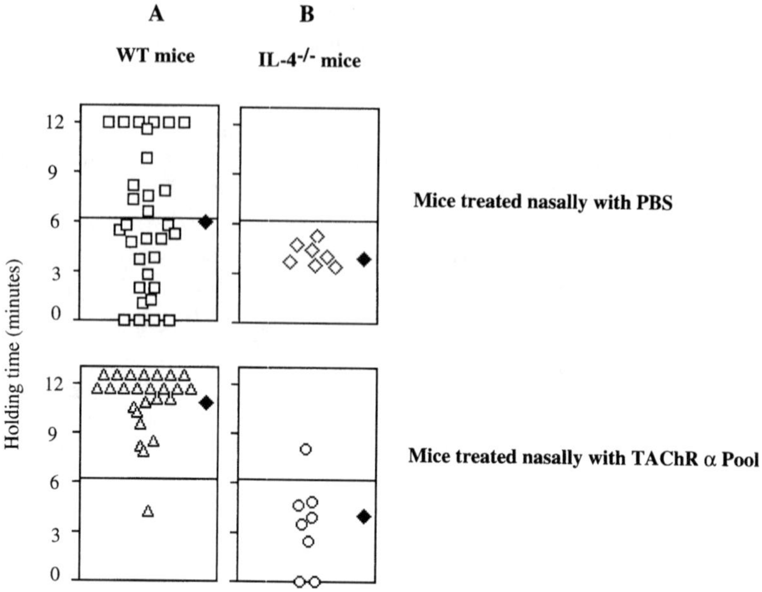

FIGURE 10. Holding time of WT **(A)** and IL-4$^{-/-}$ mice **(B)** sham-treated nasally with PBS or treated with TAChR α pool, as indicated. The *black diamonds* in each plot indicate the average holding time of that group of mice. Reprinted with the permission of *Journal of Neuroimmunology.*

The repertoire of TAChR and mouse AChR peptide sequences recognized by CD4$^+$ T cells of IL-4$^{-/-}$ and WT mice, and the intensity and time course of those responses, suggested that, when IL-4 is missing, a self-reactive anti-AChR CD4$^+$ T cell response developed.

Consistent with the results of previous studies,[91–93] the CD4$^+$ T cells of WT mice responded always to the peptides spanning the immunodominant sequence α146–169 of the TAChR, and occasionally to the subdominant epitope sequences α181–200 and α360–378. The CD4$^+$ splenocytes of IL-4$^{-/-}$ mice recognized the sequence region α146–169 most strongly and consistently. However, they also recognized a number of other peptides of the TAChR α subunit. These included the subdominant peptides α181–200 and α360–378; peptides α43–80, α111–126, α134–153, α165–184, α197–217, and α276–295; and all the peptides spanning the sequence from residue 346 to the carboxyl terminus.

The CD4$^+$ T cells of WT mice did not recognize any mouse AChR peptide sequence for the first 16 weeks after the TAChR immunization, and they had a modest response to the mouse peptide α216–235 after 24 weeks. At later times, they had a modest response to a few other mouse peptides. In contrast, the CD4$^+$ T cells of IL-4$^{-/-}$ mice had proliferative responses, which were frequently vigorous, to several mouse AChR peptides as early as 8 weeks after the TAChR immunization. At later times, they recognized a much richer repertoire of mouse α subunit peptides than the WT mice. Their responses were most diverse and intense during the first 24 weeks after the TAChR immunization. Afterwards, they were directed to a more limited peptide repertoire and were less intense than those observed at earlier times. Peptide α216–235 was recognized most frequently and strongly.

These findings further support a modulatory role of IL-4 both in the $CD4^+$ T cell response to the xenogenic TAChR and in the sensitization of self-reactive $CD4^+$ T cells, which recognize mouse AChR epitopes. The development of a chronic, self-reactive anti-AChR Ab response in IL-$4^{-/-}$ mice and the prompt sensitization of their $CD4^+$ T cells to the autologous AChR after immunization with the xenogenic TAChR suggest that IL-4 has an important role as a "gatekeeper" during immune responses to exogenous antigens potentially cross-reactive with a self-protein.

IL-4 Has a Role in the Establishment of Mucosal Tolerance to the AChR

Mucosal or systemic administration of an antigen in soluble form may down-regulate, rather than activate, the specific $CD4^+$ T cells. Those treatments prevented and even treated autoimmune diseases mediated by $CD4^+$ T cells (e.g., EAE). They are effective also in Ab-mediated diseases like EAMG.[94–98]

We investigated if nasal treatment with synthetic sequences of the TAChR α subunit that form $CD4^+$ T cell epitopes (α150–169, α181–200, α360–378) prevented EAMG in WT B6 mice.[99] We treated the mice nasally with a pool of those three epitope peptides (TAChR α pool) or with peptide α150–169 alone, before and during the immunizations with TAChR. Control mice were sham-treated with clean PBS or treated with a pool of diphtheria toxin (DTX) peptides (DTX pool). The mice treated nasally with the TAChR α pool, or with α150–169, had less frequent and less severe myasthenic weakness than the control mice (FIG. 10A). They had a reduced synthesis of anti-TAChR Abs, and a reduced T cell reactivity *in vitro* to the TAChR and to the peptides used for the nasal treatment, as compared to the control mice.

Thus, the nasal treatment with TAChR sequences forming $CD4^+$ epitopes protected the mice from EAMG, and the protection was specific for the TAChR peptides.

The reduction of the *in vitro* response to TAChR of spleen T cells from mice treated nasally with TAChR peptides was reversed by a preincubation of the T cells with IL-2. This suggests that anergy of TAChR-specific $CD4^+$ T cells is involved in the induction of nasal tolerance in EAMG. However, stimulation of modulatory Th2 cells might be another mechanism because $CD4^+$ T cells from mice treated nasally with the TAChR α pool and immunized with TAChR produced more IL-4 and IL-10 and less IL-2 than sham-tolerized mice when challenged *in vitro* with TAChR.

Another study, which demonstrated that nasal administration of the TAChR α pool did not prevent development of EAMG in IL-$4^{-/-}$ mice (FIG. 10B) or affect the synthesis of anti-TAChR Abs and of anti-TAChR IgG subclasses, supported the involvement of IL-4 in nasal tolerance.[100] Yet, the nasal treatment with the TAChR peptides had caused anergy or deletion of Th1 cells because the splenocytes of the IL-$4^{-/-}$ mice treated with the TAChR α pool had a reduced proliferative response to the TAChR and to the individual TAChR peptides used for the nasal treatment, as compared to the sham-treated mice. Also, they synthesized less IFN-γ after challenge *in vitro* with TAChR or the TAChR α pool.

Since the reduced anti-TAChR Th1 response of the peptide-treated IL-$4^{-/-}$ mice did not suffice to protect them from EAMG or to reduce the synthesis of anti-TAChR Abs, the prevention of EAMG and the reduction in the synthesis of anti-TAChR Abs observed in WT mice after nasal administration of TAChR epitopes are likely caused by activation of T regulatory (Tr) cells specific for the TAChR epitopes administered nasally, which need IL-4 for their differentiation or function.

CD4$^+$ CELLS FROM MICE TREATED NASALLY WITH TACHR PEPTIDE EPITOPES CONFER ADOPTIVE PROTECTION FROM EAMG

To test the hypothesis that TAChR-specific Tr cells can protect from EAMG, we examined whether CD4$^+$ cells from WT mice treated nasally with the TAChR α pool or with α150–169 protected IL-4$^{-/-}$ mice from EAMG.[101] Control mouse donors were sham-treated with PBS or treated with DTX pool. We prepared from their spleen a population of cells highly enriched in CD4$^+$, CD8$^-$, CD3$^+$ TCR$^+$ T cells: a

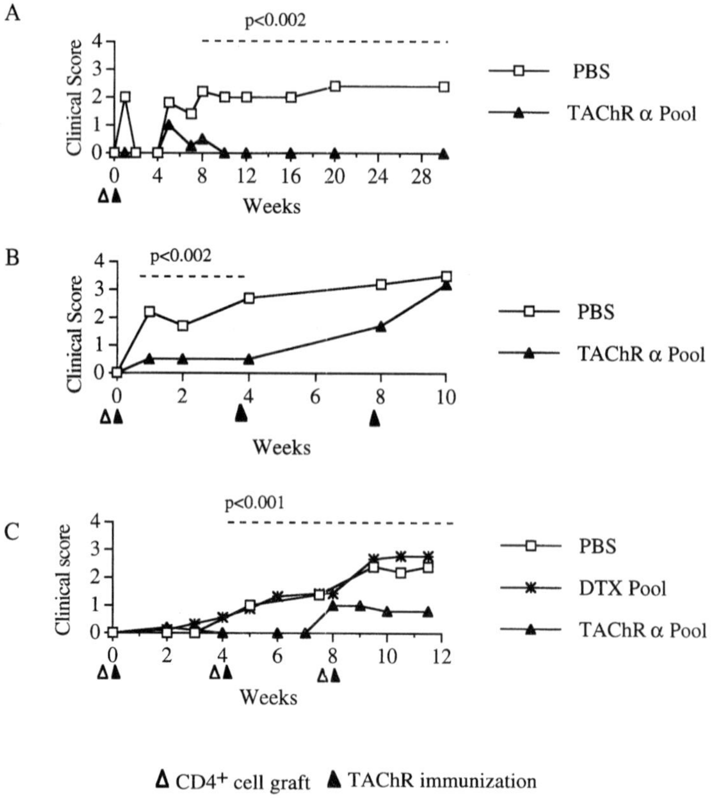

FIGURE 11. Average clinical scores of groups of IL-4$^{-/-}$ mice that received one or three grafts (*white arrowheads*) of CD4$^+$ T cells from WT mice treated nasally with the TAChR pool, DTX pool, or PBS. The mice were immunized once or three times with TAChR in Freund's adjuvant (*black arrowheads*). The clinical scores of the severity of EAMG, which are described in detail elsewhere,[100] range from grade 0 (strength of normal mice) to grade 4 (paralysis or death from EAMG). Reprinted with the permission of *Journal of Neuroimmunology*.

small percentage of the cells (5.13 ± 1.3%) expressed both the CD4 and CD25 markers. The cell preparations included $CD4^{-}CD8^{-}$ NK and NKT cells (10.9 ± 0.9% and 5.7 ± 1.7%, respectively). One graft of the $CD4^{+}$ enriched cells from WT mice treated nasally with the TAChR α pool protected IL-$4^{-/-}$ mice from EAMG induced by one TAChR injection (FIG. 11A). However, as expected from the short life span of activated $CD4^{+}$ T cells, the protective effects were not long-lived, and they were lost if, one month after the graft, the IL-$4^{-/-}$ mice received a second TAChR immunization (FIG. 11B). Repeated grafts of $CD4^{+}$ cells from WT mice treated nasally with the TAChR α pool or just with peptide α150–169, one month apart, conferred resistance to EAMG in IL-$4^{-/-}$ mice even after multiple TAChR immunizations (FIG. 11C; data for the peptide α150–169 not shown). The protection was due to TAChR-specific Tr cells because $CD4^{+}$ cells from WT mice treated nasally with DTX pool, or sham-treated with PBS, did not protect the IL-$4^{-/-}$ mice from EAMG.

IL-$4^{-/-}$ mice grafted with $CD4^{+}$ cells from WT mice treated nasally with TAChR α pool had lower serum concentrations of anti-TAChR and anti-mouse AChR Abs than IL-$4^{-/-}$ mice grafted with $CD4^{+}$ cells from donors sham-treated with PBS or treated with DTX pool. The IL-$4^{-/-}$ mice that received $CD4^{+}$ cells from PBS-treated WT mice had significantly higher concentrations of anti-TAChR IgG of the complement-fixing IgG2b and IgG2c subclasses as compared to IL-$4^{-/-}$ mice that received $CD4^{+}$ cells from WT mice treated with the TAChR α pool. The serum anti-TAChR IgG2b and IgG2c in IL-$4^{-/-}$ mice grafted with $CD4^{+}$ cells from WT mice treated with peptide α150–169 alone were slightly lower than those observed in the control group during the first two months after the beginning of the TAChR immunization, but were comparable after three months.

Purified $CD4^{+}$ cells from the spleen of WT mice treated nasally with the TAChR α pool, which did not include any NK and NKT cells, were even more effective in protecting from EAMG and in curbing the anti-TAChR Ab production than the less-purified $CD4^{+}$ cells used for the experiments summarized above. This finding is consistent with the pathogenic role of NK cells in EAMG, which has been suggested by a recent study.[102]

These findings strongly support the existence of TAChR-specific Tr cells able to prevent EAMG, which are activated by nasal exposure to the TAChR epitopes.

REFERENCES

1. CONTI-FINE, B.M. *et al.* 1997. Myasthenia Gravis: The Immunobiology of an Autoimmune Disease. Neuroscience Intelligence Unit. Landes. Austin.
2. ENGEL, A.G. 1999. The Myasthenic Syndromes. Oxford University Press. New York.
3. DRACHMAN, D.B. 1994. Myasthenia gravis. N. Engl. J. Med. **330:** 1797–1810.
4. OOSTERHUIS, H.J.G.H. 1997. Myasthenia Gravis. Groningen Neurological Press.
5. LEFVERT, A.K. & K. BERGSTROM. 1978. Acetylcholine receptor antibody in myasthenia gravis: purification and characterization. Scand. J. Immunol. **8:** 525–533.
6. VINCENT, A. & J. NEWSOM-DAVIS. 1980. Anti-acetylcholine receptor antibodies. J. Neurol. Neurosurg. Psychiatry **43:** 590–600.
7. HOHLFELD, R. *et al.* 1984. Autoimmune human T lymphocytes specific for acetylcholine receptor. Nature **310:** 244–246.
8. MELMS, A. *et al.* 1988. Thymus in myasthenia gravis: isolation of T-lymphocyte lines specific for the nicotinic acetylcholine receptor from thymuses of myasthenic patients. J. Clin. Invest. **81:** 902–908.

9. WANG, Z.Y. *et al.* 1999. Myasthenia in SCID mice grafted with myasthenic patient lymphocytes: role of $CD4^+$ and $CD8^+$ cells. Neurology **52:** 484–497.
10. AHLBERG, R. *et al.* 1994. Treatment of myasthenia gravis with anti-CD4 antibody: improvement correlates to decreased T-cell autoreactivity. Neurology **44:** 1732–1737.
11. LENNON, V.A., J.M. LINDSTROM & M.E. SEYBOLD. 1976. Experimental autoimmune myasthenia gravis: cellular and humoral immune responses. Ann. N.Y. Acad. Sci. **274:** 283–299.
12. WALDOR, M.K. *et al.* 1983. *In vivo* therapy with monoclonal anti-I-A antibody suppresses immune responses to acetylcholine receptor. Proc. Natl. Acad. Sci. USA **80:** 2713–2717.
13. CHRISTADOSS, P. & M.J. DAUPHINEE. 1986. Immunotherapy for myasthenia gravis: a murine model. J. Immunol. **136:** 2437–2440.
14. KAUL, R. *et al.* 1994. Major histocompatibility complex class II gene disruption prevents experimental autoimmune myasthenia gravis. J. Immunol. **152:** 3152–3157.
15. LISAK, R.P. *et al.* 1984. *In vitro* synthesis of antibodies to acetylcholine receptor by peripheral blood cells: role of suppressor T cells in normal subjects. Neurology **34:** 802–805.
16. LISAK, R.P. *et al.* 1986. Suppressor T cells in myasthenia gravis and antibodies to acetylcholine receptor. Ann. Neurol. **19:** 87–89.
17. YUEN, M.H. *et al.* 1995. Immunoregulatory $CD8^+$ cells recognize antigen-activated $CD4^+$ cells in myasthenia gravis patients and in healthy controls. J. Immunol. **154:** 1508–1520.
18. ZHANG, G.X. *et al.* 1995. Depletion of $CD8^+$ T cells suppresses the development of experimental autoimmune myasthenia gravis in Lewis rats. Eur. J. Immunol. **25:** 1191–1198.
19. ZHANG, G.X. *et al.* 1996. Both $CD4^+$ and $CD8^+$ T cells are essential to induce experimental autoimmune myasthenia gravis. J. Exp. Med. **184:** 349–356.
20. SHENOY, M. *et al.* 1994. Effect of MHC class I and CD8 cell deficiency on experimental autoimmune myasthenia gravis pathogenesis. J. Immunol. **153:** 5330–5335.
21. ABBAS, A.K., K.M. MURPHY & A. SHER. 1996. Functional diversity of helper T lymphocytes. Nature **383:** 787–793.
22. ROMAGNANI, S. 1997. The Th1/Th2 paradigm. Immunol. Today **18:** 263–266.
23. O'GARRA, A. 1998. Cytokines induce the development of functionally heterogeneous T helper cell subsets. Immunity **8:** 275–283.
24. SEDER, R.A. *et al.* 1998. Factors involved in the differentiation of TGF-β-producing cells from naive $CD4^+$ T cells: IL-4 and IFN-γ have opposing effects, while TGF-β positively regulates its own production. J. Immunol. **160:** 5719–5728.
25. RONCAROLO, M.G. *et al.* 2001. Type 1 T regulatory cells. Immunol. Rev. **182:** 68–79.
26. SHEVACH, E.M. 2002. $CD4^+CD25^+$ suppressor T cells: more questions than answers. Nat. Rev. Immunol. **2:** 389–400.
27. O'GARRA, A., L. STEINMAN & K. GIJBELS. 1997. $CD4^+$ T-cell subsets in autoimmunity. Curr. Opin. Immunol. **9:** 872–883.
28. LAFAILLE, J.J. 1998. The role of helper T cell subsets in autoimmune diseases. Cytokine Growth Factor Rev. **9:** 139–151
29. SOMMER, N. *et al.* 1993. Ocular myasthenia gravis: a critical review of clinical and pathophysiological aspects. Doc. Ophthalmol. **84:** 309–333.
30. CONTI-TRONCONI, B.M. *et al.* 1994. The nicotinic acetylcholine receptor: structure and autoimmune pathology. Crit. Rev. Biochem. Mol. Biol. **29:** 69–123.
31. PROTTI, M.P. *et al.* 1990. $CD4^+$ T cell response to human acetylcholine receptor subunit correlates with myasthenia gravis severity: a study with synthetic peptides. J. Immunol. **144:** 1276–1281.
32. PROTTI, M.P. *et al.* 1990. Immunodominant regions for T helper sensitization on the human nicotinic receptor subunit in myasthenia gravis. Proc. Natl. Acad. Sci. USA **87:** 7792–7796.
33. PROTTI, M.P. *et al.* 1991. Myasthenia gravis: T epitopes of the δ subunit of human muscle acetylcholine receptor. J. Immunol. **146:** 2253–2261.
34. PROTTI, M.P. *et al.* 1992. Myasthenia gravis: $CD4^+$ T epitopes on the embryonic γ subunit of human muscle acetylcholine receptor. J. Clin. Invest. **90:** 1558–1567.

35. MANFREDI, A.A. *et al.* 1992. $CD4^+$ T epitope repertoire on the human acetylcholine receptor α subunit in severe myasthenia gravis: a study with synthetic peptides. Neurology **42:** 1092–1100.
36. MANFREDI, A.A. *et al.* 1993. T helper cell recognition of muscle acetylcholine receptor in myasthenia gravis: epitopes on the γ and δ subunits. J. Clin. Invest. **92:** 1055–1067.
37. MOIOLA, L. *et al.* 1994. Epitopes on the β subunit of human muscle acetylcholine receptor recognized by $CD4^+$ cells of myasthenia gravis patients and healthy subjects. J. Clin. Invest. **93:** 1020–1028.
38. MOIOLA, L. *et al.* 1994. Myasthenia gravis: residues of the α and γ subunits of muscle acetylcholine receptor involved in formation of immunodominant $CD4^+$ epitopes. J. Immunol. **152:** 4686–4698.
39. WANG, Z.Y. *et al.* 1997. Th1 epitope repertoire on the subunit of human muscle acetylcholine receptor in myasthenia gravis. Neurology **48:** 1643–1653.
40. WANG, Z.Y. *et al.* 1998. T-cell recognition of muscle acetylcholine receptor subunits in generalized and ocular myasthenia gravis. Neurology **50:** 1045–1054.
41. WANG, Z.Y. *et al.* 2000. T cell recognition of muscle acetylcholine receptor in ocular myasthenia gravis. J. Neuroimmunol. **108:** 29–39.
42. NAVANEETHAM, D. *et al.* 2001. Human thymuses express incomplete sets of muscle acetylcholine receptor subunit transcripts that seldom include the δ subunit. Muscle Nerve **124:** 203–210.
43. CONTI-FINE, B.M. *et al.* 1998. T cell recognition of the acetylcholine receptor in myasthenia gravis. Ann. N.Y. Acad. Sci. **841:** 283–308.
44. YANG, H. *et al.* 2002. Mapping myasthenia gravis–associated T cell epitopes on human acetylcholine receptors in HLA transgenic mice. J. Clin. Invest. **109:** 1111–1120.
45. BOSMA, G.C. *et al.* 1989. The mouse mutation severe combined immune deficiency (SCID) is on chromosome 16. Immunogenetics **29:** 54–57.
46. SCHULER, W., A. SCHULER & M.J. BOSMA. 1990. Defective V-to-J recombination of T cell receptor γ chain genes in SCID mice. Eur. J. Immunol. **20:** 545–550.
47. LINDSTROM, J., D. SHELTON & Y. FUJII. 1988. Myasthenia gravis. Adv. Immunol. **42:** 233–284.
48. LENNON, V.A., J.M. LINDSTROM & M.E. SEYBOLD. 1975. Experimental autoimmune myasthenia: a model of myasthenia gravis in rats and guinea pigs. J. Exp. Med. **141:** 1365–1375.
49. FUCHS, S. *et al.* 1976. Strain differences in the autoimmune response of mice to acetylcholine receptors. Nature **263:** 329–330.
50. BERMAN, P.W. & J. PATRICK. 1980. Linkage between the frequency of muscular weakness and loci that regulate immune responsiveness in murine experimental myasthenia gravis. J. Exp. Med. **152:** 507–520.
51. HSIEH, C.S. *et al.* 1993. Development of Th1 $CD4^+$ T cells through IL-12 produced by *Listeria*-induced macrophages. Science **260:** 547–549.
52. MURPHY, E.E. *et al.* 1994. B7 and IL-12 cooperate for proliferation and IFN-γ production by mouse T helper clones that are unresponsive to B7 costimulation. J. Exp. Med. **180:** 223–231.
53. MAGRAM, J. *et al.* 1996. IL-12-deficient mice are defective in IFN-γ production and type 1 cytokine responses. Immunity **4:** 471–481.
54. DALTON, D.K. *et al.* 1993. Multiple defects of immune cell function in mice with disrupted IFN-γ genes. Science **259:** 1739–1742.
55. KARACHUNSKI, P.I. *et al.* 2000. Absence of IFN-γ or IL-12 has different effects on experimental myasthenia gravis in C57BL/6 mice. J. Immunol. **164:** 5236–5244.
56. MOIOLA, L. *et al.* 1998. IL-12 is involved in the induction of experimental autoimmune myasthenia gravis, an antibody-mediated disease. Eur. J. Immunol. **28:** 2487–2497.
57. BALASA, B. *et al.* 1997. Interferon gamma (IFN-γ) is necessary for the genesis of acetylcholine receptor–induced clinical experimental autoimmune myasthenia gravis in mice. J. Exp. Med. **186:** 385–391.
58. ZHANG, G.X. *et al.* 1999. Mice with IFN-γ receptor deficiency are less susceptible to experimental autoimmune myasthenia gravis. J. Immunol. **162:** 3775–3781.
59. CHRISTADOSS, P. *et al.* 1981. Genetic control of autoimmunity to acetylcholine receptors: role of Ia molecules. Ann. N.Y. Acad. Sci. **377:** 258–277.

60. LINDSTROM, J. *et al.* 1980. Proteolytic nicking of the acetylcholine receptor. Biochemistry **19:** 4791–4795.
61. CONTI-TRONCONI, B.M., S.M. DUNN & M.A. RAFTERY. 1982. Functional stability of *Torpedo* acetylcholine receptor: effects of protease treatment. Biochemistry **21:** 893–899.
62. GU, D. *et al.* 1995. Myasthenia gravis-like syndrome induced by expression of interferon gamma in the neuromuscular junction. J. Exp. Med. **181:** 547–557.
63. PANITCH, H.S. *et al.* 1987. Treatment of multiple sclerosis with gamma interferon: exacerbations associated with activation of the immune system. Neurology **37:** 1097–1102.
64. FERBER, I.A. *et al.* 1996. Mice with a disrupted IFN-γ gene are susceptible to the induction of experimental autoimmune encephalomyelitis (EAE). J. Immunol. **156:** 5–7.
65. WILLENBORG, D.O. *et al.* 1996. IFN-γ plays a critical down-regulatory role in the induction and effector phase of myelin oligodendrocyte glycoprotein-induced autoimmune encephalomyelitis. J. Immunol. **157:** 3223–3227.
66. WILDBAUM, G. 1998. Neutralizing antibodies to IFN-γ-inducing factor prevent experimental autoimmune encephalomyelitis. J. Immunol. **161:** 6368–6374.
67. POUSSIN, M.A. *et al.* 2000. Suppression of experimental autoimmune myasthenia gravis in IL-10 gene-disrupted mice is associated with reduced B cells and serum cytotoxicity on mouse cell line expressing AChR. J. Neuroimmunol. **111:** 152–160.
68. HAGENBAUGH, A. *et al.* 1997. Altered immune responses in IL-10 transgenic mice. J. Exp. Med. **185:** 2101–2110.
69. OSTLIE, N. *et al.* 2001. Transgenic expression of IL-10 in T cells facilitates development of experimental myasthenia gravis. J. Immunol. **166:** 4853–4862.
70. BRIERE, F. *et al.* 1994. Human IL-10 induces naive surface immunoglobulin D^+ ($sIgD^+$) B cells to secrete IgG1 and IgG3. J. Exp. Med. **179:** 757–762.
71. BRIERE, F. *et al.* 1994. IL-10 induces B lymphocytes from IgA-deficient patients to secrete IgA. J. Clin. Invest. **94:** 97–104.
72. BURDIN, N. *et al.* 1995. Endogenous IL-6 and IL-10 contribute to the differentiation of CD40-activated human B lymphocytes. J. Immunol. **154:** 2533–2544.
73. ROUSSET, F. *et al.* 1995. Long-term cultured CD40-activated B lymphocytes differentiate into plasma cells in response to IL-10, but not IL-4. Int. Immunol. **7:** 1243–1253.
74. MALISAN, F. *et al.* 1996. IL-10 induces immunoglobulin G isotype switch recombination in human CD40-activated naive B lymphocytes. J. Exp. Med. **183:** 937–947.
75. CERUTTI, A. *et al.* 1998. CD40 ligand and appropriate cytokines induce switching to IgG, IgA, and IgE and coordinated germinal center and plasmacytoid phenotypic differentiation in a human monoclonal IgM^+IgD^+ B cell line. J. Immunol. **160:** 2145–2157.
76. MACNEIL, I.A. *et al.* 1990. IL-10, a novel growth cofactor for mature and immature T cells. J. Immunol. **145:** 4167–4173.
77. CHEN, W.F. & A. ZLOTNIK. 1991. IL-10: a novel cytotoxic T cell differentiation factor. J. Immunol. **147:** 528–534.
78. YANG, G. *et al.* 1995. *In vitro* priming of tumor-reactive cytolytic T lymphocytes by combining IL-10 with B7-CD28 costimulation. J. Immunol. **155:** 3897–3903.
79. YANO, S. *et al.* 1997. T helper 2 cytokines differently regulate monocyte chemoattractant protein-1 production by human peripheral blood monocytes and alveolar macrophages. J. Immunol. **157:** 2660–2665.
80. GROUX, H. *et al.* 1998. Inhibitory and stimulatory effects of IL-10 on human $CD8^+$ T cells. J. Immunol. **160:** 3188–3193.
81. ZHANG, G.X. *et al.* 1995. Depletion of $CD8^+$ T cells suppresses the development of experimental autoimmune myasthenia gravis in Lewis rats. Eur. J. Immunol. **25:** 1191–1198.
82. ZHANG, G.X. *et al.* 1996. Both $CD4^+$ and $CD8^+$ T cells are essential to induce experimental autoimmune myasthenia gravis. J. Exp. Med. **184:** 349–356.
83. BROMBERG, J.S. 1995. IL-10 immunosuppression in transplantation. Curr. Opin. Immunol. **7:** 639–643.
84. AKDIS, C.A. & K. BLASER. 1999. IL-10-induced anergy in peripheral T cell and reactivation by microenvironmental cytokines: two key steps in specific immunotherapy. FASEB J. **13:** 603–609.

85. LLORENTE, L. *et al.* 1995. Role of IL-10 in the B lymphocyte hyperactivity and autoantibody production of human systemic lupus erythematosus. J. Exp. Med. **181:** 839–844.
86. CROSS, J.T. & H.P. BENTON. 1999. The roles of IL-6 and IL-10 in B cell hyperactivity in systemic lupus erythematosus. Inflamm. Res. **48:** 255–261.
87. HUANG, Y.M. *et al.* 1999. Increased levels of circulating acetylcholine receptor (AChR)–reactive IL-10-secreting cells are characteristic for myasthenia gravis (MG). Clin. Exp. Immunol. **118:** 304–308.
88. KUHN, R., K. RAJEWSKY & W. MULLER. 1991. Generation and analysis of IL-4 deficient mice. Science **254:** 707–710.
89. BALASA, B. *et al.* 1998. The Th2 cytokine IL-4 is not required for the progression of antibody-dependent autoimmune myasthenia gravis. J. Immunol. **161:** 2856–2862.
90. OSTLIE, N. *et al.* 2003. Absence of IL-4 facilitates development of chronic autoimmune myasthenia gravis in C57Bl/6 mice. J. Immunol. **170:** 604–612.
91. YOKOI, T. *et al.* 1987. T lymphocyte recognition of acetylcholine receptor: localization of the full T cell recognition profile on the extracellular part of the α chain of *Torpedo californica* acetylcholine receptor. Eur. J. Immunol. **17:** 1697–1702.
92. BELLONE, M. *et al.* 1991. Experimental myasthenia gravis in congenic mice: sequence mapping and H-2 restriction of T helper epitopes on the α-subunits of *Torpedo californica* and murine acetylcholine receptor. Eur. J. Immunol. **21:** 2303–2310.
93. SHENOY, M., E. GOLUZSKO & P. CHRISTADOSS. 1994. The pathogenic role of acetylcholine receptor chain epitope within 146–162 in the development of experimental autoimmune myasthenia gravis in C57BL6 mice. Clin. Immunol. Immunopathol. **73:** 338–343.
94. MILLER, A. *et al.* 1994. Orally administered myelin basic protein in neonates primes for immune responses and enhances experimental autoimmune encephalomyelitis in adult animals. Eur. J. Immunol. **24:** 1026–1032.
95. AL-SABBAGH, A. *et al.* 1996. Antigen-driven peripheral immune tolerance suppression of experimental autoimmune encephalomyelitis and collagen-induced arthritis by aerosol administration of myelin basic protein or type II collagen. Cell. Immunol. **171:** 111–119.
96. BAGGI, F. *et al.* 1999. Oral administration of an immunodominant T-cell epitope downregulates Th1/Th2 cytokines and prevents experimental myasthenia gravis. J. Clin. Invest. **104:** 1287–1295.
97. IM, S.H. *et al.* 1999. Suppression of ongoing experimental myasthenia by oral treatment with an acetylcholine receptor recombinant fragment. J. Clin. Invest. **104:** 1723–1730.
98. IM, S.H. *et al.* 2000. Role of tolerogen conformation in induction of oral tolerance in experimental autoimmune myasthenia gravis. J. Immunol. **165:** 3599–3605.
99. KARACHUNSKI, P.I. *et al.* 1997. Prevention of experimental myasthenia gravis by nasal administration of synthetic acetylcholine receptor T epitope sequences. J. Clin. Invest. **100:** 3027–3035.
100. KARACHUNSKI, P.I. *et al.* 1999. IL-4 deficiency facilitates development of experimental myasthenia gravis and precludes its prevention by nasal administration of $CD4^+$ epitope sequences of the acetylcholine receptor. J. Neuroimmunol. **95:** 73–84.
101. MONFARDINI, C. *et al.* 2002. Adoptive protection from experimental myasthenia gravis with T cells from mice treated nasally with acetylcholine receptor epitopes. J. Neuroimmunol. **123:** 123–134.
102. SHI, F.D. *et al.* 2000. Natural killer cells determine the outcome of B cell–mediated autoimmunity. Nat. Immunol. **1:** 245–251.

Immunoregulation in Experimental Autoimmune Myasthenia Gravis—about T Cells, Antibodies, and Endplates

M. DE BAETS, M. STASSEN, M. LOSEN, X. ZHANG, AND B. MACHIELS

Department of Neurology, Research Institute of Brain and Behavior, University of Maastricht, 6229 ER Maastricht, the Netherlands

ABSTRACT: Experimental autoimmune myasthenia gravis (EAMG) can be induced in a large number of animal species by active immunization (AI) AChR, by passive transfer (PT) of anti-AChR antibodies, by autologous bone marrow transplantation and cyclosporin (BMT-Cy), or spontaneously. Depending on the model used, different immunological mechanisms are operational. In the AI model, the T cell is pivotal in directing the anti-AChR antibody production towards pathogenic, that is, cross-linking and complement-fixing antibodies. Injection of anti-AChR antibodies alone suffices to induce EAMG, excluding the role of specific cell-mediated immune responses in the effector phase of the disease. Aged animals are resistant to the induction of AI and PT EAMG. This resistance is localized at the postsynaptic membrane containing more AChR-anchoring proteins, including S-laminin and rapsyn in aged animals. In BMT-CyA EAMG, a dysregulation of the immune system in the absence of immunization is capable of inducing myasthenia. The role of these animal models in relation to pathogenesis and immunotherapy is discussed.

KEYWORDS: experimental autoimmune myasthenia gravis (EAMG); animal models; T cells; B cells; AChR

INTRODUCTION

Experimental autoimmune myasthenia gravis (EAMG) can be induced in a large number of animal species by active immunization (AI) AChR, by passive transfer (PT) of anti-AChR antibodies, by autologous bone marrow transplantation and cyclosporin (BMT-Cy), or spontaneously. Depending on the model used, different immunological mechanisms are operational. In the AI model, the T cell is pivotal in directing the anti-AChR antibody production towards pathogenic, that is, cross-linking and complement-fixing antibodies. Injection of anti-AChR antibodies alone suffices to induce EAMG, excluding the role of specific cell-mediated immune responses in the effector phase of the disease. Aged animals are resistant to the induction of AI and PT EAMG. This resistance is localized at the postsynaptic membrane containing more AChR-anchoring proteins, including S-laminin and rapsyn in

Address for correspondence: M. De Baets, Department of Neurology, Institute for Neuroscience, Euron, University of Maastricht, P. O. Box 616, 6200 MD Maastricht, the Netherlands. Voice: +31-43-3875059; fax: +31-43-3877055.
mdba@sneu.azm.nl

Ann. N.Y. Acad. Sci. 998: 308–317 (2003). © 2003 New York Academy of Sciences.
doi: 10.1196/annals.1254.033

TABLE 1. EAMG models

EAMG after active immunization
Passive transfer EAMG
EAMG after bone marrow transplantation
EAMG after thymus grafting
Spontaneous myasthenia
EAMG in transgenic animals

aged animals. In BMT-CyA EAMG, a dysregulation of the immune system in the absence of immunization is capable of inducing myasthenia. The role of these animal models in relation to pathogenesis and immunotherapy is discussed (see TABLE 1).

EAMG AFTER ACTIVE IMMUNIZATION

Patrick and Lindstrom immunized rabbits with purified AChR from the electric organ of electric eels to obtain antibodies for their biochemical analysis of AChR. All animals became paralyzed and eventually died.[1] Active immunization of experimental animals (including rabbits, rats, mice, guinea pigs, monkeys, and goats) with AChR with or without adjuvant induced chronic EAMG within 30 days after immunization. The animals mount an active immune response against injected AChR. The disease is induced by antibodies cross-reacting with the animals' own AChR. In this model, many immunological aspects of MG can be studied, such as AChR processing, APC presentation, the role of MHC, T cell subsets, and cytokines (see ref. 2), as well as many nonimmune-mediated applications that are relevant to human MG.

We induced EAMG in pigs to study the pharmacokinetics of nondepolarizing muscle relaxants (rocuronium) and developed a computer model to calculate the dose of rocuronium in myasthenia. The number of AChR remaining is important for the calculation of the pharmacokinetic-dynamic relationships for rocuronium in pigs [de Haes *et al.* 2003. *Anesthesiology* **98**(1): 133–142].

PASSIVE TRANSFER EAMG

Injection of EAMG or MG serum, or monoclonal antibodies against the main immunogenic region (MIR) or against the ACh binding sites, in experimental animals induces MG within hours or days (see ref. 3). Antibodies against the ACh binding sites induce a curare-like effect within 15–30 min.[4] Anti-AChR binding site antibodies block the ligand-induced opening of the ion channel. Antibodies against the MIR induce myasthenia within 8–48 h depending on the dose and affinity of the antibody for AChR. The immunopathological mechanisms are antigenic modulation and complement-mediated focal lysis of the postsynaptic membrane for anti-MIR antibodies.[5] This passive transfer model is relevant for MG in order to study the effector phase of the disease.

EAMG AFTER BONE MARROW TRANSPLANTATION

After bone marrow transplantation (BMT), humans and experimental animals developed a graft versus host disease and occasionally MG. In a rat model originally developed by Hess and colleagues (reviewed in ref. 6), Lewis rats are lethally irradiated and rescued by a syngeneic BMT. The animals are injected with a low dose of cyclosporin A for 4 weeks. Two weeks after stopping cyclosporin A, the animals develop a scleroderma-like skin disease. In the course of these studies, we have observed two animals out of several hundred that spontaneously developed MG without injection of any antigen or adjuvant. Both rats had circulating anti-rat AChR antibodies, increased jitter and single-fiber EMG, and AChR loss (G. Bos *et al.*, unpublished observations). The mechanism of this autoimmune disease is the result of defective T cell development, including aberrant selection in the thymus and disturbed T cell balances in the periphery. Cyclosporin A is required for the intrathymic generation of autoreactive cells. Fewer cortical thymocytes are surviving positive selection and fewer medullary thymocytes are eliminated during negative selection–induced maturation arrest of the $CD4^+$ and $CD8^+$ double-positive thymocytes.[6]

This BMT model is probably relevant for MG after BMT and for the study of the role of the thymus in MG. Unfortunately, the incidence of EAMG in this model is too low for a more systematic study.

EAMG AFTER THYMUS GRAFTING

Thymus explants from MG patients with follicular hyperplasia, but not thymoma, induce MG when transplanted under the kidney capsule in SCID mice. Anti-human AChR antibodies produced by the thymic transplant cross-react with mouse AChR, which causes AChR loss and muscle weakness. The thymus contains all components to effectuate myasthenia, including AChR-expressing myoid cells, antigen-presenting cells, and T and B cells.[7,8] This MG model is relevant for the study of the role of the thymus and its cellular components.

SPONTANEOUS MYASTHENIA

MG spontaneously occurs in cats, dogs, and horses. Similar to the human disease, thymic abnormalities are seen and circulating anti-AChR antibodies can be detected by radioimmunoassay.[9] The immunological mechanisms operational in these models are probably identical to human MG. The study of spontaneous MG in animals is very relevant for human MG. Unfortunately, few animals are available for experimental studies, mostly because the owners do not like to donate their pets for scientific studies.

EAMG IN TRANSGENIC ANIMALS

Introducing or silencing immunological relevant genes in mice prior to immunization with AChR can pinpoint the role of these genes in EAMG and MG. Elimination of the genes that are relevant for APC/T cell interaction, including MHC II and CD4, results in a loss of susceptibility to disease. In the absence of a CD8 molecule, mice develop EAMG, which indicates that cytotoxic T cells are probably not involved in the pathogenesis of the disease. NKT knockout mice fail to develop EAMG.[2]

Mice transgenic for the human MHC molecule[10] are relevant for the study of the specificity of the T cell response and the susceptibility to the disease. Unfortunately, these animals do not express human T cell receptor molecules. Mice transgenic for the human IgG gene allow us to study the role of human immunoglobulins in EAMG.[11]

In another MG model, no immunization is required. Targeting the interfering γ gene to the postsynaptic membrane using the promoter of the γ subunit of AChR results in a local inflammation of the endplate and muscular weakness.[12] The animals in this model develop serum antibodies against an 87-kDa protein at the endplates, but not against AChR. Therefore, this model is not suitable for the study of MG.

IMMUNOREGULATION AT THE T CELL LEVEL

MG and EAMG are typical antibody-mediated diseases, but the production of the pathogenic antibodies by B cells depends on T helper cells. The degree of tolerance in both T and B cell compartments is dependent upon the concentration of the self-antigen in the microenvironment. If the concentration of the self-antigen, for example albumin, is high, both T and B cells are tolerant. If the concentration is low, as for thyroglobulin, only T cells are tolerant.[13] Immunization of mice with mouse thyroglobulin, which is normally circulating in nanogram amounts,[14] does not result in a T cell proliferative response. There is no tolerance if the self-antigen is not circulating in the microenvironment as is the case for AChR or myelin basic protein (MBP). Indeed, injection of nanogram amounts of syngeneic rat AChR in Lewis rats induces a vigorous immune response as judged by a T cell proliferation assay (TABLES 2 and 3).

Thus, in MG, a small amount of AChR or cross-reacting antigen is sufficient to start the immune response. When antibodies reach the endplates, the local debris of AChR antibody complexes is removed to the draining lymph nodes where the autoimmune response is maintained. The muscle cell upregulates the AChR synthesis[15] and this ensures a continuous supply of self-antigen. Immune complexes containing AChR and anti-AChR antibodies are very efficient in stimulating the immune response.[16]

T cells can be divided into T helper-one (TH1) and T helper-two cells (TH2) depending upon their cytokine profile. In EAMG mice, the pathogenic antibody response is TH1-dependent. In mice, manipulation of the balance in favor of TH2

TABLE 2. AChR-specific proliferation of immune lymph node cells

	Stimulation index		
Priming antigen	*Torpedo* AChR	Fetal calf AChR	Rat AChR
Torpedo AChR	229	24	23
Fetal calf AChR	5	100	ND
Rat AChR	1	20	20

NOTE: Cross-reaction of the proliferating response of lymph node cells from rats immunized with *Torpedo*, fetal calf, or rat AChR and stimulated with *Torpedo*, fetal calf, or rat AChR. After stimulation with syngeneic AChR, T cells are proliferating, suggesting an absence of tolerance for rat AChR. [Modified from De Baets *et al.* 1982. *J. Immunol.* **128**(5): 2228–2235.]

TABLE 3. Thyroglobulin-specific proliferation of immune lymph node cells

		Stimulation index	
Animal	Priming antigen	Bovine Tg	Mouse Tg
Guinea pig	Bovine Tg	55	0.4
	Mouse Tg	3.1	57
CBA mouse	Bovine Tg	18	2
	Mouse Tg	1.7	3

NOTE: Cross-reaction of the proliferative response of spleen lymphocytes from mice or guinea pigs immunized with bovine or mouse thyroglobulin (Tg) and stimulated *in vitro* with the same antigen. Note that T cells of mice primed with mouse Tg are tolerant for self-Tg.

cells protects against EAMG.[17] In rats, however, both TH1 and TH2 cells are able to induce pathogenic anti-AChR antibodies. Manipulation of the TH1/TH2 balance does not effect the severity of disease.[18] The different requirements for TH1-dependent responses in rats and mice can best be explained by differences in complement fixation and/or activation by antibody subclasses in rats and mice. Indeed, unlike mouse IgG subclasses, both TH1- and TH2-associated rat Ig subclasses are capable of binding complement. In humans, both TH1 and TH2 cells are able to induce the production of complement-binding antibodies.[19] It can be concluded from these studies that rat EAMG models are more relevant for the study of MG.

ANTI-AChR ANTIBODIES

The majority of anti-AChR antibodies in MG and EAMG (rat) are directed to the MIR in the α subunit. Apparently in contrast to the restricted specificity of anti-AChR antibodies, the origin of serum[20–22] and endplate antibody is polyclonal, indicating that a large population of plasma cells produce anti-AChR antibodies. Sequence analysis of monoclonal antibodies immortalized from B cells of EAMG animals reveals a high number of somatic mutations. These findings indicate that the immune response is antigen-driven and not the result of some accidental mutation. Among pathogenic antibodies, a high sequence homology (>90%) has been found, but none of these antibodies were identical.[23]

To investigate the individual contributions of anti-human AChR responses in MG, we dissected the immune response into monoclonal antibodies. A phage-display technique was used to immortalize the anti-AChR secreting clones from the thymus of myasthenic patients. Four human monoclonal antibodies were isolated by us and were seen to bind human AChR more accurately against the MIR. The antibodies were able to inhibit the binding of human MG sera to human AChR up to 80%. They were also able to protect against AChR loss by antigenic modulation induced by MG sera, making them potential therapeutic tools for patients with a myasthenic crisis. In total, 18 Fabs were isolated by three different groups. The 8 published amino acid sequences were all different.[24–26] From the published sequences for antibodies from EAMG animals and MG patients, it can be concluded that pathogenic antibodies are not structurally related. All anti-MIR antibodies that recognize a small decapeptide α67–76[27] at the top of the external side of α subunits are structurally different. Indeed, antibodies in general recognize pentapeptides, which means that they can recognize at least 5 partially overlapping epitopes by their linear amino acid structure. Moreover, the MIR, being highly conformationally dependent, expresses additional epitopes that can be recognized by their respective antibodies. The role of antibodies against non-MIR epitopes, that is, other subunits and cytoplasmic domains in the pathogenesis of myasthenia, has not been proven since only monoclonal antibodies against the MIR are capable of inducing EAMG.

REGULATORY MECHANISMS AT THE ENDPLATE

In MG and EAMG, the immunological attack is directed at the postsynaptic membrane of the neuromuscular junction, where four regulatory mechanisms aim to limit or restore the damage.

Role for Complement and Complement Regulatory Proteins

Muscle cells are able to upregulate the synthesis of complement regulatory proteins (CD55, CD59, and vitronectin) as a defensive mechanism against complement-mediated damage.[28] When anti-AChR antibodies bind to the tip of the postsynaptic folds, the classical complement pathway is activated. This results in the formation of the membrane attack complex (MAC), effecting focal lysis of the postsynaptic membrane. Complement-mediated focal lysis of the postsynaptic membrane also removes the cytoskeletal restraints on the AChRs and facilitates internalization and degradation.

In reaction to this process, decay-accelerating factor (DAF, CD55) inhibits C3 production, and CD59 inhibits the formation of MAC. Both CD55 and CD59 are produced by muscle fiber specifically at the postsynaptic membrane. DAF-deficient mice are subject to more severe EAMG than wild-type mice (H. Kaminski, this volume). Complement-deficient animals are protected against EAMG.[29,30] Rats with increased complement levels induced by the weakly virilizing anabolic steroid nandrolone showed more severe signs of passive transfer EAMG and higher loss of AChR compared to untreated EAMG animals.[31]

In view of the important role of complement in the disease and the beneficial effect of complement inhibitors in EAMG, these inhibitors or noncomplement-fixing anti-MIR antibodies could be used as therapeutic agents to rapidly reverse a myasthenic crisis.

Role of Macrophages in EAMG

In response to the antibody-mediated attack at the neuromuscular junction and the release of complement components, including C3a and C5a, macrophages migrate to the endplate region. The question is whether these macrophages are a primary cause of AChR loss in EAMG. Therefore, we depleted macrophages in rats by means of irradiation. After induction of EAMG with anti-MIR monoclonal antibody 35, muscular weakness developed to a similar extent in macrophage-depleted animals as in control animals.[32] AChR and complement depositions were similar in both groups. However, no infiltrating macrophages were seen in irradiated animals. This macrophage depletion does not interfere with the induction of acute EAMG by injection of monoclonal antibody 35. The macrophage infiltration seen in the non-depleted animals may be secondary to the focal damage at the endplate. In MG, macrophage infiltrations are present in muscle to a lesser extent, but mostly not in the vicinity of endplates. None of the inflammatory cells penetrate the muscle fiber near the endplate. In contrast, Maselli and colleagues observed some macrophages in the endplate region. Based on the results of EAMG studies, however, it seems unlikely that macrophages play a role in endplate damage because endplate-bound anti-AChR antibodies and complement deposition suffice to induce AChR loss.

AChR Neosynthesis

Induction of passive transfer EAMG results in a decrease of membrane-bound AChR levels and compensatory increase of AChR mRNA levels of all AChR subunits, as well as mRNA specific for myogenic transcription factors,[15,33] including

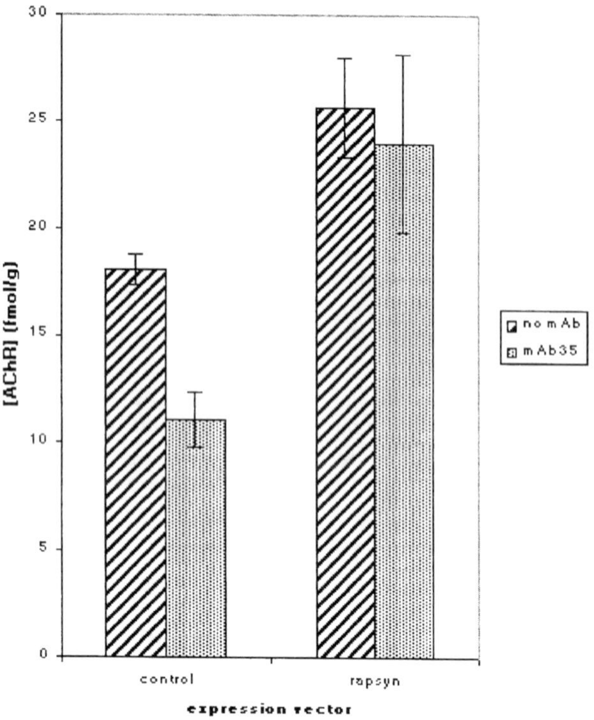

FIGURE 1. Rapsyn gene therapy in EAMG. Rat muscle fibers were electropermeabilized with a rapsyn expression vector in one tibialis anterior or with saline in the other leg. EAMG was induced by mAb 35 injection (*stippled bars*) in half of the animals at 2 weeks postgene therapy. Two days after the passive EAMG transfer, the AChR concentrations of the muscles were determined by RIA. The gene therapy–treated muscles (rapsyn) have a higher AChR concentration compared to nontreated muscles (control) due to rapsyn overexpression. Rapsyn-treated muscles of rats suffering from EAMG showed no AChR loss, in contrast to nontreated muscles of the same rats.

myogenin and MRF.[4] In very severe EAMG, a strong synaptic decrease of α and ε AChR mRNA occurs.[33]

The maintenance of high numbers of AChR at the endplate requires positive signals, including heregulins.[34] Destruction of the endplates in EAMG may interfere with positive signaling and may subsequently decrease AChR mRNA transcription. After the damage, postsynaptic membrane is restored and new AChRs are synthesized and inserted in the membrane.

Role of AChR Anchor Proteins

AChR accumulates at the top of postsynaptic folds at very high densities. Several proteins of the basal lamina and the postsynaptic skeleton are involved in maintaining AChRs at high density at the synapse. The synaptic basal lamina contains several synapse-specific molecules, including agrin and S-laminin. The postsynaptic cytoskeleton also contains AChR-anchoring proteins such as rapsyn, utrophin, etc.

Mice knocked out for anchor proteins have abnormalities in the development of the neuromuscular junction, the number of AChRs, or their clustering.[35]

In EAMG, the amount of rapsyn is decreased and the synthesis increased.[36] In our EAMG studies, we found that aged BN rats are resistant to both PT EAMG and EAMG induced by AI. The injection of mAb 35 (rat IgG1 complement fixing) does not induce muscular weakness nor clinical signs of EAMG in aged BN rats.[37] This resistance could not be explained by deficient antibody uptake, increased antibody clearance, inaccessibility of AChR for antibodies in aged animals, nor deficient complement activation or increased complement regulatory proteins.[38] The AChR degradation rates in old animals injected with mAb 35 were comparable to those of age-matched control animals. This resistance of the AChR molecules to antibody-mediated degradation most likely resides at the level of the postsynaptic membrane. Semiquantitative measurement of several proteins of the postsynaptic membrane in aged rats revealed an increase in S-laminin and rapsyn. These experiments in aged animals suggest that the susceptibility and clinical course of EAMG and possibly MG is determined not only by the level of the immune attack, but also by the rigidity and the number of AChR anchor proteins in the postsynaptic membrane.[33]

In order to test this hypothesis, we increased the expression of rapsyn in muscle fibers in young animals by injecting a rapsyn expression system under a CMV promoter into muscle fibers by means of electropermeation (technique described by Mir and colleagues[39]). Rapsyn expression was increased at the sarcolemma and the cytoplasm of transfected fibers. This increase coincides with a 40% increase of the concentration of AChR in muscle. After injection of mAb 35 (20 pmol/100 g body weight), no AChR loss was observed in the transfected muscle (musculus tibialis anterior), in contrast to a 42% loss in the nontransfected muscle. These experiments offers new therapeutic prospects for MG patients. Hyperexpression of rapsyn into ocular muscles of MG patients could induce a long-term remission of the ptosis because the electroporation of DNA results in a prolonged expression of proteins in muscle.

ACKNOWLEDGMENTS

We thank the Prinses Beatrix Fonds and L'Association Française contre les Myopathies.

REFERENCES

1. PATRICK, J. & J. LINDSTROM. 1973. Autoimmune response to acetylcholine receptor. Science **180:** 871–872.
2. CHRISTADOSS, P., M. POUSSIN & C. DENG. 2000. Animal models of myasthenia gravis. Clin. Immunol. **94:** 75–87.
3. HOEDEMAEKERS, A.C., P.J. VAN BREDA VRIESMAN & M.H. DE BAETS. 1997. Myasthenia gravis as a prototype autoimmune receptor disease. Immunol. Res. **16:** 341–354.
4. BALASS, M., Y. HELDMAN, S. CABILLY *et al.* 1993. Identification of a hexapeptide that mimics a conformation-dependent binding site of acetylcholine receptor by use of a phage-epitope library. Proc. Natl. Acad. Sci. USA **90:** 10638–10642.
5. LINDSTROM, J.M. 2000. Acetylcholine receptors and myasthenia. Muscle Nerve **23:** 453–477.
6. DAMOISEAUX, J.G.G.M.C. 2002. Cyclosporin A–induced autoimmunity in the rat: central versus peripheral tolerance. Int. J. Immunopathol. Pharmacol. **15:** 81–87.
7. SCHONBECK, S., F. PADBERG, R. HOHLFELD *et al.* 1992. Transplantation of thymic autoimmune microenvironment to severe combined immunodeficiency mice: a new model of myasthenia gravis. J. Clin. Invest. **90:** 245–250.
8. MONFARDINI, C., M. MILANI, N. OSTLIE *et al.* 2002. Adoptive protection from experimental myasthenia gravis with T cells from mice treated nasally with acetylcholine receptor epitopes. J. Neuroimmunol. **123:** 123–134.
9. SHELTON, G.D. 2002. Myasthenia gravis and disorders of neuromuscular transmission. Vet. Clin. North Am. Small Anim. Pract. **32:** 189–206.
10. YANG, H., E. GOLUSZKO, C. DAVID *et al.* 2002. Mapping myasthenia gravis–associated T cell epitopes on human acetylcholine receptors in HLA transgenic mice. J. Clin. Invest. **109:** 1111–1120.
11. STASSEN, M.H.W. *et al.* 2003. Experimental autoimmune myasthenia gravis in mice expressing human immunoglobulin loci. J. Neuroimmunol. **135:** 56–61.
12. GU, D., L. WOGENSEN, N.A. CALCUTT *et al.* 1995. Myasthenia gravis-like syndrome induced by expression of interferon gamma in the neuromuscular junction. J. Exp. Med. **181:** 547–557.
13. WEIGLE, W.O. 1980. Analysis of autoimmunity through experimental models of thyroiditis and allergic encephalomyelitis. Adv. Immunol. **30:** 159–173.
14. DE BAETS, M.H., A.M. JANSSENS, C.G. ROMBALL *et al.* 1983. A radioimmunoassay for murine thyroglobulin in serum: age-related increase of serum thyroglobulin levels in AKR/J mice. Endocrinology **112:** 1788–1795.
15. ASHER, O., W.A. KUES, V. WITZEMANN *et al.* 1993. Increased gene expression of acetylcholine receptor and myogenic factors in passively transferred experimental autoimmune myasthenia gravis. J. Immunol. **151:** 6442–6450.
16. MELMS, A., R. WEISSERT, W.E.F. KLINKERT *et al.* 1993. Specific immune complexes augment *in vitro* acetylcholine receptor–specific T-cell proliferation. Neurology **43:** 583–588.
17. MOIOLA, L., F. GALBIATI, G. MARTINO *et al.* 1998. IL-12 is involved in the induction of experimental autoimmune myasthenia gravis, an antibody-mediated disease. Eur. J. Immunol. **28:** 2487–2497.
18. SAOUDI, A., I. BERNARD, A. HOEDEMAEKERS *et al.* 1999. Experimental autoimmune myasthenia gravis may occur in the context of a polarized Th1- or Th2-type immune response in rats. J. Immunol. **162:** 7189–7197.
19. SAOUDI, A., J.C. GUERY & M. DE BAETS. 2000. Is pathogenic humoral autoimmunity a Th1 response? Immunol. Today **21:** 306–307.
20. BIONDA, A., M.H. DE BAETS, S.J. TZARTOS *et al.* 1984. Spectrotypic analysis of antibodies to acetylcholine receptors in experimental autoimmune myasthenia gravis. Clin. Exp. Immunol. **57:** 41–50.
21. LEFVERT, A.K. & K. BERGSTROM. 1978. Acetylcholine receptor antibody in myasthenia gravis: purification and characterization. Scand. J. Immunol. **8:** 525–533.
22. THOMPSON, P.A. & K.A. KROLICK. 1992. Acetylcholine receptor–reactive antibodies in experimental autoimmune myasthenia gravis differing in disease-causing potential:

subsetting of serum antibodies by preparative isoelectric focusing. Clin. Immunol. Immunopathol. **62:** 199–209.
23. GRAUS, Y.M. & M. DE BAETS. 1994. Molecular and structural characterization of anti-acetylcholine receptor antibodies in experimental autoimmune myasthenia gravis. Adv. Neuroimmunol. **4:** 457–474.
24. GRAUS, Y.F., M.H. DE BAETS *et al.* 1997. Human anti-nicotinic acetylcholine receptor recombinant Fab fragments isolated from thymus-derived phage display libraries from myasthenia gravis patients reflect predominant specificities in serum and block the action of pathogenic serum antibodies. J. Immunol. **158:** 1919–1929.
25. FARRAR, J., S. PORTOLANO, N. WILLCOX *et al.* 1997. Diverse Fab specific for acetylcholine receptor epitopes from a myasthenia gravis thymus combinatorial library. Int. Immunol. **9:** 1311–1318.
26. REY, E., M. ZEIDEL, C. RHINE *et al.* 2000. Characterization of human anti-acetylcholine receptor monoclonal autoantibodies from the peripheral blood of a myasthenia gravis patient using combinatorial libraries. Clin. Immunol. **96:** 269–279.
27. TZARTOS, S.J., T. BARKAS, M.T. CUNG *et al.* 1998. Anatomy of the antigenic structure of a large membrane autoantigen, the muscle-type nicotinic acetylcholine receptor. Immunol. Rev. **163:** 89–120.
28. HOEDEMAEKERS, A., Y. GRAUS, P. VAN BREDA VRIESMAN *et al.* 1997. Age- and sex-related resistance to chronic experimental autoimmune myasthenia gravis (EAMG) in Brown Norway rats. Clin. Exp. Immunol. **107:** 189–197.
29. LENNON, V.A., M.E. SEYBOLD, J.M. LINDSTROM *et al.* 1978. Role of complement in the pathogenesis of experimental autoimmune myasthenia gravis. J. Exp. Med. **147:** 973–983.
30. CHRISTADOSS, P. 1989. Immunogenetics of experimental autoimmune myasthenia gravis. Crit. Rev. Immunol. **9:** 247–278.
31. DE BAETS, M., H.J. VERSCHUUREN, M.R. DAHA *et al.* 1988. Effects of the rate of acetylcholine receptor synthesis on the severity of experimental autoimmune myasthenia gravis. Immunol. Res. **7:** 200–211.
32. HOEDEMAEKERS, A., Y. GRAUS, L. BEIJLEVELD *et al.* 1997. Macrophage infiltration at the neuromuscular junction does not contribute to AChR loss and age-related resistance to EAMG. J. Neuroimmunol. **75:** 147–155.
33. HOEDEMAEKERS, A., J.L. BESSEREAU, Y. GRAUS *et al.* 1998. Role of the target organ in determining susceptibility to experimental autoimmune myasthenia gravis. J. Neuroimmunol. **89:** 131–141
34. SANDROCK, A.W., S.E. DRYER, K.M. ROSEN *et al.* 1997. Maintenance of acetylcholine receptor number by neuregulins at the neuromuscular junction *in vivo*. Science **276:** 599–603.
35. GAUTAM, M. *et al.* 1999. Distinct phenotypes of mutant mice lacking agrin, MuSK, or rapsyn. Brain Res. Dev. Brain Res. **114:** 171–183.
36. ASHER, O., S. FUCHS & M.C. SOUROUJON. 1994. Acetylcholine receptor and myogenic factor gene expression in *Torpedo* embryonic development. Neuroreport **5:** 1581–1584.
37. GRAUS, Y.M.F., J.J.G.M. VERSCHUUREN, F. SPAANS *et al.* 1993. Age-related resistance to experimental autoimmune myasthenia gravis in rats. J. Immunol. **150:** 4093–4103.
38. HOEDEMAEKERS, A.C., J.J. VERSCHUUREN, F. SPAANS *et al.* 1997. Age-related susceptibility to experimental autoimmune myasthenia gravis: immunological and electrophysiological aspects. Muscle Nerve **20:** 1091–1138.
39. MIR, L.M. *et al.* 1999. High-efficiency gene transfer into skeletal muscle mediated by electric pulses. Proc. Natl. Acad. Sci. USA **96:** 4262–4267.

Circulating $CD4^+CD25^+$ and $CD4^+CD25^-$ T Cells in Myasthenia Gravis

Y. HUANG,[a,b] R. PIRSKANEN,[c] R. CISCOMBE,[a] H. LINK,[b] AND A-K. LEFVERT[a]

[a]*Immunological Laboratory, Center of Molecular Medicine, Stockholm, Sweden*

[b]*Division of Neurology, Huddinge University Hospital, Karolinska Institute, Stockholm, Sweden*

[c]*Division of Neurology, Karolinska Hospital, Stockholm, Sweden*

KEYWORDS: myasthenia gravis; regulatory T cells; cell membrane molecules; cytokines

INTRODUCTION

Murine $CD4^+CD25^+$ regulatory T (Tr) cells suppress autoaggressive immune responses. Transfer of $CD4^+CD25^+$ cells reduces the pathology in such experimental autoimmune diseases as insulin-dependent diabetes mellitus and colitis, whereas depletion of $CD4^+CD25^+$ cells results in development of systemic autoimmune diseases.[1] $CD4^+CD25^+$ cells are generated in the thymus. Recent data implicate that $CD4^+CD25^+$ cells from human blood[2] and thymus exhibit *in vitro* functions similar to murine $CD4^+CD25^+$ cells, inhibiting both Th1 and Th2 responses. The significance of $CD4^+CD25^+$ in the control of immune responses in humans has not been established. Considering the origin and potential suppressive capacities of $CD4^+CD25^+$ Tr cells, it is important to determine the frequency and functional properties of this cell subset in patients with MG.

Here, we analyzed frequencies of $CD4^+CD25^+$ Tr cells among blood mononuclear cells (MNC) and $CD4^+$ T cells in MG patients and healthy controls (HC). Phenotypic patterns and cytokine profiles of $CD4^+CD25^+$ Tr cells compared to $CD4^+CD25^-$ T cells were investigated in the two groups.

MATERIALS AND METHODS

Twenty-three patients with clinical MG and 21 HC were enrolled in the study. MNC were isolated over Ficoll-Paque by centrifugation. MNC at 10^6/mL were resuspended in culture medium. The cells were then stimulated by culturing in the presence of anti-CD3 and anti-CD28 mAb for 16 hours. For three-color staining, the

Address for correspondence: Dr. Yu-Min Huang, Division of Neurology, Huddinge University Hospital, Karolinska Institute, Stockholm, Sweden. Voice: +46-8-58582258; fax: +46-8-58587750.

yu-min.huang@neurotec.ki.se

Ann. N.Y. Acad. Sci. 998: 318–319 (2003). © 2003 New York Academy of Sciences.
doi: 10.1196/annals.1254.034

MNC were incubated with FITC-, PE- and PerCP-conjugated selected mAb. Flow cytometric analysis was performed on a FACS-caliber using CellQuest software.

RESULTS AND DISCUSSION

Circulating CD4$^+$CD25$^+$ cells from 23 MG patients and 21 age- and sex-matched HC were examined. CD4$^+$CD25$^+$ cells constitute about 8% of blood MNC and about 20% of CD4$^+$ T cells, with similar frequencies in MG and HC. Activation of blood MNC with anti-CD3 and anti-CD28 mAb upregulated the proportion of CD4$^+$CD25$^+$ cells to a similar extent in both MG and HC.

Resting CD4$^+$CD25$^+$ cells from both MG patients and HC showed an activation phenotype, reflected by augmented proportions of CD45RO$^+$ and HLA-DR$^+$ cells compared to CD4$^+$CD25$^-$ T cells. CD4$^+$CD25$^+$ cells from both groups constitutively expressed equally high levels of Fas (CD95), indicating the apoptosis proneness of this cell population.

Upon activation with anti-CD3 and anti-CD28 mAb, CD4$^+$CD25$^+$, but not CD4$^+$CD25$^-$, cells expressed CD80. Compared to activated CD4$^+$CD25$^-$ cells, activated CD4$^+$CD25$^+$ cells also contained higher proportions of cells expressing CD86, CD40L, CTLA-4, CD69, and HLA-DR. In contrast, CD4$^+$CD25$^+$ cells produced similar amounts of IL-2 and IL-10, and higher amounts of IFN-γ compared to CD4$^+$CD25$^-$ cells. These alterations were similar in MG and HC. Higher proportions of CD95 (48 ± 4% vs. 36 ± 3%; $p = 0.03$) and HLA-DR (5 ± 0.7% vs. 3 ± 0.4%; $p = 0.01$) were detected on resting CD4$^+$CD25$^-$ cells in MG compared to HC. Upon subgrouping the MG patients regarding age at MG onset, only patients with late onset MG (>40 years; $n = 9$) showed a higher proportion of HLA-DR (7 ± 1% vs. 4 ± 1%; $p < 0.01$) on CD4$^+$CD25$^-$ cells.

In conclusion, CD4$^+$CD25$^+$ Tr cells behave largely similarly in MG and HC as analyzed in this study.

REFERENCES

1. SAKAGUCHI, S. *et al.* 1995. Immunologic self-tolerance maintained by activated T cells expressing IL-2 receptor α-chains (CD25): breakdown of a single mechanism of self-tolerance causes various autoimmune diseases. J. Immunol. **160:** 1151–1164.
2. DIECKMANN, D. *et al.* 2001. *Ex vivo* isolation and characterization of CD25$^+$CD4$^+$ T cells with regulatory properties from human blood. J. Exp. Med. **193:** 1303–1310.

Rationale for a T Cell Receptor Peptide Therapy in Myasthenia Gravis

F. JAMBOU,[a] M. MENESTRIER,[a] I. KLINGEL-SCHMITT,[a] S. CAILLAT-ZUCMAN,[b] A. AÏSSAOUI,[a] S. BERRIH-AKNIN,[a] AND S. COHEN-KAMINSKY[a]

[a]*CNRS UMR 8078, IPSC, Université Paris XI, Hôpital Marie Lannelongue, Le Plessis-Robinson, France*

[b]*Service d'Immunologie Clinique, Hôpital Necker, Paris, France*

KEYWORDS: T cell receptor peptide therapy; myasthenia gravis

INTRODUCTION

From studies in experimental autoimmune encephalomyelitis (EAE) and multiple sclerosis (MS), it is admitted that the natural tendency in autoimmune conditions to develop focused antigen-specific responses that overuse certain T cell receptor (TCR) V region segments prompts the induction of anti-TCR-specific T cells[1] and antibodies[2,3] that can inhibit the pathogenic T cells and promote recovery from disease. This natural regulatory network can be manipulated by injecting synthetic peptide vaccines that correspond to segments of the overexpressed V gene. The prerequisites for the development of a TCR peptide vaccine in myasthenia gravis (MG) are the identification of pathogenic T cells causing the disease and using preferentially one TCR Vβ gene. We have identified in HLA-DR3 MG patients a pathogenic subpopulation of thymic T cells expressing the Vβ5.1 TCR gene,[4,5] providing a rationale for searching for an anti-TCR-mediated regulation. We therefore searched for anti-TCR antibodies in the sera of MG patients in the absence of prior T cell or TCR vaccination.

METHODS

Patients

MG patients were young patients presenting a recent disease (<40 years) with a hyperplastic thymus and a high rate of anti-AChR antibody titer (>10 nM)—severe generalized disease. Healthy controls came from the Centre de Transfusion Sanguine. In addition, we tested sera from patients with other clearly defined auto-

Address for correspondence: Sylvia Cohen-Kaminsky, CNRS UMR 8078–Remodelage Tissulaire et Fonctionnel: Signalisation et Physiopathologie, IPSC, Université Paris XI, Hôpital Marie Lannelongue, 133 avenue de la Résistance, 92350 Le Plessis-Robinson, France. Voice: +33-1-40-94-29-94; fax: +33-1-46-30-45-64.
sylvia.kaminsky@ccml.u-psud.fr

Ann. N.Y. Acad. Sci. 998: 320–323 (2003). © 2003 New York Academy of Sciences.
doi: 10.1196/annals.1254.035

TABLE 1. Anti-Vβ antibody levels in MG patients and controls

	HLA-DR3 MG patients			Non-HLA-DR3 MG patients			Healthy controls		
	n	Mean titer ± SEM	Median	*n*	Mean titer ± SEM	Median	*n*	Mean titer ± SEM	Median
Anti-Vβ5.1	21	305.5 ± 48.7	250	19	156.8 ± 15.9	145	14	83 ± 8.8	92.5
Anti-Vβ6.7	9	16.1 ± 6.1	10	5	53.00 ± 9.7	55	6	55.00 ± 24.7	35
Anti-Vβ14	9	35 ± 9.6	30	5	10 ± 0	10	6	10 ± 0	10

antibodies other than anti-AChR antibodies. Patients on corticosteroid treatment are excluded from the study.

TCR Peptides

Vβ peptides were chosen regarding their immunogenicity predicted by Epiplot and Antheprot softwares. TCR Vβ5.1 peptide (TPGQGLQFLFEYFSETQRNKG) contained a portion of Fr2 and all CDR2 regions according to the nomenclature of IMGT. Peptide controls contain the CDR2 region of the TCR Vβ6.7 (PGKGLR-LIYYSVAAALTDKG) and TCR Vβ14 (VMGKEIKFLLHFVKESKQDES) chains not thought to be involved in MG and chosen regarding their expression level, compared to Vβ5.1 expression level, in peripheral blood T cells.

Anti-TCR Antibody Assay

Anti-Vβ TCR antibodies were assayed on serially diluted sera by the ELISA method using Vβ peptides. The titer is defined as the reciprocal of the dilution at which the optical density value is 0.2. The value is obtained by interpolation on the linear portion of the curve.

RESULTS AND DISCUSSION

Using the TCR Vβ5.1 CDR2 peptide, higher levels of anti-Vβ5.1 antibodies were detected in MG patients' sera than in healthy controls (FIG. 1). This difference between MG patients and healthy controls is statistically significant ($p < 0.0003$). These antibodies are disease-specific as their titers proved to be significantly lower in patients with other autoimmune syndromes ($p < 0.01$). There is a difference in the anti-Vβ5.1 antibody titer between HLA-DR3 MG patients and non-HLA-DR3 MG patients (FIG. 1), which is statistically significant ($p < 0.04$), further supporting the link between the HLA-DR3 context and the Vβ5.1-expressing T cell. These antibodies are Vβ5.1-specific as there is no significant recognition of analogous CDR2 peptide from the Vβ6.7 and Vβ14 sequences even in HLA-DR3 cases (TABLE 1), and binding

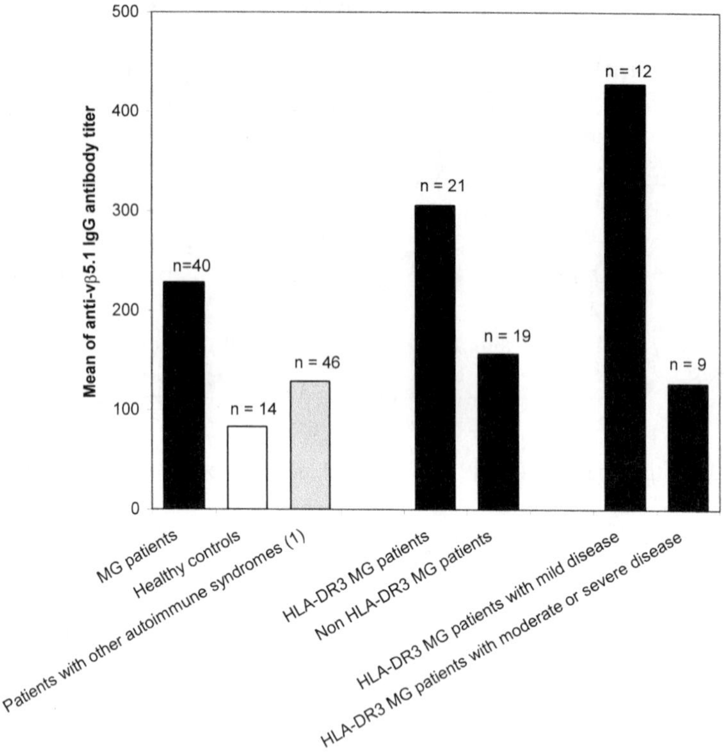

FIGURE 1. Anti-Vβ5.1 IgG antibody levels in MG patients and controls. [(1)]Other autoimmune syndromes: stiff man syndrome, Lambert-Eaton myasthenic syndrome, Miller Fisher syndrome, Guillain-Barré syndrome, paraneoplastic disease, or acquired neuromyotonia.

is inhibited by preincubation with Vβ5.1 CDR2 peptide (not shown). More interestingly, HLA-DR3 MG patients with mild (class II, MGFA classification) disease versus moderate or severe (class III and IV) disease showed elevated anti-Vβ5.1 antibody titers ($p < 0.0004$) (FIG. 1), suggesting that these anti-Vβ5.1 antibodies may have a protective role.

Our data show that, without any previous vaccination against the TCR, HLA-DR3 MG patients produce an increased level of circulating specific anti-Vβ5.1 antibodies of the IgG class that (1) is restricted to the AChR autoimmune response and (2) varies in the course of the disease and is correlated to a less severe disease or to clinical improvement in follow-up studies (not shown). These observations establish that MG patients spontaneously present an active and dynamic immune regulation process involving protective anti-Vβ5.1 antibodies. This induced anti-TCR regulatory network may be fashioned to target the excess of pathogenic Vβ5.1-expressing T cells and may not be sufficient to stop a chronic exacerbated autoimmune process, supporting the need to be boosted with a TCR peptide as vaccine.

ACKNOWLEDGMENTS

This research was supported by grants from the AFM (Association Française contre les Myopathies), the CNRS (Centre National de la Recherche Scientifique), the CNAMTS (Caisse Nationale d'Assurance Maladie des Travailleurs Salariés), and the European Community (QOL-2000-01918 and QLK3CT-2001-00225). F. Jambou was a recipient of a doctoral grant from the AFM.

REFERENCES

1. KUMAR, V. & E. SERCARZ. 1999. Distinct levels of regulation in organ-specific autoimmune diseases. Life Sci. **65:** 1523–1530.
2. VANDENBARK, A.A. *et al.* 1996. T cell receptor peptides in treatment of autoimmune disease: rationale and potential. J. Neurosci. Res. **43:** 391–402.
3. VANDENBARK, A.A. *et al.* 1996. Treatment of multiple sclerosis with T-cell receptor peptides: results of a double-blind pilot trial. Nat. Med. **2:** 1109–1115.
4. TRUFFAULT, F. *et al.* 1997. Altered intrathymic T-cell repertoire in human myasthenia gravis. Ann. Neurol. **41:** 731–741.
5. AÏSSAOUI, A. *et al.* 1999. Prevention of autoimmune attack by targeting specific T cell receptor in a SCID mice model of myasthenia gravis. Ann. Neurol. **46:** 559–567.

Antibodies in Myasthenia Gravis and Related Disorders

ANGELA VINCENT,[a] JOHN McCONVILLE,[a] MARIA ELENA FARRUGIA,[a] JOHN BOWEN,[a] PAUL PLESTED,[a] TERESA TANG,[a] AMELIA EVOLI,[b] IAN MATTHEWS,[a] GARY SIMS,[c] PAOLA DALTON,[a] LESLIE JACOBSON,[a] AGATA POLIZZI,[a] FRANS BLAES,[a] BETHAN LANG,[a] DAVID BEESON,[a] NICK WILLCOX,[a] JOHN NEWSOM-DAVIS,[a] AND WERNER HOCH[d]

[a]*Neurosciences Group, Department of Clinical Neurology, Weatherall Institute of Molecular Medicine, John Radcliffe Hospital, Oxford OX3 9DS, United Kingdom*

[b]*Department of Neurology, Catholic University of Rome, Rome, Italy*

[c]*Department of Immunology and Bacteriology, Western Infirmary, Glasgow, United Kingdom*

[d]*Department of Biology and Biochemistry, University of Houston, Houston, Texas, USA*

Abstract: Acetylcholine receptor (AChR) antibodies are present in around 85% of patients with myasthenia gravis (MG) as measured by the conventional radioimmunoprecipitation assay. Antibodies that block the fetal form of the AChR are occasionally present in mothers who develop MG after pregnancy, especially in those whose babies are born with arthrogryposis multiplex congenita. The antibodies cross the placenta and block neuromuscular transmission, leading to joint deformities and often stillbirth. In these mothers, antibodies made in the thymus are mainly specific for fetal AChR and show restricted germline origins, suggesting a highly mutated clonal response; subsequent spread to involve adult AChR could explain development of maternal MG in those cases who first present after pregnancy. In the 15% of "seronegative" MG patients without AChR antibodies (SNMG), there are serum factors that increase AChR phosphorylation and reduce AChR function, probably acting via a different membrane receptor. These factors are not IgG and could be IgM or even non-Ig serum proteins. In a proportion of SNMG patients, however, IgG antibodies to the muscle-specific kinase, MuSK, are present. These antibodies are not found in AChR antibody-positive MG and are predominantly IgG4. MuSK antibody positivity appears to be associated with more severe bulbar disease that can be difficult to treat effectively.

Keywords: myasthenia gravis; arthrogryposis multiplex congenita; fetal acetylcholine receptor; adult acetylcholine receptor; muscle-specific kinase; MuSK; seronegative myasthenia; muscle atrophy; disease severity

Address for correspondence: Dr. A. Vincent, Neurosciences Group, Weatherall Institute of Molecular Medicine, John Radcliffe Hospital, Oxford OX3 9DS, United Kingdom. Voice: +44-1865-222321; fax: +44-1865- 222402.
angela.vincent@imm.ox.ac.uk

Ann. N.Y. Acad. Sci. 998: 324–335 (2003). © 2003 New York Academy of Sciences.
doi: 10.1196/annals.1254.036

INTRODUCTION

Antibodies to acetylcholine receptors (AChRs) and their effects on AChR number and function have now been recognized for almost 30 years. However, their characterization and the increasing recognition of other antigenic targets are still adding to our knowledge and understanding of different forms of myasthenia gravis (MG). Here, we will summarize some recent findings.

ACHR ANTIBODIES

AChR antibodies continue to provide the mainstay of the diagnosis of MG as they have for 20 years. In laboratories worldwide, they are measured by immunoprecipitation of ^{125}I-α-bungarotoxin-labeled AChR, but there have been several recent attempts to provide nonradioactive assays. For instance, Gotti *et al.*[1] immobilized fetal calf AChR on ELISA plates with a monoclonal antibody and were able to detect antibodies in the majority of patients with MG, including some who were negative with the radioimmunoprecipitation assay. Another approach has been to use a nonradioactive labeled bungarotoxin. An assay using europium, a time-dependent fluorescence emitter, may be promising and shows a strong correlation with the radioimmunoprecipitation assay.[2]

It may also be possible to use recombinant polypeptides rather than the whole AChR. This has been avoided in the past because of concerns that many antibodies bind to the whole AChR molecule rather than to the independent subunits. Though undoubtedly true, the possibility of expressing appreciable amounts of α subunits or α/ε dimers for a nonradioactive ELISA assay should be further explored. Many MG antibodies bind to the main immunogenic region (MIR), which is predominantly located on the α subunit, and some antibodies bind to the other subunits or perhaps to MIR epitopes that are dependent on the adjacent subunits.[3] If assays using recombinant polypeptides are developed, as seems likely now that good expression systems are being developed,[4,5] it will be important to determine the proportion of MG patients who are positive with such an assay, as well as how well the results correlate with the radioimmunoprecipitation assay.

ANTIBODIES TO FETAL ACHRS IN MOTHERS OF BABIES WITH ARTHROGRYPOSIS

A small number of women with MG have had babies born with arthrogryposis multiplex congenita (AMC). We previously showed that the AChR antibodies in these cases are directed mainly toward the fetal isoform of the AChR and strongly inhibit its function.[6–8] Moreover, after injection of the serum antibodies into pregnant mice, the offspring may show many of the features of AMC—joints fixed in abnormal positions, scoliosis, altered cranial morphology, and occasionally CNS abnormalities.[9] Thus, AMC associated with MG is a maternal antibody-mediated condition directed against a fetal antigen.

To find out more about these antibodies, we took thymic cells from two women with AMC babies, who had not been diagnosed as having MG until after the second and fourth affected pregnancies, respectively, and extracted the cDNAs. The immunoglobulin heavy and light chain cDNAs were cloned and recombined to form a combinatorial expression library (as in Farrar *et al.*[10]). The recombined Fabs were expressed in *E. coli*, and those capable of binding AChR were identified by binding of ^{125}I-α-BuTx-labeled AChR. The AChR-binding Fabs were characterized and sequenced.

All the Fab heavy chains were derived from heavily mutated sequences, and two sets of Fabs showed evidence of evolution from highly mutated progenitors.[11] All of these antibodies, with only one exception, were highly specific for fetal AChR (FIG. 1) and did not bind appreciably to adult AChR. The exception was an antibody that bound to both adult and fetal AChR and was shown to be specific for the β subunit. Thus, in contrast to the antibodies cloned similarly from other MG patients,[10,12] those cloned from mothers of AMC babies who had developed MG after pregnancy were highly fetal-specific.

(a)

(b)

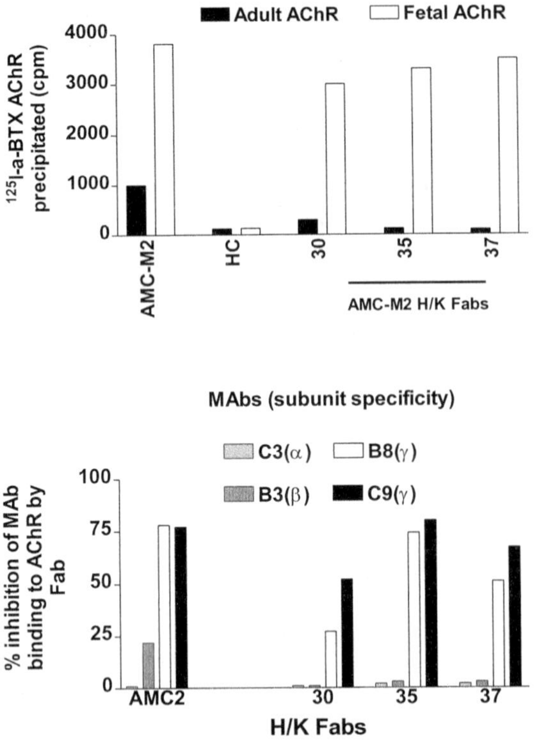

FIGURE 1. Fetal-specific Fab antibodies cloned from AMC-M2. Examples of three Fabs showing high specificity for fetal AChR over adult AChR **(a)**, and competition with monoclonal antibodies (Mabs) that bind to the different subunit **(b)**. Only one Fab, from one other AMC mother, out of over 20 Fabs studied, bound to an epitope on adult AChR. H/K: heavy chain kappa light chain. (For further details, see ref. 11.)

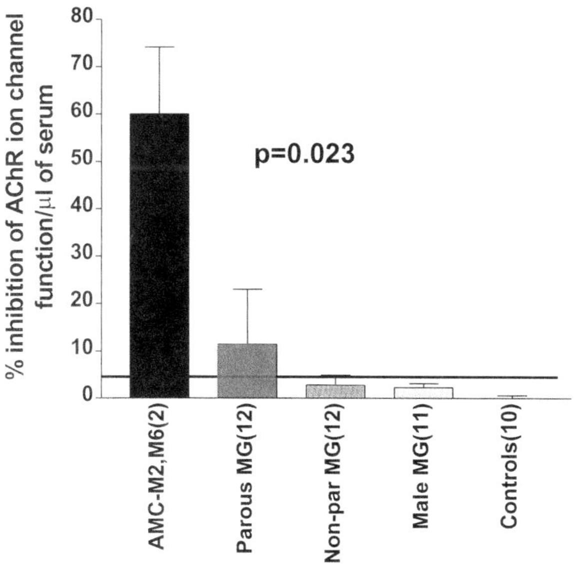

FIGURE 2. Fetal specificity of antibodies in parous women. Sera from parous MG women contain more antibodies capable of inhibiting the function of fetal AChR than those from women who develop MG before pregnancy (non-par MG). The antibodies were measured by inhibition of AChR function in TE671 cells as previously described.[11]

These studies led us to ask whether the fetus itself induces antibodies against fetal AChRs and whether, if so, some women develop MG as a result of immunization against fetal cells. We studied sera from 12 women who had developed MG following pregnancy and compared those findings with sera from women with onset before pregnancy. There was a significantly higher level of fetal-inhibitory AChR antibodies in the parous mothers compared with the nonparous mothers (FIG. 2). [11]

Often, the diagnosis of the mother is not made until after the birth of affected babies; in at least one well-studied case, the mother remains asymptomatic,[8] presumably because her antibodies do not bind appreciably to adult AChR. This means that these antibodies should be looked for in other women with AMC babies, irrespective of whether they have clinical MG. We have studied over 200 sera from women with histories of one to six affected pregnancies. Only a small proportion of the women had histories of MG; however, among the remaining mothers, AChR antibodies were found in only two individuals (1%). One mother had only one affected baby, and the other had her last three pregnancies affected. Interestingly, though, a proportion of the mothers without AChR antibodies had serum antibodies binding to different neonatal mouse tissues, particularly muscle and peripheral nerve (Dalton, Clover, and Vincent, in preparation), suggesting that they have developed other antibodies that might be involved in causing AMC.

ANTIBODIES TO ADULT AChR IN OCULAR MYASTHENIA GRAVIS AND AN ANTIBODY-MEDIATED SLOW-CHANNEL SYNDROME

Antibodies that bind preferentially to fetal AChR, but that do not block its function, are relatively common, even in women who develop MG before pregnancy, probably because the fetal isoform is expressed on myoid cells in the thymus.[13] However, it is clear that a minority of patients with MG, often those with low total AChR antibody levels, have antibodies with a preference for the adult form. These antibodies may escape detection if only denervated muscle or TE671 cell lines are used for the diagnostic assay. Use of cell lines that have been transfected to express the ε subunit ensures that antibodies to adult AChR will be detected.[14] This applies particularly to patients with ocular MG who often have low AChR antibodies; in this subset, the AChR antibody positivity increased significantly when adult AChR was used.[14,15]

One case of MG associated with antibodies that were highly specific for adult AChR has been described. A female patient who responded clinically to plasma exchange, and whose plasma IgG transferred disease to mice, had antibodies that bound only to the adult isoform. Interestingly, her physiological defects were more similar to those seen in the genetic disorder, the slow-channel syndrome, than to those in typical MG.[16] This suggests that, by analogy with the genetic slow-channel syndrome mutations, the antibodies may increase ACh affinity for the AChR or bind to a site that slows the rate of channel closure (see Engel *et al.* and Beeson *et al.*, this volume).

LATE-ONSET MYASTHENIA GRAVIS AND AChR ANTIBODIES IN THE ELDERLY

It is increasingly clear that MG is not only a disease of younger individuals, particularly women, but that there is a higher proportion of individuals over the age of 50, many of them male.[17,18] A survey of all antibody assays performed in the United Kingdom over the period 1997–1999 shows an annual rate of positive AChR antibodies of approximately 1000/year, of which the great majority are thought to be new cases. The results from sera referred to Oxford for testing over a 3-year period (1997–1999) are shown in FIGURE 3. Approximately 1000 samples were positive for AChR antibodies, and more than 650 were from patients over the age of 50 years. In smaller studies of individual patients, these late-onset MG (LOMG) patients are found to have a raised incidence of antibodies to ryanodine receptor and titin,[19] and to interferon-α and IL-12 antibodies.[20,21] These similarities between LOMG and thymoma cases are discussed by Skeie and by Aarli (see this volume).

SERONEGATIVE MYASTHENIA GRAVIS

A variable proportion of MG patients do not have antibodies to the AChR as determined by the radioimmunoprecipitation assay. These patients, who are usually termed seronegative MG (SNMG), have been the focus of several studies that will be summarized here.

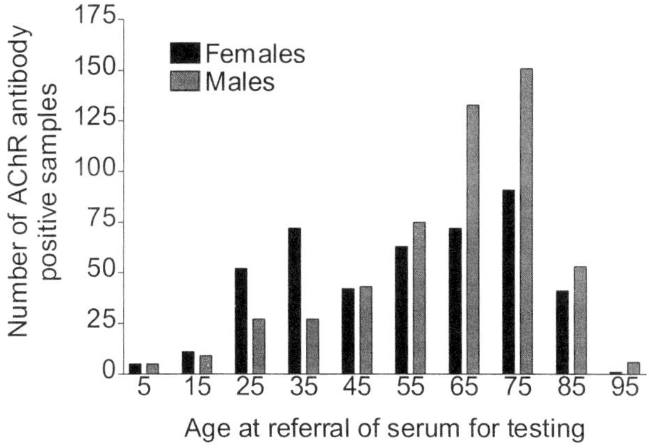

FIGURE 3. Frequency distribution for the age at referral for sera positive for acetylcholine receptor antibody. All samples from patients in the United Kingdom sent to Oxford over a 3-year period are included.

SNMG patients clearly have a humorally mediated disorder since they improve clinically with plasma exchange, and injection of their IgG or Ig fractions into mice results in defects in neuromuscular transmission.[22–24] We have studied the effects of these plasma factors on AChR function in the TE671 cell line, which expresses many features of cultured muscle cells.

A NON-IgG FACTOR IN SNMG PLASMAS AFFECTS AChR FUNCTION

We used a ^{22}Na uptake assay to look at AChR function[25] after incubating the cells in the SNMG and control plasmas. During a 1-min incubation in 0.5–1.0 mM carbamylcholine, the cells take up ^{22}Na, but the uptake reaches a plateau within 1 min, probably because of desensitization of the AChRs. This plateau was lower and was reached more quickly in the presence of 8 of the 12 SNMG plasmas studied, suggesting that they increase the rate of desensitization of the AChRs.[26] Similar observations had been found after addition of calcitonin gene–related peptide (CGRP), which binds to a G protein–linked receptor leading to protein kinase A activation.[27] Thus, we hypothesize that the SNMG plasmas were reducing AChR function by binding to a receptor distinct from the AChR, and activating an intracellular pathway leading to AChR phosphorylation (as summarized in FIG. 4).

To investigate phosphorylation of the AChR, the TE671 cells were preincubated in ^{32}P-containing physiological solution followed by addition of three SNMG and two healthy control plasmas. The incorporation of ^{32}P into the AChRs was measured by immunoprecipitation by a monoclonal antibody to human AChR and counting of the radioactivity in the precipitate. ^{32}P uptake into AChR in cells incubated in medium alone was subtracted. AChR phosphorylation was significantly increased by each of the three SNMG plasmas tested, which were those that had the most substantial effects on AChR function.[26]

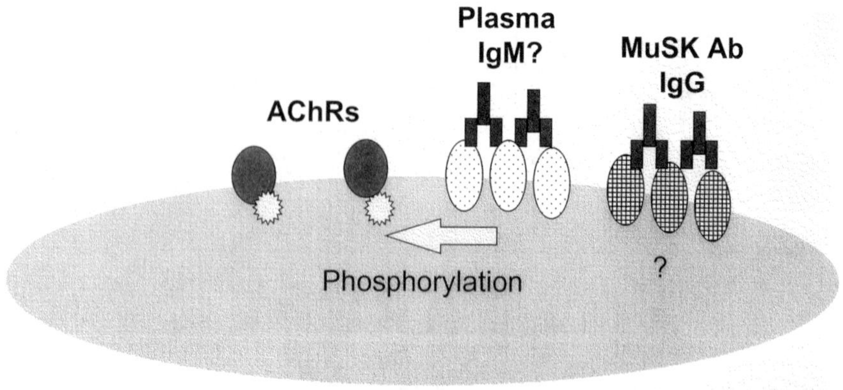

FIGURE 4. Scheme to illustrate how SNMG plasmas appear to affect AChR function in TE671 cells by increasing phosphorylation. The active factor is not in the purified IgG fraction and is therefore not MuSK antibody. It may be an IgM or even a non-Ig.

A feature of the hypothesis is that the SNMG plasmas should bind to a receptor distinct from the AChR, leading to activation of an intracellular pathway. To address this issue, we measured AChR opening frequency by single-channel recordings within a cell patch, while applying the SNMG plasmas outside the patch pipette. In order to reproduce the conditions present in the ^{22}Na uptake assay, we added 1 mM carbamylcholine after the SNMG plasmas. A reduction in AChR channel-opening frequency was found with two SNMG plasmas, but not with the third.[26]

These results provided support for the hypothesis, but as reported previously[27] the SNMG factor that inhibits AChR function in these assays is not an IgG antibody. It copurified with IgM in an earlier study,[25] but we have not been able to unequivocally demonstrate that the inhibitory activity is due to an IgM, and the possibility that a non-Ig factor is involved should also be considered.

IgG ANTIBODIES BINDING TO MuSK

SNMG can be passively transferred from a mother to her baby,[28] suggesting that there must also be IgG antibodies present in some patients. To look for IgG antibodies, we incubated the TE671 cells in plasmas from SNMG patients, AChR antibody–positive (SPMG) patients, and healthy controls, and used the fluorescence-activated cell sorter (FACS) to quantify IgG binding. The results of the SNMG plasmas were bimodal. About 50% showed strong IgG binding to the TE671 cells, higher than that achieved with SPMG samples.[29] Interestingly, some of the IgG-positive samples were from patients whose plasmas did not affect AChR function (see above), suggesting that the IgG antibodies and non-IgG factors are unrelated. These results suggested that the IgG antibodies were binding to a target on the TE671 cells that could have been the AChR or another muscle cell surface antigen. To exclude unequivocally the former possibility, we tested binding to human embryonic kidney

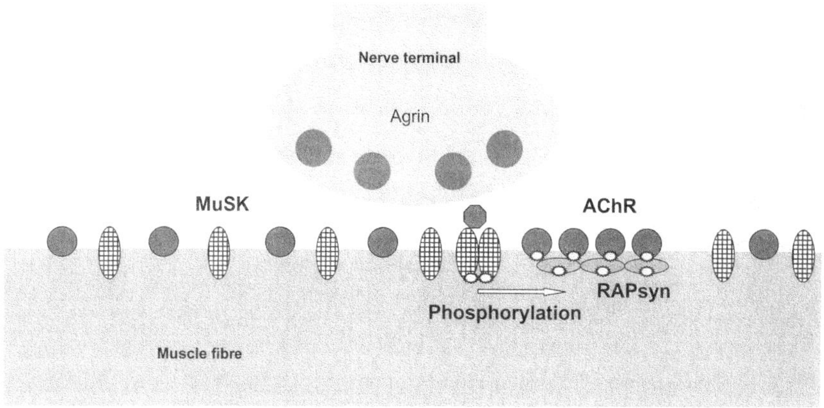

FIGURE 5. Scheme of MuSK pathway to illustrate how the agrin/MuSK pathway induces AChR clustering during development. Sera or plasmas from MuSK antibody-positive SNMG patients inhibit agrin-induced clustering in cultured C2C12 cells,[32] suggesting that they may interfere with the function of MuSK at the adult neuromuscular junction. Since the antibodies are predominantly IgG4, it is unlikely that complement binding plays a role.

cells that had been transfected to express human AChR. There was strong binding of IgG from SPMG patients, but none from the SNMG patients.[29]

These results indicated that a proportion of SNMG sera contained antibodies to a non-AChR antigen that was present on TE671 cells, but not on human embryonic kidney cells. A possible candidate antigen was the muscle-specific receptor kinase, MuSK. MuSK is present in TE671 cells and is also found at the neuromuscular junction. During development, it plays an essential role in orchestrating the agrin-dependent clustering of AChRs and other components that make up the postsynaptic architecture of the neuromuscular junction[30,31] (see FIG. 5).

We tested SNMG sera for binding to MuSK by immunofluorescence on COS cells expressing full-length MuSK and by ELISA using the extracellular domain of MuSK bound to microtiter plates. With both techniques, a high proportion of the SNMG plasmas bound to MuSK, compared with none of the healthy controls or other disease controls. Strikingly, SPMG sera from both thymoma MG and non-thymoma MG patients failed to bind to MuSK, indicating that the two forms of MG are distinct conditions.[32] An immunoprecipitation assay using human recombinant MuSK radiolabeled with ^{125}I has now been established and the results are highly similar (FIG. 6) (McConville, Newsom-Davis, Beeson, and Vincent, in preparation). Moreover, the binding of antibodies to MuSK correlates with the binding to the TE671 cells, indicating that the target for IgG antibodies on this cell line[29] is almost certainly MuSK (as illustrated in FIG. 4).

A question arises as to how these antibodies cause the symptoms of myasthenia. One possibility is that the antibodies bind complement and cause loss of AChR-containing postsynaptic membrane, similar to the known action of AChR antibodies.[33] However, the MuSK antibodies were found to be predominantly in the IgG4 subclass, which does not activate complement (McConville, Newsom-Davis, Beeson, and Vincent, in preparation).

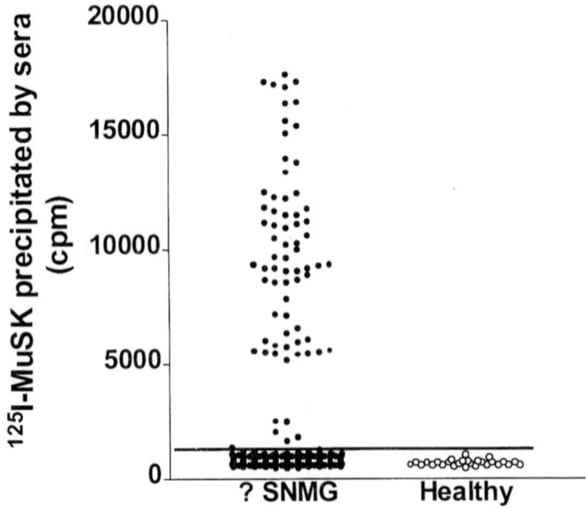

FIGURE 6. Radioimmunoprecipitation assay for MuSK antibodies. Illustration of results from 267 SNMG sera sent for testing; 64 sera gave clearly positive values. Some of these sera were from patients with well-established SNMG who were positive for MuSK antibodies;[32] others were being tested for the first time.

Another possible explanation is that the antibodies alter the function of MuSK at the adult neuromuscular junction. The plasmas were applied to the mouse C2C12 cell line, which expresses the components necessary for agrin-induced AChR clustering. If agrin is added, the AChRs, which are normally fairly evenly distributed on the cell surface, are clustered into dense spots that can be detected by use of rhodamine-labeled α-bungarotoxin. The SNMG plasmas that contained MuSK antibodies were able to inhibit agrin-dependent AChR clustering substantially.[32] Moreover, in the absence of added agrin, they caused a modest clustering of AChR, suggesting that they are able to cross-link and activate MuSK on the cell surface. Therefore, it is possible that the antibodies interfere with the function of MuSK at the adult neuromuscular junction, perhaps leading to reduced clustering of AChRs and reduced stability of the postsynaptic membrane architecture.[32]

CLINICAL ASSOCIATIONS OF MUSK ANTIBODIES

MuSK antibodies have now been detected in many patients with SNMG, but the proportion of positive patients is somewhat lower than that reported in 2001.[32] This may be because the samples originally tested were from SNMG patients who had undergone plasma exchange and who were usually at the more severe end of the clinical spectrum.

To investigate clinical expression of disease in SNMG patients (from the United Kingdom and Italy) with or without MuSK antibodies, we retrospectively analyzed the clinical notes from 23 patients with MuSK antibodies, 25 patients without MuSK antibodies, and 50 SPMG patients. We assessed their MGFA grades and expressed this measurement on a linear scale from 1 to 8 (corresponding to MGFA I, IIA, IIB, IIIA, IIIB, IVA, IVB, V). The ages at onset of disease and duration of follow-up were not significantly different, but the patients who were subsequently shown to be MuSK antibody-positive had significantly more disease at final follow-up (Bowen, Farrugia, Newsom-Davis, Evoli, and Vincent, unpublished results). Thus, even with conventional immunosuppression, MuSK antibody-positive SNMG patients appear to do less well than MuSK antibody-negative SNMG or AChR antibody-positive SPMG patients. These results are preliminary, the numbers are still small, and we are extending the study to patients from more centers in Europe and the United States.

SUMMARY AND CONCLUSIONS

Fetal-specific antibodies are a rare, but potentially preventable cause of AMC in babies. The antibodies appear to be restricted in their germline origin and may be induced by AChR from the fetus itself. Other antibodies that bind to developing tissues are present in a proportion of mothers of AMC babies who do not have AChR antibodies. Therefore, the role of maternal antibodies to fetal proteins in developmental conditions should be further investigated, particularly if the condition recurs in consecutive pregnancies.

Seronegative MG is a distinct disease from AChR antibody-positive MG and appears to exist in at least two forms. A proportion of patients have IgG antibodies to the muscle-specific kinase, MuSK. These antibodies do not bind complement and may alter the ability of MuSK to maintain the high density of AChRs at the neuromuscular junction. Patients with these antibodies may have more bulbar symptoms[23] and be relatively difficult to treat effectively. By contrast, other SNMG patients do not have MuSK antibodies; however, in several cases studied, their plasma reduces AChR function in cell culture assays, probably by increasing its desensitization rate. The plasma factor that causes these changes is not an IgG antibody and may be an IgM or even another plasma factor.

REFERENCES

1. Gotti, C. *et al.* 1997. Detection of antibody classes and subpopulations in myasthenia gravis patients using a new nonradioactive enzyme immunoassay. Muscle Nerve **20:** 800–808.
2. Ricny, J., L. Simkova & A. Vincent. 2002. Determination of anti-acetylcholine receptor antibodies in myasthenic patients by use of time-resolved fluorescence. Clin. Chem. **48:** 549–554.
3. Fostieri, E., D. Beeson & S.J. Tzartos. 2000. The conformation of the main immunogenic region on the alpha-subunit of muscle acetylcholine receptor is affected by neighboring receptor subunits. FEBS Lett. **481:** 127–130.
4. Alexeev, T. *et al.* 1999. Physicochemical and immunological studies of the N-terminal domain of the *Torpedo* acetylcholine receptor alpha-subunit expressed in *Escherichia coli*. Eur. J. Biochem. **259:** 310–319.
5. Psaridi-Linardaki, L. *et al.* 2002. Expression of soluble ligand- and antibody-binding extracellular domain of human muscle acetylcholine receptor alpha subunit in yeast *Pichia pastoris*: role of glycosylation in alpha-bungarotoxin binding. J. Biol. Chem. **277:** 26980–26986.
6. Vincent, A. *et al.* 1995. Arthrogryposis multiplex congenita with maternal autoantibodies specific for a fetal antigen. Lancet **346:** 24–25.

7. RIEMERSMA, S. *et al.* 1996. Association of arthrogryposis multiplex congenita with maternal antibodies inhibiting fetal acetylcholine receptor function. J. Clin. Invest. **98:** 2358–2363.
8. BRUETON, L.A. *et al.* 2000. Asymptomatic maternal myasthenia as a cause of the Pena-Shokeir phenotype. Am. J. Med. Genet. **92:** 1–6.
9. JACOBSON, L. *et al.* 1999. An animal model of antibody-mediated neurodevelopmental disease: arthrogryposis multiplex congenita caused by antibodies to fetal acetylcholine receptor. J. Clin. Invest. **103:** 1031–1038.
10. FARRAR, J. *et al.* 1997. Diverse Fab specific for acetylcholine receptor epitopes from a myasthenia gravis thymus combinatorial library. Int. Immunol. **9:** 1311–1318.
11. MATTHEWS, I., G. SIMS *et al.* 2002. Antibodies to acetylcholine receptor in parous women with myasthenia: evidence for immunization by fetal antigen. Lab. Invest. **82:** 1407–1417.
12. GRAUS, Y.F. *et al.* 1997. Human anti-nicotinic acetylcholine receptor recombinant Fab fragments isolated from thymus-derived phage display libraries from myasthenia gravis patients reflect predominant specificities in serum and block the action of pathogenic serum antibodies. J. Immunol. **158:** 1919–1929.
13. SCHLUEP, M. *et al.* 1987. Acetylcholine receptors in human myoid cells *in situ*: an immunohistological study. Ann. Neurol. **22:** 212-222.
14. BEESON, D. *et al.* 1996. A transfected human muscle cell line expressing the adult subtype of the human muscle acetylcholine receptor for diagnostic assays in myasthenia gravis. Neurology **47:** 1552–1555.
15. MACLENNAN, C. *et al.* Acetylcholine receptor expression in human extraocular muscles and their susceptibility to myasthenia gravis. Ann. Neurol. **41:** 423–431.
16. WINTZEN, A.R. *et al.* 1998. Acquired slow channel syndrome: a form of myasthenia gravis with prolonged open time of the acetylcholine receptor channel. Ann. Neurol. **44:** 657–664.
17. SCHON, F., M. DRAYSON & R.A. THOMPSON. 1996. Myasthenia gravis and elderly people. Age Ageing **25:** 56–58.
18. SOMNIER, F.E. 1996. Myasthenia gravis. Dan. Med. Bull. **43:** 1–10.
19. ROMI, F. *et al.* 2000. The severity of myasthenia gravis correlates with the serum concentration of titin and ryanodine receptor antibodies. Arch. Neurol. **57:** 1596–1600.
20. MEAGER, A. *et al.* 1997. Spontaneous neutralising antibodies to interferon-α and interleukin-12 in thymoma-associated autoimmune disease. Lancet **350:** 1596–1597.
21. BUCKLEY, C. *et al.* 2001. Do titin and cytokine antibodies in MG patients predict thymoma or thymoma recurrence? Neurology **57:** 1579–1582.
22. MOSSMAN, S., A. VINCENT & J. NEWSOM-DAVIS. 1986. Myasthenia gravis without acetylcholine-receptor antibody: a distinct disease entity. Lancet **i:** 116–118.
23. EVOLI, A. *et al.* 1996. Clinical heterogeneity of seronegative myasthenia gravis. Neuromuscul. Disord. **6:** 155–161.
24. BURGES, J. *et al.* 1990. A myasthenia gravis plasma immunoglobulin reduces miniature endplate potentials at human endplates *in vitro*. Muscle Nerve **13:** 407–413.
25. YAMAMOTO, T. *et al.* 1991. Seronegative myasthenia gravis: a plasma factor inhibiting agonist induced acetylcholine receptor function co-purifies with IgM. Ann. Neurol. **30:** 550–557.
26. PLESTED, C.P. *et al.* 2002. AChR phosphorylation and indirect inhibition of AChR function in seronegative MG. Neurology **59:** 1682–1688.
27. PLESTED, C.P., J. NEWSOM-DAVIS & A. VINCENT. 1998. Seronegative myasthenia plasmas and non-IgG fractions transiently inhibit nAChR function. Ann. N.Y. Acad. Sci. **841:** 501–504.
28. MIER, A.K. & C.W.H. HAVARD. 1985. Diaphragmatic myasthenia in mother and child. Postgrad. Med. J. **61:** 725–727.
29. BLAES, F. *et al.* 2000. IgG from "seronegative" myasthenia gravis patients binds to a muscle cell line, TE671, but not to human acetylcholine receptor. Ann. Neurol. **47:** 504–510.
30. HOCH, W. 1999. Formation of the neuromuscular junction: agrin and its unusual receptors. Eur. J. Biochem. **265:** 1–10.

31. LIYANAGE, Y. *et al.* 2001. The agrin/muscle specific kinase pathway: new targets for autoimmune and genetic disorders at the neuromuscular junction. Muscle Nerve **25:** 4–16.
32. HOCH, W. *et al.* 2001. Autoantibodies to the receptor tyrosine kinase MuSK in patients with myasthenia gravis without acetylcholine receptor antibodies. Nat. Med. **7:** 365–368.
33. ENGEL, A.G. & K. ARAHATA. 1987. The membrane attack complex of complement at the endplate in myasthenia gravis. Ann. N.Y. Acad. Sci. **505:** 326–332.

Differences between the ϵ and γ Subunits of the Acetylcholine Receptor (AChR) May Be Significant in Autoimmune Myasthenia Gravis

SAMIA RAGHEB AND ROBERT P. LISAK

Department of Neurology, Wayne State University School of Medicine, Detroit, Michigan 48201, USA

KEYWORDS: myasthenia gravis; acetylcholine receptor; epitope

Autoimmune myasthenia gravis (MG) is a disease in which a wayward immune response targets the nicotinic acetylcholine receptor (AChR).[1] Because of the antibody-mediated pathology, MG is classified as a B cell–mediated autoimmune disease. T cells do not appear to be directly involved in AChR damage; however, both arms of the immune system contribute to the pathogenesis of MG.[2]

The AChR is composed of two α, one β, one δ, and either a γ or an ε subunit. The ε subunit is found in innervated adult skeletal muscle, whereas the γ subunit is found in denervated adult skeletal muscle and in fetal AChR. The thymus, which is not normally innervated by somatic motor neurons, has the fetal form of the AChR that contains the γ subunit rather than the ε subunit.[3]

Because the α subunit is immunodominant for B cells and T cells, synthetic peptides corresponding to antigenic sites on the α subunit have been used to identify the antigenic repertoire of T cells in MG. We previously examined the *in vitro* proliferative response of peripheral blood mononuclear cells (PBMC) to the α peptides: 65–82, 125–163, 256–269, and 386–411. We found that individual patients responded to more than one peptide, indicating that the T cell response is heterogeneous. Furthermore, no differences were observed in the immune response of MG patients and healthy subjects to any of the α epitopes tested. PBMC from nonmyasthenic subjects were also stimulated to proliferate by the same α peptides to which MG patients responded. These were healthy subjects who did not exhibit any signs or symptoms of MG and who did not have detectable serum anti-AChR antibodies. Serial studies of the immune response of individual patients to the α peptides suggest that epitope spread does occur over time. Our data show that patients may initially respond to the α peptide 125–163; subsequently, they also respond to 65–82 and 386–411; finally, they also respond to the transmembrane peptide 256–269.

Address for correspondence: Samia Ragheb, Ph.D., Department of Neurology, Wayne State University, 3128 Elliman Building, 421 East Canfield Avenue, Detroit, MI 48201. Voice: 313-577-7594; fax: 313-577-7552.

sragheb@med.wayne.edu

Ann. N.Y. Acad. Sci. 998: 336–338 (2003). © 2003 New York Academy of Sciences.
doi: 10.1196/annals.1254.037

TABLE 1. The six peptides synthesized

Peptide		
I	ε	IRRHDGDSAGGPGETD
II	γ	MLLDEAAPAEEAGHQK
III	ε	PPEIPRAASPPRRASSLGLLLRA
IV	γ	PVAVQDAHPRLQNGSSSGWPITAG
V	ε	TWTATLCQNLGAAAPE
VI	γ	LVRAALEKLEKGPESGQSPEWCGSLKQAAPA

Immune responses against other AChR subunits have not been examined as carefully as those against the α subunit. The differential expression of the γ and ε subunits in thymic and muscle AChR, respectively, may be highly significant to the pathogenesis of MG. ε and γ subunit synthetic peptides were tested for their capacity to stimulate PBMC *in vitro*. On the basis of published amino acid sequences of calf ε and γ subunits,[4] peptides were selected from regions with little sequence homology to the α subunit. Furthermore, to distinguish between ε and γ epitopes, peptides were selected from regions where there was little sequence homology between the ε and γ subunits. Three regions were selected representing amino acids 194–209, 343–366, and 389–419. Six peptides (3ε and 3γ, TABLE 1) were synthesized commercially to >95% purity. We determined the *in vitro* proliferative response of PBMC isolated from MG patients ($n = 36$; 12 M, 24 F) and healthy nonmyasthenic subjects ($n = 22$; 10 M, 12 F) to these peptides; as a negative control, cells were cultured without stimulation; as a positive control, cells were cultured with mitogen, tetanus toxoid, and the α peptides previously tested. The proliferative response was determined by measuring tritiated thymidine uptake by PBMC. The mean cpm ± SD of triplicate wells was calculated. A stimulation index of ≥3 was considered a positive response. As in our previous studies, no differences were observed in the proliferative response of MG patients and healthy subjects to mitogen, tetanus toxoid, or the α peptides.

PBMC from MG patients were stimulated by the ε and γ subunit peptides, although the proliferative response was weaker than that to the α subunit peptides. Of the 36 patients with MG, 16 had not received any immunosuppressive treatment at the time of study. The number of patients with a positive response to each peptide was as follows—peptide I: 7/16 (44%); II: 7/16 (44%); III: 2/16 (13%); IV: 2/16 (13%); V: 3/16 (19%); and VI: 11/16 (69%). PBMC from most healthy nonmyasthenic subjects did not respond. The number of healthy subjects who gave a positive response was as follows—peptide I: 0/22 (0%); II: 2/22 (9%); III: 0/22 (0%); IV: 1/22 (5%); V: 0/22 (0%); and VI: 7/22 (32%). Healthy subjects who responded showed reactivity to only γ subunit peptides. None of the healthy subjects responded to the three ε subunit synthetic peptides tested. This is in contrast to studies with α subunit peptides, where it was found that MG patients and healthy nonmyasthenic subjects responded to the same epitopes with equal magnitude. Differences between the ε and γ subunits of the AChR may be important in the immunopathogenesis of MG because only MG patients respond to epitopes that are unique to the ε subunit. Future studies will determine the relative importance of the immune response to the ε subunit in the pathogenesis of autoimmune MG.

REFERENCES

1. Patrick, J. & J. Lindstrom. 1973. Autoimmune response to acetylcholine receptors. Science **180:** 871–872.
2. Ragheb, S. & R.P. Lisak. 1994. The immunopathogenesis of acquired (autoimmune) myasthenia gravis. *In* Handbook of Myasthenia Gravis and Myasthenic Syndromes, pp. 239–276. Dekker. New York.
3. Geuder, K.I., A. Marx, V. Witzemann *et al.* 1992. Pathogenetic significance of fetal-type acetylcholine receptors on thymic myoid cells in myasthenia gravis. Dev. Immunol. **2:** 69–75.
4. Takai, T., M. Noda, M. Mishina *et al.* 1985. Cloning, sequencing, and expression of cDNA for a novel subunit of acetylcholine receptor from calf muscle. Nature **315:** 761–764.

Use of Peptide:HLA Class II Complexes to Study Specific T Cells in Autoimmune Myasthenia Gravis

UDAY KISHORE,[a] WEI ZHANG,[a] LOUISE CORLETT,[a] PATRICK WATERS,[a] NICOLAS GLAICHENHAUS,[b] AND NICK WILLCOX[a]

[a]*Neurosciences Group, Weatherall Institute of Molecular Medicine, John Radcliffe Hospital, University of Oxford, Oxford OX3 9DS, United Kingdom*

[b]*Centre National de la Recherche Scientifique, University of Nice–Sophia Antipolis, Valbonne, France*

KEYWORDS: early-onset myasthenia gravis; antibody-mediated diseases; acetylcholine receptor epitopes

INTRODUCTION

Early-onset myasthenia gravis (EOMG) is a T helper cell (Th)–dependent, autoantibody-mediated disorder, which has strong genetic associations with the HLA haplotype DR3-B8.[1] The pathogenic Th must recognize acetylcholine receptor (AChR) epitopes presented by HLA class II molecules on antigen-presenting cells (APC). Current evidence suggests that the Th cells are less heterogeneous than the specific B cells and thus more suitable for selective immunotargeting.

The "minor" class II allele HLA-DR52a (DRB3*0101) is the presenting molecule for an AChR epitope (ε201–219) recognized by Th cloned from three of four EOMG patients.[2] Interestingly, DR52a belongs specifically to the DR3-B8 haplotype rather than to the DR3-B18.[1] This may explain why B8 associates more strongly with EOMG than with DR3 itself, and is consistent with a pathogenic role for the Th that recognizes the AChR ε201–219 epitope.

To assess systematically the potential dominance and pathogenicity of the corresponding Th in a wider range of patients and controls, we have generated soluble peptide-linked DR52a molecules (ε201–215:DR52a) attached to an IgG2a Fc framework. Since monomeric peptide:HLA-DR molecules have low affinities for the T cells' receptor (TcR), we multimerized the ε201–215:DR52a dimer after cross-linking with fluorescent protein A. The resulting multimers (probably tetramers) bind much more avidly to the Th and label the clone specifically. These results suggest that the expressed DR molecules are correctly folded and loaded with peptide, and therefore are suitable for further characterization of Th in MG patients.

Address for correspondence: Nick Willcox, Neurosciences Group, Weatherall Institute of Molecular Medicine, John Radcliffe Hospital, University of Oxford, Oxford OX3 9DS, United Kingdom. Voice: +44-1865-222325; fax: +44-1865-222402.
nick.willcox@imm.ox.ac.uk

Ann. N.Y. Acad. Sci. 998: 339–342 (2003). © 2003 New York Academy of Sciences.
doi: 10.1196/annals.1254.038

METHODS

Expression plasmids encoding the extracellular domains (deleted transmembrane domains) of invariant α and DR52a β chains were fused to acidic/basic leucine zipper sequences, followed by addition of a sequence encoding the C_H2 and C_H3 domains of murine IgG2a.[3] For the β chain plasmid, a DNA sequence coding for the peptide ε201–215 (ENGEWAIDFCPGVIR) was covalently attached by a 10-residue spacer and a thrombin cleavage site to the amino-terminus of the DR52a β chain. The two plasmids were used to transfect *Drosophila* S2 cells, and stable transfectants were selected and induced for expression. The secreted ε201–215:DR52a dimers were purified by affinity chromatography using L243 monoclonal antibody (mAb) or protein A. The dimers were multimerized via the murine IgG2a Fc region with Alexa 488–coupled protein A.

RESULTS

The ε201–215:DR52a dimer was secreted by transfected S2 cells (150–200 μg per 100 mL culture). The expressed product bound to a protein A–Sepharose column, confirming an intact Fc scaffold. It also bound to immobilized L243, a conformation- and DRα chain–specific mAb. When adsorbed to microtiter wells,

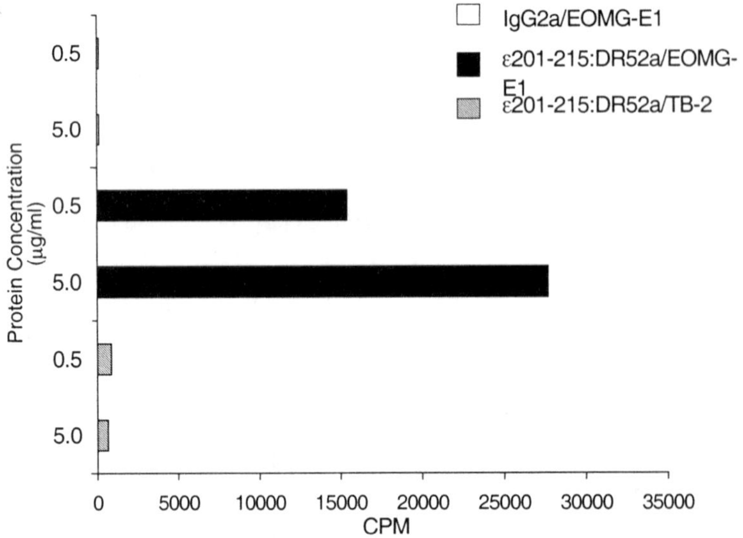

FIGURE 1. Direct stimulation of clone EOMG-E1 by solid-phase ε201–215:DR52a dimer. The dimer was coated onto a microtiter plate in phosphate-buffered saline (PBS) overnight. After blocking with PBS + 2% BSA and washing, clonal Th were added to the wells and allowed to proliferate for 48 h; they were then pulsed with ^{3}H-thymidine. Murine IgG2a and clone TB-2 were used as control protein and Th clone, respectively.

these IgG-like dimers stimulated the relevant Th clone (EOMG-E1) efficiently in the absence of APC (FIG. 1), suggesting the presence of epitope, correctly loaded within the DR molecule. Stimulation was maximal at 2×10^{-8} M and half-maximal at 2×10^{-9} M in the presence of APC, but undetectable with another clone (TB-2) that recognizes α146–160:DR52a. The ε201–215:DR52a dimers, multimerized with Alexa 488–labeled protein A, bound well to the homologous cells, giving a peak at least ten times brighter than the background with the unrelated clone (data not shown). They usually give low backgrounds on control blood T cells; we are now staining blood and thymic cells from patients.

DISCUSSION

The pathogenic autoantibodies to AChR depend on specific Th: if these recognize a restricted range of dominant epitopes, they may prove to be the most suitable targets for selective immunotherapy.[1] In EOMG patients, we have recently found an apparently dominant Th epitope (ε201–219) that is presented by a susceptibility molecule, HLA-DR52a (DRB3*0101).[2] This epitope is processed from adult ($\alpha_2\beta\delta\varepsilon$), but not fetal ($\alpha_2\beta\delta\gamma$) AChR and has a typical DR52a-binding motif (^{205}Trp at p1 and ^{208}Asp at p4). This underrecognized DR52a allele belongs to the strongly predisposing HLA-DR3-B8 haplotype and it is even more prevalent (~70%) in EOMG than the better known DR3, which has a related motif. So far, our clones from EOMG patients are clearly Th1 and could induce the typical pathogenic complement-activating antibodies. Use of ε201-215:DR52a multimers should help assess both the apparent dominance and pathogenicity of the recurring epitope in a wider range of patients and controls.[3]

After establishing the validity of these multimers with a panel of Th clones, we will use them to examine the frequency and heterogeneity of the corresponding Th serially in a wide range of patients and controls; we will also especially evaluate their pathogenic/regulatory potential by focusing on their *in vivo* persistence, thymic localization, surface phenotype/activation state, cytokine profile, and helper activity. We will also assess peptide:HLA-DR molecules and their multimers as novel weapons for specifically inducing tolerance by engaging TcR without costimulation.[4]

This versatile technology should have broad applications to other Th-dependent disorders, wherever immunodominant epitopes are known.[5] It should be particularly suitable in antibody-mediated diseases, including allergies, where target molecules have proved easier to identify than in the more intensively studied Th-mediated examples, but where pervasive weapons will be required *in vivo* for specifically treating disseminated responses.[6]

ACKNOWLEDGMENTS

This work was supported by the Muscular Dystrophy Campaign, the Myasthenia Gravis Association, and the European Commission (Contract No. QLK3-CT-2001-00225).

REFERENCES

1. VINCENT, A., J. PALACE & D. HILTON-JONES. 2001. Myasthenia gravis. Lancet **357:** 2122–2128.
2. HILL, M., D. BEESON *et al.* 1999. Early-onset myasthenia gravis: a recurring T-cell epitope in the adult-specific acetylcholine receptor ε subunit presented by the susceptibility allele HLA-DR52a. Ann. Neurol. **45:** 224–231.
3. MALHERBE, L., C. FILIPPI *et al.* 2000. Selective activation and expansion of high-affinity $CD4^+$ T cells in resistant mice upon infection with *Leishmania major*. Immunity **13:** 771–782.
4. NICOLLE, M.W., B. NAG *et al.* 1994. Specific tolerance to an acetylcholine receptor epitope induced *in vitro* in myasthenia gravis $CD4^+$ lymphocytes by soluble major histocompatibility complex class II–peptide complexes. J. Clin. Invest. **93:** 1361–1369.
5. MCMICHAEL, A.J. & A. KELLEHER. 1999. The arrival of HLA class II tetramers. J. Clin. Invest. **104:** 1669–1670.
6. FERLIN, W., N. GLAICHENHAUS & E. MOUGNEAU. 2000. Present difficulties and future promise of MHC multimers in autoimmune exploration. Curr. Opin. Immunol. **12:** 670–675.

Pathogenesis of Myositis and Myasthenia Associated with Titin and Ryanodine Receptor Antibodies

GEIR OLVE SKEIE, FREDRIK ROMI, JOHAN A. AARLI, PÅL TORE BENTSEN, AND NILS ERIK GILHUS

Department of Neurology, University of Bergen, Bergen, Norway

ABSTRACT: Some myasthenia gravis (MG) patients have antibodies against skeletal muscle antigens in addition to the acetylcholine receptor (AChR). Two major antigens for these antibodies are the Ca^{2+} release channel of the sarcoplasmic reticulum, the ryanodine receptor (RyR), and titin, a gigantic filamentous muscle protein essential for muscle structure, function, and development. RyR and titin antibodies are found in MG patients with a thymoma and in a proportion of late-onset MG, and they correlate with severe MG disease. The RyR antibodies recognize a region near the N-terminus important for channel regulation. They inhibit Ca^{2+} release from sarcoplasmic reticulum *in vitro*. There is electrophysiological evidence for a disordered excitation-contraction coupling in MG patients. The presence of titin antibodies, which bind to key regions near the A/I junction and in the central I-band, correlates with myopathy in MG patients. However, so far, there is no direct evidence that antibodies against the intracellular antigens RyR and titin are pathogenic *in vivo*.

KEYWORDS: myasthenia gravis; acetylcholine receptor; ryanodine receptor; titin; antibodies

INTRODUCTION

Myasthenia gravis (MG) is an autoimmune disease of the neuromuscular junction characterized by an increased fatigability of skeletal muscle. Antibodies against the nicotinic acetylcholine receptor (AChR), binding at the muscle endplate, cause focal muscle membrane damage and an accelerated rate of AChR degradation.[1] There is no correlation between AChR antibody levels and degree of muscle weakness. This may be due to a heterogeneity of AChR antibodies regarding epitope specificity or to the presence of antibodies against other functionally important muscle antigens.

The process of muscle contraction is complex and involves nerve-muscle transmission, muscle membrane excitation, and signal transmission to sarcoplasmic reticulum (SR), Ca^{2+} release from SR, activity of the contractile proteins, and SR reuptake of Ca^{2+}. MG patients have in their sera circulating antibodies against key proteins in several of these processes. There are electrophysiological reports of both

Address for correspondence: Dr. Geir Olve Skeie, Department of Neurology, Haukeland University Hospital, N-5021 Bergen, Norway. Voice: +47-55-97-50-45; fax: +47-55-97-51-65. gske@haukeland.no

Ann. N.Y. Acad. Sci. 998: 343–350 (2003). **© 2003 New York Academy of Sciences.**
doi: 10.1196/annals.1254.039

disordered excitation-contraction coupling and myopathy in skeletal muscle of MG patients as well as reports of myositis unrelated to the endplates.[2–6] The muscle weakness in MG may therefore be more complex than a mere neuromuscular block due to AChR antibodies.

In the early 1960s, sera from MG patients with thymoma were shown to stain skeletal muscle in a striational pattern.[7] In 1990, these antibodies were found to react with the giant muscle protein titin.[8] Another set of non-AchR antibodies bound to unidentified protein antigens in SR membranes. Mygland *et al.* showed that these antibodies stained a high-molecular-weight protein that was identified as the Ca^{2+} release channel of SR: the ryanodine receptor (RyR).[9] Both proteins occur only intracellularly. To be able to interact with their targets, the RyR and titin antibodies thus have to cross the sarcolemma. Whether antibodies against intracellular molecules can have pathogenic significance *in vivo* is still controversial. However, antibodies are able to penetrate the cell membrane and have been found intracellularly bound to their target antigens.[10] This has not been examined for the titin and RyR antibodies. In a study by Beutner *et al.*, it is stated that human striational antibodies were found bound to muscle biopsies from MG patients.[11] This indicates that the non-AChR antibodies are able to bind to their targets also *in vivo*. Both titin and RyR are vital muscle proteins and, if the antibodies reach their targets, one would predict a severe effect on muscle development and function.

TITIN

Titin (connectin) is the third most abundant protein in skeletal and cardiac muscle. It is the largest single-chain protein identified, predicted to consist of around 27,000 amino acids with a molecular mass of about 3000 kDa.[12] Ninety percent of titin's mass is contained in a repetitive structure comprising 244–297 copies of two different 100-residue repeats resembling two well-known superfamily motifs, 112–165 immunoglobulin (Ig)–like domains and 132 fibronectin (FN3)–like domains.[12] The titin filament extends along the entire sarcomere from the Z-disc to the M-line and is >1 mm long.[13] A-band titin is composed of regular arrangements of a series of 43-nm-long repeats, matching exactly the 43-nm intervals where myosin-binding protein C is found bound to titin. Titin interacts also with several other muscle proteins. The pattern of interaction correlates closely with the known locations of these proteins within the sarcomere, and thus together with titin's highly ordered structure suggest that titin plays an important role in sarcomere assembly.[12]

The I-band titin consists of tandemly arranged Ig repeats of variable number. There are additional unique sequences, the largest of which is a region rich in Pro (P), Glu (E), Val (V), and Lys (K), the so-called PEVK domain. As titin is stretched, the PEVK region is thought to extend by unfolding. Another unique sequence in the cardiac isoform is called N2-B, which also extends by unfolding.[14] Titin provides axial continuity between the two filament systems in order to provide resting tension; on the other hand, titin keeps the thick filaments in register in the center of the sarcomere, thus enabling the direct sliding of the thick and thin filaments upon contraction. It acts like a spring and is responsible for building up passive resistance to stretch. Four different titin regions working in series give rise to the mechanical properties of titin.[15] During the initial stretching of the sarcomere, there will be a straightening of the Ig domain regions without building up much tension. When the Ig repeat chain is straightened, more tension is needed to increase the sarcomere length, which occurs by unfolding the PEVK part of titin. The exact tertiary structure of PEVK titin and how this part of titin unfolds is not well characterized. In cardiac muscle, the PEVK region is relatively short, and the N2-B region contributes more to the extensibility and elasticity.[14] At such sarcomere lengths (until the Ig chain straightened, PEVK/N2-B unfolded), the sarcomere will build up passive tension, and the force needed to increase sarcomere length increases exponentially. The titin filaments will at this stage spring back to their original position if released. This represents the elasticity at physiological sarcomere lengths. To increase sarcomere lengths even further, much more force is needed to unfold single Ig modules. When the force is released, these modules will not spring back into position at once. Unfolding of Ig modules may serve as a safety mechanism to maintain the mechanical integrity of the sarcomere even at overstretch, allowing the filaments to hold together and restore sarcomere function.

TITIN ANTIBODIES

There is a complex domain architecture near the junction of the I-band and A-band. Interestingly, most experimental animals, immunized with whole titin, produce antibodies against this region. By immunoscreening a cardiac muscle cDNA library with pooled MG sera, this sequence near the A/I-junction of titin was found to be the main immunogenic region (MIR) on titin for spontaneously produced autoantibodies in both humans and dogs with myasthenia gravis (MG). This region was therefore named myasthenia gravis titin 30 kDa (MGT-30).[16] Using immunofluorescence microscopy on stretched single myofibrils from both skeletal and cardiac muscle, antibodies against additional titin epitopes were identified, indicating epitope spreading.[17] These antibodies stained central I-band epitopes located between the N1- and N2-line of titin, a region that consists of homologous, tandemly arranged Ig domains and that is differentially expressed; in cardiac muscle, only 15 domains are present, whereas up to 68 such modules can be present in skeletal muscle.[12] This contrasts with the MIR region, which is constitutively expressed in striated muscle. About 40% of titin antibody–positive patients had sera reacting with additional I-band epitopes from skeletal muscle, whereas only a single serum reacted with the I-band of cardiac muscle, which explains why the I-band epitope was not discovered by Gautel *et al.*,[16] who used a cardiac muscle library for screening.

Titin antibodies produced by a thymoma-derived B cell clone had the same specificity as those found in the serum of the same patient. The antibodies contained somatic mutations, suggesting that the antibody response was a specific antigen-driven immune response.[18] The presence of titin antibodies correlates with MG severity.[19] Titin antibody–positive MG patients benefit less from thymectomy than MG patients without titin antibodies.

The presence of titin antibodies correlates positively with myopathy in MG, as defined with QEMG, showing shortening of motor unit potentials (MUP) and increased polyphasic MUP. No denervation was found and there was no association with the decremental response. Muscle biopsy showed abnormal and small fibers scattered randomly throughout the sections. Necrotic or targeted fibers were not present. There were no ragged red fibers, and connective tissue and vessels appeared normal.[5] A coexistence of myopathy and disturbed neuromuscular transmission in titin antibody–positive MG patients may explain their more severe muscle weakness. The mechanisms for the development of MG myopathy remain unclear, but titin is important for myofibrillogenesis and sarcomere structure and elasticity. Another potential mechanism for the increased MG severity in titin-positive patients is the cell-mediated immune response against titin. Some thymoma MG patients with titin antibodies have a myositis that cannot be explained by their AChR antibodies, as the T cell deposits occur far from the neuromuscular junction. Titin antibody–positive MG patients have circulating peripheral blood mononuclear cells that respond with cell proliferation when cultured with MGT-30 (MIR titin).[20] The culture supernatant contained IL-4 in a low concentration. Using ELISpot, both titin-reactive IFN-γ-secreting Th1 cells and titin-reactive IL-4-secreting Th2 cells were identified.[21]

RYANODINE RECEPTOR (RyR)

RyR is the Ca^{2+} release channel of the SR.[22] It is a transmembrane protein composed of four homologous subunits arranged around a central pore. The amino acid sequence of the RyR shows extensive homology across species, especially in the COOH-terminal transmembrane segments,[23] which have some sequence homology also with the transmembrane regions of the AChR.[24] There are separate genes for skeletal muscle RyR (RyR1), cardiac muscle RyR (RyR2), and brain RyR (RyR3). The mRNAs encode proteins of 4872 (RyR3)–5037 (RyR1) amino acids with a molecular weight of about 565. RyR is located at the terminal cisternae of the SR at the triad junction where the communications between T-tubule invaginations of the sarcolemma and SR occur.[25] The amino terminus and central parts of the molecule are hydrophilic and believed to form the cytoplasmic foot that interacts with the dihydropyridine receptor (DHPR), the voltage sensor of the T-tubuli. The RyR has a crucial role in excitation-contraction coupling in skeletal muscle.[26] Sarcolemmal depolarization will spread longitudinally along the sarcolemma and transversely down the T-tubuli, which are junctionally associated with the terminal cisternae of the SR by the foot structures at the triadic junction. Excitation-contraction coupling in skeletal muscle involves a direct link among the DHPR, the voltage sensor, and the RyR.[27] A charge movement in the DHPR is transmitted via a polypeptide loop to the RyR, resulting in channel opening, Ca^{2+} release from the terminal cisternae, and muscle contraction. In cardiac muscle, the mechanism is different as the activation of the DHPR voltage sensor causes a Ca^{2+} influx, which in turn causes RyR opening (Ca^{2+}-dependent Ca^{2+} release).

RyR ANTIBODIES

The RyR antibodies are closely associated with thymoma MG.[9] MG patient RyR antibodies bind to both the skeletal and cardiac form of the RyR.[28] RyR antibody–positive patients have more severe MG symptoms.[29] They usually have generalized muscle weakness with prominent bulbar symptoms and often weakness of respiratory muscles, requiring assisted ventilation. The RyR antibodies are mainly of the IgG1 and IgG3 subclass[30] and can activate complement.[31] This is interesting as the presence of RyR antibodies in MG patients correlates to cardiac disease with sudden death. AChR antibodies cannot explain the cardiac involvement since nicotinic AChRs are not found in the heart.

The RyR antibodies circulating in MG patients with thymoma inhibit ryanodine binding to the RyR. This inhibition is concentration-dependent. The ryanodine binding is inhibited even at very high ryanodine concentrations, indicating a high antibody affinity for the receptor.[32] A reciprocal competition between the RyR antibodies and ryanodine for binding to the RyR exists since preincubating the RyR with ryanodine inhibits binding of RyR antibodies in Western blots.[32] Measuring the binding of [^{3}H]ryanodine to SR membranes is a well-established method for investigating RyR function *in vitro*.[22] This binding depends on the conformational opening state of the ion channel and thus reflects the Ca^{2+} release activity. The inhibition of ryanodine binding by RyR antibodies from MG patients indicates that the antibodies affect Ca^{2+} release from SR by causing conformational changes that close the RyR ion channel.

RyR antibodies from MG patients cause a marked inhibition of 4-chloro-*m*-cresol-induced Ca^{2+} release from isolated terminal cisternae fractions.[33] The RyR antibodies reacting with the MIR region were responsible for this effect since the inhibition of Ca^{2+} release disappeared when these RyR antibodies were removed from the IgG fraction. The MIR for MG patient RyR antibodies is located near the N-terminus (residues 799–1172) of the RyR.[33] Some sera also react with a shorter and more centrally located region (residues 2595–2935). The MIR region is probably essential for RyR function and regulation since it is overlapping with the RyR region (922–1220) known to bind and interact with the DHPR.[34,35] The RyR antibodies are thus able to interfere with the interaction between RyR and DHPR, which in turn would inhibit opening of the RyR channel and subsequently inhibiting Ca^{2+} release.

MG patients with RyR antibodies inhibiting ryanodine binding have a more severe disease than patients with RyR antibodies that do not inhibit ryanodine binding,[32] suggesting a correlation between symptom severity and the antibody effect on the RyR *in vitro*. If the antibodies reach their target, one would predict a severe effect on excitation-contraction coupling and muscle contraction. Excitation-contraction coupling seems to be affected in some MG patients,[2–4] and there are circumstantial evidence for an *in vivo* effect of RyR. A rat strain with spontaneous thymomas, muscular weakness, and fatigability resembling MG has electrophysiological signs of a defective excitation-contraction coupling; they have RyR antibodies, but no detectable AChR antibodies.[36] RyR-positive MG patients have circulating Th1 and Th2 cells (Bentsen *et al.*, unpublished), which could, in theory, contribute to the autoimmune myositis seen in some MG patients, particularly with thymoma.

CLINICAL USEFULNESS OF TITIN AND RyR ANTIBODIES

The titin antibody assay is clinically useful since 95% of thymoma MG patients have antibodies reacting with the titin MIR epitope. When combining the titin antibody assay with CT scanning of the thymus, the titin antibodies have a near 100% specificity of detecting a thymoma.[37] When titin antibodies are not present, the CT scan provides no additional information.[38]

RyR antibodies are found in about 75% of thymoma MG patients and are more specific for thymoma than the titin antibodies that occur in about 50% of all late-onset MG patients, also without a thymoma. The combination of titin and RyR antibody testing gives a 95% sensitivity and specificity and a 70% positive predictive value for a thymoma in MG.[38] RyR antibodies are found more often in patients with an invasive/malignant thymoma.[39] The presence of RyR antibodies in thymoma MG patients should thus make the surgeon more careful when removing the thymoma, choosing a technique that assures complete removal of a potentially invasive thymoma.

As the presence of titin and RyR antibodies correlates with MG severity, the antibody status is useful when assessing disease prognosis, treatment, and follow-up. The presence of titin/RyR antibodies makes a positive thymectomy effect more unlikely.[40]

ACKNOWLEDGMENT

This work was supported by the Unger-Vetlesen Medical Fund.

REFERENCES

1. Lindstrom, J., D. Schelton & Y. Fujii. 1988. Myasthenia gravis. Adv. Immunol. **42:** 233–284.
2. Nielsen, V.K., O.B. Paulson, J. Rosenkvist *et al.* 1982. Rapid improvement of myasthenia gravis after plasma exchange. Ann. Neurol. **11:** 160–169.
3. Pagala, M., N.V. Nandakumar, S.A.T. Venkatachari *et al.* 1990. Responses of intercostal muscle biopsies from normal subjects and patients with myasthenia gravis. Muscle Nerve **13:** 1012–1022.
4. Pagala, M., N.V. Nandakumar, S.A.T. Venkatachari *et al.* 1993. Mechanisms of fatigue in normal intercostal muscle and muscle from patients with myasthenia gravis. Muscle Nerve **16:** 911–921.
5. Somnier, F.E., G.O. Skeie, J.A. Aarli *et al.* 1999. EMG evidence of myopathy and the occurrence of titin autoantibodies in patients with myasthenia gravis. Eur. J. Neurol. **6:** 1–9.
6. Aarli, J.A. 1998. Inflammatory myopathy in myasthenia gravis. Curr. Opin. Neurol. **11:** 233–234.
7. Strauss, A.J.L. & P.G. Kemp. 1967. Serum autoantibodies in myasthenia gravis and thymoma: selective affinity for I-bands of striated muscle as a guide to identification of antigen(s). J. Immunol. **99:** 945–953.
8. Aarli, J.A., K. Stefansson, L.S.G. Marton *et al.* 1990. Patients with myasthenia gravis and thymoma have in their sera IgG autoantibodies against titin. Clin. Exp. Immunol. **82:** 284–288.
9. Mygland, Å., O.B. Tysnes, R. Matre *et al.* 1992. Ryanodine receptor autoantibodies in myasthenia gravis patients with a thymoma. Ann. Neurol. **32:** 589–591.
10. Alarcon-Segovia, D., A. Ruiz-Arguelles & L. Llorente. 1996. Broken dogma: penetration of autoantibodies into living cells. Immunol. Today **17:** 163–164.
11. Beutner, E.H., G. Fazekas, A. Scott *et al.* 1966. Direct fluorescent antibody studies of gamma globulin localization in muscle of patients with myasthenia gravis. Ann. N.Y. Acad. Sci. **135:** 588–600.
12. Labeit, S. & B. Kolmerer. 1995. Titins: giant proteins in charge of muscle ultrastructure and elasticity. Science **270:** 293–296.
13. Furst, D.O., M. Osborn, R. Nave *et al.* 1988. The organization of titin filaments in the half-sarcomere revealed by monoclonal antibodies in immunoelectron microscopy: a

map of ten non-repetitive epitopes starting at the Z-line extends close to the M-line. J. Cell Biol. **106:** 1563–1572.
14. LINKE, W., D.E. RUDY, T. CENTNER *et al.* 1999. I-band titin in cardiac muscle is a three-element molecular spring and is critical for maintaining thin filament structure. J. Cell Biol. **146:** 631–644.
15. MARSZALEK, P.I., H. LU, H. LI *et al.* 1999. Mechanical unfolding intermediates in titin modules. Nature **402:** 100–103.
16. GAUTEL, M., A. LAKEY, P.D. BARLOW *et al.* 1993. Titin antibodies in myasthenia gravis: identification of a major immunogenic region of titin. Neurology **43:** 1581–1585.
17. LUEBKE, E., A. FREIBURG, G.O. SKEIE *et al.* 1998. Striational autoantibodies in myasthenia gravis patients recognize I-band titin epitopes. J. Neuroimmunol. **81:** 98–108.
18. WILLIAMS, C.L., J.E. HAY, T.W. HUIATT *et al.* 1992. Paraneoplastic IgG striational autoantibodies produced by clonal thymic B cells and in serum of patients with myasthenia gravis and thymoma react with titin. Lab. Invest. **66:** 331–336.
19. SKEIE, G.O., Å. MYGLAND, J.A AARLI *et al.* 1995. Titin antibodies in patients with late-onset myasthenia gravis: clinical correlations. Autoimmunity **20:** 99–105.
20. SKEIE, G.O., J.A. AARLI, R. MATRE *et al.* 1997. Titin antibody positive myasthenia gravis patients have a cellular immune response against the main immunogenic region of titin. Eur. J. Neurol. **4:** 131–137.
21. SKEIE, G.O., P.T. BENTSEN, A. FREIBURG *et al.* 1998. Cell mediated immune response against titin in myasthenia gravis: evidence for the involvement of Th1 and Th2 cells. Scand. J. Immunol. **47:** 76–81.
22. CORONADO, R., J. MORRISSETTE, M. SUKHAREVA *et al.* 1994. Structure and function of ryanodine receptors. Am. J. Physiol. **266:** c1485–c1504.
23. ZORZATO, F., J. FUJII, K. OTSU *et al.* 1990. Molecular cloning of DNA encoding human and rabbit forms of the Ca^{2+} release channel (ryanodine receptor) of skeletal muscle sarcoplasmic reticulum. J. Biol. Chem. **265:** 2244–2256.
24. TAKESHIMA, H., S. NISHIMURA, T. MATSUMOTO *et al.* 1989. Primary structure and expression from complementary DNA of skeletal muscle ryanodine receptor. Nature **339:** 439–445.
25. INUI, M., A. SAITO & S. FLEISCHER. 1987 Isolation of the ryanodine receptor from cardiac sarcoplasmic reticulum and identity with the feet structures. J. Biol. Chem. **262:** 15637–15642.
26. TAKESHIMA, H., I. MASAMITSU, H. TAKEKURA *et al.* 1994. Excitation-contraction uncoupling in mice lacking functional skeletal muscle ryanodine-receptor gene. Nature **369:** 556–559.
27. TANABE, T., K. BEAN, B.A. ADAMS *et al.* 1990. Region of the skeletal muscle dihydropyridine receptor critical for excitation-contraction coupling. Nature **346:** 567–569.
28. MYGLAND, Å., O.B. TYSNES, R. MATRE *et al.* 1994 Anti-cardiac ryanodine receptor antibodies in thymoma associated myasthenia gravis. Autoimmunity **17:** 327–331.
29. MYGLAND, Å., J.A. AARLI, R. MATRE *et al.,* 1994. Ryanodine receptor antibodies related to severity of thymoma-associated myasthenia gravis. J. Neurol. Neurosurg. Psychiatry **57:** 843–846.
30. MYGLAND, Å., O.B. TYSNES, J.A. AARLI *et al.* 1993. IgG subclass distribution of ryanodine receptor autoantibodies in patients with myasthenia gravis and thymoma. J. Autoimmun. **6:** 507–515.
31. ROMI, F., G.O. SKEIE, J.A. AARLI *et al.* 2000. Complement activation by titin and ryanodine receptor autoantibodies in myasthenia gravis: a study of IgG subclasses and clinical correlation. J. Neuroimmunol. **111:** 169–176.
32. SKEIE, G.O., P.K. LUNDE, O.M. SEJERSTED *et al.* 1998 Myasthenia gravis sera containing anti-ryanodine receptor antibodies inhibit binding of [^{3}H]-ryanodine to sarcoplasmic reticulum. Muscle Nerve **21:** 329–335.
33. SKEIE, G.O., Å. MYGLAND, S. TREVES *et al.* 2003. Ryanodine receptor antibodies in myasthenia gravis: epitope mapping and effect on calcium release *in vitro*. Muscle Nerve **27:** 81–89.
34. LEONG, P. & D.H. MACLENNAN. 1998. A 37-amino acid sequence in the skeletal muscle ryanodine receptor interacts with the cytoplasmic loop between domains II and III in the skeletal muscle dihydropyridine receptor. J. Biol. Chem. **273:** 7791–7794.

35. LEONG, P. & D.H. MACLENNAN. 1998. The cytoplasmic loops between domains II and III and domains III and IV in the skeletal muscle dihydropyridine receptor bind to a contiguous site in the skeletal muscle ryanodine receptor. J. Biol. Chem. **273:** 29958–29964.
36. IWASA, K., K. KOMAI & M. TAKAMORI. 1998. Spontaneous thymoma rat as a model for myasthenic weakness caused by anti-ryanodine receptor antibodies. Muscle Nerve **21:** 1655–1660.
37. VOLTZ, R.D., W.C. ALBRICH, A. NAGELE *et al.* 1997. Paraneoplastic myasthenia gravis: detection of anti-MGT30 (titin) antibodies predicts thymic epithelial tumor. Neurology **49:** 1454–1457.
38. ROMI, F., G.O. SKEIE, J.A. AARLI *et al.* 2000. Muscle autoantibodies in subgroups of myasthenia gravis patients. J. Neurol. **247:** 369–375.
39. SKEIE, G.O., E. BARTOCCIONI, A. EVOLI *et al.* 1996. Ryanodine receptor antibodies are associated with severe myasthenia gravis. Eur. J. Neurol. **3:** 136–140.
40. ROMI, F., N.E. GILHUS, J.E. VARHAUG *et al.* 2002. Thymectomy vs. non-thymectomy in late-onset myasthenia gravis in correlation with muscle autoantibodies. Eur. J. Neurol. **9:** 55–61.

Antibodies in Sera of Patients with Late-Onset Myasthenia Gravis Recognize the PEVK Domain of Titin

MIRTA MIHOVILOVIC,[a] EMMA CIAFALONI,[a]
JENNIFER BUTTERWORTH-ROBINETTE,[a] JIAN-PING JIN,[b]
JANICE MASSEY,[a] AND DONALD B. SANDERS[a]

[a]*Division of Neurology, Duke University Medical Center, Durham, North Carolina 27710, USA*

[b]*Department of Physiology and Biophysics, Case Western Reserve University, Cleveland, Ohio 44106, USA*

KEYWORDS: **titin; myasthenia gravis; thymic neoplasia; thymic histopathology**

INTRODUCTION

Antibodies directed to a recombinant peptide carrying the main immunogenic region of human titin are found in 70%[1] to 97%[2] of myasthenia gravis (MG) patients that present with thymic neoplasia, 34% to 50%[3] of late-onset MG, and in a smaller percentage of patients that present with thymic atrophy[1–3] or thymic hyperplasia.[3] MG sera, however, also bind to epitopes directed to other antigenic regions of titin.[4] Studies with a peptide located within the PEVK domain of human skeletal muscle titin showed that 21% of randomly selected MG patients have reactivity toward this antigen.[5] Here, we report a study on titin PEVK-binding antibody activity associated with late-onset MG. The study compares the expression of antibodies directed to the PEVK peptide, striational antigens, and myofibrils in late-onset MG. Thirty MG patients and sex/age-matched controls were studied. Among the MG patients, 8 had known thymic pathology.

METHODS

Production and purification of PEVK recombinant peptide and ELISAs were done as previously reported.[5] In brief, IgG and IgM anti-PEVK peptide activities were established using goat anti-human peroxidase conjugates (Sigma Chemical, St. Louis, MO) as secondary antibodies; sera were used at a dilution of 1/200, noncoated wells served as blanks for PEVK peptide–coated wells, and ELISA plates were

Address for correspondence: Mirta Mihovilovic, Division of Neurology, Duke University Medical Center, Durham, NC 27710. Voice: 919-684-0063; fax: 919-684-6514.
mihov001@mc.duke.edu

Ann. N.Y. Acad. Sci. 998: 351–355 (2003). **© 2003 New York Academy of Sciences.**
doi: 10.1196/annals.1254.040

developed using the TMB Microwell Peroxidase Substrate System as recommended by the supplier (Kirkegaard & Perry Laboratories, Gaithersburg, MD). Serum samples were run in triplicate, and the extent of binding was determined by subtracting OD readings of noncoated wells from those coated with PEVK peptide. Baseline for the assays was obtained using pooled normal sera with PEVK binding activity lower than 0.200 OD units. Samples producing OD readings higher than three standard deviations (SD) above the baseline were considered positive.

Rat myofibrils were prepared as previously described by Reedy *et al.*[6] Immunostaining was done as described earlier for immunocytological assays[7] using aliquots of 0.1 mL of the myofibril preparations fixed to glass slides through partial evaporation followed by 3.7% paraformaldehyde treatment for 30 min at room temperature. Antibody Ti102, which recognizes an A/I junction epitope in the I-48 motif of titin, was used as positive control.[8]

Anti-striational antibody determinations were done in the Neuroimmunology Laboratory at Mayo Clinic (Rochester, MN).[9]

RESULTS AND CONCLUSIONS

Thirty patients between the ages of 43 and 83 were part of the study. Four had thymoma and 28 were receiving immunosuppression; 6 of the immunosuppressed patients were exclusively receiving azathioprine (aza) and 1 was exclusively receiving cyclosporine (cya). The severity of MG ranged from purely ocular to moderately severe generalized (TABLE 1). At the time of sampling, 19 patients showed striational-binding antibody activity and 16 myofibril-binding activity; of these, 13 had both activities and 8 had neither. Seven sera (23%) reacted with the recombinant peptide (activity between 0.239 and 1.025 relative units; see TABLE 1); 6 had IgG that bound to the peptide and 1 had IgM. Two of 30 sex/age-matched controls had moderate IgG PEVK peptide–binding activity (0.329 and 0.464 relative units), indicating that autoimmune responses to the PEVK titin peptide were not exclusively associated with late-onset MG.

Two out of 6 samples that showed PEVK peptide–binding activity did not show striational titers. These results indicate that not all epitopes present in the titin recombinant peptide were present in the striational antigen preparation. It is possible that the titin peptide epitopes are susceptible to degradation during striational antigen purification or that conformational differences between the recombinant and striational antigen preparations account for these results. Samples that recognize the PEVK peptide had striational titers ranging from 240 to 30,720.

Two of the PEVK peptide–binding samples had antibodies that bound to the rat myofibrils, but the binding pattern did not conform to interactions taking place between MG antibodies and the PEVK domain of titin. The MG myofibrillar-binding pattern, found in 15 of 16 MG-positive samples, highlights the A/I junction and the M line of stretched myofibrils. In a fully stretched myofibril (3.5 μm sarcomere length), it is expected that PEVK peptide–binding antibodies will bind toward the middle of the I band and move toward the Z line as the myofibril contracts. It is possible that sequence or conformational differences between the recombinant peptide of human origin and fixed rat myofibrils account for these results. Alternatively, recombinant peptide epitopes engaged in MG antibody binding are not readily accessible on

TABLE 1. Titin PEVK peptide–, striational-, and myofibril-binding antibodies in late-onset MG

Age of Onset	Age at Study	Sex	Class at Study[a]	Worse Class[a]	Thymect	Rx at Study	Striational Ab titers	Myofibril Staining IgG	Myofibril Staining IgM	PEVK ELISA[d] IgG	PEVK ELISA[d] IgM
78	82	F	IIA	IIIB	na	aza	3,840	+[b]	+/-[c]	-	-
75	**80**	**F**	**IIA**	**IIA**	**na**	**mestinon**	**neg**	**-**	**-**	**1.000**	**-**
74	78	M	I	I	na	aza/prednisone	480	-	-	-	-
73	72	F	IIIB	IIIB	na	aza/prednisone	1,920	+[b]	-	-	-
73	74	M	IIB	IIIB	na	aza/prednisone	960	-	-	-	-
72	**82**	**F**	**IIA**	**IVB**	**na**	**aza/prednisone**	**7,680**	**-**	**-**	**1.025**	**-**
72	72	M	I	I	na	mestinon	7,680	+[b]	-	-	-
71	**77**	**M**	**I**	**IIA**	**na**	**aza**	**30,720**	**+[b]**	**-**	**0.320**	**-**
70	83	M	IIA	IVA	na	prednisone	neg	-	+/-[c]	-	-
70	72	M	IIA	IIIA	na	aza	neg	-	-	-	-
70	75	M	I	IIIB	na	aza	30,720	+[b]	-	-	-
70	75	F	PR	I	na	prednisone	neg	-	-	-	-
68	83	F	IIA	IIA	na	prednisone	neg	-	-	-	-
67	75	F	IIA	IIIB	na	prednisone	480	+[b]	-	-	-
67	71	M	PR	IIA	na	aza/prednisone	neg	-	-	-	-
65	73	M	IIA	IIIB	atrophic	cya/prednisone	neg	+[b]	-	-	-
64	65	M	I	I	na	aza/prednisone	neg	-	-	-	-
63	74	M	IIB	IVB	na	aza/prednisone	3,840	+[b]	-	-	-
61	68	F	IVA	IVA	na	prednisone	neg	-	-	-	-
61	61	F	IIB	IIB	Mal.thym	aza/prednisone	480	+[b]	-	-	-
60	61	M	PR	IIIA	na	prednisone	120	-	-	-	-
60	**64**	**M**	**PR**	**IIA**	**na**	**prednisone**	**3,840**	**+[b]**	**-**	**0.556**	**-**
57	62	M	I	IVB	atrophy	cya/prednisone	480	+/-[b]	-	-	-
57	63	M	I	IIB	na	aza	neg	+[b]	-	-	-
57	**64**	**M**	**I**	**IIB**	**na**	**cya**	**15,360**	**+[b]**	**-**	**-**	**0.317**
56	65	M	IIA	IIIB	atrophy	aza/prednisone	3,840	+[b]	-	-	-
54	55	M	I	IIIB	thymoma	cya/prednisone	3,840	+[b]	-	-	-
53	**60**	**M**	**I**	**IIA**	**thymoma**	**aza/prednisone**	**240**	**-**	**-**	**0.293**	**-**
50	**58**	**M**	**PR**	**IIA**	**atrophic**	**prednisone**	**neg**	**-**	**-**	**0.446**	**-**
42	43	F	IIB	IIB	thymoma	aza	480	-	-	-	-

[a]Clinical status given as MGFA class.[12] [b]Antibody binding to the A/I junction and M line (typical pattern of MG IgG binding to myofibrils). [c]Antibody binding to the A band. [d]ELISA results in relative units. For data normalization, two MG sera showing high IgG or IgM antibody-binding activity for the PEVK peptide were used as positive controls; control corresponds to a sample used in an earlier assay.[5] MG-negative samples had IgG and IgM titers of <0.173 and <0.123 relative units, respectively. Highlighted samples are those that showed PEVK peptide–binding activity that was three SD above the normal pooled sera baseline (see METHODS).

myofibrils. Interestingly, our control antibody Ti102 mimics the predominant MG myofibrillar-staining pattern. Ti102 was developed by immunization with a cloned rat cardiac titin fragment[8] and recognizes the I-48 Ig-like motif of titin.[10] It is known to bind strongly to the A/I junction as shown by electron microscopy.[11] Since the Ti102 epitope is located within an Ig motif with similarities to other Ig motifs in the titin filament, we hypothesize that Ti102 may also recognize Ig domains present in the M line of stretched myofibrils. In contracted sarcomeres, overlapping structures may mask this binding epitope.

Histopathology of the thymus was available for 8 out of 30 patients; of these, one serum from 4 patients with thymoma and one serum from 4 patients with atrophic thymi showed PEVK peptide–binding activity (TABLE 1). These observations are in agreement with earlier results obtained using a randomized MG patient population in which PEVK peptide–binding activity was found in 21% of patients with no correlation observed between this activity and thymic pathology.[5]

It is also important to indicate that, in the course of the study, we have found that 2 out of 6 transplant patients (not shown) present with PEVK peptide–binding activity. These samples have the highest IgM responses and show modest or no IgG-binding activity. Considering that, in response to an immunizing antigen, B cell–mediated production of IgM precedes IgG production, our observations suggest that 20% of the late-onset MG population (6 out of 30 patients) shows a "chronic" autoimmune response toward the PEVK domain titin peptide.

In summary, PEVK domain–binding antibodies are present in 23% of late-onset MG patients, but their binding activity does not correlate with disease severity or thymic histopathology, nor with striational-binding or myofibrillar-binding activities. Taken together, our results indicate that the humoral autoimmune response in MG varies greatly among patients. Further studies are needed to investigate the participation of different titin epitopes in the breakdown of tolerance that leads to autoimmune responses characteristic of MG. In this context, it is important to keep in mind that PEVK peptide–binding antibodies were present in 7% of sex/age-matched controls.

ACKNOWLEDGMENT

We wish to acknowledge the support of the Deane Laboratory.

REFERENCES

1. VOLTZ, R.D. *et al.* 1997. Paraneoplastic myasthenia gravis: detection of anti-MGT30 (titin) antibodies predicts thymic epithelial tumor. Neurology **49:** 1454–1457.
2. GAUTEL, M. *et al.* 1993. Titin antibodies in myasthenia gravis: identification of a main immunogenic region of titin. Neurology **43:** 1581–1585.
3. YAMAMOTO, A.M. *et al.* 2001. Anti-titin antibodies in myasthenia gravis: tight association with thymoma and heterogeneity of nonthymoma patients. Arch. Neurol. **58:** 885–890.
4. LUBKE, E. *et al.* 1998. Striational autoantibodies in myasthenia gravis patients recognize I-band titin epitopes. J. Neuroimmunol. **81:** 98–108.
5. MIHOVILOVIC, M. *et al.* 1998. Sera from myasthenia gravis patients recognize the PEVK domain of titin. Ann. N.Y. Acad. Sci. **841:** 538–541.
6. REEDY, M.K. *et al.* 1981. Thick myofilament mass determination by electron scattering measurements with the scanning transmission electron microscope. J. Muscle Res. Cell Motil. **2:** 45–64.

7. Mihovilovic, M. *et al.* 1997. Thymocytes and cultured thymic epithelial cells express transcripts encoding α-3, α-5, and β-4 subunits of neuronal nicotinic acetylcholine receptors: preferential transcription of the α-3 and β-4 genes by immature CD4+8+ thymocytes. J. Neuroimmunol. **79:** 176–184.
8. Jin, J-P. 1995. Cloned rat cardiac titin class I and class II motifs: expression, purification, characterization, and interaction with F-actin. J. Biol. Chem. **270:** 6908–6916.
9. Griesmann, G.E. *et al.* 2002. Autoantibody profiles of myasthenia gravis and Lambert-Eaton myasthenic syndrome. *In* Manual of Clinical and Laboratory Immunology. Sixth edition, pp. 1005–1012. ASM Press. Washington, D.C.
10. Labeit, S. & B. Kolmerer. 1995. Titins: giant proteins in charge of muscle ultrastructure and elasticity. Science **270:** 293–296.
11. Trombitas, K. *et al.* 1995. The mechanically active domain of titin in cardiac muscle. Circ. Res. **77:** 856–861.
12. Jaretzki, A. *et al.* 2000. Myasthenia gravis: recommendations for clinical research standards. Neurology **55:** 16–23.

Identification of Disease-Specific Autoantibodies in Seronegative Myasthenia Gravis

EMANUELA BARTOCCIONI,[a] MARIAPAOLA MARINO,[a] AMELIA EVOLI,[b] MARCUS A. RUEGG,[c] FLAVIA SCUDERI,[a] AND CARLO PROVENZANO[a]

[a]*Institute of General Pathology, Catholic University, 00168 Rome, Italy*

[b]*Institute of Neurology, Catholic University, 00168 Rome, Italy*

[c]*Biozentrum, University of Basel, CH-4051 Basel, Switzerland*

KEYWORDS: myasthenia gravis; muscle-specific kinase; MuSK; seronegative myasthenia; autoantibody; autoimmunity

Ten to 15% of patients with myasthenia gravis (MG) do not have anti-AChR antibodies (seronegative MG; SNMG). Much evidence demonstrated that these subjects have circulating pathogenic autoantibodies directed against muscle antigens other than the AChR and that plasma or purified IgG from these patients can transfer the neuromuscular transmission defect to mice.[1,2] Recent studies demonstrated that IgG from some SNMG patients bind to a surface antigen distinct from the AChR on the TE671 rhabdomyosarcoma cell line;[3] moreover, serum antibodies against the muscle-specific receptor tyrosine kinase (MuSK) were detected in these subjects.[4] On clinical ground, it was reported that some SNMG patients show a distinct clinical picture, characterized by prevalent involvement of bulbar muscles.[5] Using a cytofluorimetric assay similar to Blaes' one, we studied a large MG population and correlated the laboratory findings with clinical data: we found a high frequency of positive results in SNMG, while TE671-specific immunoreactivity was nearly absent in anti-AChR positive MG (SPMG) patients.[6] To define the candidate antigen, we analyzed immunoreactivity of 21 SNMG sera by immunoprecipitation of biotinylated membrane proteins from TE671 cells: the IgGs from 15 out of 21 SNMG patients identified a band of about 110 kDa that was absent in the immunoprecipitates from SPMG and control sera. When these immunoprecipitates were probed with an anti-MuSK antiserum, this p110 band was recognized by the anti-MuSK antibodies in all of these 15 sera (FIG. 1). FIGURE 2 shows the anti-MuSK-specific immunoreactivity distribution in patients and controls. Each of these MuSK-positive patients has a

Address for correspondence: Dr. Emanuela Bartoccioni, Institute of General Pathology, Catholic University, Largo Francesco Vito 1, 00168 Rome, Italy. Voice: +39-06-30154914; fax: +39-06-3386446.
ebartoc@rm.unicatt.it

Ann. N.Y. Acad. Sci. 998: 356–358 (2003). **© 2003 New York Academy of Sciences.**
doi: 10.1196/annals.1254.041

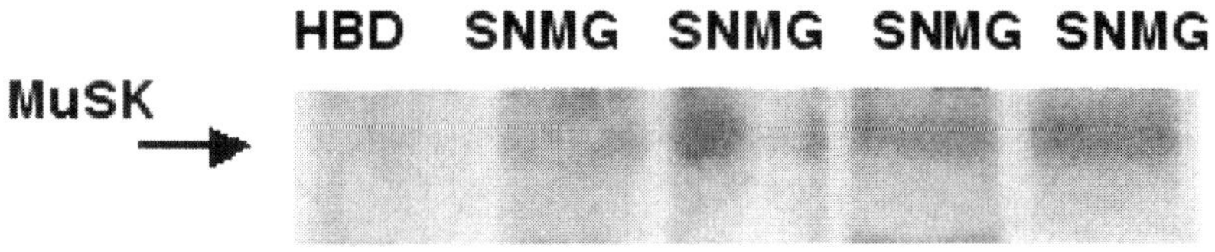

FIGURE 1. Demonstration of the presence of MuSK protein in TE671 membrane proteins immunoprecipitated by SNMG patient sera; no MuSK protein is present in the immunoprecipitates by HBD control sera.

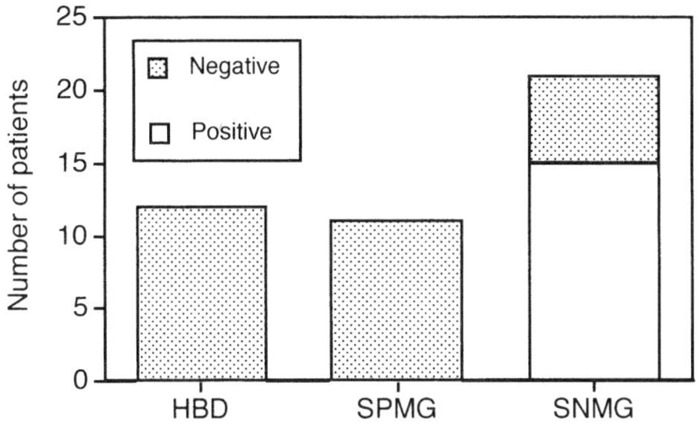

FIGURE 2. Distribution of the anti-MuSK immunoreactivity as detected by the immunoprecipitation and blotting assay.

clinical picture characterized by severe involvement of ocular and bulbar muscles, high incidence of respiratory crises, and unsatisfactory response to pyridostigmine.

CONCLUSIONS

Experimental and clinical data have long supported the view that the anti-AChR negative form of myasthenia gravis is a disease entity distinct from the anti-AChR positive one.[1] Moreover, distinctive clinical features have been reported in a subgroup of these patients.[5]

MuSK is a synapse tyrosine kinase involved in agrin-induced AChR clustering. Our findings, although not formally proving that anti-MuSK antibodies induce this form of MG, constitute an additional support to the identification of the pathogenic autoantibodies; moreover, the strong association of MuSK immunoreactivity with distinctive clinical features represents a relevant contribution to the identification and definition of SNMG as a new disease entity. Understanding the mechanism of action will not only open new therapeutic perspectives, but will also foster our understanding of synapse formation and maintenance.

REFERENCES

1. Mossman, S., A. Vincent & J. Newsom-Davis. 1986. Myasthenia gravis without acetylcholine receptor antibody: a distinct disease entity. Lancet **1:** 116–119.
2. Provenzano, C., O. Arancio, A. Evoli *et al.* 1988. Familial autoimmune myasthenia gravis with different pathogenetic antibodies. J. Neurol. Neurosurg. Psychiatry **51:** 1228–1230.
3. Blaes, F., D. Beeson, P. Plested *et al.* 2000. IgG from "seronegative" myasthenia gravis patients binds to a muscle cell line, TE671, but not to human acetylcholine receptor. Ann. Neurol. **47:** 504–510.
4. Hoch, W., J. McConville, S. Helms *et al.* 2001. Auto-antibodies to the receptor tyrosine kinase MuSK in patients with myasthenia gravis without acetylcholine receptor antibodies. Nat. Med. **7:** 365–368.
5. Evoli, A., A.P. Batocchi, M. Lo Monaco *et al.* 1996. Clinical heterogeneity of seronegative myasthenia gravis. Neuromuscul. Disord. **6:** 155–161.
6. Scuderi, F., M. Marino, L. Colonna *et al.* 2002. Anti-P110 autoantibodies identify a subtype of "seronegative" myasthenia gravis with prominent oculo-bulbar involvement. Lab. Invest. **82:** 1139–1146.

Muscle and Neuronal Autoantibody Markers of Thymoma

Neurological Correlations

STEVEN VERNINO[a] AND VANDA A. LENNON[a,b,c]

Departments of [a]Neurology, [b]Immunology, and [c]Laboratory Medicine and Pathology, Mayo Clinic, Rochester, Minnesota 55905, USA

KEYWORDS: thymoma; CRMP-5; potassium channel; myasthenia gravis; encephalitis; autonomic

Thymoma is well known for its association with autoimmune phenomena, particularly myasthenia gravis (MG).[1–3] Antibodies specific for skeletal muscle antigens are a common serological marker of thymoma, but the prevalence of antibodies against neuronal autoantigens in patients with thymoma has not been documented.

In a retrospective study of patients with thymoma (167 patients) or thymic carcinoma (5 patients), we evaluated neurological correlations and the frequency of muscle and neuronal autoantibodies. Serological studies included evaluation of muscle and neuronal ganglionic acetylcholine receptor (AChR), striational, voltage-gated potassium channel, and neuronal cytoplasmic and nuclear antibodies, including CRMP-5-IgG.[4]

MG was the most common neurological disorder in this study group. Females predominated among patients with MG (64%), but there was no significant sex predominance among thymoma patients without MG. Thirty-six patients had a neurological disorder other than MG. These included myositis, neuromuscular hyperexcitability, limbic encephalitis, autonomic neuropathy, and gastrointestinal dysmotility. MG coexisted with another neurological disorder in 23 of these 36 patients. Thirteen patients had a nonneurological autoimmune disorder, including pure red cell aplasia, pemphigus, and vitiligo.

Muscle AChR antibodies were found in all thymoma patients with MG and in a majority of patients without MG (TABLE 1). Patients with thymoma and MG typically had striational antibodies and high levels of AChR-modulating antibodies (73% had antibodies that caused more than 90% loss of AChR). Striational antibodies were detected in 76% of patients with a diagnosis of MG and in 18% of patients without clinical evidence of MG.

Address for correspondence: Steven Vernino, Department of Neurology, Mayo Clinic, 200 First Street SW, Rochester, MN 55905. Voice: 507-284-8726; fax: 507-284-1814.
verns@mayo.edu

Ann. N.Y. Acad. Sci. 998: 359–361 (2003). © 2003 New York Academy of Sciences.
doi: 10.1196/annals.1254.042

TABLE 1. Muscle autoantibody frequency with thymoma or thymic carcinoma

Patients		Muscle AChR antibodies				
Clinical subgroup	No.	Binding	Modulating	Blocking	Striational	Any muscle antibody
MG only[a]	92	100%[c]	99%[c]	64%[c]	74%[c]	100%[c]
Other neurological disorder with MG	23	100%[d]	100%[d]	48%[d]	87%[d]	100%[d]
Other neurological disorder without MG	13	54%	62%	15%	31%	69%
Uncomplicated thymoma[b]	44	30%	34%	9%	14%	52%

[a]No other neurological disorder. Includes 4 with pemphigus, 1 lupus, and 1 idiopathic thrombocytopenic purpura.
[b]No evidence of MG or other paraneoplastic disorder.
[c]Seroprevalence significantly higher than patients without MG; $p < 0.0001$ (χ^2 test).
[d]Seroprevalence significantly higher than neurological disorders without MG; $p < 0.001$.

TABLE 2. Neuronal autoantibody frequency with thymoma or thymic carcinoma

Patients					
Clinical subgroup	No.	Ganglionic AChR antibody	Potassium channel antibody	CRMP-5-IgG	Any neuronal antibody
MG only	92	9%[b]	11%[b]	17%[b]	32%[b]
Other neurological disorder (± MG)[a]	36	19%	33%[c]	31%[c]	67%[c]
Uncomplicated thymoma	44	11%	14%	7%	25%

[a]Twenty-three also had MG.
[b]No difference in seroprevalence compared to patients without MG.
[c]Seroprevalence significantly higher than patients without a paraneoplastic disorder or with MG alone; $p < 0.05$ (χ^2 test).

One or more neuronal autoantibodies were found in 37% of all thymoma patients, in 25% of those without a paraneoplastic neurological complication, and in 67% of patients with neurological disorders other than MG (TABLE 2). Potassium channel antibodies and CRMP-5-IgG were the most frequently encountered neuronal autoantibodies and were most frequent in patients with neurological disorders other than MG.

This study documents that neuronal autoantibodies complement muscle AChR and striational antibodies as serological markers of thymoma.

REFERENCES

1. SOUADJIAN, J.V. *et al.* 1974. The spectrum of diseases associated with thymoma. Arch. Intern. Med. **134:** 374–379.
2. LEWIS, J.E. *et al.* 1987. Thymoma: a clinicopathologic review. Cancer **60:** 2727–2743.
3. VERNINO, S. *et al.* 1999. Myasthenia, thymoma, presynaptic antibodies, and a continuum of neuromuscular hyperexcitability. Neurology **53**(6)**:** 1233–1239.
4. YU, Z. *et al.* 2001. CRMP-5 neuronal autoantibody: marker of lung cancer and thymoma-related autoimmunity. Ann. Neurol. **49:** 146–154.

Susceptibility of Ocular Tissues to Autoimmune Diseases

HENRY J. KAMINSKI,[a,b] ZHUYI LI,[c] CHELLIAH RICHMONDS,[a]
ROBERT L. RUFF,[a,b] AND LINDA KUSNER[a]

[a]*Department of Neurology,* [b]*Department of Neurosciences, Case Western Reserve University, University Hospitals of Cleveland, Louis Stokes Cleveland Veterans Affairs Medical Center, Cleveland, Ohio, USA*

[c]*Department of Neurology, Tang Du Hospital, Xi'an, Shaanxi, China*

ABSTRACT: The orbital tissues may form a unique immunological environment, as evidenced by autoimmune disorders that specifically target orbital tissues, particularly myasthenia gravis (MG) and Graves' ophthalmopathy (GO). The reasons for the preferential susceptibility are likely to be multiple, based on the interplay of molecular and physiological properties of extraocular muscles (EOM), the unique requirements of the ocular motor system, and the specific autoimmune pathology. Of general importance, even a minor loss of EOM force generation will sufficiently misalign the visual axes to produce dramatic symptoms, and proprioceptive feedback is limited to overcome such a deficit. Particular to MG, EOM synapses appear susceptible to neuromuscular blockade, the autoimmune pathology differs between ocular and generalized MG patients, and the influence of complement regulatory factors may be less prominent in preventing damage at EOM neuromuscular junctions. GO pathogenesis is poorly understood, but shared epitopes of orbital fibroblasts, EOM, and thyroid could lead to specific autoimmune targeting of these tissues. The differential response of orbital fibroblasts to cytokines may be a key factor in disease development. Greater appreciation of the immunologic environment of orbital tissues may lead to therapies specifically designed for orbital autoimmune diseases.

KEYWORDS: extraocular muscle; myasthenia gravis; Graves' ophthalmopathy; autoimmunity

INTRODUCTION

The anterior chamber of the eye, which allows prolonged survival of transplanted foreign tissue, has long been known to be an immune-privileged site.[1] The other orbital tissues, the extraocular muscles (EOM), orbital connective tissue, and fat also may form a unique immunological environment. The basis of this statement is (1) the differential expression of immunologically important genes and proteins within

Address for correspondence: Henry J. Kaminski, M.D., Department of Neurology, University Hospitals of Cleveland, 11100 Euclid Avenue, Cleveland, OH 44106. Voice: 216-368-0250; fax: 216-368-0249.
hjk3@po.cwru.edu

**Ann. N.Y. Acad. Sci. 998: 362–374 (2003). © 2003 New York Academy of Sciences.
doi: 10.1196/annals.1254.043**

orbital tissues, (2) the response of orbital tissue to immune modulators, and (3) the differential involvement of the orbit by autoimmune disorders. This discussion focuses on two disorders that preferentially target the orbit: myasthenia gravis (MG) and Graves' ophthalmopathy (GO). There are several reasons for the EOM to be susceptible to MG, most not related to immune factors, and these are also reviewed. The final section discusses the most common autoimmune disorder of orbital contents, GO. Here, insights into the pathology of the disease are less well defined, but speculation is provided for targeting of orbital tissue. The first section provides a detailed discussion of the EOM to form a basis to understand their preferential involvement by MG.

EXTRAOCULAR MUSCLES AND THE REQUIREMENTS OF THE OCULAR MOTOR SYSTEM

The ocular motor system has specific requirements for its muscles in the generation of eye movements.[2,3] The six muscles of each eye must be perfectly coordinated to maintain alignment of the visual axes (FIG. 1) either looking straight ahead, to the side, or when the eyes are in motion. An array of eye movements is appreciated. The eyes may move relatively slowly, as during the pursuit of an object of interest of low velocity, or extremely rapidly during a saccade that redirects gaze, as when a threatening event appears in one's peripheral field of view. Additional classes of eye movements include vergence movements (which uncouple the visual axes during convergence), the vestibular-ocular reflex, the optokinetic reflex (which rotates the

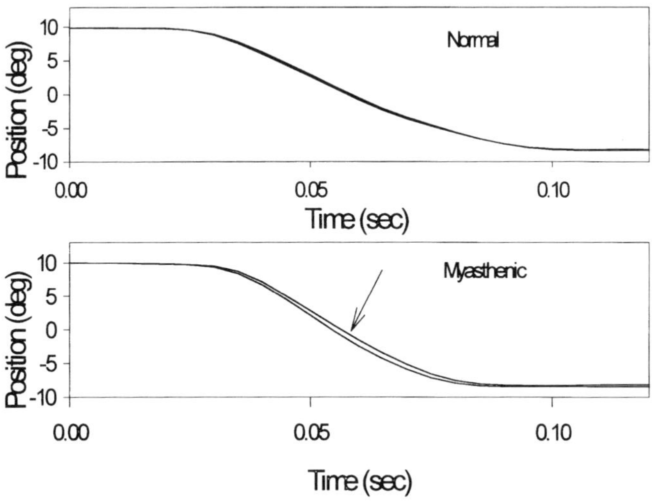

FIGURE 1. Comparison of vertical saccades in a normal subject (*top*) and a mildly affected myasthenic (*bottom*). The normal subject shows perfectly conjugate saccades, but the myasthenic shows a faster movement by the right eye (the difference in eye speed is evident at the *arrow*).

eyes to compensate for motion of the visual world), and nystagmus quick phases (which are similar to saccades, but are used to reset eye position to prevent the vestibular-ocular or optokinetic reflexes from carrying the eyes beyond the limits of comfort during rotation).[3]

The ocular motor neurons deliver the brain's message in a fashion distinct from that of spinal and bulbar motor neurons. There is a specific relationship between motor neuron firing frequency and eye position. The activity levels of the ocular motor neurons are extremely rapid compared to other motor neurons whether during a rapid movement or in an "off-position". During a saccade, firing frequencies are on the order of 400–600 Hz. In contrast, a spinal motor neuron achieves momentary stimulation rates of 150 Hz during a rapid limb movement. Further, ocular motor neurons are never silent.

EOM differ profoundly from other skeletal muscles to such an extent that the muscles should be placed in a distinct allotype, as are smooth and cardiac muscle. Gene expression studies in rats and mice using microarray or serial analysis of gene expression identify significant numbers of differentially expressed genes in EOM ranging in number from approximately 100 to 350 genes.[4–7] The studies uniformly indicate expression differences compared to other skeletal muscle of genes involved in intermediary metabolism, excitation-contraction coupling, sarcomeric organization, and transcriptional regulation.

EOM differentially express immune-related genes, suggesting that their susceptibility and response to autoimmune disorders may differ from other skeletal muscle.[8] Decay accelerating factor (Dafl), a membrane-bound complement regulatory gene, is expressed at low levels in EOM. The complement regulators serve to protect cells from spontaneous deposition of complement, which could lead to cell injury.[9] Those complement regulatory proteins found on the surface of cells are thought to be ubiquitously expressed; their distribution in skeletal muscle, however, has not been studied in detail. A circulating complement regulator (complement factor H–related protein) gene is expressed at high levels in EOM, although it has not been established whether skeletal muscle was the source of the gene transcript or other cells within the tissue.

In keeping with the requirements set by the ocular motor neurons, EOM have rapid contractile speeds and high fatigue resistance.[10,11] The EOM are highly vascular and have high densities of mitochondria, which contribute to their fatigue resistance *in vivo*.[12–15] Genomic profiles also indicate that metabolic pathways are optimized for glucose by uptake from the blood and utilization by the Krebs cycle and oxidative phosphorylation.[5,8] Such a pattern is seen in fatigue-resistant muscle of hummingbirds. EOM generate low levels of force (even when normalized for their small fiber size) compared to other skeletal muscles, which serve moving the eye well because the globe has a very low load (why the EOM generate such low levels of force is not known).[16]

The basic fiber-type classification of skeletal muscle into type 1 and 2 fibers cannot be applied to EOM. Six distinct muscle fiber-types based on anatomic location, histochemical staining, and innervational pattern are appreciated in EOM.[6,12] EOM are divided into a global region, adjacent to the globe, and an orbital region, next to the bony orbit (FIG. 2). The global region inserts into the globe, but the orbital layer has recently been appreciated to attach to a connective tissue and smooth muscle pulley system, which serves to define the path of force of an individual muscle.[17,18]

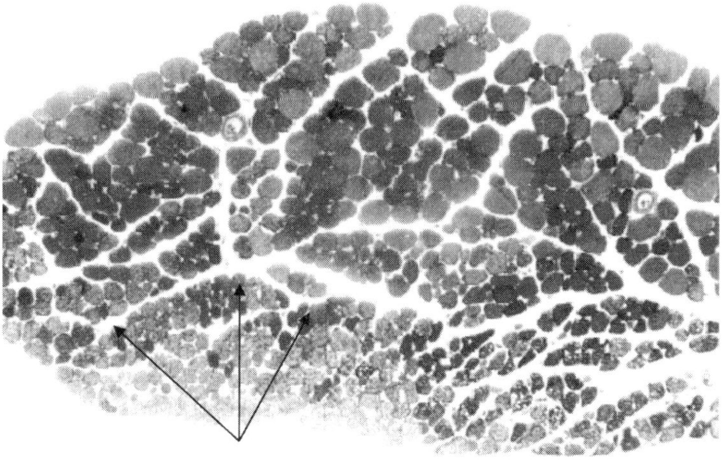

FIGURE 2. Horizontal section of a mouse EOM. The orbital region in this plane is small and restricted to the area crossed by the *arrows*. The *arrowheads* are at the border with much larger global region. Also note the significant vascularity of the EOM.

The majority of EOM fibers are singly innervated fibers (SIF) and share similar endplate morphology with other skeletal muscles having a single en plaque neuromuscular junction, although synaptic folds are less complex (FIG. 3). Again similar to other muscles, these fibers when stimulated produce a synchronized contraction and propagate an action potential. Certain SIF have greater contraction speeds and fatigue resistance (with associated higher mitochondrial content) than the twitch fibers of other skeletal muscles. The ocular motor neurons innervating the SIF lie within the three ocular motor neuron nuclei of the brain stem.[19]

About 20% of EOM fibers are innervated at multiple points, the multiply innervated fibers (MIF). Existence of these fibers was thought to be limited largely to EOM, tensor tympani, and stapedius; however, studies of humans indicate that MIF are found also in laryngeal muscles and the tongue.[20] In mammalian EOM, two MIF are present, one in each of the anatomic regions. The global MIF has en grappe endplates along its length and contracts in a graded or "tonic" fashion. The en grappe endplates compose a significantly smaller surface area of the muscle and have shallow synaptic folds compared to the en plaque endplates, which are similar in morphology to endplates of other skeletal muscle. The orbital MIF has multiple, small en grappe endplates at its ends and a single en plaque endplate at its center. These fibers contract in a graded fashion in the region of the en grappe endplates and in a twitch pattern around the en plaque endplates.[21] The motor neurons innervating the MIF lie in the periphery of ocular motor nuclei and are innervated by premotor neurons that control smooth pursuit, vergence, and gaze holding. This pattern of innervation suggests that these fibers are likely to serve a proprioceptive role, although their precise function in generation of eye movements has not been defined.[19,22]

Synaptic folds serve to increase the safety factor for neuromuscular transmission by increasing the density of acetylcholine receptors (AChR) and concentrating

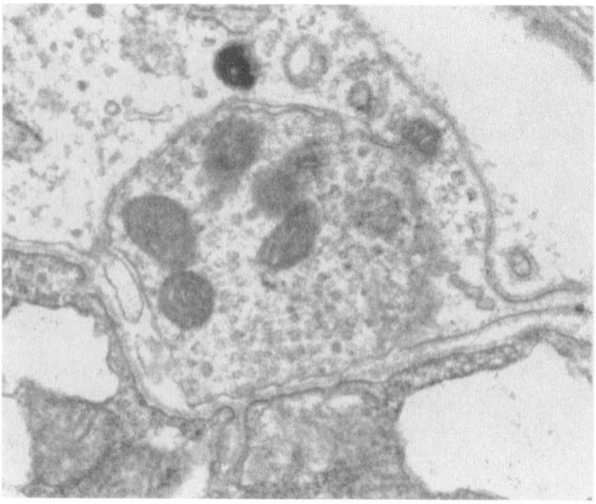

FIGURE 3. Neuromuscular junction of an EOM SIF. Appreciate the lack of synaptic folds.

current onto the depths where concentrations of sodium channels are found.[23] Their simplification at SIF junctions of EOM suggests a lower safety factor. Thus, despite the rapid motor neuron firing frequencies that these junctions experience, they perform reliably within a narrow range of tolerance. Despite the ultrastructural uniqueness of the EOM junctions, the protein scaffold that underlies the EOM junctions, whether en grappe or en plaque, does not differ significantly from that of other skeletal muscles.[24] Known signaling pathways that control development and maintenance of the junction also do not distinguish junctions. A further curious observation is that the MIF and certain SIF junctions express the fetal isoform of the AChR in the mature state.[25–28] The fetal AChR has a longer open time and lower conductance, which would effect the endplate potential time course and amplitude. The fetal AChR also has a greater calcium conductivity compared to the adult receptor and perhaps it could serve an intracellular signaling function. The function of the fetal AChR at EOM junctions has not been studied.

Given the high firing frequencies of ocular motor neurons, there may be need for reconsideration in how the EOM SIF and their motor neurons interact. For other skeletal muscles, the neuromuscular junction is a slave synapse. Every time a nerve fires, the muscle normally generates a suprathreshold endplate potential that leads to an action potential (see Ruff, this volume). In contrast, the MIF appear not to generate action potentials and do not have safety factors. Therefore, the size of the summed endplate depolarizations probably controls the amount of calcium released internally and hence force development. It may also be that the SIF do not fire in a slave-like manner. The high firing rates of EOM motor neurons have two physiological implications: (1) the endplate potentials would sum (unless the endplate potential decay at the EOM SIF junctions is much faster than at other skeletal muscle junctions at which the endplate potential would not be completely gone in a few milliseconds) and (2) the muscle action potentials are likely to be generated faster than the muscle membrane could follow (the action potentials would be expected to be generated within the relative refractory period of the last action potential). Perhaps the EOM fibers respond more like central nervous system synapses or other peripheral targets. If so, then the size of the postsynaptic response would be proportional to the motor neuron firing frequency, and the frequency of firing of the EOM fibers would in turn depend upon the size of the generator potential. Except at a low firing rate, the EOM fibers would not be "twitching"; they would generate a fused contraction force (tetanic-like in manner). In this manner, the EOM fibers would generate a more graded force response in which, when active, they would be firing continually and their firing rates would then dictate the force the muscle generates. The brain would "learn" the contractile properties of the EOM and develop firing patterns for EOM that would compensate for any existent fatigue and result in steady force output. The contractile apparatus may be optimized for consistency rather than absolute force magnitude, which would be consistent with gene expression profiles that suggest the structure of the contractile apparatus of EOM SIF differs fundamentally from that of other skeletal muscles. If this conceptualization were true, the motoneuron firing frequency would more finely control force than is true for other skeletal muscle. The "size principle" that exists for other skeletal muscle may not apply. Force would be controlled by the motor neuron firing rates rather than by having additional motor units recruited to generate additional force. Such a formulation is in keeping with the observation that ocular motor neuron firing frequency correlates with eye position.

SUSCEPTIBILITY TO MYASTHENIA GRAVIS

Weaknesses of the EOM and the levator palpebrae are the initial signs of MG in the majority of patients, ultimately occurring in nearly all patients, and may remain restricted to these muscles in 10–15% of patients.[29] The apparent preferential clinical involvement of EOM to MG could have a simple explanation.[30,31] Their dysfunction leads to the dramatic symptom of double or blurred vision.[3] Such problems are usually not ignored and patients seek out medical attention early in the course of the illness. Because of the precision required in maintaining alignment of the visual axes, even a minor reduction of force generation produces visual abnormalities. In contrast, a small reduction in force generation of a limb muscle may not be readily appreciated and is often ignored by patient and physician. Although some proprioceptive feedback in ocular motor control appears to be present, its role in maintaining ocular alignment by control of muscle force generation is unlikely to be as important as in other skeletal muscles. Thus, the recruitment of additional motor units when reduced force generation is perceived in a limb muscle would not occur in EOM (see above discussion). More complex factors contribute to the common involvement of EOM by neuromuscular transmission disorders.

Following from the discussion in the last section, anatomical characteristics are a factor in their susceptibility to neuromuscular transmission block. These fibers have less prominent synaptic folds and therefore one would predict fewer AChR and sodium channels on the postsynaptic membrane.[12] A reduction in AChR, sodium channels, and quantal content would reduce the safety factor predisposing EOM to neuromuscular transmission failure. However, the EOM miniature endplate potential amplitudes are similar to those of leg muscle junctions, indicating that AChR density is similar at these synapses.[32]

Certain multi-innervated fibers of EOM are similar to reptile tonic and intermediate fibers that have tonic contractile characteristics, with the functional consequence that force generation is directly proportional to the membrane depolarization caused by the endplate potential. Therefore, a safety factor does not exist for tonic fibers and any reduction of endplate potential induced by a loss of AChR would decrease contractile force of these fibers.[13,21] Also, the neuromuscular junctions have a scarcity to a complete absence of junctional folds. These structures in singly innervated fibers serve to increase the concentration of AChR and to concentrate current onto the depths of the folds where sodium channels are highly concentrated. Repetitive stimulation leads to a relative reduction of ACh release from the nerve terminal. At a normal junction, this is inconsequential because of a high safety factor, but at a myasthenic junction the safety factor is reduced. The EOM junctions that are subjected to high rates of stimulation would be expected to be particularly susceptible to a reduced safety factor, especially if they normally function with low or no safety factor.

The common observation of ocular weakness in other disorders of neuromuscular transmission further supports that physiological factors contribute to EOM involvement. Congenital myasthenias have a propensity for manifesting with ptosis and double vision. The same is true of botulism. Even with botulinum toxin administration for treatment of craniofacial dystonias, ocular misalignment may occur. Botulinum toxin effects appear to involve an initial effect related to blockade of the neuromuscular junction and a delayed effect due to specific orbital SIF atrophy.[33–35] The specific degeneration of these EOM fibers is surprising because EOM do not show significant morphological alteration with denervation.[36,37] In contrast to MG, Lambert-Eaton syndrome manifests with only mild to moderate ptosis, and eye movement disturbances are not as prominent.[38] Miniature endplate potential frequency is greater at EOM junctions, indicating greater calcium influx to the nerve terminal,[32] and this property may be relatively protective from the defect produced by Lambert-Eaton syndrome.

The autoimmune process of patients with ocular myasthenia does differ from patients with generalized disease. Ocular myasthenia patients have lower levels of AChR autoantibodies, and the majority are seronegative.[39,40] The intensities of T cell responses to AChR epitopes of ocular myasthenia patients are lower than that of generalized patients and they fluctuate over time.[41] The combination of mild autoimmune disease and physiologic susceptibility may be the explanation for the existence of purely ocular myasthenia. Patients with purely ocular myasthenia may not develop general disease because these patients may have residual regulatory mechanisms that suppress the autoimmune reaction. T cells (CD4+) may not be sufficiently activated to drive a pathogenic antibody response.[41] Although EOM is unique in its expression of the fetal AChR at the neuromuscular junctions,[25,27] there is no evidence that there is specific immunological targeting of the receptor by the autoimmune disease.[41–43]

There is a differential expression of complement regulatory genes in EOM.[8] We have found that some of these proteins are concentrated at the neuromuscular junction and increase their expression in the skeletal muscle of mice with experimental autoimmune MG (Li and Kaminski, unpublished observations). However,

EOM junctions appear not to show this increase in expression. Mice lacking the Dafl gene are exceptionally sensitive to experimental autoimmune MG.[44] This observation strongly suggests that an additional reason for EOM susceptibility to MG would be reduced protective mechanisms to complement-mediated tissue injury, especially when disease activity is relatively low.

The discussion has thus far ignored the levator palpebrae (LP), the elevator of the lid. The reason for the frequency of levator involvement in MG is not as easily understood as that of the EOM. The muscle shares embryological origin and innervation with the superior rectus, but otherwise is markedly different from the muscles involved in ocular motility.[12,34,45] The levator has no anatomic division and it has four muscle fiber types, with three similar to the three global SIF of EOM and a separate slow-twitch fiber. The levator fibers have twitch characteristics and some are highly fatigue-resistant, based on histological appearances, but there are no MIF. Several factors may contribute to levator involvement by MG. Nonimmune disorders of neuromuscular transmission also have a predilection for producing ptosis, suggesting that physiological reasons are likely to exist for their susceptibility to neuromuscular transmission failure. The levator fibers are under constant neuronal stimulation during eye opening. This makes neuromuscular fatigue more likely to occur compared to other skeletal muscles. The junctional folds of LP endplates are also sparse as in EOM.[45] This suggests a lower AChR number and a reduction in safety factor, making LP more susceptible to the effects of the autoimmune-induced AChR loss seen in MG.

GRAVES' OPHTHALMOPATHY

Graves' ophthalmopathy (GO) is a chronic inflammatory condition of orbital tissue and often is associated with autoimmune thyroid disease.[46,47] Patients manifest proptosis, usually painful and restricted eye movements. Severe exophthalmos is associated with prominent chemosis and eyelid edema, and may produce blindness from optic nerve compression. No involvement of skeletal muscle beyond the EOM occurs. Ophthalmopathy occurs in only 5% of patients with Graves' disease; subclinical disease, however, is detected by imaging studies in 90% of patients. Among patients with orbital tissue involvement, most are hyperthyroid, but hypothyroidism or no thyroid dysfunction may be evident.

The pathology is enlargement of orbital contents, including the muscles, to several times their normal size. A cellular infiltrate of macrophages, T cells, and some B cells is characteristic.[47,48] The lymphocytes and macrophages that infiltrate retroocular connective tissue secrete cytokines, which induce cell proliferation, glycosaminoglycan synthesis by orbital fibroblasts, and recruitment of adipose precursor cells. The hydrophylic glycosaminoglycans, predominantly hyaluronic acid and chondroitin sulfate, accumulate and bind water, leading to profound tissue swelling.[49–51] The EOM fibers become separated by the increase in glycosaminoglycans and extracellular fluid; the EOM fibers, however, remain intact. As the disease progresses, edema and increased fibrous tissue may produce tissue hypoxia, injuring surrounding cells, including muscle fibers. Fibers may degenerate,[52] but this occurs at late stages. Some studies do not identify prominent inflammation and little muscle fiber damage, but this could be a function of sampling and disease stage.[53]

The inflammatory process is driven by T cells in response to an antigen that has yet to be firmly identified. The pathogenesis of ophthalmopathy may be related to an immune-mediated process involving a shared antigen between thyroid and orbital protein.[54,55] In Graves' disease, thyroid-stimulating antibodies are thought to initiate immune-mediated destruction of the thyroid and thyrotoxicosis.[56] Some of these antibodies are thought to cross-react with orbital tissues, suggesting a direct link between the thyroid disease and the ophthalmopathy. The orbital fibroblasts are presently the leading candidates for harboring the antigenic target, but some studies indicate EOM epitopes are bound by Graves' sera. Orbital fibroblasts (but not fibroblasts from other locations) are recognized in an MHC class I–restricted manner by T cells obtained from orbital tissue of Graves' patients. EOM extracts are not. The leading autoantigenic target is the thyroid-stimulating hormone receptor (TSHr). Low levels of TSHr gene expression are identified in orbital tissue, including EOM,[57] and immunoreactivity of the TSHr is found in orbital fibroblasts.[58,59] Cultured orbital fibroblasts in the presence of thyroid-stimulating hormone express TSHr.[47] Severe Graves' disease usually only occurs among patients with high circulating TSHr antibodies; however, in general, there is not a tight correlation with clinical status. Antibodies in patients with ophthalmopathy have been found to react with EOM and retroorbital connective tissue.[60–62] These do not correlate with disease severity and are likely to be secondary phenomena of inflammation.[63,64] Another factor that may direct the immune response to the orbit is that there are interconnections between the lymphatic drainage of the thyroid and the orbit. Consequently, orbital tissue may be exposed to high concentrations of thyroglobulin and its antithyroid autoantibodies.[65] Variations in lymphatic anatomy could then account for the frequent asymmetry of ocular involvement.

In contrast to MG, the involvement of complement as a disease effector mechanism has not been established. Activated complement components are found in orbital connective tissue, but not in all patient biopsies.[66–68] Sera of patients with GO do not induce complement-mediated lysis of isolated EOM or orbital fibroblasts using *in vitro* assays.[67] The response of orbital fibroblasts to cytokines that are expressed by orbital-infiltrating T cells of GO may influence complement activation. In contrast to all other cell types, Daf expression is not increased by tumor necrosis factor (TNF) K in orbital fibroblasts.[69] However, Daf expression is upregulated by TNF-β. The cytokine expression profile of GO T cells has not been firmly established; some investigators have reported a T_H1-type profile (IL-2, IFN-γ, TNF-K), others a T_H2 profile (IL-4, IL-5, IL-10), and others a mixed picture.[46] Depending on the cytokine profile and response of orbital fibroblasts (or other target cells), there may be more or less complement activation.

Autoimmune thyroid disease and MG appear to share some characteristics. A proportion of patients with MG has thyroid dysfunction, and rarely GO and MG present simultaneously. GO patients with MG have a significantly greater prevalence of ophthalmopathy without coincident hyperthyroidism. Among patients with Graves' disease and ocular MG, ophthalmopathy may be more commonly found than among those with Graves' disease and generalized MG. The results suggest a preferential association between the ocular manifestations of Graves' disease and MG, which may be due to immunological cross-reactivity against common autoimmune targets in the eye muscle as well as to a common genetic background.[70]

CONCLUSIONS

MG and GO are two diseases that may produce widespread disease: in the one case, other skeletal musclc; and in the other, the thyroid gland as well as the pretibial dermis; they also have propensity for specific involvement of orbital tissues. Other inflammatory conditions, orbital myositis and idiopathic orbital inflammation, exclusively damage EOM and other orbital tissue, but the inflammatory myopathies, which diffusely involve skeletal muscle and may involve the heart, spare the EOM. The conceptualization of the orbit as a unique immune environment is in its infancy, and this summary has only been able to provide indirect support of this hypothesis.

ACKNOWLEDGMENTS

The Office of Research and Development, the Medical Research Service of the Department of Veterans Affairs, and the National Institutes of Health (Grant Nos. EY-13238 and P30 EY-11373) supported this work.

REFERENCES

1. STREILEIN, J.W. *et al.* 2002. Immunobiology and privilege of neuronal retina and pigment epithelium transplants. Vision Res. **42**: 487–495.
2. KAMINSKI, H.J. & R.J. LEIGH, Eds. 2002. Neurobiology of Eye Movements. Vol. 956. N.Y. Acad. Sci. New York.
3. LEIGH, R.J. & D.S. ZEE. 1999. The Neurology of Eye Movements. Davis. Philadelphia.
4. ANDRADE, F.H., A.P. MERRIAM & J.D. PORTER. 2002. Extraocular muscle gene expression and function after dark rearing. Ann. N.Y. Acad. Sci. **956:** 391–393.
5. FISCHER, M.D. *et al.* 2002. Expression profiling reveals metabolic and structural components of extraocular muscles. Physiol. Genomics **9:** 71–84.
6. PORTER, J.D. 2002. Extraocular muscle: cellular adaptations for a diverse functional repertoire. Ann. N.Y. Acad. Sci. **956:** 7–16.
7. CHENG, G. & J.D. PORTER. 2002. Transcriptional profile of rat extraocular muscle by serial analysis of gene expression. Invest. Ophthalmol. Visual Sci. **43**: 1048–1058.
8. PORTER, J.D. *et al.* 2001. Extraocular muscle is defined by a fundamentally distinct gene expression profile. Proc. Natl. Acad. Sci. USA **98:** 12062–12067.
9. MIWA, T. & W.C. SONG. 2001. Membrane complement regulatory proteins: insight from animal studies and relevance to human diseases. Int. Immunopharmacol. **1:** 445–459.
10. LYNCH, G.S., B.R. FRUEH & D.A. WILLIAMS. 1994. Contractile properties of single skinned fibres from the extraocular muscles, the levator and superior rectus, of the rabbit. J. Physiol. **475:** 337–346.
11. FRUEH, B.R. *et al.* 1994. Contractile properties and temperature sensitivity of the extraocular muscles, the levator and superior rectus, of the rabbit. J. Physiol. **475:** 327–336.
12. SPENCER, R.F. & J.D. PORTER. 1988. Structural organization of the extraocular muscles. *In* Neuroanatomy of the Oculomotor System, pp. 33–79. Elsevier. Amsterdam.
13. RUFF, R.L. *et al.* 1989. Ocular muscles: physiology and structure-function correlations. Bull. Soc. Belg. Ophthalmol. **237:** 321–352.
14. WOOTEN, G.F. & D.J. REIS. 1972. Blood flow in extraocular muscle of cat. Arch. Neurol. **26:** 350–352.
15. WILCOX, L.M. *et al.* 1981. Comparative extraocular muscle blood flow. J. Exp. Zool. **215:** 87–90.
16. RICHMONDS, C.R. & H.J. KAMINSKI. 2001. Nitric oxide synthase expression and nitric oxide effects on contractility in rat lateral rectus. FASEB J. **15:** 1764–1770.

17. DEMER, J.L. 2002. The orbital pulley system: a revolution in concepts of orbital anatomy. Ann. N.Y. Acad. Sci. **956:** 17–32.
18. DEMER, J.L., S.Y. OH & V. POUKENS. 2000. Evidence for active control of rectus extraocular muscle pulleys. Invest. Ophthalmol. Visual Sci. **41**: 1280–1290.
19. BÜTTNER-ENNEVER, J. *et al.* 2001. Motoneurons of twitch and nontwitch extraocular muscle fibers in the abducens, trochlear, and oculomotor nuclei of monkeys. J. Comp. Neurol. **438:** 318–335.
20. HAN, Y. *et al.* 1999. Slow tonic muscle fibers in the thyroarytenoid muscles of human vocal folds: a possible specialization for speech. Anat. Rec. **256:** 146–157.
21. JACOBY, J., D.J. CHIARANDINI & E. STEFANI. 1989. Electrical properties and innervation of fibers in the orbital layer of rat extraocular muscles. J. Neurophysiol. **61:** 116–125.
22. BÜTTNER-ENNEVER, J. *et al.* 2002. Modern concepts of brainstem anatomy: from extraocular motoneurons to proprioceptive pathways. Ann. N.Y. Acad. Sci. **956:** 75–84.
23. WOOD, S.J. & C.R. SLATER. 2001. Safety factor at the neuromuscular junction. Prog. Neurobiol. **64:** 393–429.
24. KHANNA, S. & J.D. PORTER. 2002. Conservation of synapse-signaling pathways at the extraocular muscle neuromuscular junction. Ann. N.Y. Acad. Sci. **956:** 394–396.
25. HORTON, R.M., A.A. MANFREDI & B.M. CONTI-TRONCONI. 1993. The "embryonic" gamma subunit of the nicotinic acetylcholine receptor is expressed in adult extraocular muscle. Neurology **43:** 983–986.
26. KAMINSKI, H.J. *et al.* 1995. The γ-subunit of the acetylcholine receptor is not expressed in the levator palpebrae superioris. Neurology **45:** 516–518.
27. KAMINSKI, H.J., L.L. KUSNER & C.H. BLOCK. 1996. Expression of acetylcholine receptor isoforms at extraocular muscle endplates. Invest. Ophthalmol. Visual Sci. **37:** 345–351.
28. MISSIAS, A.C. *et al.* 1996. Regulation of the acetylcholine receptor gamma subunit gene in developing skeletal muscle: analysis with subunit-specific antibodies, transgenic mice, and cultured cells. Dev. Biol. **179:** 223.
29. GROB, D. *et al.* 1987. The course of myasthenia gravis and therapies affecting outcome. Ann. N.Y. Acad. Sci. **505:** 472–499.
30. KAMINSKI, H.J. *et al.* 2002. Differential susceptibility of the ocular motor system to disease. Ann. N.Y. Acad. Sci. **956:** 42–54.
31. UBOGU, E.E. & H.J. KAMINSKI. 2002. Preferential involvement of extraocular muscle by myasthenia gravis. Neuroophthalmology **25:** 219–228.
32. MOSIER, D.R., L. SIKLÓS & S. APPEL. 2000. Resistance of extraocular motoneuron terminals to effects of amyotropic lateral sclerosis sera. Neurology **54:** 252–255.
33. STAHL, J. *et al.* 1998. Clinical evidence of extraocular muscle fiber-type specificity of botulinum toxin. Neurology **51:** 1093–1099.
34. PORTER, J.D., S. STREBECK & N.F. CAPRA. 1991. Botulinum-induced changes seen in monkey eylid muscle: comparison with changes seen in extraocular muscle. Arch. Ophthalmol. **109:** 396–404.
35. SPENCER, R.F. & K.W. MCNEER. 1987. Botulinum toxin paralysis of adult monkey extraocular muscle: structural alterations in orbital, singly innervated muscle fibers. Arch. Ophthalmol. **105:** 1703–1711.
36. PORTER, J.D., L.A. BURNS & E.J. MCMAHON. 1989. Denervation of primate extraocular muscle: a unique pattern of structurral alterations. Invest. Ophthalmol. Visual Sci. **30:** 1894–1908.
37. CHRISTIANSEN, S.P. *et al.* 1993. Type specific changes in fiber morphometry following denervation of caninine extraocular muscle. Exp. Mol. Pathol. **56:** 87–95.
38. O'NEILL, J.H., N.M.F. MURRAY & J. NEWSOM-DAVIS. 1988. The Lambert-Eaton myasthenic syndrome: a review of 50 cases. Brain **111:** 577–596.
39. ODA, K. & Y. ITO. 1981. Myasthenia gravis: antibodies to acetylcholine receptor in ocular myasthenia gravis. J. Neurol. **225:** 251–258.
40. LIMBURG, P.C. *et al.* 1983. Anti-acetylcholine receptor antibodies in myasthenia gravis. I. Relation to clinical parameters in 250 patients. J. Neurol. Sci. **58:** 357–370.
41. WANG, Z. *et al.* 2000. T-cell recognition of muscle acetylcholine receptor in ocular myasthenia gravis. J. Neuroimmunol. **108:** 29–39.

42. MACLENNAN, C. *et al.* 1997. Acetylcholine receptor expression in human extraocular muscles and their susceptibility to myasthenia gravis. Ann. Neurol. **41:** 423–431.
43. KAMINSKI, H. & R. RUFF. 1997. Ocular muscle involvement by myasthenia gravis. Ann. Neurol. **41:** 419–420.
44. LIN, F. *et al.* 2002. Enhanced susceptibility to myasthenia gravis in the absence of decay-accelerating factor protection. J. Clin. Invest. **110:** 1269–1274.
45. PORTER, J.D., L.A. BURNS & P.J. MAY. 1989. Morphological substrate for eyelid movements: innervation and structure of primate levator palpebrae superioris and obicularis oculi muscles. J. Comp. Neurol. **287:** 64–81.
46. BAHN, R. 2000. Understanding the immunology of Graves' ophthalmopathy. Endocrinol. Metab. Clin. North Am. **29:** 287–296.
47. HEUFLEDER, A.E. 2000. Pathogenesis of ophthalmopathy in autoimmune thyroid disease. Rev. Endocr. Metab. Dis. **1:** 87–95.
48. MCGREGOR, A.M. 1998. Has the target autoantigen for Graves' ophthalmopathy been found? Lancet **352:** 595–596.
49. SMITH, T., R.S. BAHN & C.A. GORMAN. 1989. Connective tissue, glycosaminoglycans, and diseases of the thyroid. Endocr. Rev. **10:** 366–391.
50. HUFNAGEL, T.J. *et al.* 1984. Immunohistochemical and ultrastructural studies on the exenterated orbital tissues of a patient with Graves' disease. Ophthalmology **91:** 1411–1419.
51. FELLS, P. 1978. Orbital pathology. *In* The Thyroid, pp. 660. Harper & Row. New York.
52. WEETMAN, A.P. *et al.* 1989. Immunohistochemical analysis of the retrobulbar tissues in Graves' ophthalmopathy. Clin. Exp. Immunol. **75:** 222–227.
53. TALLSTEDT, L. & R. NORBERG. 1988. Immunohistochemical staining of normal and Graves extraocular muscle. Invest. Ophthalmol. Visual Sci. **29:** 175–184.
54. YAMADA, M., A.W. LI & J.R. WALL. 2000. Thyroid-associated ophthalmopathy: clinical features, pathogenesis, and management. Crit. Rev. Clin. Lab. Sci. **37:** 523–549.
55. WALL, J. 1995. Extrathyroidal manifestations of Graves' disease. J. Clin. Endocrinol. Metab. **80:** 3427–3429.
56. WALL, J. *et al.* 1991. Thyroid-associated ophthalmopathy—a model for the association of organ-specific autoimmune disorders. Immunol. Today **12:** 150–153.
57. MAJOR, B., A. CURES & A. FRAUMAN. 1997. The full length and splice variant thyrotropin receptor is expressed exclusively in skeletal muscle of extraocular origin: a link to the pathogenesis of Graves' ophthalmopathy. Biochem. Biophys. Res. Commun. **230:** 493–496.
58. BAHN, R.S. *et al.* 1998. Thyrotropin receptor expression in cultured Graves' orbital preadipocyte fibroblasts is stimulated by thyrotropin. Thyroid **8:** 193–196.
59. BAHN, R.S. *et al.* 1998. Thyrotropin receptor expression in Graves orbital adipose/connective tissue: potential autoantigen in Graves ophthalmopathy. J. Clin. Endocrinol. Metab. **83:** 998–1002.
60. AHMAN, A. *et al.* 1987. Antibodies to porcine eye muscle in patients with Graves ophthalmopathy: identification of serum immunoglobins directed against unique determinants by immunoblotting and enzyme-linked immunosorbent assay. J. Clin. Endocrinol. Metab. **64:** 454–460.
61. HIROMATSU, Y. *et al.* 1988. A thyroid cytotoxic antibody that cross-reacts with an eye muscle cell surface antigen may be the cause of thyroid associated ophthalmopathy. J. Clin. Endocrinol. Metab. **67:** 565–570.
62. SCHIFFERDECKER, E. *et al.* 1989. Re-evaluation of eye muscle autoantibody determination in Graves' ophthalmopathy: failure to detect a specific antigen by use of enzyme-linked immunosorbent assay, indirect immunofluorescence, and immunoblotting techniques. Acta Endocrinol. (Copenh.) **121:** 643–650.
63. KADLUBOWSKI, M., W.J. IRVINE & A.C. ROWLAND. 1986. The lack of specificity of ophthalmic immunoglobulins in Graves' disease. J. Clin. Endocrinol. Metab. **63:** 990–995.
64. GUNJI, K. *et al.* 1999. A 63 kDa skeletal muscle protein associated with eye muscle inflammation in Graves' disease is identified as the calcium binding protein calsequestrin. Autoimmunity **29:** 1–9.
65. KRISS, J. 1975. Studies on the pathogenesis of Graves ophthalmopathy (with some related observations regarding therapy). Recent Prog. Horm. Res. **31:** 3533.

66. ANTONELLI, A. *et al.* 1996. IgG, IgA, and C3 deposits in the extra-thyroidal manifestations of autoimmune Graves' disease: their *in vitro* solubilization by intravenous immunoglobulin. Clin. Exp. Rheumatol. **14**(suppl. 15)**:** S31–S35.
67. DILLON, J. *et al.* 1989. Failure to detect complement-mediated antibody-dependent cytotoxicity against human orbital tissue cells in the serum of patients with thyroid-associated ophthalmopathy. Autoimmunity **5:** 125–132.
68. ROSEN, C.E. *et al.* 1992. Immunohistochemical evidence for C3bi involvement in Graves ophthalmopathy. Ophthalmology **99:** 1325–1331.
69. COCUZZI, E.T. *et al.* 2001. Upregulation of DAF (CD55) on orbital fibroblasts by cytokines: differential effects of TNF-beta and TNF-alpha. Curr. Eye Res. **23:** 86–92.
70. MARINO, M. *et al.* 2000. Increased frequency of euthyroid ophthalmopathy in patients with Graves' disease associated with myasthenia gravis. Thyroid **10:** 799–802.

Induction of Myasthenia Gravis in HLA Transgenic Mice by Immunization with Human Acetylcholine Receptors

HUAN YANG,[a] ELZBIETA GOLUSZKO,[a] CHELLA DAVID,[b] DAVID K. OKITA,[c] BIANCA CONTI-FINE,[c] TEH-SHENG CHAN,[a] MATHILDE A. POUSSIN,[a] AND PREMKUMAR CHRISTADOSS[a]

[a]*Department of Microbiology and Immunology, University of Texas Medical Branch, Galveston, Texas 77555-1070, USA*

[b]*Department of Immunology, Mayo Clinic, Rochester, Minnesota 55905, USA*

[c]*Department of Biochemistry, Molecular Biology, and Biophysics, University of Minnesota, Minneapolis–St. Paul, Minnesota 55108, USA*

ABSTRACT: We utilized HLA transgenic mice to identify the dominant epitopes on the human (H)–AChR α subunit. The cytoplasmic H-AChR peptide α320–337 was the dominant T cell epitope for DQ8, DR3, and DQ8×DQ6 F1 mice. The H-AChR-immunized HLA-DQ8, DR3, DQ8×DR3 F1 and DQ8×DQ6 F1 mice developed clinical EAMG, whereas HLA-DQ6 mice were less susceptible.

KEYWORDS: myasthenia gravis (MG); experimental autoimmune myasthenia gravis (EAMG); AChR; HLA transgenic mice

INTRODUCTION

Myasthenia gravis (MG) and experimental autoimmune myasthenia gravis (EAMG) are T cell–dependent, antibody (Ab)–mediated diseases.[1] In EAMG, the immune response gene at the I-A subregion controls Th cell recognition of AChR.[2] MG is associated with polymorphism (certain alleles) of the HLA-DQ genes.[3] HLA B8 and HLA DR3 are linked to MG in Caucasians. On the other hand, the DQ6 allele has been suggested to be negatively associated with MG. Raju *et al.* immunized HLA-DQ8, DQ6, and DR3 transgenic mice with *Torpedo californica* AChR (T-AChR) in CFA and found DQ8 and DR3 mice developed EAMG, while DQ6 mice had reduced susceptibility to EAMG.[4,5] An epitope in the T-AChR α-chain 146–162 peptide was shown to be involved in EAMG pathogenesis. Administration of a high dose of the T-α146–162 peptide significantly prevented EAMG development.[6]

Address for correspondence: Premkumar Christadoss, M.D., Department of Microbiology and Immunology, University of Texas Medical Branch, Galveston, TX 77555-1070. Voice: 409-772-5857; fax: 409-747-6869.
pchrista@utmb.edu

Ann. N.Y. Acad. Sci. 998: 375–378 (2003). © 2003 New York Academy of Sciences.
doi: 10.1196/annals.1254.044

In this study, we utilized the HLA transgenic mice to identify the dominant epitopes on the human (H)–AChR α subunit. The cytoplasmic H-AChR peptide α320–337 was the dominant T cell epitope for DQ8, DR3, and DQ8×DQ6 F1 mice. H-AChR-immunized HLA-DQ8, DR3, DQ8×DR3 F1 and DQ8×DQ6 F1 mice developed clinical EAMG, whereas HLA-DQ6 mice were less susceptible.

MATERIALS AND METHODS

Mice

Transgenic mice deficient in the mouse MHC class II molecules, which express only functional human HLA-DQ8, DQ6, or DR3 genes in the C57BL/10 background, were used for this study.[7]

Human AChR and Peptides

H-AChR was purified from the TE671 cell line, which expresses H-AChR, by neurotoxin affinity column.[8,9] The overlapping peptides spanning most of the H-AChR α-subunit sequence were synthesized by parallel synthesis.[10,11]

Induction and Clinical/Immunopathological Evaluation of EAMG

The methods of induction and clinical evaluation of EAMG were done according to previously published methods.[6,8]

Mapping the T Cell Epitopes on the H-AChR α-Subunit

DQ8, DQ6, DR3, and DQ8×DQ6 F1 transgenic mice were immunized with 20 μg of H-AChR in CFA. After 7 days, pooled draining (popliteal and inguinal) LNC at 4×10^5 cells in 200 μL were exposed in triplicate to each of the overlapping synthetic H-AChR-α (H-α) subunit peptides (40 μg/mL) and H-AChR (0.5 μg/mL) and PBS. Lymphocyte proliferation was evaluated as previously described.[6,8]

RESULTS AND DISCUSSION

H-AChR-Immunized HLA-DQ8, DR3, DQ8×DR3 F1, and DQ8×DQ6 F1 Mice Developed Clinical EAMG

After the third immunization, 75% DQ8 and DR3 mice and 80% DQ8×DR3 F1 mice developed clinical EAMG (from grade 1 to 3), but only 25% DQ6 mice developed low-grade clinical EAMG. The H-AChR and H-α320–337 specific lymphocyte proliferation was significantly reduced from DQ6 mice versus those from DQ8, DR3, and DQ8×DQ6 F1 mice.[12] DQ8×DQ6 F1 mice developed clinical EAMG with an incidence and severity similar to those of DQ8 mice, suggesting one MG-susceptible HLA-DQ allele in a heterozygote could be sufficient for full expression of MG.

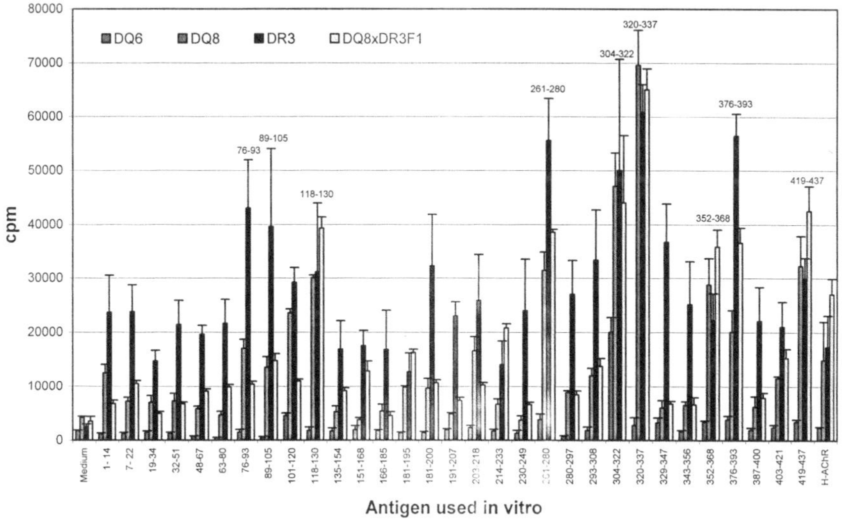

FIGURE 1. T cell epitope mapping on the H-AChR α subunit in DQ6, DQ8, DR3 transgenic mice and DQ8×DQ6 F1 mice immunized with H-AChR. Mice were immunized with H-AChR (20 μg) in CFA. Seven days later, draining LNC (popliteal and inguinal) were exposed to each of the overlapping synthetic H-AChR-α subunit peptides (40 μg/mL) and H-AChR (0.5 μg/mL), and ^{3}H-incorporation determined. The error bars are standard error.

Peptide H-α320–337 Was Most Strongly Recognized by T Cells of H-AChR-Immunized DQ8, DR3, and DQ8×DQ6 F1 Mice

The sequence α320–337 was a dominant T cell epitope in DQ8, DR3, and DQ8×DQ6 F1 mice. Peptide α304–322 and α419–437 were subdominant epitopes in DQ8 mice. H-AChR-immunized T cells of DR3 mice responded well to numerous peptides of the H-AChR α-subunit, with α320–337 as one of the dominant peptides. H-AChR-immune T cells from DQ6 mice responded moderately to peptide α304–322. H-AChR-immune T cells from DQ8×DQ6 F1 mice responded to almost all of the peptides recognized by H-AChR-immune T cells from DQ8 mice (FIG. 1).[12] Several studies have mapped the T cell epitopes on the different H-AChR α-subunits using H-AChR-specific CD4$^+$ derived from MG patients.[10] Those studies demonstrated that the sequence α320–337 was recognized by several MG patients.[11] H-AChR-immune T cells of DQ8, DR3, and DQ8×DQ6 F1 mice responded dominantly to the H-α320–337 peptide. The sequence H-α320–337 might form a promiscuous epitope, recognized by T cells of MG patients with different HLA-DQ or DR alleles, besides the DQ8 and DR3 alleles. The finding that this peptide is frequently recognized by CD4$^+$ cells of MG patients, irrespective of their class II haplotype,[10,11] supports this possibility. If peptide H-α320–337 induces T cell tolerance amelioration of EAMG in HLA transgenic mice, this H-α320–337 peptide could be used for antigen-specific tolerance induction in human MG.

ACKNOWLEDGMENTS

This study was supported by the MDA, NIH-A1049995, and a Texas Higher Education Coordinating Board Advanced Technology Program Grant (to P. Christadoss) and by NIH: NINDS NS 23919 (to B. Conti-Fine). Huan Yang was an MG Foundation Osserman/Sosin/McClure postdoctoral fellow and is now an MDA Neuromuscular Disease Research Career Award recipient. Mathilde Poussin was an MDA Neuromuscular Disease Research Career Award recipient.

The full paper of this study was published in reference 12. Permission has been obtained from the Copyright Clearance Center, Inc., to republish this article.

REFERENCES

1. Christadoss, P., M. Poussin & C. Deng. 2000. Animal models of myasthenia gravis. Clin. Immunol. **94:** 75–87.
2. Christadoss, P., J.M. Lindstrom, R.W. Melvold *et al.* 1985. Mutation at I-A beta chain prevents experimental autoimmune myasthenia gravis. Immunogenetics **21:** 33–38.
3. Bell, J., L. Rassenti, S. Smoot *et al.* 1986. HLA-DQ beta-chain polymorphism linked to myasthenia gravis. Lancet **1:** 1058–1060.
4. Raju, R., W.Z. Zhan, P. Karachunski *et al.* 1998. Polymorphism at the HLA-DQ locus determines susceptibility to experimental autoimmune myasthenia gravis. J. Immunol. **160:** 4169–4174.
5. Raju, R., E.G. Spack & C.S. David. 2001. Acetylcholine receptor peptide recognition in HLA DR3-transgenic mice: *in vivo* responses correlate with MHC-peptide binding. J. Immunol. **167:** 1118–1124.
6. Wu, B., C. Deng, E. Goluszko *et al.* 1997. Tolerance to a dominant T cell epitope in the acetylcholine receptor molecule induces epitope spread and suppresses murine myasthenia gravis. J. Immunol. **159:** 3016–3023.
7. Taneja, V. & C.S. David. 1998. HLA transgenic mice as humanized mouse models of disease and immunity. J. Clin. Invest. **101:** 921–926.
8. Wu, B., E. Goluszko & P. Christadoss. 1997. Experimental autoimmune myasthenia gravis in the mouse. *In* Current Protocols of Immunology. Vol. 3, pp. 8.1–8.16. Wiley. New York.
9. Luther, M.A., R. Schoepfer, P. Whiting *et al.* 1989. A muscle acetylcholine receptor is expressed in the human cerebellar medulloblastoma cell line TE671. J. Neurosci. **9:** 1083–1096.
10. Protti, M.P., A.A. Manfredi, C. Straub *et al.* 1990. $CD4^+$ T cell response to human acetylcholine receptor α subunit in myasthenia gravis: a study with synthetic peptides. J. Immunol. **144:** 1276–1281.
11. Manfredi, A., M.H. Yuen, L. Moiola *et al.* 1994. Human acetylcholine receptor presentation in myasthenia gravis: DR restriction of autoimmune T epitopes and binding of synthetic receptor sequences to DR molecules. J. Immunol. **152:** 4165–4174.
12. Yang, H., E. Goluszko, C. David *et al.* 2002. Mapping myasthenia gravis–associated T cell epitopes on human acetylcholine receptors in HLA transgenic mice. J. Clin. Invest. **109:** 1111–1120.

Production and Characterization of a T Cell Receptor Transgenic Mouse Recognizing the Immunodominant Epitope of the *Torpedo californica* Acetylcholine Receptor

ALEXEI MIAGKOV,[a] ADRIAN A. LOBITO,[b] BINGZHI YANG,[a] MARCELA F. LOPES,[b] ROBERT N. ADAMS,[a] GREGORY R. PALARDY,[b] MICHELE M. JOHNSON,[b] HUGH I. McFARLAND,[b] MICHAEL J. LENARDO,[b] AND DANIEL B. DRACHMAN[a]

[a]*Department of Neurology, Johns Hopkins School of Medicine, Baltimore, Maryland, USA*

[b]*National Institute of Allergy and Infectious Diseases, National Institutes of Health, Bethesda, Maryland, USA*

KEYWORDS: transgenic mice; immunodominant epitope; T cells; TAChR

INTRODUCTION

In patients with MG and animals with EAMG, the pathogenic antibody response to AChR is T cell–dependent.[1] In C57BL/6 (B6) mice, the majority of $CD4^+$ T cells respond to an immunodominant epitope derived from the α subunit of TAChR, comprising amino acids 146–162 (Tα146–162).[2] Mice expressing transgenic T cell receptors specific for the immunodominant epitope of TAChR might be utilized to analyze several important issues regarding the pathogenesis and treatment of MG:

(1) We wondered how a marked increase of the T cells specific for the Tα146–162 epitope would influence anti-AChR antibody production and the disease process in mice.
(2) The availability of a model with large numbers of AChR-specific T cells will be invaluable in the testing of novel immunotherapeutic strategies.
(3) A transgenic mouse model for EAMG could be used to study disease pathogenesis in conjunction with the plethora of available mice with genetically altered immune properties.
(4) A transgenic model with a highly restricted AChR-specific T cell repertoire should facilitate investigation of the role of T cells in providing help for the heterogeneous AChR antibody repertoire in MG and EAMG.

Address for correspondence: Alexei Miagkov, Department of Neurology, Johns Hopkins School of Medicine, Baltimore, MD 21287. Voice: 410-614-4276; fax: 410-955-1961.
miagkov@earthlink.net

**Ann. N.Y. Acad. Sci. 998: 379–383 (2003). © 2003 New York Academy of Sciences.
doi: 10.1196/annals.1254.045**

CREATION OF THE TRANSGENIC MICE

To generate transgenic mice, we cloned the functionally rearranged variable regions of the T cell receptor (TCR) α (Vα8) and β (Vβ6) chain genes from a T cell hybridoma that had previously been developed to recognize the Tα146–162 epitope[3] and inserted them into appropriate transgenic vectors for expression of the TCR chains in T lymphocytes.[4] The resulting constructs were used to generate one Vα founder mouse and one Vβ founder mouse on a B6 background. The founders were crossbred to establish αβ double-transgenic mice.

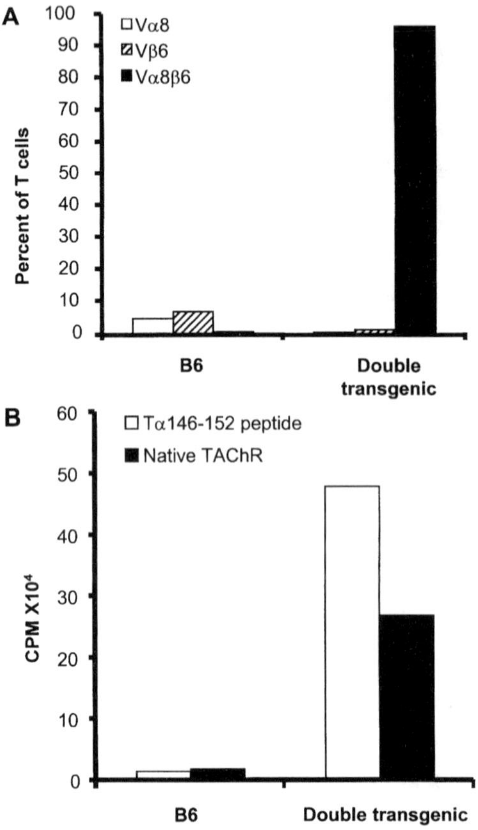

FIGURE 1. **(A)** Percentage of transgenic T cells in peripheral blood. Flow cytometry shows that more than 90% of $CD3^+$ cells from transgenic mice express Vα8 and Vβ6 TCR subunits on their T cells. **(B)** T cells from transgenic mice respond strongly to Tα146–162 peptide or native TAChR. Lymph node cells were incubated with either Tα146–162 peptide (1 mg/mL) or native TAChR (10 mg/mL) for 72 h. Proliferative response was determined by $[^3H]$-thymidine incorporation. Results are expressed as CPM.

PHENOTYPIC AND FUNCTIONAL CHARACTERIZATION OF TRANSGENIC LYMPHOCYTES

Flow cytometric analysis revealed that >90% of the $CD3^+$ T cells from lymph nodes of the αβ double-transgenic mice expressed the transgenic α and β TCR chains (FIG. 1A). Stimulation of lymph node cells from αβ transgenic mice, using either the Tα146–162 peptide or intact purified TAChR, produced strong proliferative responses (FIG. 1B). Unexpectedly, peripheral blood lymphocytes (PBLs) from αβ transgenic mice showed a marked, but variable, decrease in the percentage of B cells, ranging from <2% to >50% of PBLs, compared to a mean of 55% in wild-type B6 mice.

IN VIVO STUDIES IN TRANSGENIC MICE

We immunized groups of wild-type B6 mice and unselected αβ transgenic mice with TAChR in complete Freund's adjuvant (CFA) followed by a boost at 4 weeks. Antibody levels were significantly lower in αβ transgenic mice: <50% of the levels present in B6 mice. To test the possibility that the decreased anti-TAChR antibody levels in αβ transgenic mice resulted from the B cell deficiency, we selected αβ transgenic mice with relatively high B cell counts. The "selected" αβ transgenic mice, and age- and sex-matched B6 mice, were immunized and boosted twice with either TAChR or an unrelated control antigen, KLH. We found that the levels of anti-TAChR antibodies in these "selected" αβ transgenic mice were equal to those in the wild-type B6 mice. In contrast, the antibody response to the control antigen, KLH, was significantly lower in KLH-immunized "selected" αβ transgenic mice as compared to KLH-immunized wild-type B6 mice. We concluded that this limitation was due to the lack of variability in the T cell repertoire: Since >95% of the T cells in the transgenic mice are specific for TAChR, it is likely that there were not sufficient KLH-specific T cells to provide optimum help for production of anti-KLH antibodies.

TRANSGENIC MICE HAVE AN ENHANCED TH1-TYPE IMMUNE RESPONSE TO TACHR

In B6 mice, production of the IgG2c isotype of immunoglobulins is dependent on help from the Th1 subpopulation of T cells, while production of IgG1 is dependent on Th2 cells. We measured the isotypes of anti-TAChR antibodies from the TAChR immunized "selected" mice. The ratio of IgG2c to IgG1 was strikingly and significantly higher in the αβ double-transgenic mice as compared to control B6 mice. This anti-AChR isotype profile strongly suggests an enhanced Th1-type immune response to TAChR in αβ transgenic mice.

CLINICAL MANIFESTATIONS OF EAMG

The αβ transgenic mice did not spontaneously develop EAMG. Thus, the presence of even large numbers of TAChR-specific T cells did not by itself induce EAMG. EAMG occurred only after immunization with TAChR. Although the percentage of mice affected with EAMG and the severity of their clinical manifestations varied in different experiments (as is well known to occur in mice[5]), our overall experience indicated that the effects of immunization with TAChR gave similar clinical results in the αβ transgenic mice and the wild-type B6 mice. To evaluate EAMG further in αβ transgenic mice and B6 mice that were immunized with AChR, we measured the free AChR content in their carcasses[6] and compared the results with free AChR in the carcasses of mice immunized with control KLH. We found a significant reduction of free AChR in both αβ transgenic and B6 mice immunized with TAChR compared to those immunized with control KLH. However, there were no significant differences between the αβ transgenic mice and B6 mice that had been immunized with TAChR.

CONCLUSIONS

We have developed transgenic mice to analyze T cell reactivity towards the immunodominant epitope of TAChR in the B6 mouse model of MG. More than 90% of T cells express transgenic receptors. These mice show robust T cell responses to both the Tα146–162 peptide and native TAChR. Many of the TCR transgenic mice had significantly, but variably, reduced numbers of B cells, both in the periphery and in the lymphoid organs. The reduction in B cells is a new phenotypic characteristic of these transgenic mice that has not been reported previously in TCR transgenic mice. Immunization of transgenic mice selected to have relatively higher numbers of peripheral B cells resulted in anti-TAChR antibody levels equal to those observed in B6 mice. The antibody isotype profile in these mice suggests a Th1 phenotype response to TAChR. This model system offers a new approach for analyzing events in EAMG antibody production and the role of reactivity towards Tα146–162. Further, it should provide a valuable resource to give insight into the pathogenesis of EAMG and will aid in the design of specific treatments for EAMG, MG, and other autoimmune disorders.

REFERENCES

1. LENNON, V.A., J.M. LINDSTROM & M.E. SEYBOLD. 1976. Experimental autoimmune myasthenia gravis: cellular and humoral immune responses. Ann. N.Y. Acad. Sci. **274:** 283–289.
2. OSHIMA, M., T. YOKOI, P. DEITIKER & M.Z. ATASSI. 1998. T cell responses in EAMG-susceptible and non-susceptible mouse strains after immunization with overlapping peptides encompassing the extracellular part of *Torpedo californica* acetylcholine receptor alpha chain: implication to role in myasthenia gravis of autoimmune T-cell responses against receptor degradation products. Autoimmunity **27:** 79–90.
3. YAHG, B., K.R. MCINTOSH & D.B. DRACHMAN. 1998. How subtle differences in MHC class II affect the severity of experimental myasthenia gravis. Clin. Immunol. Immunopathol. **86:** 45–58.
4. KOUSKOFF, V., K. SIGNORELLY, C. BENOIST & D. MATHIS. 1995. Cassette vectors directing expression of T cell receptor genes in transgenic mice. J. Immunol. Methods **180:** 273–280.
5. LINDSTROM, J.M. 1999. Experimental autoimmune myasthenia gravis: induction and treatment. *In* Myasthenia Gravis and Myasthenic Disorders, pp. 111–130. Oxford University Press. London/New York.

6. LINDSTROM, J.M., B.L. EINARSON, V.A. LENNON & M.E. SEYBOLD. 1976. Pathological mechanisms in experimental autoimmune myasthenia gravis: immunogenicity of syngeneic muscle acetylcholine receptor and quantitative extraction of receptor and antibody-receptor complexes of muscles of rats with experimental autoimmune myasthenia gravis. J. Exp. Med. **144:** 726–738.

Epitope Repertoire of Th1 and Th2 Cells Reactive with the Mouse Muscle AChR α Subunit in C57Bl/6 Mice

WEI WANG,[a] MONICA MILANI,[a] DAVID OKITA,[a] NORMA OSTLIE,[a] AND BIANCA M. CONTI-FINE[a,b,c]

[a]*Department of Biochemistry, Molecular Biology, and Biophysics,*
[b]*Department of Pharmacology, University of Minnesota, Minneapolis, Minnesota 55455, USA*

KEYWORDS: C57Bl/6 mice; T cells; Th1; Th2; myasthenia gravis; experimental autoimmune myasthenia gravis; epitope

Antibodies (Abs) to the muscle acetylcholine receptor (AChR) cause the symptoms of myasthenia gravis (MG) and experimental autoimmune MG (EAMG).[1,2] Anti-AChR CD4$^+$ T helper cells have an important role in MG and EAMG pathogenesis because they modulate the anti-AChR Ab synthesis. CD4$^+$ T cells include Th1 and Th2 cells. Th1 and Th2 cells, and the cytokines they secrete, have different roles in EAMG. Th1 cells induce synthesis of pathogenic anti-AChR Abs that fix complement.[3,4] In contrast, Th2 cells may curb EAMG development by secreting anti-inflammatory cytokines and promoting the synthesis of Abs that do not bind complement.[3,4]

Most anti-AChR Ab and CD4$^+$ T cells recognize epitopes formed by the AChR α subunit.[1,5] In this study, we have identified the sequence regions of the mouse AChR α subunit, which form epitopes recognized by CD4$^+$ Th1 and Th2 cells in C57Bl/6 mice (see FIG. 1).

We have used 32 overlapping synthetic peptides, which were usually 20 residues long and overlapped by 5 residues, and spanned the mouse AChR α subunit sequence. We have described previously their synthesis and characterization.[6,7] We indicate each peptide with the symbol α and two numbers, which refer to the position of the first and last peptide residue on the subunit sequence.

We used C57Bl/6 mice genetically deficient in IL-4 (IL-4$^{-/-}$) or IL-12 (IL-12$^{-/-}$) as the source of Th2 and Th1 cells, respectively. We used also wild-type (WT) C57Bl/6 mice. To obtain a broad assessment of the epitope repertoire, including "cryptic" epitopes, we immunized the mice with pools of the synthetic peptide

Address for correspondence: Wei Wang, Department of Biochemistry, Molecular Biology, and Biophysics, 321 Church St. SE, 6-155 Jackson Hall, Minneapolis, MN 55455. Voice: 612-624-3790. wangx241@umn.edu
[c]Previously known as Bianca M. Conti-Tronconi.

Ann. N.Y. Acad. Sci. 998: 384–387 (2003). © 2003 New York Academy of Sciences.
doi: 10.1196/annals.1254.046

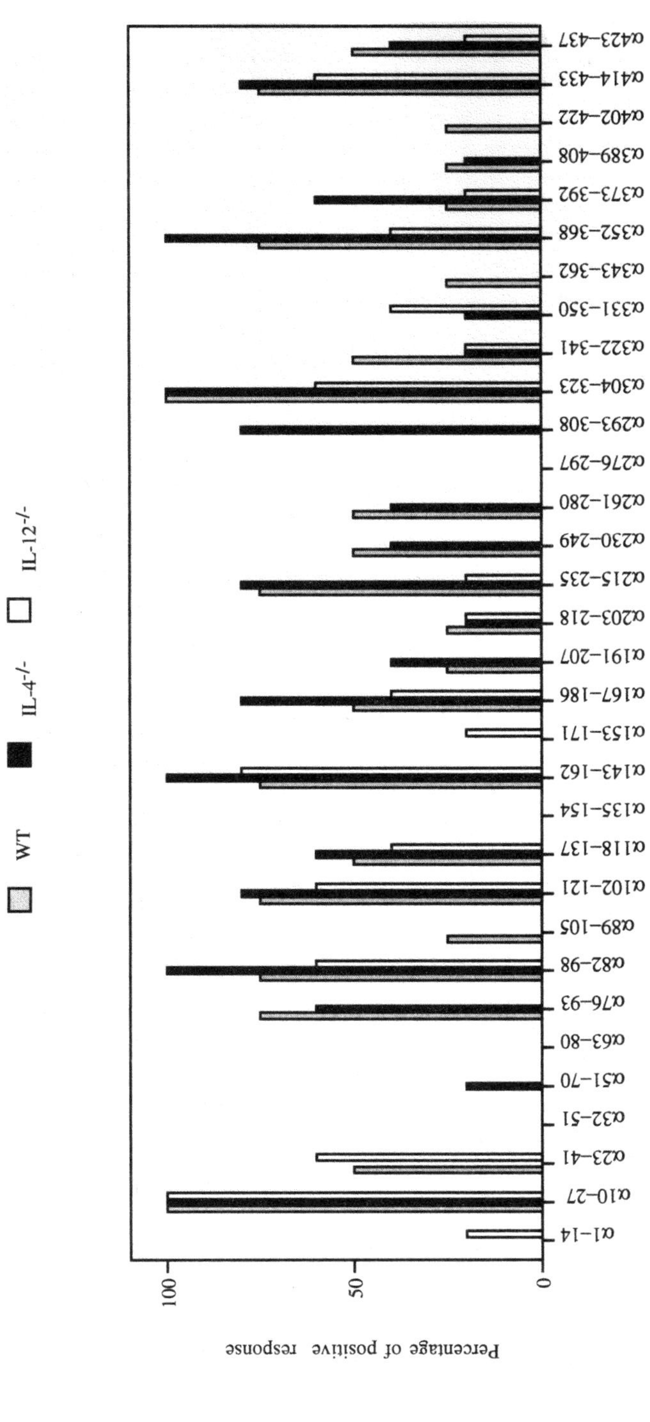

FIGURE 1. Percentage of positive response of the sequence regions of the mouse AChR α subunit.

spanning the α subunit.[7] We grouped the peptides in 4 equimolar pools (8 peptides/pool) dissolved in PBS, and we immunized each mouse subcutaneously three times with a volume of pool solution containing 10 μg of each peptide, emulsified in an equal volume of Freund's adjuvant. Three to 14 days after the last immunization, we obtained cells from the spleens and inguinal lymph nodes of 3 identically treated mice and removed the $CD8^+$ cells, as we described previously.[8] We have identified the peptide sequences recognized by the remaining $CD4^+$ T cells in 3-day proliferation assays, which we described previously,[9] using the individual peptides as stimulants. Negative controls were cells cultured in the absence of any antigen or with a 20-residue peptide unrelated to the AChR sequence. We evaluated the rate of cell proliferation from the incorporation of [^{3}H]thymidine, and we expressed the results as a stimulation index (the ratio between the average cpm of antigen-stimulated cultures and the average cpm from the negative control cultures).

The $CD4^+$ T cells from all 3 strains recognized many subunit peptide sequences. Several peptides elicited strong proliferative responses (peptides comprising residues α10–27, α82–98, α102–121, α118–137, α143–161, α304–323, and α352–368). A few other peptides elicited modest, yet significant and consistent responses (α167–186, α215–234, and α414–433).

$CD4^+$ T cells of IL-$4^{-/-}$ mice (i.e., by Th1 cells) recognized all but one of the peptides recognized by the $CD4^+$ T cells of WT mice. Peptide α23–41 was recognized in 50% or more experiments by the $CD4^+$ T cells of WT and IL-$12^{-/-}$ mice, but never by those of IL-$4^{-/-}$ mice. This suggests that Th2 cells might uniquely recognize an epitope within those residues. The $CD4^+$ T cells from IL-$12^{-/-}$ mice (i.e., Th2 cells) did not recognize several peptides (α76–93, α230–249, α261–280, and α293–308), which elicited frequent and sometimes substantial responses in the other 2 strains. This suggests that Th1 cells might uniquely recognize epitopes within those sequence regions. FIGURE 1 reports the frequency with which the different peptides elicited a significant response ($p < 0.01$ as determined by Student's t test), which yielded SI > 1.5 in different, independent experiments (5 each for the IL-$4^{-/-}$ and IL-$12^{-/-}$ mice, 4 for the WT mice) that we carried out with $CD4^+$ T cells from the 3 mice strains.

Among the sequence regions that appear to form epitopes recognized by Th1, but not by Th2 cells, residues α76–93 are close to the sequence region α67–76, which contributes to the so-called MIR, a set of overlapping epitopes recognized by abundant and highly pathogenic anti-AChR Ab.[1,2,9] This raises the possibility that the AChR sequence α76–93 may be especially important for sensitization of anti-AChR $CD4^+$ T cells with high pathogenic potential.

REFERENCES

1. CONTI-FINE, B.M. *et al.* 1997. Myasthenia Gravis: The Immunobiology of an Autoimmune Disease. Landes Co. Austin, TX.
2. LINDSTROM, J.M. 2000. Acetylcholine receptors and myasthenia. Muscle Nerve **3:** 453–477.
3. O'GARRA, A. 1998. Cytokines induce the development of functionally heterogeneous T helper cell subsets. Immunity **8:** 275–283.
4. KARACHUNSKI, P.I. *et al.* 2000. Absence of IFN-γ or IL-12 has different effects on experimental myasthenia gravis in C57BL/6 mice. J. Immunol. **164:** 5236–5244.
5. DRACHMAN, D.B. 1994. Myasthenia gravis. N. Engl. J. Med. **330:** 1797–1810.

6. MANFREDI, A.A. *et al.* 1992. $CD4^+$ T-epitope repertoire on the human acetylcholine receptor alpha subunit in severe myasthenia gravis: a study with synthetic peptides. Neurology **42:** 1092–1100.
7. BELLONE, M. *et al.* 1993. Cryptic epitopes on the nicotinic acetylcholine receptor are recognized by autoreactive $CD4^+$ cells. J. Immunol. **151:** 1025–1038.
8. OSTLIE, N. *et al.* 2001. Transgenic expression of IL-10 in T cells facilitates development of experimental myasthenia gravis. J. Immunol. **166:** 4853–4862.
9. TZARTOS, S.J. *et al.* 1991. The main immunogenic region (MIR) of the nicotinic acetylcholine receptor and the anti-MIR antibodies. Mol. Neurobiol. **5:** 1–29.

Epitope Spreading to Hidden Cytoplasmic Regions of the Acetylcholine Receptor in Experimental Autoimmune Myasthenia Gravis

TALI FEFERMAN,[a] SIN-HYEOG IM,[a] SARA FUCHS,[a]
AND MIRIAM C. SOUROUJON[a,b]

[a]*Department of Immunology, Weizmann Institute of Science, Rehovot 76100, Israel*

[b]*Open University of Israel, Tel Aviv 61392, Israel*

KEYWORDS: EAMG; autoantibodies/autoimmunity; epitope spreading; tolerance

INTRODUCTION

The autoimmune disease, myasthenia gravis (MG), and its animal model, experimental autoimmune myasthenia gravis (EAMG), develop as a result of a B cell–mediated T cell–dependent attack on the acetylcholine receptor (AChR). Even though the antibody response to AChR is heterogeneous, a large portion of the autoimmune response in myasthenia is directed toward the extracellular domain of the α-subunit of AChR. We have previously reported on an additional highly immunogenic region within the cytoplasmic region of the AChR α-subunit.[1] Antibodies to cytoplasmic regions have been found also in sera of myasthenic patients.[2,3] Such antibodies are probably not involved in the elicitation of myasthenia, but may have a role in the sustaining of the autoimmune response in the process of epitope or determinant spreading.[4]

We wanted to test the possibility that although the autoimmune attack in myasthenia is first elicited against exposed epitopes of the AChR, in the course of disease progression, a tolerance breakage leads to the elicitation of an immune response toward hidden cytoplasmic regions of the autoantigen. This is hard to follow in MG patients since they seek medical help when their disease is already full-blown. The classical animal model also does not permit testing of this hypothesis since EAMG is induced by injecting the entire *Torpedo* AChR molecule. We have thus designed an experimental system in which we induced EAMG in rats by a recombinant fragment that corresponds to the extracellular portion of the mammalian AChR α-subunit and is native in its conformation. We then followed changes in the specificities of anti-AChR antibodies that develop at different times after disease induction.

Address for correspondence: Dr. Sara Fuchs, Department of Immunology, Weizmann Institute of Science, Rehovot 76100, Israel. Voice: +972-8-9342618; fax: +972-8-9344141.
sara.fuchs@weizmann.ac.il

Ann. N.Y. Acad. Sci. 998: 388–390 (2003). **© 2003 New York Academy of Sciences.**
doi: 10.1196/annals.1254.047

METHODS

EAMG was induced by injecting rats with CFA or with 500 μg of fragment TRX-Hα1–210, corresponding to the extracellular portion of the human AChR α-subunit fused to thioredoxin. The rat antibody responses to extracellular and cytoplasmic fragments were analyzed by Western blot at 3-week intervals. MAb198, directed to the MIR within the extracellular region of the AChR α-subunit, was used to ensure the identification of this fragment. Response to the cytoplasmic region of AChR α-subunit, represented by the fragment Hα301–406, was monitored by binding to a polyclonal antibody to residues 351–368 within the cytoplasmic region.

Determination of AChR-specific IgG isotypes was performed by overlaying the blots, after the reaction with the rat sera, with biotinylated mouse monoclonal antibodies to specific rat IgG isotypes.

RESULTS AND DISCUSSION

Rats were injected with the fragment that corresponds to TRX-Hα1–210 and their antibody response to it and toward a fragment that corresponds to the large cytoplasmic loop of the human AChR α-subunit fused to dihydrofolate reductase (DHFR-Hα301–406).

Rats first develop antibodies to the injected extracellular portion only, but later also develop antibodies to the intracellular hidden cytoplasmic loop of the α-subunit (Hα301–406). The development of antibodies to the cytoplasmic region was correlated with severe myasthenia. The humoral response to the injected extracellular portion encompassed all IgG isotypes, whereas the immune response to the cytoplasmic region consisted of IgG2a antibodies only. Namely, breakage of tolerance led to the elicitation of a typical Th1-regulated immune response toward newly exposed epitopes of the autoantigen. We propose that a similar intramolecular epitope spreading takes place during the natural elicitation of myasthenia.

In view of these findings, we plan to test whether induction of tolerance to recombinant fragments corresponding to cytoplasmic regions of AChR has a suppressive effect on the course of EAMG.

ACKNOWLEDGMENTS

This work was supported by grants from the Muscular Dystrophy Association of America (MDA), the Association Française Contre les Myopathies (AFM), and the European Commission (EC) (Nos. QLG1-CT-2001-10918 and QLRT-2001-00225).

REFERENCES

1. SOUROUJON, M.C., D. NEUMANN, S. PIZZIGHELLA *et al.* 1986. Localization of a highly immunogenic region on the acetylcholine receptor α-subunit. Biochem. Biophys. Res. Commun. **135:** 82–89.

2. Wang, Z-Y., D.K. Okita, J.R. Howard & B. Conti-Fine. 1998. Th1 cells of myasthenia gravis patients recognize multiple epitopes on the muscle AChR α subunit. Ann. N.Y. Acad. Sci. **841:** 329–333.
3. Tzartos, S.J. & M. Remoundos. 1999. Detection of antibodies directed against the cytoplasmic region of the human acetylcholine receptor in sera from myasthenia gravis patients. Clin. Exp. Immunol. **116:** 146–152.
4. Vanderlugt, C. & S.D. Miller. 2002. Epitope spreading in immune-mediated disease: implications for immunotherapy. Nat. Rev. Immunol. **2:** 85–95.

Immunization with Rat-, but Not Torpedo-Derived 97–116 Peptide of the AChR α-Subunit Induces Experimental Myasthenia Gravis in Lewis Rat

FULVIO BAGGI,[a] ANDREA ANNONI,[a] FEDERICA UBIALI,[a] RENATO LONGHI,[b] MONICA MILANI,[c] RENATO MANTEGAZZA,[a] FERDINANDO CORNELIO,[a] AND CARLO ANTOZZI[a]

[a]*Immunology and Muscular Pathology Unit, National Neurological Institute "Carlo Besta", 20133 Milan, Italy*

[b]*IBRM, CNR, 20133 Milan, Italy*

[c]*Department of Biochemistry, Molecular Biology, and Biophysics, University of Minnesota, St. Paul, Minnesota 55108, USA*

KEYWORDS: myasthenia gravis; Lewis rat; antigen-specific therapies

INTRODUCTION

Experimental autoimmune myasthenia gravis (EAMG) is routinely induced by a single immunization with Torpedo AChR, and the immunodominant T cell epitope has been mapped to the sequences 97–112 and 100–116 of the AChR α-subunit.[1,2] T cells from EAMG rats respond not only to Torpedo α97–116 peptide (DGDFAI-VHMTKLLLDYTGKI), but also to rat α97–116 (DGDFAIVKFTKVLLDYTGHI). Moreover, T cell lines specific for rat and Torpedo 97–116 peptides were successfully isolated and cultured long-term. The aim of the study is to test whether the rat peptide (self-antigen) can induce EAMG in Lewis rats.

METHODS

Female Lewis rats (6–8 weeks) were immunized in the hind foot pads with peptide (50 μg/200 μL) in CFA and boosted on day 30 with peptide/IFA. Control EAMG animals were immunized with 50 μg of purified TAChR in CFA. Peptides were synthesized using f-moc chemistry on an Applied Biosystems 431A automated peptide synthesizer, and their quality was confirmed by HPLC and mass spectrometry.

Address for correspondence: Fulvio Baggi, Immunology and Muscular Pathology Unit, National Neurological Institute "Carlo Besta", via Celoria 11, 20133 Milan, Italy. Voice: +39-02-2394369; fax: +39-02-70633874.
baggi@istituto-besta.it

Ann. N.Y. Acad. Sci. 998: 391–394 (2003). © 2003 New York Academy of Sciences.
doi: 10.1196/annals.1254.048

Muscle fatigability was evaluated by repetitive paw grips on the cage grid. EAMG evaluation was performed as follows: grade 0, normal strength; grade 1, mildly decreased activity and weak grip; grade 2, signs of weakness at rest; grade 3, moribund; grade 4, dead. Disease was further confirmed by Tensilon test and repetitive nerve stimulation. Anti-rat AChR antibodies were assayed by conventional radioimmunoprecipitation methods. Rat sera were incubated with $[^{125}I]\alpha$-bungarotoxin-labeled rat AChR; antibody-AChR complexes were precipitated with rabbit anti-rat IgG. The pellets were washed twice with PBS 0.5%/Triton X-100 and radioactivity counted. Serum samples incubated with rat AChR preincubated in excess of cold α-BTX (nonspecific binding) were subtracted from test samples. Muscle AChR content was determined by incubation of Triton X-100 muscle crude extract with $[^{125}I]\alpha$-BTX (4 h, RT). Muscle extracts were transferred on DE-81 DEAE disks, washed twice with PBS 0.5%/Triton X-100, and radioactivity counted. The aspecific binding was subtracted from each sample by parallel tubes preincubated with cold α-BTX. Direct ELISA technique was used to measure antipeptide antibodies. Dynex Immulon 4HBX 96-well plates were coated with peptides (5 μg/well) and blocked with PBS/0.05% Tween-20/1% BSA. Pooled rat sera (0.5 μL, diluted with PBS/Tween20) were added, incubated for 2 h, and followed by rabbit anti-rat IgG-HRP conjugate. Optical density was measured at 450 nm.

RESULTS

The onset of EAMG and disease progression in Lewis rats immunized with rat or Torpedo 97–116 peptides, and with purified TAChR as positive control, were evaluated by measurement of body weight and clinical score (FIG. 1). Three separate experiments were performed, and signs of EAMG occurred in 72% (13 out of 18) of rats immunized with rat 97–116 peptide, while no sick animals were found in Torpedo 97–116 immunized groups (0 out of 14). TAChR induced EAMG in 100% (10 out

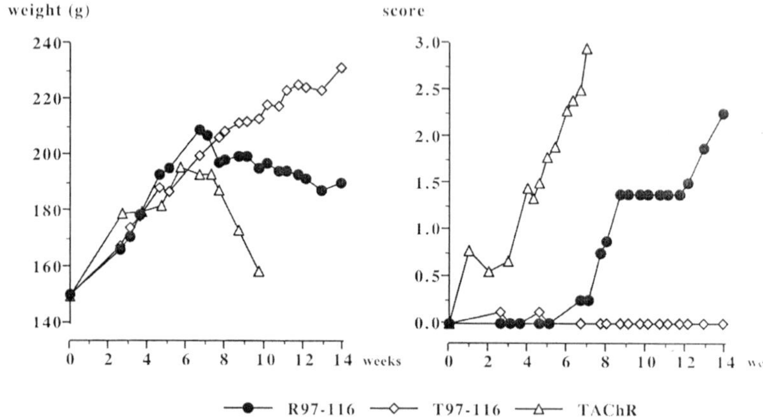

FIGURE 1. Body weight and clinical score of EAMG induced by rat-, Torpedo-peptide 97–116, and Torpedo AChR. See text for details.

of 10) of immunized rats. Typical growth rates are shown in FIGURE 1 (left panel). The weight of Torpedo 97–116 immunized rats (*open diamond*) was similar to non-immunized animals, while TAChR (*open triangle*) and rat 97–116 (*solid circle*) immunized groups began to lose body weight at 6–8 weeks after immunization, with a slower loss of weight in rat 97–116 induced EAMG compared to TAChR induced EAMG. The mean clinical score at the end of the experiments (FIG. 1, right panel) was 2.5 ± 0.35 in rat 97–116 immunized rats (*solid circle*) and 3 ± 0.26 in TAChR-immunized rats (*open triangle*). Only rats immunized with the self-peptide, but not with the Torpedo sequence, showed clinical signs of EAMG, although with a different time course compared to that induced by TAChR. IgG antibodies against both peptides were found in all animals (FIG. 2, top). On the contrary, pathogenic anti-rat AChR antibodies were significantly increased in animals immunized with rat peptide compared to those with the Torpedo sequence (16.8 vs. 2.2 pmol/mL). Muscle AChR content in muscles from rat 97–116 immunized animals was reduced compared to normal control muscles (9.3 ± 2.1 and 36.5 ± 4.2 pmol/100 g, respectively) and was similar to that of EAMG control rats. AChR content in the muscles

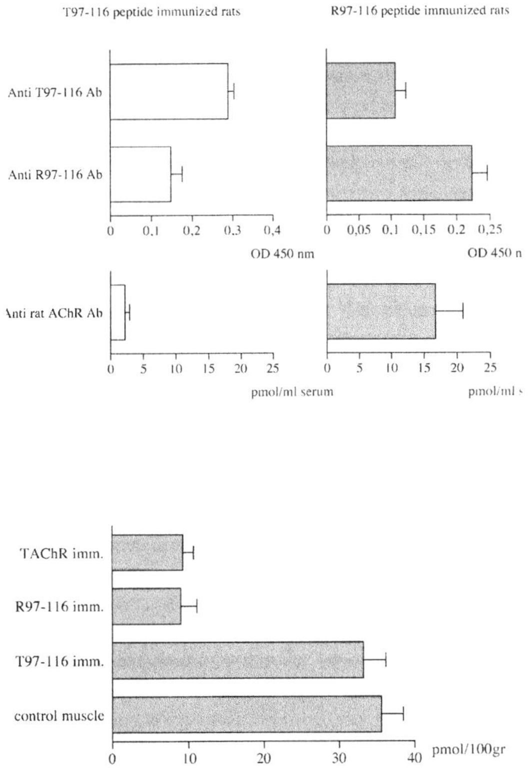

FIGURE 2. (Top) Antipeptide and anti-rat AChR antibodies in peptide-immunized animals. **(Bottom)** Muscle AChR content.

from T97–116 immunized rats was similar to normal control muscles (33.6 ± 2.9 and 36.5 ± 4.2 pmol/100 g, respectively) (FIG. 2, bottom).

CONCLUSIONS

Immunodominant AChR-derived T cell epitopes have been described in human MG as well as in EAMG, but their role in disease induction or maintenance is not completely defined. Recently, a peptide corresponding to sequence 129–145 of the AChR α-subunit able to induce EAMG in rats was described.[3] This epitope was identified and characterized in rats immunized with the recombinant fragment 1–210 of the human α-subunit. On the contrary, Torpedo 97–116 epitope, derived from TAChR immunized rats,[1,2] does not induce EAMG, as shown by our results. Lewis rats were immunized with two peptides corresponding to the T cell immunodominant epitope 97–116 of the AChR α-subunit: one peptide derived from the rat AChR sequence and the other from Torpedo AChR. Breakdown of tolerance to self-AChR, leading to EAMG induction, was seen only in rats treated with the rat peptide. EAMG was confirmed by clinical, electrophysiological (repetitive nerve stimulation), and immunological evidence, and responded to the Tensilon test. Lewis rats immunized with Torpedo-derived 97–116 peptide did not develop EAMG, even in animals that received a further peptide boost (data not shown). Although these peptides correspond to immunodominant T cell epitopes, antibodies (IgG type) against both peptides were induced. High levels of anti-rat AChR antibodies were detected in animals immunized with the rat peptide; moreover, only these animals had reduced muscle AChR content. Our data suggest that EAMG can be induced by immunization with a single peptide of the self-rat AChR (emulsified in CFA only for immunization and without additional adjuvants, such as *Bordetella pertussis*) and that this sequence is recognized by both T and B cells. Rat and Torpedo 97–116 sequences differ only in four residues, and these amino acids may be critical in the induction of EAMG in Lewis rats. This region (as well as region 129–145) derived from self-AChR, and able to induce EAMG, might constitute a crucial target for developing antigen-specific therapies in myasthenia gravis.

REFERENCES

1. FUJII, Y. & J. LINDSTROM. 1988. Specificity of the T cell immune response to acetylcholine receptor in experimental autoimmune myasthenia gravis: response to subunits and synthetic peptides. J. Immunol. **140:** 1830–1837.
2. ZHANG, Y.S. *et al.* 1990. Identification of T-cell epitopes of autoantigens using recombinant proteins: studies on experimental autoimmune myasthenia gravis. Immunology **71:** 538–543.
3. YOSHIKAWA, H. *et al.* 1997. A 17-mer self-peptide of acetylcholine receptor binds to B cell MHC class II, activates helper T cells, and stimulates autoantibody production and electrophysiologic signs of myasthenia gravis. J. Immunol. **159:** 1570–1577.

Effect on T Cell Recognition and Immunogenicity of Alanine-Substituted Peptides Corresponding to 97–116 Sequence of the Rat AChR α-Subunit

FULVIO BAGGI,[a] ANDREA ANNONI,[a] FEDERICA UBIALI,[a] RENATO LONGHI,[b] RENATO MANTEGAZZA,[a] FERDINANDO CORNELIO,[a] AND CARLO ANTOZZI[a]

[a]*Immunology and Muscular Pathology Unit, National Neurological Institute "Carlo Besta", 20133 Milan, Italy*

[b]*IBRM, CNR, 20133 Milan, Italy*

KEYWORDS: T cell recognition; immunogenicity; alanine-substituted peptides

INTRODUCTION

The dominant TAChR epitope in Lewis rats is represented by the sequence 97–116 of the α-subunit.[1,2] Animals immunized with Torpedo-derived 97–116 peptide do not show clinical signs of the disease, while EAMG can be induced by immunization with a peptide corresponding to region 97–116 of rat AChR α-subunit (see Baggi *et al.*, this volume). Comparison between rat and Torpedo 97–116 sequences revealed only four differences (K104H, F105M, V108L, H115K), but only one residue differentiates rat and human sequences (D111Q). Each of these amino acid residues might be relevant for immune recognition of rat 97–116 peptide and hence induction of EAMG. To test this hypothesis, rat and Torpedo 97–116 specific T cell lines were raised and their epitope specificity was studied with peptides corresponding to rat, Torpedo, and human sequences, as well as with five alanine-substituted peptides (K104A, F105A, V108A, D111A, H115A) derived from the rat 97–116 sequence.

METHODS

Female Lewis rats, 6–8 weeks of age, were immunized in hind foot pads with 50 μg peptide in CFA. Peptides corresponding to region 97–116 of the AChR α-subunit were synthesized using f-moc chemistry on an Applied Biosystems 431A automated peptide synthesizer, and the quality of each peptide was confirmed by

Address for correspondence: Fulvio Baggi, Immunology and Muscular Pathology Unit, National Neurological Institute "Carlo Besta", via Celoria 11, 20133 Milan, Italy. Voice: +39-02-2394369; fax: +39-02-70633874.
baggi@istituto-besta.it

Ann. N.Y. Acad. Sci. 998: 395–398 (2003). **© 2003 New York Academy of Sciences.**
doi: 10.1196/annals.1254.049

analytical reverse-phase HPLC and mass spectrometry. Alanine-substituted peptides were synthesized on the basis of the rat 97–116 sequence.

Peptide sequences are the following:

αAChR 97–116 sequence

Rat	**DGDFAIVKFTKVLLDYTGHI**
Human	**DGDFAIVKFTKVLLQYTGHI**
Torpedo	**DGDFAIVHMTKLLLDYTGKI**

Ala-analogue peptides

K104A	**DGDFAIVAFTKVLLDYTGHI**
F105A	**DGDFAIVKATKVLLDYTGHI**
V108A	**DGDFAIVKFTKALLDYTGHI**
D111A	**DGDFAIVKFTKVLLAYTGHI**
H115A	**DGDFAIVKFTKVLLDYTGAI**

T cell lines were isolated from lymph nodes and cultured in RPMI-1640 medium plus 1% normal rat serum, and stimulated with 5 μg/mL of rat or Torpedo 97–116. T cell lines were maintained by restimulation with the appropriate peptide every 15 days and expanded with IL-2 every 3–4 days thereafter. For the proliferation assay, 3×10^4 T cells were cocultured in triplicates with irradiated splenic cells (2×10^5 per well) plus peptide(s). Concanavalin-A was used at 2 μg/mL as positive control. After 72 h, 1 μCi of [^{3}H]thymidine was added to each well. The plates were harvested after 16 h. Competition experiments with V108A peptide were performed as follows: splenic APC were incubated with V108A peptide for 2 h at 37°C, treated with mitomycin C (50 μg/mL) for 20 min at 37°C, and washed twice. T cells (3×10^4) were cocultured in triplicates with V108A-pulsed APC (2×10^5 per well) plus rat 97–116 peptide (2 and 10 μg/mL) in RPMI-1640 medium with 1% normal rat serum. After 72 h, 1 μCi of [^{3}H]thymidine was added to each well. The plates were harvested after 16 h.

RESULTS

The rat 97–116 peptide of the AChR α-subunit is a T cell immunodominant epitope and can induce EAMG in Lewis rats. T cell lines grown from rat or Torpedo 97–116 peptide immunized rats gave a different pattern of response when challenged with rat, Torpedo, or human 97–116 peptide (FIG. 1). The rat 97–116 T cell line responded equally well to both rat and human sequences and was able to respond also to Torpedo 97–116 peptide, although partially (left panel). On the contrary, the Torpedo 97–116 specific T cell line responded exclusively to Torpedo 97–116 peptide (right panel). The observed differences in antigen recognition suggested that we test our rat 97–116 specific T cell line against a panel of alanine-substituted peptides, derived from the rat sequence (FIG. 2, left panel). Removal of K104 and F105 reduced T cell proliferation, and the strongest nonstimulatory effect was observed when the T cell line was challenged with V108A peptide: alanine replacement of valine at

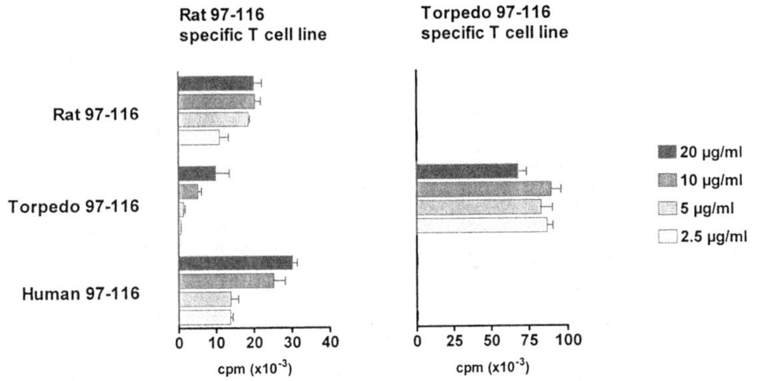

FIGURE 1. *In vitro* proliferative response of peptide-specific T cell lines to rat, Torpedo, and human sequence 97–116.

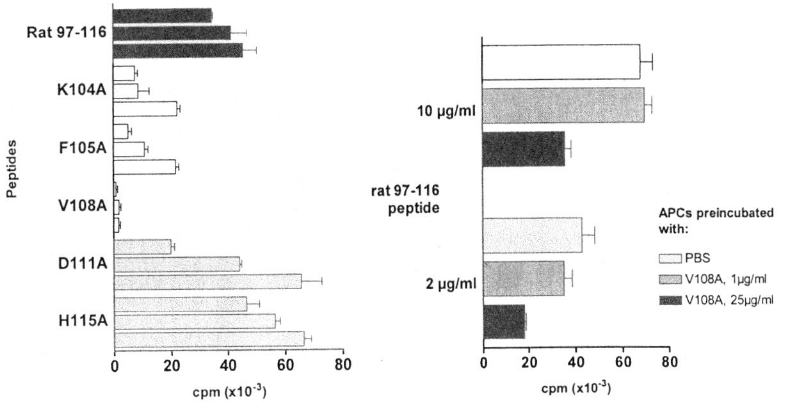

FIGURE 2. (Left) Proliferation of the rat 97–116 specific T cell line against alanine-substituted peptides. **(Right)** Proliferation of the rat 97–116 specific T cell line after APC preincubation with peptide V108A.

position 108 completely abrogated the specific T cell response. On the contrary, substitution of residues D111 and H115 with alanine caused more efficient stimulation of the rat 97–116 T cell line. Preliminary studies on the relative affinity of peptide V108A (nonresponder) for presenting MHC molecules were conducted by preincubating splenic APC with different concentrations of V108A peptide followed by classical proliferation experiments (FIG. 2, right panel). We observed a partial reduction in the response of the rat 97–116 specific T cell line when APC were preincubated with the high concentration (25 μg/mL) of V108A, and the effect was not reversed by increasing rat 97–116 concentration (10 μg/mL).

CONCLUSIONS

The definition of the T cell epitope and the relevant residues contained within the rat sequence 97–116 is crucial to understanding the events leading to EAMG induction by this peptide. The four amino acid residues that differ between rat (myasthenogenic sequence) and Torpedo (nonmyasthenogenic sequence) simplified the search of residues with different affinity/specificity for MHC binding and TCR interaction. The T cell line raised against Torpedo 97–116 peptide is highly specific for this peptide and does not recognize the rat sequence nor any of the alanine-substituted peptides. On the contrary, the T cell line selected with rat 97–116 peptide fully responds to human- and rat-derived 97–116 peptides, and partially to Torpedo-derived 97–116 peptide. These data suggest that the absence of cross-reactivity showed by the Torpedo 97–116 T cell line implies that these lymphocytes cannot be stimulated by rat AChR in the animal, and hence cannot be "self-maintained" *in vivo* once the immunizing antigen has been cleared. On the contrary, the observed cross-reactivity of the rat specific T cell line suggested the use of ala-substituted peptides to modulate the antigen-specific response. Indeed, rat 97–116 T cell proliferation is significantly reduced when challenged with K104A and F105A peptides, and abrogated with V108A-substituted peptide, while removal of D111 and H115 does not affect T cell proliferation. Moreover, the partial inhibition of the T cell response by V108A peptide competition experiments suggests the potential modulatory properties of this peptide on the response *in vitro* and possibly sensitization to AChR *in vivo*. The observed T cell responses by ala-substituted peptides might be the consequence of changes in those residues involved in MHC binding or in TCR contact. The RT1.B^l anchor motif consists of a nonamer sequence with four major anchor positions.[3] In this paper, the authors suggest that residues V103, M105, T106, L108, and D111 are relevant for Torpedo 100–116 peptide interaction with rat MHC class II molecule. V103, T106, and D111 are present in the rat sequence, while M105 and L108 are replaced by F and V, respectively (anyway both residues are accepted in the putative binding motif). We can speculate that the other residues that are different between rat and Torpedo 97–116 sequences, namely K104 and H115, might contact TCR, affecting antigen recognition and the T cell response. On the other hand, the conservative replacement of the V108A peptide might explain the absence of the T cell response not fully confirmed by the blocking experiment. This study suggests that alanine-substituted peptides might be used for antigen-specific tolerization studies of EAMG induced by the rat 97–116 peptide.

REFERENCES

1. Fujii, Y. & J. Lindstrom. 1988. Specificity of the T cell immune response to acetylcholine receptor in experimental autoimmune myasthenia gravis: response to subunits and synthetic peptides. J. Immunol. **140:** 1830–1837.
2. Zhang, Y.S. *et al.* 1990. Identification of T-cell epitopes of autoantigens using recombinant proteins: studies on experimental autoimmune myasthenia gravis. Immunology **71:** 538–543.
3. Reizis, B. *et al.* 1996. The peptide binding specificity of the MHC class II I-A molecule of the Lewis rat, RT1.B^l. Int. Immunol. **8:** 1825–1832.

Characterization of a Fully Human IgG1 Reconstructed from an Anti-AChR F_{ab}

MAURICE H. W. STASSEN,[a] BARBIE M. MACHIELS,[a] EFROSINI FOSTIERI,[b] SOCRATES J. TZARTOS,[b] SONIA BERRIH-AKNIN,[c] EUGÈNE BOSMANS,[d] PAUL W. H. I. PARREN,[e] AND MARC H. DE BAETS[a]

[a]*Brain and Behavior Institute, University of Maastricht, NL-6200 MD Maastricht, the Netherlands*

[b]*Department of Biochemistry, Hellenic Pasteur Institute, Athens, Greece*

[c]*Hospital Marie Lannelongue, Paris, France*

[d]*DiaMed-Eurogen, Tessenderlo, Belgium*

[e]*Department of Immunology, Scripps Research Institute, La Jolla, California 92037, USA*

KEYWORDS: **myasthenia gravis; acetylcholine receptor; antigenic modulation; F_{ab}; IgG1**

In myasthenia gravis (MG), autoantibodies directed to the acetylcholine receptor (AChR) cause disturbed neurotransmission, either by hindrance of ACh binding or by decrease of functional AChR, resulting in muscle weakness. The two mechanisms that lead to AChR loss are complement-mediated focal lysis of the postsynaptic membrane and increased internalization of AChR by antibody-mediated receptor cross-linking (antigenic modulation). The human antigen-binding fragment (F_{ab}) 637 was previously isolated from a phage-display library, derived from an MG patient's thymus.[1] F_{ab}637 is highly specific for the human AChR's major immunogenic region (MIR) and is a potential *in vivo* protective agent against pathogenic MG antibodies. Because of its monovalent binding capacity, F_{ab}637 prevents antigenic modulation; and because of its anti-MIR specificity, F_{ab}637 competes with the majority of MG antibodies. *In vitro* experiments have shown that F_{ab}637 blocks antigenic modulation by MG patient sera, without interfering with receptor function.

In order to increase the *in vivo* half-life, we produced a completely human, full-size IgG1 isotype variant of F_{ab}637 (IgG637), by cloning the coding sequences of its light-chain (LC) and heavy-chain variable domain (V_H) in a single mammalian expression vector, pIgG1. The V_H was genetically fused in pIgG1 to the human γ1

Address for correspondence: Maurice H. W. Stassen, Brain and Behavior Institute (Box 38), University of Maastricht, P. O. Box 616, NL-6200 MD Maastricht, the Netherlands. Voice: +31-43-3881021; fax: +31-43-3671096.
m.stassen@np.unimaas.nl

Ann. N.Y. Acad. Sci. 998: 399–400 (2003). **© 2003 New York Academy of Sciences.**
doi: 10.1196/annals.1254.050

constant domains, resulting in an expression cassette of a fully human heavy chain (HC). The LC and HC cistrons, including immunoglobulin leader peptides, were controlled by CMV promoters. Chinese hamster ovary (CHO) cells were transfected with pIgG1-637, and stable monoclonal cell lines were established. Hollow fiber cultures of a stable transfectant yielded 50 mg of protein G–purified IgG637 per liter. IgG637, as well as Alexa488-conjugated IgG637, was able to precipitate the human AChR in a radioimmunoassay comparable to $F_{ab}637$. The titer of IgG637 was greater than 48 μM anti-AChR antibody per mg purified Ig. A hybrid receptor of human α and *Torpedo* β, γ, and δ subunits was also recognized, but not the *Torpedo* AChR or a peptide of the first 210 amino acids of the human α subunit. Immunohistochemical staining of monkey muscles clearly showed costaining of Alexa488-conjugated IgG637 with rhodamine-conjugated α-bungarotoxin. FACS analysis of IgG637 on the human embryonic AChR-expressing TE671 cells gave a half log-scale shift after amplification.

These data indicate the preservation of specificity after the F_d to HC reconstruction. This finding is similar to our previous study where $F_{ab}637$ was changed into a single-chain variable fragment (scF_v).[2] The reconstructed human anti-AChR IgG1-637 is an addition to the few existing MG monoclonal antibodies that have been isolated directly as full-size immunoglobulins from MG patients. The pIgG1-637–transfected CHO cells are excellent for large-scale production of IgG637. This could serve as a more constant source of reference antibody, for example, in diagnostic radioimmunoassays, as compared to patient-derived polyclonals. Point mutations and/or modifications of the glycosylation could change IgG637 from a pathogenic into a therapeutic. Although F_{ab} fragments have proven to protect against antigenic modulation,[3,4] their short half-life is a major drawback for potential therapeutic applications. Altering IgG637 in an IgG4-like bispecific molecule, with monovalent anti-AChR binding and no complement-activating capacities, could be a prolonged half-life alternative to F_{ab} treatment.

REFERENCES

1. GRAUS, Y.F., M.H. DE BAETS, P.W. PARREN *et al.* 1997. Human anti-nicotinic acetylcholine receptor recombinant Fab fragments isolated from thymus-derived phage display libraries from myasthenia gravis patients reflect predominant specificities in serum and block the action of pathogenic serum antibodies. J. Immunol. **158:** 1919–1929.
2. MENG, F., M.H.W. STASSEN, S. SCHILLBERG *et al.* 2002. Construction and characterization of a single-chain antibody fragment derived from thymus of a patient with myasthenia gravis. Autoimmunity **35:** 125–133.
3. TOYKA, K.V., B. LOWENADLER, K. HEININGER *et al.* 1980. Passively transferred myasthenia gravis: protection of mouse endplates by Fab fragments from human myasthenic IgG. J. Neurol. Neurosurg. Psychiatry **43:** 836–840.
4. PAPANASTASIOU, D., K. POULAS, A. KOKLA & S.J. TZARTOS. 2000. Prevention of passively transferred experimental autoimmune myasthenia gravis by Fab fragments of monoclonal antibodies directed against the main immunogenic region of the acetylcholine receptor. J. Neuroimmunol. **104:** 124–132.

Roles of Complex Gangliosides at the Neuromuscular Junction

R. W. M. BULLENS,[a,b] G. M. O'HANLON,[c] E. WAGNER,[c] P. C. MOLENAAR,[b] KOICHI FURUKAWA,[d] KEIKO FURUKAWA,[d] J. J. PLOMP,[a,b] AND H. J. WILLISON[c]

Departments of [a]Neurology and [b]Neurophysiology, Leiden University Medical Center, Leiden, the Netherlands

[c]University Department of Neurology, Southern General Hospital, Glasgow, Scotland

[d]Department of Biochemistry, Nagoya University School of Medicine, Nagoya, Japan

KEYWORDS: **complex gangliosides; neuromuscular junction (NMJ); Miller Fisher syndrome (MFS)**

INTRODUCTION

Neuronal membranes, in particular at synapses, are highly enriched in gangliosides, a diverse family of sialylated glycosphingolipids. On the basis of *in vitro* studies on the effects of exogenous gangliosides, it has been hypothesized that gangliosides, especially complex ones, modulate neurotransmitter release. Furthermore, they are believed to act as cell-surface receptors for clostridial botulinum neurotoxins at the neuromuscular junction (NMJ) and as primary autoantigenic targets of antiganglioside antibodies associated with paralytic neuropathies. We have tested these hypotheses directly using mice lacking endogenous complex gangliosides due to deletion of the gene coding for β1,4-GalNAc-transferase (GalNAcT).[1]

METHODS

Mice were obtained through breeding with heterozygous GalNAcT null-mutant mice. Microelectrode measurements were performed at diaphragm NMJs *in vitro* using standard equipment. We recorded miniature endplate potentials (MEPPs) and endplate potentials (EPPs) upon stimulation of the phrenic nerve. To prevent muscle action potentials and contraction, muscle Na^+ channels were blocked with μ-conotoxin-GIIIB. The quantal content, that is, the number of ACh quanta released per nerve impulse, was calculated from MEPP and EPP amplitudes. We tested the effect of Miller Fisher syndrome (MFS)–associated anti-GQ1b antibodies with added normal serum as a complement source and that of 2 ng/mL botulinum toxin type A.

Address for correspondence: Dr. J. J. Plomp, Ph.D., Department of Neurophysiology, Leiden University Medical Center, P. O. Box 9604, Wassenaarseweg 62, 2300 RC Leiden, the Netherlands. Voice: +31-71-527-6208; fax: +31-71-527-6782.
j.j.plomp@lumc.nl

Ann. N.Y. Acad. Sci. 998: 401–403 (2003). © 2003 New York Academy of Sciences.
doi: 10.1196/annals.1254.051

TABLE 1. Induction of the α-latrotoxin-like effects (increase in MEPP frequency) at NMJs of GalNAcT$^{-/-}$ and control mice (N = 3–6) by specific antiganglioside mouse monoclonal antibodies and MFS serum

		MEPP frequency (s^{-1})	
Antibody	Specificity	Control (wild-type/heterozygous)	GalNAcT$^{-/-}$
EM6	GQ1b	30.12 ± 9.89	0.73 ± 0.06
CGG2	GD3	0.86 ± 0.10	14.18 ± 3.65
CGM3	GQ1b/GD3	85.70 ± 9.82	89.03 ± 13.69

NOTE: Normal value of MEPP frequency before antibody/complement treatment is in the range of 0.25–1.0 s^{-1}.

RESULTS

At normal conditions (2 mM Ca^{2+}, 20°C), presynaptic ACh release evoked by 0.3 or 40 Hz nerve stimulation, as well as the frequency and amplitude of MEPPs (i.e., spontaneous release), did not differ between wild-type and knockout NMJs. Treatment of wild-type NMJs with botulinum neurotoxin type A readily induced a drastic reduction of nerve stimulation–evoked ACh release (quantal content) and MEPP frequency to about 1–2% of their values obtained without the toxin. In contrast, quantal content and MEPP frequency of GalNAcT$^{-/-}$ NMJs were unchanged by the botulinum neurotoxin. Serum from MFS patients contains autoantibodies against the complex ganglioside GQ1b. MFS serum (1:2), as well as a monospecific anti-ganglioside GQ1b mouse IgM monoclonal antibody (EM6, 50 μg/mL) induced a complement-dependent α-latrotoxin-like effect (which has been described in detail previously[2] and is characterized by a dramatic increase of MEPP frequency) in wild-type NMJs, but failed to do so at GalNAcT$^{-/-}$ NMJs (TABLE 1). Conversely, a monospecific anti-GD3 monoclonal IgG antibody (CGG2, 50 μg/mL) had no effect at wild-type NMJs, but readily induced α-latrotoxin-like effects at GalNAcT$^{-/-}$ NMJs. A bispecific anti-GQ1b/GD3 monoclonal IgM antibody (CGM3, 50 μg/mL) induced the α-latrotoxin-like effects at NMJs of both genotypes.

CONCLUSIONS

Our studies demonstrate that complex gangliosides are functionally redundant for synaptic function under physiological conditions, but form receptors for botulinum neurotoxin type A and neuropathy-associated autoantibodies at the NMJ. It has been shown that the level of the simple ganglioside GD3 is increased in brains of GalNAcT$^{-/-}$ mice.[3] This seems also the case at motor nerve terminals, in view of our observation that monospecific anti-GD3 antibodies induce α-latrotoxin-like effects only at GalNAcT$^{-/-}$ NMJs. On the basis of the observed effects of specific anti-ganglioside antibodies, we conclude that the complex ganglioside GQ1b is indeed the primary antigenic target for MFS-related anti-GQ1b antibodies that induce the α-latrotoxin-like effects at the NMJ, and that high levels of the simple ganglioside GD3 can substitute for GQ1b in mediating this effect.

ACKNOWLEDGMENT

This work was supported by the Prinses Beatrix Fonds, Grant No. MAR62-0210.

REFERENCES

1. BULLENS, R.W.M., G.M. O'HANLON, E. WAGNER *et al.* 2002. Complex gangliosides at the neuromuscular junction are membrane receptors for autoantibodies and botulinum neurotoxin, but redundant for normal synaptic function. J. Neurosci. **22:** 6876–6884.
2. PLOMP, J.J., P.C. MOLENAAR, G.M. O'HANLON *et al.* 1999. Miller Fisher anti-GQ1b antibodies: alpha-latrotoxin-like effects on motor end plates. Ann. Neurol. **45:** 189–199.
3. TAKAMIYA, K., A. YAMAMOTO, K. FURUKAWA *et al.* 1996. Mice with disrupted GM2/GD2 synthase gene lack complex gangliosides, but exhibit only subtle defects in their nervous system. Proc. Natl. Acad. Sci. USA **93:** 10662–10667.

Role of Munc18-1 in Synaptic Plasticity at the Myasthenic Neuromuscular Junction

M. S. SONS,[a] M. VERHAGE,[b] AND J. J. PLOMP[a]

[a]*Departments of Neurology and Neurophysiology, Leiden University Medical Center, Leiden, the Netherlands*

[b]*Center for Neurogenomics and Cognition Research (CNCR), Vrije Universiteit Amsterdam, Amsterdam, the Netherlands*

Keywords: myasthenia gravis; neuromuscular junction; acetylcholine receptor density; toxin-induced myasthenia gravis; Munc18-1

INTRODUCTION

In myasthenia gravis (MG), the decreased acetylcholine (ACh) receptor density at the neuromuscular junction (NMJ) is partly compensated for by an increase of presynaptic ACh release.[1] The underlying mechanism remains largely unknown, but might involve retrograde signals from muscle fiber to motor nerve terminal, acting on the exocytotic proteins that regulate transmitter secretion. A crucial step in regulated secretion is the formation of a complex consisting of syntaxin, SNAP25, and synaptobrevin/VAMP, which is highly regulated by a number of proteins, among which are sec/Munc18-like proteins. Sec/Munc18-like proteins are essential for neurotransmitter secretion in *Drosophila*, *C. elegans*, and mice,[2] and for vesicle fusion in yeast. Munc18-1–deficient mice lack prenatal neurotransmission and die upon birth. Heterozygous Munc18-1 null-mutant mice are viable and have a 50% protein level. Earlier, we found that ACh release at NMJs of 2-month-old heterozygous Munc18-1 mice is reduced by about 25%, but that this reduction becomes less pronounced at later ages (Sons and Plomp, unpublished results), suggesting age-dependent adaptation of the ACh release mechanism to the 50% Munc18-1 protein level. Munc18-1 might also be of importance in processes of synaptic adaptation. Therefore, we investigated the possible involvement of Munc18-1 in the upregulation of ACh release at myasthenic NMJs.[3]

Address for correspondence: Dr. J. J. Plomp, Ph.D., Department of Neurophysiology, Leiden University Medical Center, P. O. Box 9604, Wassenaarseweg 62, 2300 RC Leiden, the Netherlands. Voice: +31-71-527-6208; fax: +31-71-527-6782.
j.j.plomp@lumc.nl

**Ann. N.Y. Acad. Sci. 998: 404–406 (2003). © 2003 New York Academy of Sciences.
doi: 10.1196/annals.1254.052**

METHODS

Groups ($N = 5–6$) of 4-month-old Munc18-1 heterozygous and wild-type mice were used. We applied a model of MG, toxin-induced myasthenia gravis (TIMG), previously described in rats.[2] In TIMG, ACh receptors at the NMJ are reduced by α-bungarotoxin injection (4 weeks, 1–1.2 μg toxin per 48 h). Control mice received saline. Mice were sacrificed, and hemidiaphragms with the phrenic nerves were dissected. With standard microelectrode equipment, we analyzed NMJ synaptic function. We recorded miniature endplate potentials (MEPPs) and endplate potentials (EPPs) upon stimulation of the phrenic nerve (0.3 and 40 Hz). To prevent muscle action potentials and contraction, muscle Na^+ channels were blocked with μ-conotoxin-GIIIB. The quantal content, that is, the number of ACh quanta releases per nerve impulse, was calculated from MEPP and EPP amplitudes.

RESULTS

Both low-rate stimulation-evoked (0.3 Hz) and spontaneous ACh release (MEPP frequency) at Munc18-1 heterozygous NMJs were not different from wild type. However, we found a slightly increased depression of EPP amplitude at high-rate (40 Hz) stimulation (i.e., 26%, compared to 16% in the wild-type, $p < 0.01$). TIMG treatment induced a reduction of the mean MEPP amplitude of about 65% at NMJs of both Munc18-1 heterozygous and wild-type mice (FIG. 1), reflecting an equal reduction of postsynaptic sensitivity to ACh. We found compensatory increase in

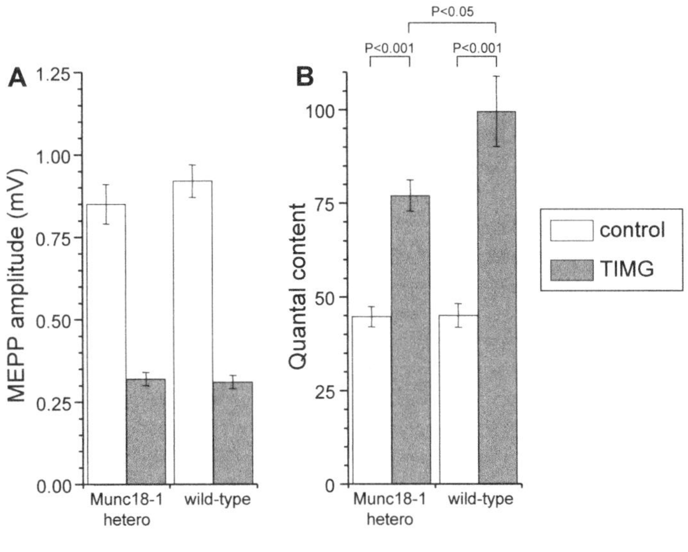

FIGURE 1. Effects of toxin-induced myasthenia gravis (TIMG) on MEPP amplitude **(A)** and quantal content **(B)** at NMJs in Munc18-1 heterozygous and wild-type mice.

quantal content, as previously demonstrated in rat and human MG NMJs.[1] However, this phenomenon was much less pronounced at Munc18-1 heterozygous NMJs (68% increase vs. 125% at wild-type NMJs, $p < 0.05$).

DISCUSSION

One suggested role for Munc18-1 is that it makes presynaptic transmitter vesicle fusion ready, thereby increasing the pool that is directly available for release. The observed increased rundown of ACh release at 40-Hz stimulation at NMJs of heterozygous Munc18-1 mice, apparently due to an incapability to maintain the readily releasable pool, supports such a role. The finding that Munc18-1 heterozygous NMJs are less capable of developing a compensatory increase in ACh release under TIMG conditions indicates that Munc18-1 is involved in the underlying mechanism of this form of synaptic plasticity. Our results suggest that Munc18-1 increases the readily releasable pool of ACh vesicles in TIMG so that more transmitter is released. A retrograde factor from the myasthenic postsynapse might stimulate presynaptic Munc18-1 activity. This might involve a signaling cascade that affects the phosphorylation state of Munc18-1, which is shown to be highly important for its function.[4]

ACKNOWLEDGMENT

This work was supported by the Netherlands Organization for Scientific Research NWO, Grant No. 903-42-073.

REFERENCES

1. Plomp, J.J., G.T. Van Kempen, M.B. De Baets *et al.* 1995. Acetylcholine release in myasthenia gravis: regulation at single end-plate level. Ann. Neurol. **37:** 627–636.
2. Verhage, M., A.S. Maia, J.J. Plomp *et al.* 2000. Synaptic assembly of the brain in the absence of neurotransmitter secretion. Science **287:** 864–869.
3. Molenaar, P.C., B.S. Oen, J.J. Plomp *et al.* 1991. A non-immunogenic myasthenia gravis model and its application in a study of transsynaptic regulation at the neuromuscular junction. Eur. J. Pharmacol. **196:** 93–101.
4. de Vries, K.J., A. Geijtenbeek, E.C. Brian *et al.* 2000. Dynamics of Munc18-1 phosphorylation/dephosphorylation in rat brain nerve terminals. Eur. J. Neurosci. **12:** 385–390.

The Epidemiology of Myasthenia Gravis

LAWRENCE H. PHILLIPS II

Department of Neurology, University of Virginia, Charlottesville, Virginia 22908, USA

ABSTRACT: Population-based studies of the epidemiology of myasthenia gravis (MG) have been conducted for over 50 years. Over that time, there has been a clear trend towards an increase in the reported prevalence of the disease. In recent years, there has also been an interest in determining a reasonably accurate estimate of the number of MG patients in the United States. Current estimates place the prevalence at a high value of about 20 per 100,000. The year 2000 U.S. population estimate is slightly less than 280 million. A crude estimate of the number of MG patients derived from the population estimate and the reported prevalence from selected populations indicates that there are between 53,000 and 59,900 patients in the United States at this time. The age and ethnic distributions in the United States are evolving from those that were present when the majority of the population-based studies were done, and the distribution of severity of the disease may also have changed. Future studies of the epidemiology of MG should take these factors into account, and further research into the economic and quality-of-life impact of the disease in the population is needed.

KEYWORDS: epidemiology; myasthenia gravis (MG); population

Myasthenia gravis (MG) is an uncommon disease. Neurologists with busy clinical practices often encounter only a handful of patients with the disease in their entire careers. The small number of patients with MG has hindered research into effective targeted therapies for the disease since funding agencies and the pharmaceutical industry do not perceive there to be a market with enough size to warrant large investment. One consequence has been that treatment innovations for MG have lagged behind other diseases. Most of the newer therapies for MG have been "borrowed" from treatments devised for other diseases. Frustration with this situation has led some within the MG community in the United States to suggest that a large-scale effort be devoted to more intensive epidemiological research in an attempt to identify additional numbers of patients with the disease.

When considering where epidemiological research in MG should go in the future, one should first determine what is already known. If additional studies are to be done, how and where should efforts be directed? A considerable number of studies based on populations in various locations in the United States as well as increasingly diverse areas throughout the world have been done. From these studies, we have

Address for correspondence: L. H. Phillips II, M.D., Department of Neurology, University of Virginia, Box 800394, Charlottesville, VA 22908. Voice: 434-924-5361; fax: 434-982-1850.
lhp3n@virginia.edu

Ann. N.Y. Acad. Sci. 998: 407–412 (2003). **© 2003 New York Academy of Sciences.**
doi: 10.1196/annals.1254.053

learned that MG is a disease with worldwide distribution. There are, however, some large populations that have been surveyed incompletely (e.g., in China and sub-Saharan Africa) or not at all (e.g., in South America and Australia). If there were ethnic or geographic differences in the occurrence or natural history of the disease, study of some of these populations would be important.

What do we know from the available data? My colleagues and I performed a population-based study of the epidemiology of MG in locations in Virginia in the 1980s.[1] When we did the background research for that study, it became clear from the published data on the epidemiology of MG that the prevalence of the disease was trending upwards over time. In 1996, we did a detailed analysis of the literature to establish that, in fact, there had been an increase in the reported prevalence of MG over the preceding 40 years that exceeded what would have been expected from a corresponding increase in incidence.[2] We postulated that the rise in prevalence was a consequence of several factors, including improved case identification, prolonged survival with the disease due to increasingly effective therapy, and aging of the population at risk. From this data, I was also able to make an estimate that the total number of patients with MG in the United States was somewhere between 20,000 and 70,000.[3]

Since the data upon which this estimate was based are now nearly a decade old, has the epidemiology of MG changed in any way? Is there any indication that the evolving natural history of the disease has altered the numbers of patients with MG in any substantial way? If the answer to either of these questions is positive, there may be a need for further classical population-based epidemiological surveys in the United States as well as other countries. In this study, I have updated my previous examination of the world's literature on population-based studies of the epidemiology of MG. My goal is to determine whether or not the previously noted trend of increasing prevalence has continued and to produce an updated estimate of the actual number of patients with MG in the United States.

METHODS

Using our previous publication on the subject[2] as a starting point, I identified all reports in the world literature of population-based studies of the epidemiology of MG. In addition to the reports that were included in the previous study, I performed a MEDLINE search using the search terms of MG, epidemiology, prevalence, incidence, and mortality for the period from 1989 through 2002. Additional non-indexed publications were identified from bibliographic references in the publications found from the MEDLINE search. Publications were included if they were based on a population survey and reported a point prevalence rate.

In most reports, the actual number of cases was noted; however, where they were not, they were estimated by multiplying the population by the rate. Confidence intervals (CIs) for rates were calculated from tables prepared by Schoenberg.[4] In this method, the rate is considered to be the mean of a Poisson distribution, and 95% CIs are derived from the tables based on the number of patients from which the rate is derived.

U.S. population estimates were obtained from U.S. Bureau of the Census figures.[5] The population estimates are derived from projections of the 1990 census data because the data for the 2000 census were not available at the time of the preparation of this study.

The prevalence trends over time were analyzed in two ways. First, I performed a linear regression of the date of the study against the reported prevalence rate. A 95% prediction line was fitted to the regression line to define its upper and lower limits. Second, a weighted mean prevalence rate for each decade was calculated. This incorporated the size of the populations studied by summing the number of patients identified in each decade of the study and dividing it by the total of the populations surveyed for that decade. This calculation produces a weighted mean prevalence rate for each decade. The rate of increase in the mean prevalence was further highlighted by calculating a risk ratio for each decade by dividing each rate by the rate obtained for the earliest decade of the study (1950–1959). This is expressed as the relative rate.

RESULTS

In our 1996 study, we found reports of 37 prevalence rates from 29 locations. An additional 13 rates were reported in the interval since that time, bringing the total number of studies for this analysis to 50.[6–15] The most recent report, from British Columbia, indicated a prevalence estimate of 20.4 per 100,000.[15] This is the highest rate yet reported. In addition, a "lifetime prevalence rate" for MG of 40 per 100,000 was reported for a population in London, United Kingdom.[16] This rate was not included in the present calculations because it is a different type of measurement.

When the rates are plotted against the year of study, the regression fitted to the values continues to have a positive slope (FIG. 1). The 95% prediction bands include the rate reported by Isbister and colleagues.[15] The weighted mean prevalence rates per decade have also continued to rise (FIG. 2 and TABLE 1).

The previous estimate of the number of patients with MG in the United States was based on the prevalence rate we obtained from the Virginia study.[3] At the time, the

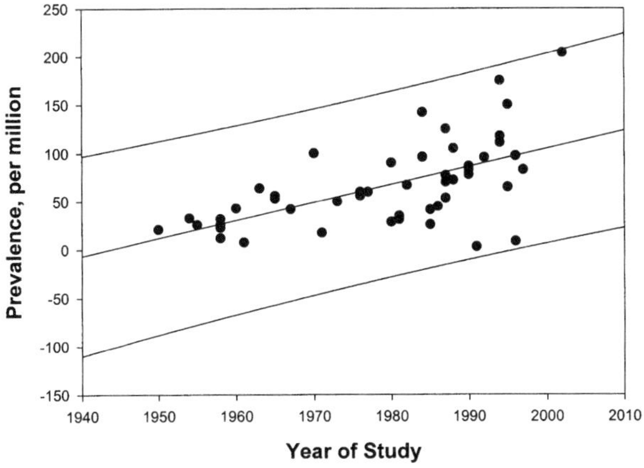

FIGURE 1. A plot of point prevalence rate against year of study is shown. The regression line has a correlation coefficient of 0.59. The 95% prediction lines are also plotted.

TABLE 1. Weighted mean prevalence by decade

	1950–1959	1960–1969	1970–1979	1980–1989	1990–present
Prevalence[a]	22.2	25.1	58.2	58.2	93.9
CI[b]	18.7–26.3	22.7–27.7	54.6–61.9	54.6–61.9	88.2–99.9
Relative rate	1.0	1.1	2.6	2.6	4.2

[a]Rate expressed per million population.
[b]Confidence interval (95%).

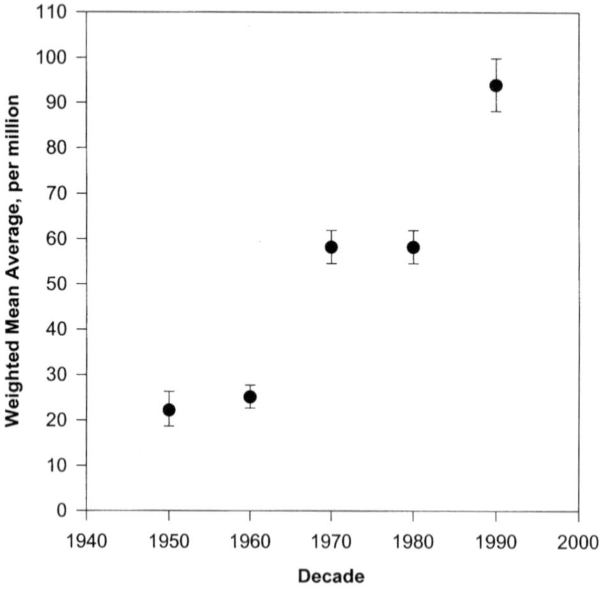

FIGURE 2. The weighted mean prevalence rates for each decade are shown with 95% confidence intervals.

rate of 14.2 per 100,000 represented the highest prevalence rate yet reported. Since that time, additional higher rates have been reported on various populations, and the highest to date is 20.4 per 100,000.[15] The 95% confidence interval for this rate is 19.2–21.7. An estimate of the number of patients in the entire country can be made by multiplying a rate by the 2000 population estimate of 276,059,000. If we consider the weighted mean rate for 1990–present to be a reliable estimate, the number of patients in the United States would be 25,922 (95% CI of 24,348–27,598). If we use the rate quoted by Isbister and colleagues,[15] the estimated number of patients would be 56,316 (95% CI of 53,003–59,904).

DISCUSSION

Several observations can be made from the accumulated body of epidemiological data for MG. It is clear from the present analysis that the reported prevalence of the disease continues to rise. The probable reasons for this increase are likely those noted above. We can take some satisfaction from the fact that, in addition to improved diagnostic accuracy and increasing longevity of the population in general, patients with MG are living longer. Our present treatments must have some impact on prolonging survival with the disease, and this is reflected in an increase in the number of people living with the disease at any one time (i.e., the prevalence).

It is equally clear, however, that the total number of patients with MG is still relatively small. I previously estimated that the number of patients with the disease in 1995 would be just over 38,000.[3] The present estimate of up to 59,000 patients in 2000 indicates that, although the trend is clearly upwards, the total number continues to fall into the category of a rare disease. How then might these data be used to advocate for our patients with funding agencies and pharmaceutical companies?

Although epidemiological studies are being done in increasing numbers, the populations being studied have been in locations other than the United States. The last reported prevalence on a population in this country was the one we reported from Virginia in 1984.[1] The only other more recent North American study was the British Columbia study, reported only in abstract form to date.[15] Most of the remainder of recent studies have been on European populations. If there are any ethnic or racial differences in the occurrence or natural history of MG, the studies reported to date are unlikely to have discovered them. There is at least some indication of a higher incidence and prevalence among African-Americans in the Virginia population.[1] Since there is increasing ethnic diversity in the United States population, further research into the patterns of diseases such as MG should be done. We cannot just assume that a largely Hispanic population, for example, will have the same disease frequency and natural history as does a largely Caucasian one.

Another fruitful area of emphasis for epidemiological research in MG may be related to evolving disease severity patterns. Some clinicians who deal with large populations of patients with MG feel that the number of patients with ocular-only disease (class I MGFA classification[17]) seems to be increasing in recent years. If there are increasing numbers of patients who have the restricted form of the disease, the design of future treatment trials should take this into account.

Lastly, even though MG may not be a major public health problem in terms of the numbers of patients affected, it is surely a disease that has major financial impact. There is only one study that has examined the quality of life for patients with MG, and it did not address the economic impact of the disease.[18] A population-based study that assessed this issue would help clarify the true impact of the disease.

In summary, although the number of patients with MG in the United States continues to rise, it is still a rare disease. Further research into the demographic and economic impact of the disease in the population in this country is needed.

REFERENCES

1. PHILLIPS, L.H., J.C. TORNER, M.S. ANDERSON *et al.* 1992. The epidemiology of myasthenia gravis in central and western Virginia. Neurology **42:** 1888–1893.

2. PHILLIPS, L.H. & J.C. TORNER. 1996. Epidemiologic evidence for a changing natural history of myasthenia gravis. Neurology **47:** 1233–1238.
3. PHILLIPS, L.H. 1994. The epidemiology of myasthenia gravis. Neurol. Clin. North Am. **12:** 263–271.
4. SCHOENBERG, B.S. 1983. Calculating confidence intervals for rates and ratios: simplified method utilizing tabular values based on the Poisson distribution. Neuroepidemiology **2:** 257–265.
5. UNITED STATES BUREAU OF THE CENSUS. 2002. Resident population estimates of the United States by age and sex: April 1, 1990 to July 1, 1999, with short-term projection to November 1, 2000 [http://eire.census.gov/popest/archives/national/nation2/intfile2-1.txt]. [Accessed March 5, 2002.]
6. KRYIALLIS, K., A.H. HRISTOVA & L.T. MIDDLETON. 1995. What is the real epidemiology of myasthenia gravis [abstract]? Neurology **45**(suppl. 4)**:** A351–A352.
7. CISNEROS, A.D., R.S. LUIS, R. LÉON *et al.* 1996. Algunos aspectos epidemiológicos de la miastenia gravis en Cuba. Rev. Neurol. (Barcelona) **24:** 435–439.
8. VILLAGRA-COCCO, A. & P. VILLAGRA-COCCO. 1997. Prevalencia de la miastenia gravis en la isla de La Palma. Rev. Neurol. (Barcelona) **25:** 2068–2069.
9. AIELLO, I., M. PASTORINO, S. SOTGIU *et al.* 1997. Epidemiology of myasthenia gravis in northwestern Sardinia. Neuroepidemiology **16:** 199–206.
10. ZIVADINOV, R., A. JURJEVIC, K. WILLHEIM *et al.* 1998. Incidence and prevalence of myasthenia gravis in the county of the Coast and Gorski kotar, Croatia, 1976 through 1996. Neuroepidemiology **17:** 265–272.
11. GUIDETTI, D., R. SABADINI, M. BONDAVALLI *et al.* 1998. Epidemiological study of myasthenia gravis in the province of Reggio Emilia, Italy. Eur. J. Epidemiol. **14:** 381–387.
12. ROBERTSON, N.P., J. DEANS & D.A.S. COMPSTON. 1998. Myasthenia gravis: a population-based epidemiological study in Cambridgeshire, England. J. Neurol. Neurosurg. Psychiatry **65:** 492–496.
13. LAVRNIC, D., M. JAREBINSKI, V. RAKOCEVIC-STOJANOVIC *et al.* 1999. Epidemiological and clinical characteristics of myasthenia gravis in Belgrade, Yugoslavia (1983–1992). Acta Neurol. Scand. **100:** 168–174.
14. HOLTSEMA, H., J. MOURIK, R.E. RICO *et al.* 2000. Myasthenia gravis on the Dutch Antilles: an epidemiological study. Clin. Neurol. Neurosurg. **102:** 195–198.
15. ISBISTER, C.M., P.J. MACKENZIE, D. ANDERSON *et al.* 2002. Co-occurrence of multiple sclerosis and myasthenia gravis in British Columbia: a population-based study [abstract]. Neurology **58**(suppl. 3)**:** A185–A186.
16. MACDONALD, B.K., O.C. COCKERELL, A.S. SANDER *et al.* 2000. The incidence and lifetime prevalence of neurological disorders in a prospective community-based study in the UK. Brain **123:** 665–676.
17. JARETZKI, A., R.J. BAROHN, R.M. ERNSTOFF *et al.* 2000. Myasthenia gravis: recommendations for clinical research standards. Neurology **55:** 16–23.
18. PAUL, R.H., J.M. NASH, R.A. COHEN *et al.* 2001. Quality of life and well-being of patients with myasthenia gravis. Neurology **24:** 512–516.

Myasthenia Gravis (MG): Epidemiological Data and Prognostic Factors

RENATO MANTEGAZZA,[a] FULVIO BAGGI,[a] CARLO ANTOZZI,[b]
PAOLO CONFALONIERI,[b] LUCIA MORANDI,[b] PIA BERNASCONI,[a]
FRANCESCA ANDREETTA,[a] ORNELLA SIMONCINI,[a]
ANGELA CAMPANELLA,[b] ETTORE BEGHI,[c] AND FERDINANDO CORNELIO[b]

[a]*Immunology and Muscular Pathology Unit,* [b]*Department of Neuromuscular Diseases, National Neurological Institute "Carlo Besta", 20133 Milan, Italy*

[c]*Istituto di Ricerche Farmacologiche "Mario Negri", 20133 Milan, Italy*

Abstract: Data from 756 myasthenic patients were analyzed for diagnostic criteria, clinical aspects, and therapeutic approaches. The patients were followed up at our institution from 1981 to 2001. Clinical evaluation was performed according to the myasthenia gravis score adopted at our clinic. Clinical features of each patient (comprising demographic, clinical, neurophysiological, immunological, radiological, and surgical data, as well as serial myasthenia gravis scores) were filed in a relational database containing more than 7000 records. Clinical efficacy and variables influencing outcome were assessed by life-table methods and Cox proportional hazards regression analysis. Complete stable remission, as defined by the Task Force of the Medical Scientific Advisory Board of the Myasthenia Gravis Foundation of America, was the end point for good prognosis. Four hundred and ninety-nine patients (66%) were female and 257 (34%) were male. Mean follow-up was 55.1 ± 48.1 months. Onset of symptoms peaked in the third decade in females, whereas the male distribution was bimodal with peaks in the third and sixth decades. Modality of myasthenia gravis presentation was as follows: ocular, 39.3%; generalized, 28.5%; bulbar, 31.3%; and respiratory, 0.8%. Thymectomy was carried out on 63.7% of our patients by different approaches: (1) transcervical; (2) transsternal; (3) video-thoracoscopic mini-invasive surgery. The last approach has been preferentially used in more recent years and accounted for 62.4% of the thymectomized myasthenia gravis population. Univariate analysis and Kaplan-Meier analysis showed that variables such as sex (female), age at onset (below 40 years), thymectomy, and histological diagnosis of thymic hyperplasia were significantly associated with complete stable remission, whereas on multivariate analysis only age at onset below 40 years and thymectomy were confirmed.

Keywords: myasthenia gravis (MG); diagnosis; database; prognostic factor

Address for correspondence: Renato Mantegazza, Immunology and Muscular Pathology Unit, National Neurological Institute "Carlo Besta", via Celoria 11, 20133 Milan, Italy. Voice: +39-022394372; fax: +39-0270633874.
rmantegazza@istituto-besta.it

Ann. N.Y. Acad. Sci. 998: 413–423 (2003). © 2003 New York Academy of Sciences.
doi: 10.1196/annals.1254.054

INTRODUCTION

Myasthenia gravis (MG) is a rare disease whose prevalence is between 50 and 125 persons within a population of 1 million. MG may manifest in any race, at any age, and in either sex.[1] Incidence peaks below 40 years for women and above 60 years for men, but an increase in the prevalence over the past 45 years has been reported.[2,3] Whether this increase is related to the general trend of aging or to different factors remains to be elucidated.

Since the early 1980s, a large cohort of myasthenic patients was identified through a multicenter Italian network and defined in terms of demographic, clinical, and prognostic features.[4,5] However, the data reported from that cohort were retrospective and possibly confounded by the lack of standardized methods for data collection and by the heterogeneity of the sources of cases.

Since then, our group has developed a database for tracking MG patients, and the database includes a myasthenia gravis score (MGS), which accounts for weakness and fatigability; demographic, clinical, neurophysiological, immunological, radiological, and surgical data; and prospective MGS evaluations.[6] The MGS has been used systematically in both inpatients and outpatients, and the database has been updated, providing a file of more than 7000 records containing most of the clinical data useful for the prognostic evaluation of our MG population.

MATERIALS AND METHODS

Population

Seven hundred fifty-six MG outpatients or inpatients seen at our center between 1981 and 2001 were included in this study. A diagnosis of MG was made according to clinical, pharmacological, and electrophysiological criteria.[7] The anti-acetylcholine receptor (anti-AChR) antibody titer was assayed by an immunoprecipitation method using the human AChR as antigen.[8] Clinical evaluation of the patients was performed according to the MGS adopted at our clinic, as previously reported (TABLE 1).[6] The system provides a numerical score for muscular strength and resistance. Four different disability levels are recognized: ocular, generalized, bulbar, and respiratory. The patients' outcomes were determined by comparison of pretreatment and last checkup scores. Patients' clinical records were filed in the MG patients' database (FIG. 1). All patients were diagnosed and followed up by the same neurologists (R.M., C.A., P.C., L.M., and F.C.) involved in this study. An example of the clinical follow-up of a single patient is illustrated in FIGURE 2.

End Points and Statistical Analysis

The rate of remission (R) was used as the end point to evaluate the outcome and prognostic features in our MG population.[9] The impact of variables potentially affecting outcome was assessed by life-table analysis using the Kaplan-Meier survival curves, the log-rank function to comparisons, and the Cox proportional hazards function for multivariate analysis. Data are expressed as odds ratios (ORs) with 95% confidence intervals (CIs) in univariate and multivariate analyses.[10,11] Where applica-

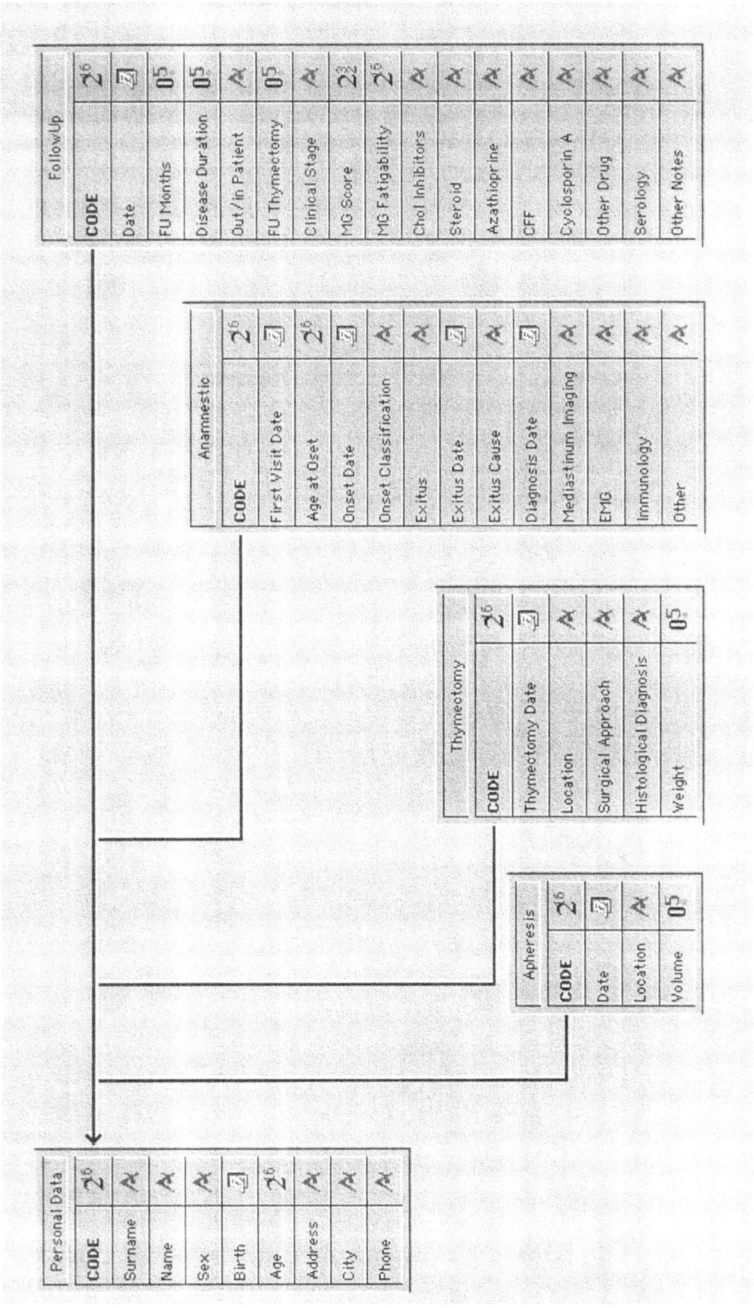

FIGURE 1. MG patient database structured on a relational software. Each box contains the records relative to the different clinical aspects filed in the database.

TABLE 1. MG score system

Ocular level	
0	Normal
1	Paretic nystagmus and/or blurred vision and/or provoked ptosis
2	Diplopia in one or two cardinal directions and/or monolateral ptosis
3	Diplopia in primary position and/or bilateral ptosis
4	Monolateral or bilateral ophthalmoplegia
Generalized level	
Facial muscles	
0	Normal
10	Orbicularis oculi and/or oris are weak, but can overcome outside resistance and snarl or smile
20	Orbicularis oculi and/or oris are weak and cannot overcome outside resistance
30	Lagophthalmos and/or orbicularis oris plegia
Anterior head and neck flexor muscles	
0/10/20/30/40/50	(Graded according to an inverted MRC grading scale)
Abdominal muscles	
0	Normal
10	Ability to flex the vertebral column with hands clasped behind the head
20	Ability to flex the vertebral column with forearms folded across the chest
30	Ability to flex the vertebral column with forearms extended forward
40	Ability to flex the cervical spine with forearms extended forward
50	Inability to curl the trunk
Deltoid muscles	
0/10/20/30/40/50	(Graded according to an inverted MRC grading scale)
Lower extremity muscles	
0	More than 15 squats
10	6–14 squats
20	1–5 squats
30	Squats with aid of the hands
40	Rising from a normal chair
50	Inability to rise from a normal chair
Bulbar level	
Chewing	
0	Normal
1000	Weakness of masseters against resistance
2000	Ptosis of the jaw
Tongue	
0	Normal

TABLE 1. MG score system (*Continued*)

1000	Inability to press the tip against cheek and/or inability to curl the tongue and reach the upper lip frenulum
2000	Inability to protrude the tongue
Swallowing	
0	Normal
1000	Dysphagia and/or necessity for soft foods
20,000	Impossible; nasal tube feeding
Phonation	
0	Normal
1000	Slight nasal voice
2000	Severe nasal voice, but speech still intelligible
3000	Speech difficult to understand
Respiratory level	
0	Normal
200,000	Vital capacity between 15 and 25 mL/kg body weight
500,000	Impossible; artificial ventilation
Total score ...	***Fatigability***
	Upper limbs (normal value: > 120) ...
	Lower limbs (normal value: > 120) ...

ble, the χ^2 test and Student's *t* test were used; *p* values lower than 0.05 were considered significant. All analyses were performed using the Statview statistical software, release 5.0 (Abacus Concepts, Berkeley, CA).

RESULTS

The main demographic and clinical features of the sample are depicted in TABLE 2. Seven hundred fifty-six MG patients were included in this study. Four hundred ninety-nine (66%) of the patients were female and 257 (34%) were male. Age at onset, evaluated by decades, revealed the following distribution: for females, one peak in the third decade; for males, a wider distribution showing two peaks, one in the third decade and the other in the sixth decade (FIG. 3). Median age at onset was 32.6 years (range: 2–82 years). Age at onset was less than 40 years in 62% of the patients and over 40 years in 38%. Clinical status at MG onset was as follows: 297 (39.3%) with ocular symptoms, 215 (28.5%) with generalized MG, 237 (31.3%) with bulbar MG, and 7 (0.8%) with respiratory symptoms. A positive decremental response to low-frequency repetitive stimulation (the Desmedt test) was observed in 75.9% of the patients. Five hundred fifty-three (73.2%) patients were positive to anti-AChR antibody testing at diagnosis; serum samples were not available in 17 patients (2.2%). Mean duration of MG at the time of diagnosis was 11.7 months (range: 0.5–492). Clinical status of MG at maximal worsening was as follows: 130 (17.2%) with ocular symptoms, 173 (22.8%) with generalized MG, 337 (44.7%)

TABLE 2. Main clinical features of 756 Italian MG patients

Variable	% of females	% of males	Total number of patients (%)
Sex	66	34	756 (100)
Age at onset			
< 40 years	69.7	47.2	469 (62)
> 40 years	30.3	52.8	287 (38)
Onset: clinical status			
Ocular	38	41.9	297 (39.3)
Generalized	30	25.7	215 (28.5)
Bulbar	31.5	31	237 (31.3)
Respiratory	0.5	1.4	7 (0.8)
EMG			
Positive	63.7	36.3	574 (75.9)
Anti-AChR Ab at diagnosis			
Positive	72.7	74.2	553 (73.2)
Deaths	46.2	53.8	26 (3.4)
Clinical status at maximal worsening			
Ocular	48.1	51.9	130 (17.2)
Generalized	65.8	34.2	172 (22.8)
Bulbar	64.1	35.9	338 (44.7)
Respiratory	64.9	35.1	116 (15.3)
Clinical status at last observation			
Free of symptoms	54.5	52.5	407 (58.3)
Ocular	5.9	5.5	44 (5.8)
Generalized	32.9	36.4	258 (34.1)
Bulbar	6.6	5.5	48 (6.3)

with bulbar MG, and 116 (15.3%) with respiratory symptoms. At the last follow-up visit, 407 (53.8%) patients were symptom-free, 258 (34.1%) were affected with a generalized MG, 48 (6.3%) were affected with a bulbar MG, and 44 (5.8%) were affect with an ocular form

A total of 26 (3.4%) MG patients died (12 females and 14 males): 9 for causes related to MG, 9 because of malignancies, and 8 for other medical problems. The mean follow-up for the whole group was 55.1 ± 48.1 months (range: 0.5–354); presurgery follow-up was 30.2 ± 46.7 months (range: 0.5–309).

Cholinesterase inhibitors, prednisone, and azathioprine, as single drugs, were given in 28.8%, 66.9%, and 4.6% of patients, respectively. The association of prednisone and azathioprine was used in 32% of our patients. The use of cyclofosfamide and cyclosporin A was 1.8% and 2.7%, respectively.

Thymectomy was performed in 481 patients (63.7%); 155 of these (32.3%) were operated on by a transsternal approach, 21 (4.3%) by a transcervical approach, 300 (62.4%) by a video-thoracoscopic approach (VATET), and 5 (1.1%) by other

A EL 18-04-1974

Cod. 2 Timect. SI 20-11-1987 Sedute PEX 0 Durata Malattia 16 anni 11 mesi

Nr	Data	Sede	Punt	Sec	Prel	Mst	MstR	Cortisone ON	Cortisone OFF	Tipo	Aza	CCF	CyA	☐	Outcome 1°	Outcome prec	Altri farm.
4	27-11-1986	R	27263	0	0	360	0	75	75	Delta	0	0	0	0	W	W	
5	3-12-1986	R	4133	6	0	360	0	75	75	Delta	0	0	0	0	W	I	
6	11-12-1986	R	3133	8	0	360	0	75	75	Delta	0	0	0	0	U	U	
7	4-02-1987	A	1080	70	0	360	0	75	75	Delta	0	0	0	0	I	I	
8	13-06-1987	A	1090	70	0	360	0	75	65	Delta	0	0	0	0	I	U	SI
9	4-08-1987	A	100	30	0	360	0	110	30	Delta	0	0	0	0	MI	I	
10	27-09-1987	R	24111	0	1152	360	0	120	120	Delta	0	0	0	0	W	W	
11	17-10-1987	R	2091	28	0	360	0	110	0	Delta	0	0	0	0	U	MI	
12	17-11-1987	R	4173	0	1251	360	180	90	10	Delta	0	0	0	0	W	W	
13	24-11-1987	R	1053	20	0	360	180	90	10	Delta	0	0	0	0	I	I	
14	1-12-1987	R	2141	18	0	360	180	90	10	Delta	0	0	0	0	U	U	
15	9-02-1988	A	50	140	1462	480	180	70	10	Delta	0	0	0	0	MI	MI	
16	26-04-1988	A	60	85	1669	360	130	70	0	Delta	0	0	0	0	MI	U	SI
17	22-07-1988	A	60	150	1885	240	90	60	0	Delta	0	0	0	0	MI	U	
18	24-05-1989	A	20	140	0	240	0	45	0	Delta	0	0	0	0	MI	I	
19	2-08-1989	A	50	170	0	180	0	40	0	Delta	0	0	0	0	MI	U	
20	4-10-1989	A	40	155	0	180	0	35	0	Delta	0	0	0	0	MI	U	
21	13-12-1989	A	50	145	0	180	0	30	0	Delta	0	0	0	0	MI	U	
22	13-12-1989	A	50	145	0	180	0	30	0	Delta	0	0	0	0	MI	U	
23	7-02-1990	A	20	155	0	180	0	25	0	Delta	0	0	0	0	MI	I	
24	4-04-1990	A	30	145	0	180	0	20	0	Delta	0	0	0	0	MI	U	
25	6-06-1990	A	20	165	0	180	0	17.5	0	Delta	0	0	0	0	MI	U	
26	25-07-1990	A	20	150	0	120	0	15	0	Delta	0	0	0	0	MI	U	
27	19-09-1990	A	50	180	0	120	0	12.5	0	Delta	0	0	0	0	MI	U	
28	18-11-1990	A	50	165	0	45	0	10	0	Delta	0	0	0	0	MI	U	
29	13-02-1991	A	40	150	3671	120	0	7.5	0	Delta	0	0	0	0	MI	U	
30	10-04-1991	A	40	140	0	60	0	7.5	0	Delta	0	0	0	0	MI	U	
31	5-06-1991	A	40	130	0	60	0	5	0	Delta	0	0	0	0	MI	U	
32	9-10-1991	A	50	140	0	180	0	2.5	0	Delta	0	0	0	0	MI	U	
33	18-03-1992	A	60	150	0	120	0	2.5	0	Delta	0	0	0	0	MI	U	
34	18-03-1992	A	40	150	0	60	0	2.5	0	Delta	0	0	0	0	MI	U	
35	15-07-1992	A	50	95	5269	120	0	0	0		0	0	0	0	MI	U	
36	25-11-1992	A	50	160	0	240	0	0	0		0	0	0	0	MI	U	
37	12-05-1993	A	60	140	0	240	0	0	0		0	0	0	0	MI	U	
38	10-11-1993	A	50	80	7134	240	0	0	0		0	0	0	0	MI	U	
39	18-05-1994	A	50	120	7964	240	0	0	0		0	0	0	0	MI	U	
40	25-10-1995	A	20	140	0	240	0	0	0		0	0	0	0	MI	I	
41	5-06-1996	A	50	100	0	300	0	0	0		0	0	0	0	MI	U	
42	16-07-1997	A	43	80	0	450	0	0	0		0	0	0	0	MI	U	
43	20-10-1999	A	42	75	0	600	0	0	0		0	0	0	0	MI	U	
44	19-01-2000	A	80	140	0	600	0	0	0		100	0	0	0	MI	U	
45	31-05-2000	A	32	180	0	600	0	0	0		150	0	0	0	MI	I	
46	28-03-2001	A	52	165	0	480	0	0	0		150	0	0	0	MI	U	

FIGURE 2. Example of a myasthenic patient follow-up series as derived by the MG patient database. The list is printable automatically after each clinical visit.

techniques. Since February 1994, it has been routine to use VATET as the initial approach; in only 13 out of 300 patients for whom VATET was proposed did technical problems in performing thymectomy via VATET result in thymectomies being given via a transsternal approach. Histological diagnoses in our thymectomized MG population were as follows: involuted thymus in 137 (28.5%), hyperplastic thymus in 220 (45.8%), and thymoma in 124 (25.7%) (TABLE 1).

The cumulative probability of achieving *R* in the whole MG population is shown in FIGURE 4. Life-table analyses of MG patients are shown in FIGURE 5. These analyses take into account sex, age at onset, thymectomy (yes or no), type of surgery, time to surgery, thymus histology, clinical classification of MG at onset, and positivity for anti-AChR antibodies. A significantly greater probability of achieving *R* was associated with female sex (FIG. 5A), age at onset below 40 years (FIG. 5B), thymectomy (FIG. 6A), type of surgery (FIG. 6B), and histological diagnosis of thymic

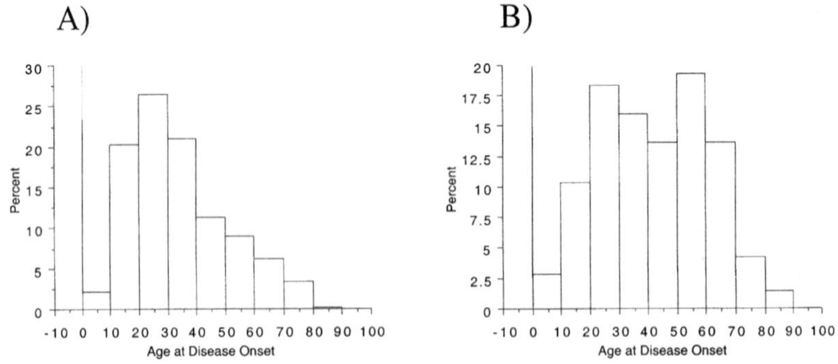

FIGURE 3. Age at onset, in decades, for **(A)** female MG patients and **(B)** male MG patients. Altogether, 756 MG patients were followed up from 1981 to 2001.

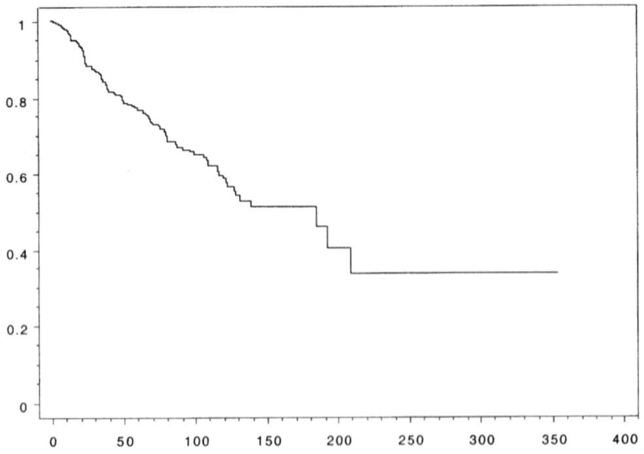

FIGURE 4. Kaplan-Meier analysis of remission in the 756 Italian MG patients included in the study.

hyperplasia (FIG. 6D). Clinical classification at onset (FIG. 5C), seronegativity to AChR antibodies (FIG. 5D), and time to surgery (FIG. 6C) had no influence on achievement of *R*.

Univariate Analysis

MG patients with age at onset below 40 years had a significantly higher probability of achieving *R* (OR: 2.59; 95% CI: 0.166–4.04; $p < 0.0001$) as did female patients (OR: 1.55; 95% CI: 1.67–2.26; $p = 0.02$). Thymectomy significantly improved the probability of achieving *R* (OR: 2.17; 95% CI: 1.46–3.24; $p < 0.0001$); the surgical approach seems to influence the probability of achieving *R* as the transsternal

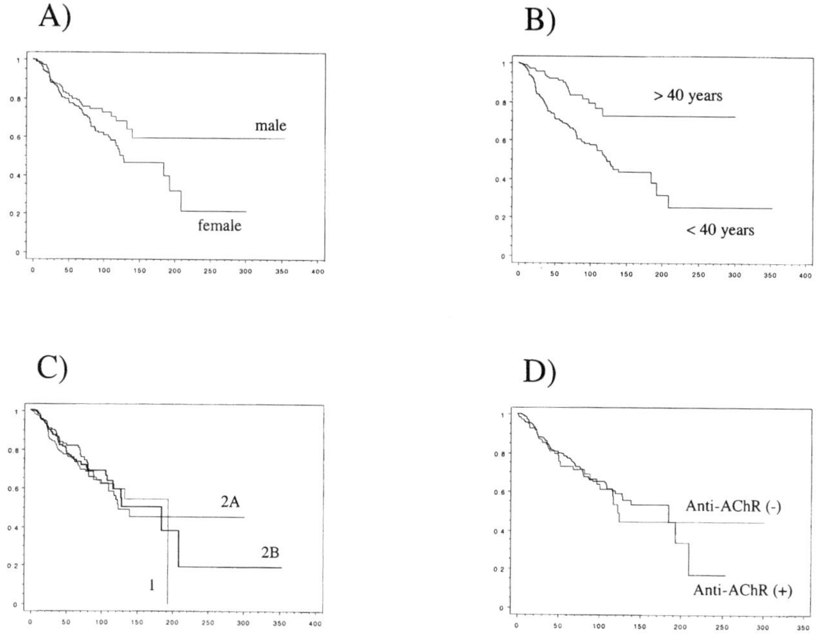

FIGURE 5. Kaplan-Meier analysis of remission according to **(A)** sex ($p = 0.04$), **(B)** age at onset ($p < 0.0001$), **(C)** clinical status at onset (p = not significant), and **(D)** anti-AChR antibody detection (p = not significant). The statistical analysis relied on the log-rank test.

approach was significantly different from VATET (OR: 0.36; 95% CI: 0.24–0.56; $p < 0.0001$). The histological diagnosis of thymic hyperplasia was significantly associated with *R* (OR: 4.32; 95% CI: 2.35–7.95), whereas thymoma was not (OR: 1.61; 95% CI: 0.60–4.31). A time from onset to surgery of less than 12 months (OR: 0.98; 95% CI: 0.67–1.47), an absence of anti-AChR antibody (OR: 1.12; 95% CI: 0.77–1.63), and the clinical stage at onset were not associated with *R*.

Multivariate Analysis

The variables significantly associated with *R* in the univariate analysis were used in a multivariate model. The results showed that the only variables maintaining statistical significance were an age at onset below 40 years and thymectomy (TABLE 3).

TABLE 3. Multivariate analysis of the odds of complete remission by age at onset, sex, and thymectomy

Variable	Odds ratio	Confidence interval	*p* value
Onset < 40 years	2.32	1.47–3.65	0.0003
Sex (female)	1.16	0.80–1.68	0.42
Thymectomy (yes)	1.63	1.08–2.45	0.02

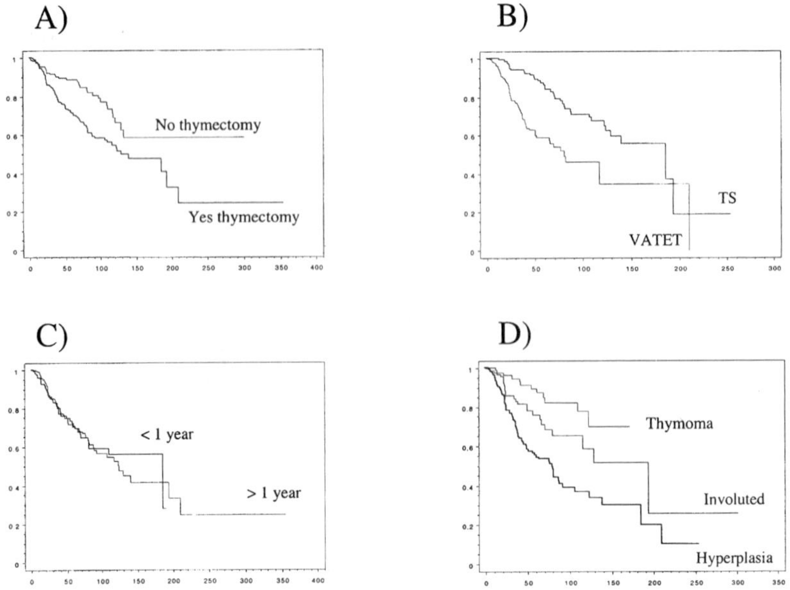

FIGURE 6. Kaplan-Meier analysis of remission according to **(A)** thymectomy ($p = 0.0003$), **(B)** type of surgery ($p < 0.0001$), **(C)** time to surgery (p = not significant), and **(D)** thymus histology ($p < 0.0001$).

DISCUSSION

In this study, we present epidemiological and prognostic features of an Italian MG population collected at a single center from 1981 through 2001. The main characteristics of this study are as follows: (1) a homogeneous diagnostic and clinical follow-up protocol that stems from the adoption and systematic use of the simple and reliable MGS system developed at our institution; (2) a life-table analysis that was permitted by a prospective evaluation and a computerized archive of MG patients; (3) a homogeneous therapeutical approach on the drug usage and surgical aspects.

A preponderance of females has been observed in our MG population; the same finding has been made in most of the other epidemiological studies on MG. As far as the age at onset is concerned, we have detected a peak age at onset in the third decade among females, whereas among males a wider distribution was noticed, with one peak appearing in the third decade and one appearing in the sixth, the latter probably due to a higher incidence of males with thymoma. Around 40% of our cases started with ocular symptoms; the generalized and the bulbar forms of the disease accounted for the remaining 60% of cases. At maximal worsening, 60% of the patients had either bulbar or respiratory symptoms; it is interesting to note that the ocular form accounted for 17% of cases at maximal worsening. These results are in line with those already reported.[2]

We have noticed in our MG population an overall mortality of about 3.4% and a mortality due to MG of about 1.2%. This rate is different from that already reported[4] and may be related to the intensive use of therapeutic plasma exchange, a procedure we performed ourselves.[12]

Our patients' mean follow-up was 55.1 ± 48.1 months, a period long enough to make reliable conclusions on the possibility of achieving remission, the end point adopted in the present study and used according to suggestions from the Task Force of the Medical Scientific Advisory Board of the Myasthenia Gravis Foundation of America.[9] Choosing *R* as the end point, we have also analyzed possible prognostic factors associated with remission. The univariate analysis and the Kaplan-Meier curves were concordant in assigning positive values to the following variables: female sex, young age at onset (below 40 years), thymectomy, the most radical surgical approach (in our hands shifting from transsternal to VATET), and a histological diagnosis of thymic hyperplasia. It is important to note that also patients seronegative for anti-AChR antibodies have a significant possibility of reaching remission, which can be the outcome of the disease independently from the clinical presentation of MG and the time to surgery. The multivariate analysis showed that the variables significantly associated with *R* were an age at onset below 40 years and thymectomy.

In conclusion, we have identified the main prognostic factors leading to *R* in our series of patients. However, it must be emphasized that a considerable proportion of patients are still symptomatic, showing a significant neurological handicap at the end of the follow-up period. Research efforts should be much more concentrated on these patients so that the immunological factors underlying a negative outcome may be elucidated.

REFERENCES

1. Oosterhuis, H.J.G.H. 1997. Clinical aspects and epidemiology. *In* Myasthenia Gravis, pp. 17–48. Groningen Neurological Press. Groningen.
2. Grob, D., N.G. Brunner & T. Namba. 1981. The natural course of myasthenia gravis and effect of therapeutic measures. Ann. N.Y. Acad. Sci. **377:** 652–669.
3. Phillips, L.H. & J.C. Torner. 1996. Epidemiological evidence for a changing natural history of myasthenia gravis. Neurology **47:** 1233–1238.
4. Mantegazza, R. *et al.* 1990. A multicentre follow-up study of 1152 patients with myasthenia gravis in Italy. J. Neurol. **237:** 339–344.
5. Beghi, E. *et al.* 1991. Prognosis of myasthenia gravis: a multicenter follow-up study of 844 patients. J. Neurol. Sci. **106:** 213–220.
6. Mantegazza, R. *et al.* 1988. Azathioprine as a single drug or in combination with steroids in the treatment of myasthenia gravis. J. Neurol. **235:** 449–453.
7. Younger, D.S., B.B. Worrall & A.S. Penn. 1997. Myasthenia gravis: historical perspective and overview. Neurology **48**(suppl. 5)**:** S1–S7.
8. Beeson, D., L. Jacobson, J. Newsom-Davis & A. Vincent. 1996. A transfected human muscle cell line expressing the adult type of the human muscle acetylcholine receptor for diagnostic assays in myasthenia gravis. Neurology **47:** 1552–1555.
9. Task Force of the Medical Scientific Advisory Board of the Myasthenia Gravis Foundation of America. 2000. Myasthenia gravis: recommendations for clinical research standards. Neurology **55:** 16–23.
10. Kaplan, E.L. & P. Meier. 1958. Nonparametric estimation for incomplete observations. J. Am. Stat. Assoc. **53:** 457–481.
11. Cox, D.R. 1972. Regression model and life tables. J. R. Stat. Soc. **B34:** 187–220.
12. Antozzi, C. *et al.* 1991. A short plasma exchange protocol is effective in severe myasthenia gravis. J. Neurol. **238:** 103–107.

Myasthenia Gravis in Individuals over 40

JOHAN A. AARLI, FREDRIK ROMI, GEIR OLVE SKEIE, AND NILS ERIK GILHUS
Department of Neurology, University of Bergen, Bergen, Norway

ABSTRACT: Myasthenia gravis (MG) in individuals over 40 years of age comprises three groups: early-onset MG with prolonged disease duration, late-onset MG with thymoma, and late-onset of nonthymomatous MG. The clinical features do not differ between the three groups, except that early-onset patients with prolonged disease duration usually have a less severe disease. More than 60% of our MG patients are now more than 50 years of age, often with disease onset after age 40. Although 2 out of the 3 patients in Erb's original description had onset of myasthenic symptoms after age 40, this was apparently infrequent in 1879, when the disease was first identified. Onset of MG after age 40 is now common. For example, in our material, 88/184 (47.8%) had onset of MG after age 40. Eighteen (20.5%) had a thymoma. The female:male ratio in the early-onset group was 2.4:1, whereas it was 1:1.1 among those with onset after age 40. There was no human leukocyte antigen association for MG with thymoma. Antibodies to the acetylcholine receptor were detected in 88% of sera from nonthymomatous MG and in 100% of those with late-onset MG with thymoma. Antibodies to titin were found in sera from 85.7% of MG patients with thymoma (all age groups) and in 58% of nonthymomatous MG with late onset and acetylcholine receptor antibodies. Late-onset, nonthymomatous MG comprises two subgroups, one corresponding to delayed early onset and one immunologically similar to that seen in patients with MG and thymoma.

KEYWORDS: myasthenia gravis; acetylcholine receptor; ryanodine receptor; titin; thymus; thymoma; epidemiology

INTRODUCTION

Myasthenia gravis (MG) in individuals over age 40 comprises three groups: early-onset MG with prolonged disease duration, late-onset MG with thymoma, and late-onset nonthymomatous MG. Erb[1] first described the disease in 1878. He reported 3 patients, aged 30, 47, and 55 years, who had developed ptosis, bulbar paresis, and weakness of the neck muscles and had a fluctuating course of the disease. This was the first detailed description of a new syndrome, and there can be no doubt that they all suffered from MG. By 1900, when Campbell and Bramwell[2] surveyed the literature and added 1 case of their own, they were able to collect 60 cases, only 3 of which corresponded to patients who were more than 50 years of age at disease onset. In his review on MG from 1893, Goldflam[3] argued that a high age at onset (55 years) was less compatible with MG, but did not exclude the diagnosis. In 1903, Laquer[4] reported

Address for correspondence: Johan A. Aarli, Department of Neurology, Haukeland University Hospital, N-5021 Bergen, Norway. Voice: +47-55-97-50-69; fax: +47-55-97-51-65.
johan.a.aarli@helse-bergen.no

Ann. N.Y. Acad. Sci. 998: 424–431 (2003). © 2003 New York Academy of Sciences.
doi: 10.1196/annals.1254.055

a case of MG with thymoma, and Weigert[5] postulated a causal relation between the thymic neoplasm and the neuromuscular disease.

Epidemiology

The first indications of heterogeneity of MG were based upon epidemiological studies. Campbell and Bramwell[2] pointed out that the ages at which the sexes are attacked are different and that the average age at onset is 24 years for women and 35 for men. Simpson *et al.*[6] found that 49% of the female patients, but only 23% of the males, had onset of MG before the age of 30. The corresponding figures found by Schwab and Leland[7] were 62% of the women and 27% of the men. The majority of male patients in both studies were over 60 years. However, Simpson *et al.* also observed a bimodal pattern for males. When they grouped the patients according to the age at MG onset, the males showed one group with a peak age at onset at 25–35 years and another at 60–70 years. They could not observe a similar bimodal pattern for the female patients. Osserman and Genkins,[8] who presented data from 1200 MG patients, also found a much higher peak age at MG onset in men, 61–70 years, compared to 21–30 years in women.

Storm-Mathisen[9] reported a first peak age at MG onset in women at 20–29 years followed by a second at 70–79. She did not detect any similar peak age at onset among young males. Similar findings were also reported by Christensen *et al.*[10] Osterman,[11] who examined 213 MG patients between 1974 and 1988 (127 females and 86 males), found a bimodal age at onset for both sexes. For females, the peaks were at 25–30 and 70–80 years. For men, the peaks were at 40–50 and 70–80 years. Somnier *et al.*,[12] who examined the age- and sex-specific incidence, were the first to explicitly report a bimodal appearance for both sexes with a peak age at onset located in the early-onset group and another peak for late-onset MG. They found that early onset of MG in men was approximately 10 years later than in females. However, the peak for late onset of MG was located at the same age for both sexes, between 70 and 80 years. These figures correspond to those determined by Osterman.[11] Recent studies show that there is one group of MG patients with female predominance and peak age at onset of 20–30 years (early onset), and another with a slight predominance of males and a later age at onset (late onset). Thymoma can be found in MG patients from both age groups, but it is much more common in the late-onset group.

Why 40?

Compston *et al.*[13] used 40 years of age as an arbitrary division in the nontumor cases and found a significant association between presentation at less than 40 years and females, and conversely between presentation at more than 40 years of age and males.

Christensen *et al.*,[10] who studied the epidemiology of MG in western Denmark, included data from 290 patients. They found that the incidence rate in women showed a bimodal pattern, with a second peak in the 70–79 age group. The incidence rate was lower in the 40–49 age group than in the 30–39 and 50–59 age groups. In men, the incidence rate increased slightly after 40 years of age, but more so after age 50.

Somnier *et al.*,[12] who had reported a bimodal appearance for both sexes, suggested the use of 50 years of age as a dividing line between early- and late-onset MG. We also found lower rates of age at onset in the 40–49 age group than in the 30–39 and

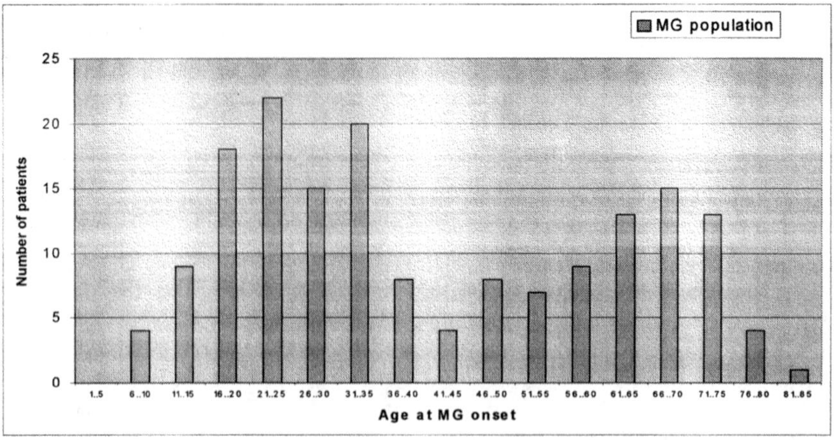

FIGURE 1. The distribution of age at onset of 170 consecutive nonthymomatous MG patients. Each vertical bar shows the number of patients that had an age at onset within a given 5-year period.

50–59 age groups. On the basis of the recent data, we therefore recommend using 50 years of age as a dividing line between early- and late-onset MG (FIG. 1). This should better reflect any pathogenetic differences.

ARE THERE CLINICAL DIFFERENCES BETWEEN EARLY-ONSET AND LATE-ONSET MG?

The neuromuscular symptoms in patients with late-onset MG do not differ from those observed in patients with early-onset MG, except that the disease is likely to be more severe in patients in whom MG develops after the age of 50 years. Donaldson *et al.*,[14] who compared 110 patients who were younger than 50 at diagnosis with 55 patients who were 50 or older at diagnosis, found that the presenting symptoms were not statistically different in younger and older populations, although ocular signs alone were less common and bulbar signs more common in the older group. The percentage of older patients who progressed to severe disease was significantly greater than the percentage of younger patients who progressed to serious disease.

Associated Autoimmune Diseases

Several studies have shown that MG patients have an increased incidence of other diseases with autoimmune features, such as rheumatoid arthritis, systemic lupus erythematosus, Hashimoto's thyroiditis, and pernicious anemia. In some cases, these disorders have developed first and MG later, although MG in other patients was the first manifestation of an autoimmune disorder. Christensen *et al.*[15] found that patients with associated autoimmune diseases were slightly younger than patients without such diseases, but the difference was not significant. However, in the majority of their patients, the onset of the associated autoimmune disease occurred before the diagnosis of MG.

Early-Onset MG with Prolonged Disease Duration

Any population of MG patients over age 40 will have a group of patients who developed MG when they were young and who have lived with the disease for many years, some with a full or partial remission. A few of them have had an operation for a thymoma, but most of them have nonthymomatous MG with a female:male ratio near 3:1. Christensen *et al.*[16] showed that the survival of younger patients is not significantly different from the corresponding age-matched population. The female to male ratio in the early-onset group was 2.4:1, whereas it was 1.1:1 among those with onset after age 40. In our material, the female to male ratio in late-onset, nonthymomatous MG is 1:1.1.

Thymoma and MG

Thymoma is much more common among patients with late-onset MG. In our material, 88/184 (47.8%) had onset of MG after age 40. Eighteen of the patients (20.5%) had a thymoma. Patients with nonthymomatous MG never or almost never develop cardiac symptoms. Cardiac disease, however, is not uncommon in patients with thymoma and MG.[17] The condition has been termed "Herzmyasthenia" or myasthenia of the heart.[4]

Late-Onset Nonthymomatous MG

Newsom-Davis and colleagues[18] reported a male:female ratio of 3:1 in MG patients with thymus involution and onset after age 40, compared to 1:3 in patients with early onset. Somnier *et al.*[12] found twice as many men as women among MG patients with onset after age 50. They raised the hypothesis that late-onset MG may be a disease different from early-onset MG.

IMMUNOLOGICAL FINDINGS

Immunological data are important indicators in the differential diagnosis between MG with thymoma and late-onset, nonthymomatous MG.[19] They comprise antibodies to the acetylcholine receptor (AChR), titin, and the ryanodine receptor (RyR); tumor necrosis factor (TNF) polymorphism; and HLA data.

AChR Antibodies

Compston *et al.*[13] found that patients with onset of MG after age 40 and thymus involution had low levels of AChR antibodies, compared with patients with thymus hyperplasia and with thymoma. This work was later extended by Newsom-Davis and *et al.*,[18] who confirmed the findings.

Limburg *et al.*[20] and Mantegazza *et al.*[21] also found evidence for an association between AChR antibody levels and age at onset. Limburg *et al.*[20] reported that late onset was associated with low anti-AChR antibody titers and the presence of antibodies to striated muscle. Young and old patients with early onset had the same levels of AChR antibodies. Patients without thymoma and age at onset above 40 years had the lowest values. All studies agreed that MG with thymoma had higher concentrations of AChR antibodies than those with thymus involution. However, Lindstrom *et al.*[22] were unable to find any correlation with age. They did not differentiate between thymoma and nonthymoma cases. Because thymoma usually has a late onset and presents with high concentrations of AChR antibodies, the results of these studies cannot be directly compared. Somnier *et al.*[12] found a nonsignificantly lower concentration of AChR antibodies in late-onset MG, but again thymoma cases were not excluded. The data may thus concede that the AChR antibody concentration is lower in cases with late-onset MG than it is in early-onset and thymoma-associated MG. We have also confirmed these findings and found that patients with early-onset MG had significantly higher AChR antibody concentrations than patients with late onset.[23]

The AChR antibody titers, however, correspond poorly with the severity of the disease. AChR antibodies accelerate the degradation and produce blockade of the receptors, but this functional ability does not correlate with the total concentration of antibodies. There is a close correspondence between the functional antibody activity and the clinical manifestations of the disease.[24]

Titin Antibodies

In 1990, we demonstrated that titin is a major antigenic determinant for cross-striational antibodies and that 20% of patients with late-onset, nonthymomatous MG have such antibodies.[25,26] Titin antibodies occur very infrequently in sera of patients with early-onset MG.[23,27] Their pathogenetic relevance is unclear, but the severity of the MG correlates with the serum concentration of titin (and RyR) antibodies.[27]

Yamamoto *et al.*[28] have confirmed that titin antibodies serve as a useful marker for the presence of a thymoma in MG patients below the age of 60. What may be even more interesting is that the presence of such antibodies in nonthymomatous MG patients reveals a heterogeneity in late-onset MG: one group characterized by a broad antimuscle immune response, including both titin and AChR, and another group preferentially associated with the HLA-A3, B7, and DRw2 antigens representing a delayed early onset of the disease and with a selective AChR immune response.[28]

We found titin antibodies in sera of 85.7% of MG patients with thymoma (all age groups) and in 58% of nonthymomatous MG with late onset and detectable AChR antibodies.[23]

The production of antibodies to titin is not caused by AChR antibody-mediated muscle cell destruction because titin antibodies do not appear in the sera of patients with long-standing, early-onset MG and thymus hyperplasia. The mechanisms for titin antibody production must therefore be different from those related to AChR antibody production.

RyR Antibodies

Some MG patients also have antibodies to the calcium release channels (RyR) of the sarcoplasmic reticulum. The RyR is located at the terminal cisternae at the site of its communication with the invaginating T-tubule of the sarcolemma. The epitope is near the transmembrane assembly site. Mygland *et al.*[29,30] found such antibodies in about half of the thymoma patients. RyR antibodies have also been detected in a few patients with late-onset MG, but so far neither in sera of patients with early-onset MG nor in sera from healthy individuals. Their pathogenetic relevance is unclear, but *in vitro* studies have shown that RyR antibodies from MG patients inhibit calcium release from isolated terminal cisternae fractions. It is possible that the RyR antibodies interfere with the interaction between the RyR and the receptor, which may inhibit opening of the RyR channel and subsequent calcium release.[31]

TNF Polymorphism

MG patients with titin antibodies are most often homozygous for tumor necrosis factor-α and tumor necrosis factor-β alleles, specifically, the TNFA*T1 and TNFB*2 alleles, whereas the presence of the TNFA*T2 and TNFB*1 alleles correlates with early-onset MG and the absence of titin antibodies.[32]

HLA Data

Patients with early-onset, nonthymomatous MG and thymus hyperplasia are often DR3 positive. Patients with thymoma and MG do not seem to have a specific HLA profile, but are very seldom DR3 positive. Giraud *et al.*[33] recently evaluated the association of HLA with MG in 656 MG patients and confirmed that MG with thymus hyperplasia was positively associated with DR3 and negatively associated with DR7. Conversely, patients with titin antibodies had an increase of DR7 and a decrease of DR3. Giraud *et al.* also found that DR7 was not associated with MG and thymoma despite the high prevalence of titin antibodies in this form of MG. They concluded, therefore, that the mechanism for titin antibody production in MG patients with thymoma must be different in MG patients without thymoma.

HETEROGENEITY IN LATE-ONSET NONTHYMOMATOUS MG

A nonthymomatous MG patient with disease onset after age 40 represents one out of two subgroups of MG. This heterogeneity may have a genetic basis. One subgroup consists of patients who have all the criteria of early-onset MG apart from age, a high frequency of nonmuscle autoantibodies, and concomitant autoimmune disease with no antibodies to titin or RyR. This subgroup may represent the same form of MG as that seen in early-onset MG with thymus hyperplasia ("delayed early onset" MG, type I). Patients with this type of MG have an increased frequency of the extended A1-B8-DR3 haplotype. This kind of MG may occur at any age, but is more common among individuals in their third and fourth decades.

The other subgroup (type II) is different. It is equally common among men and women. The patients may have a more severe disease, have a broader range of antibodies to striated muscle (but seldom other autoantibodies), often express HLA DR7, and respond less well to thymectomy.[33,34]

REFERENCES

1. Erb, W. 1879. Zur Casuistik der bulbären Lähmungen. Über einen neuen, wahrscheinlich bulbären Symptomencomplex. Arch. Psychiatrie **9:** 336–350.
2. Campbell, H. & E. Bramwell. 1900. Myasthenia gravis. Brain **23:** 277–366.
3. Goldflam, S. 1893. Über einen scheinbar heilbaren bulbärparalytischen Symptomencomplex mit Betheiligung der Extremitäten. Dtsch. Z. Nervenheilkd. **4:** 312–352.
4. Laquer, L. 1903. Ueber die Erb'sche Krankheit (myasthenia gravis). Neurol. Zentralbl. **20:** 594–597.
5. Weigert, C. 1903. Patologisch-anatomischer Beitrag zur Erb'schen Krankheit (myasthenia gravis). Neurol. Zentralbl. **20:** 597–601.
6. Simpson, J.F., M.R. Westerberg & K.R. Magee. 1966. Myasthenia gravis: an analysis of 295 cases. Acta Neurol. Scand. **42**(suppl. 23)**:** 1–27.
7. Schwab, R.S. & C.C. Leland. 1953. Sex and age in myasthenia gravis as critical factors in incidence and remission. J. Am. Med. Assoc. **153:** 1270–1273.
8. Osserman, K.E. & G. Genkins. 1971. Studies in myasthenia gravis: a review of a twenty-year experience in over 1200 patients. Mt. Sinai J. Med. **38:** 497–537.
9. Storm-Mathisen, A. 1984. Epidemiology of myasthenia gravis in Norway. Acta Neurol. Scand. **70:** 274–284.
10. Christensen, P.B. *et al.* 1993. Incidence and prevalence of myasthenia gravis in western Denmark: 1975 to 1989. Neurology **43:** 1779–1783.
11. Osterman, P. 1990. Current treatment of myasthenia gravis. *In* Progress in Brain Research, pp. 151–161. Elsevier Science. Oxford.
12. Somnier, F.E., N. Keiding & O.B. Paulson. 1991. Epidemiology of myasthenia gravis in Denmark: a longitudinal and comprehensive population survey. Arch. Neurol. **48:** 733–739.
13. Compston, D.A.S. *et al.* 1980. Clinical, pathological, HLA-antigen, and immunological evidence for disease heterogeneity in myasthenia gravis. Brain **103:** 579–601.
14. Donaldson, D.H. *et al.* 1990. The relationship of age to outcome in myasthenia gravis. Neurology **40:** 786–790.
15. Christensen, P.B. *et al.* 1995. Associated autoimmune diseases in myasthenia gravis: a population-based study. Acta Neurol. Scand. **91:** 192–195.
16. Christensen, P.B. *et al.* 1998. Mortality and survival in myasthenia gravis: a Danish population based study. J. Neurol. Neurosurg. Psychiatry **64:** 78–83.
17. Aarli, J.A. 1994. Myasthenia gravis and thymoma. *In* Handbook of Myasthenia Gravis and Myasthenic Syndromes, pp. 207–224. Dekker. New York.
18. Newsom-Davis, J., A. Vincent & N. Willcox. 1982. Acetylcholine receptor antibody: clinical and experimental aspects. *In* Receptors, Antibodies, and Disease. Ciba Foundation Symposium. Vol. 90, pp. 225–247. Pitman. London.
19. Aarli, J.A. 1997. Late onset myasthenia gravis. Eur. J. Neurol. **4:** 203–209.
20. Limburg, P.C. *et al.* 1983. Anti-acetylcholine receptor antibodies in myasthenia gravis. I. Relation to clinical parameters in 250 patients. J. Neurol. Sci. **58:** 357–370.
21. Mantegazza, R. *et al.* 1998. Anti-AChR antibody: relevance to diagnosis and clinical aspects of myasthenia gravis. Ital. J. Neurol. Sci. **9:** 141–145.
22. Lindstrom, J.M. *et al.* 1976. Antibody to acetylcholine receptor in myasthenia gravis: prevalence, clinical correlates, and diagnostic value. Neurology **26:** 1054–1059.
23. Romi, F. *et al.* 2000. Muscle autoantibodies in subgroups in myasthenia gravis patients. J. Neurol. **247:** 369–375.
24. Drachman, D.B. *et al.* 1982. Functional activities of autoantibodies to acetylcholine receptors and the clinical severity of myasthenia gravis. N. Engl. J. Med. **307:** 769–775.
25. Aarli, J.A. *et al.* 1990. Patients with myasthenia gravis and thymoma have in their sera IgG autoantibodies against titin. Clin. Exp. Immunol. **82:** 284–288.
26. Gautel, M. *et al.* 1993. Identification of a major immunogenic region of titin. Neurology **43:** 1581–1585.
27. Skeie, G.O. *et al.* 1995. Titin antibodies in patients with late onset myasthenia gravis: clinical correlations. Autoimmunity **20:** 99–104.

28. YAMAMOTO, A.M. *et al.* 2001. Anti-titin antibodies in myasthenia gravis: tight association with thymoma and heterogeneity of nonthymoma patients. Arch. Neurol. **58:** 885–890.
29. MYGLAND, Å. *et al.* 1992. Ryanodine receptor autoantibodies in myasthenia gravis patients with thymoma. Ann. Neurol. **32:** 589–591.
30. MYGLAND, Å. *et al.* 1994. Ryanodine receptor autoantibodies related to the severity of thymoma associated myasthenia gravis. J. Neurol. Neurosurg. Psychiatry **57:** 843–846.
31. SKEIE, G.O. *et al.* 2001. Autoimmunity against the ryanodine receptor in myasthenia gravis. Acta Physiol. Scand. **171:** 379–384.
32. SKEIE, G.O. *et al.* 1999. TNFA and TNFB polymorphism in myasthenia gravis. Arch. Neurol. **56:** 457–461.
33. GIRAUD, M. *et al.* 2001. Linkage of HLA to myasthenia gravis and genetic heterogeneity depending on anti-titin antibodies. Neurology **57:** 1555–1560.
34. ROMI, F. *et al.* 2002. Thymectomy and anti-muscle autoantibodies in late-onset myasthenia gravis. Eur. J. Neurol. **9:** 55–61.

Standards of Measurements in Myasthenia Gravis

RICHARD J. BAROHN

Department of Neurology, University of Kansas Medical Center, Kansas City, Kansas 66160, USA

ABSTRACT: In 1997, the Medical Scientific Advisory Board of the Myasthenia Gravis Foundation of America formed a Task Force to develop classification and outcome measures for myasthenia gravis (MG). The goal of the Task Force was to achieve uniformity in recording and reporting clinical trials and outcomes research. The Task Force met frequently over a three-year period, obtained input from national and international experts, and produced a consensus document on recommendations for MG clinical research standards. In this article, the essential elements of the Task Force's recommendations will be summarized. In addition, several other MG measurement tools that are in various stages of development are mentioned.

KEYWORDS: myasthenia gravis (MG); recommendations; measurement

INTRODUCTION

In 1997, the Medical Scientific Advisory Board (MSAB) of the Myasthenia Gravis Foundation of America (MGFA) formed a Task Force to develop classification and outcome measures for myasthenia gravis (MG). The goal of the Task Force was to achieve uniformity in recording and reporting clinical trials and outcomes research. The moving force behind this project was a thoracic surgeon, Alfred Jaretzki III, who was to become the chair of the Task Force. Jaretzki, who had published extensively with his colleagues at Columbia Presbyterian Medical Center on thymectomy for MG,[1,2] was concerned that outcome data from various centers regarding thymectomy outcomes could not be easily compared because of the lack of universally accepted measurement tools. Once the group met, it became clear that this shortcoming was not only true for the thymectomy literature, but for all MG clinical research. Through Jaretzki's initiative and continuous efforts, the Task Force met frequently over a three-year period, obtained input from national and international experts, and produced a consensus document on recommendations for MG clinical research standards.[3]

Address for correspondence: Richard J. Barohn, M.D., Department of Neurology, University of Kansas Medical Center, 3901 Rainbow Boulevard, Kansas City, Kansas 66160-7314. Voice: 913-588-6094; fax: 913-588-6948.
rbarohn@kumc.edu

Ann. N.Y. Acad. Sci. 998: 432–439 (2003). © 2003 New York Academy of Sciences.
doi: 10.1196/annals.1254.056

The Task Force realizes these recommendations will require revisions and modifications. To this end, the MSAB of the MGFA has established a standing Clinical Research Standards Review Committee.

In this article, the essential elements of the Task Force's recommendations will be summarized. In addition, several other MG measurement tools that are in various stages of development are briefly mentioned.

CLINICAL CLASSIFICATION OF MG

Clinicians have struggled with devising an adequate classification system for MG for over 40 years. In 1958, Osserman and colleagues[4,5] proposed placing patients in five groups—I: localized (ocular); II: generalized (mild or moderate); III: acute fulminating; IV: late severe; and V: muscle atrophy. A separate category for neonatal and juvenile forms was created. Osserman and Genkins divided group II into A

TABLE 1. MGFA clinical classification

Class	Clinical signs
I	Any ocular muscle weakness. May have weakness of eye closure. All other muscle strength is normal.
II	Mild weakness affecting other than ocular muscles. May also have ocular muscle weakness of any severity.
IIa	Predominantly affecting limb or axial muscles or both. May also have lesser involvement of oropharyngeal muscles.
IIb	Predominantly affecting oropharyngeal or respiratory muscles or both. May also have lesser or equal involvement of limb or axial muscles or both.
III	Moderate weakness affecting other than ocular muscles. May also have ocular muscle weakness of any severity.
IIIa	Predominantly affecting limb or axial muscles or both. May also have lesser involvement of oropharyngeal muscles.
IIIb	Predominantly affecting oropharyngeal or respiratory muscles or both. May also have lesser or equal involvement of limb or axial muscles or both.
IV	Severe weakness affecting other than ocular muscles. May also have ocular muscle weakness of any severity.
IVa	Predominantly affecting limb and/or axial muscles. May also have lesser involvement of oropharyngeal muscles.
IVb	Predominantly affecting oropharyngeal or respiratory muscles or both. May also have lesser or equal involvement of limb or axial muscles or both.
V	Defined by intubation, with or without mechanical ventilation, except when employed during routine postoperative management. The use of a feeding tube without intubation places the patient in class IVb.

NOTE: From ref. 3 with permission.

(mild) and B (moderate) subdivisions and dropped the muscle atrophy group.[6] Various "modified Osserman criteria" were suggested over the years, and some new schemes were developed.[1,7–11]

When the Task Force began meeting, it became clear that the group should tackle the difficult topic of MG classification, even though it did not bear directly on research outcome measures. The Task Force used the term "class" for the five broad subdivisions (TABLE 1) and recognized that these classes are ultimately subjective—even two clinical experts in MG might not always be able to agree on whether a patient has mild or moderate generalized MG. A patient with class I ocular MG can have orbicularis oculi weakness, but any other axial, limb, or oropharyngeal weakness placed the patient in one of the generalized classes. The Task Force appreciated that some patients with MG have selective bulbar musculature involvement; thus, separate subclasses under classes II, III, and IV are designated "a" if the predominant weakness is limb/axial or "b" if the predominant weakness is oropharyngeal/respiratory. A patient requiring intubation is placed in class V. Use of a feeding tube without intubation placed the patient in category IVb. The most severe class that the patient has experienced is considered the "maximum severity designation" and this should be used as an historical point of reference. The Task Force recommended that this MGFA clinical classification system replace others now in use. The Task Force also recognized that this classification system cannot be used as an outcome measure in clinical trials (see below), but should be used to identify subgroups of patients who share distinct clinical features, particularly with regard to entry into clinical research trials.

QUANTITATIVE MG SCORE

The current quantitative MG scoring system (QMG Score) is an expansion and modification of the tool developed by Besinger *et al.*[12,13] (TABLE 2). The original scoring system consisted of 8 items, each graded 0 to 3, with 3 being the most severe. Tindall *et al.*[14,15] expanded the scale to 13 items and used the scale as the primary efficacy measurement in two cyclosporine trials. Barohn *et al.*[16] replaced some of the subjective items with quantifiable measures, performed interrater reliability testing, and determined that approximately 17 patients would be needed in each arm of a placebo-controlled study. This version of the QMG Score was utilized as the primary end point in trials of intravenous immunoglobulin in MG.[17] The Task Force recommended that the QMG Score be used in prospective studies of therapy for MG. In addition, the Task Force encouraged proposals to improve and validate the QMG Score.

A demonstration video and manual that explain how to perform the QMG Score are available from the MGFA.[18] The QMG Score takes approximately 20 minutes to perform by a well-trained evaluator.

MGFA MG THERAPY STATUS

For MG patients enrolled in many types of clinical studies, it is appropriate for the treatment regimen to be defined. The Task Force recommended that categories listed in the MGFA MG Therapy Status should be utilized for this purpose (TABLE 3). The duration of the status, dose of medications, and treatment schedules should be included. The designation of a particular therapy status is most useful when used in conjunction with the MGFA Postintervention Status (below).

TABLE 2. Quantitative MG score for disease activity

Test item	None	Mild	Moderate	Severe
Grade	0	1	2	3
Double vision on the lateral gaze right or left (circle one), s	61	11–60	1–10	Spontaneous
Ptosis (upward gaze), s	61	11–60	1–10	Spontaneous
Facial muscles	Normal lid closure	Complete, weak, some resistance	Complete, without resistance	Incomplete
Swallowing 4 oz. water (1/2 cup)	Normal	Minimal coughing or throat clearing	Severe coughing/choking or nasal regurgitation	Cannot swallow (test not attempted)
Speech after counting aloud from 1 to 50 (onset of dysarthria)	None at 50	Dysarthria at 30–49	Dysarthria at 10–29	Dysarthria at 9
Right arm outstretched (90° sitting), s	240	90–239	10–89	0–9
Left arm outstretched (90° sitting), s	240	90–239	10–89	0–9
Vital capacity, % predicted	≥80	65–79	50–64	<50
Right-hand grip, kgW				
Men	≥45	15–44	5–14	0–4
Women	≥30	10–29	5–9	0–4
Left-hand grip, kgW				
Men	≥35	15–34	5–14	0–4
Women	≥25	10–24	5–9	0–4
Head lifted (45° supine), s	120	30–119	1–29	0
Right leg outstretched (45° supine), s	100	31–99	1–30	0
Left leg outstretched (45° supine), s	100	31–99	1–30	0
		*Total QMG score (range, 0–39)*___		

NOTE: From ref. 3 with permission.

TABLE 3. MGFA MG therapy status

NT	No therapy
SPT	Status postthymectomy (record type of resection)
CH	Cholinesterase inhibitors
PR	Prednisone
IM	Immunosuppression therapy other than prednisone (define)
PE(a)	Plasma exchange therapy, acute (for exacerbations or preoperatively)
PE(c)	Plasma exchange therapy, chronic (used on a regular basis)
IG(a)	IVIg therapy, acute (for exacerbations or preoperatively)
IG(c)	IVIg therapy, chronic (used on a regular basis)
OT	Other forms of therapy (define)

NOTE: From ref. 3 with permission.

MGFA POSTINTERVENTION STATUS

The clinical state for patients is defined in the MGFA Postintervention Status (TABLE 4) and this assessment can be used at any time after the designated follow-up or therapy period in an MG study. This determination must be made by a clinician skilled in the evaluation of MG patients. In particular types of studies (e.g., the effect of thymectomy), the MGFA Postintervention Status may be the most important aspect of outcome determination. The MGFA Postintervention Status defines complete and pharmacologic remission and various categories of minimal manifestations. Patients requiring cholinesterase inhibitor cannot be in pharmacological remission. However, a patient can be in remission and still have subclinical orbicularis oculi weakness. Regarding the Improved, Unchanged, and Worse categories in the Change of Status section, the Task Force recommended that the status be determined in terms of change in the QMG Score.

OTHER MG MEASUREMENT TOOLS

MG–Activity of Daily Living Profile (MG-ADL)

The MG-ADL is an 8-point questionnaire that focuses on symptoms that occur in MG patients.[19] In this functional status instrument, each response is graded 0 (normal) to 3 (most severe). A nurse, technician, or physician asks the patient the 8 questions and records the responses. The test can be administered in less than 10 minutes. The MG-ADL has been shown to correlate well with the QMG Score and can serve as a secondary efficacy of measurement in clinical trials. The MG-ADL is not a quality-of-life (QOL) scale, and the Task Force recognized that a disease-specific MG QOL instrument needs to be developed.[3]

TABLE 4. MGFA postintervention status

Complete stable remission (CSR)	The patient has had no symptoms or signs of MG for at least 1 year and has received no therapy for MG during that time. There is no weakness of any muscle on careful examination by someone skilled in the evaluation of neuromuscular disease. Isolated weakness of eyelid closure is accepted.
Pharmacological remission (PR)	The same criteria as for CSR, except that the patient continues to take some form of therapy for MG. Patients taking cholinesterase inhibitors are excluded from this category because their use suggests the presence of weakness.
Minimal manifestations (MM)	The patient has no symptoms of functional limitations from MG, but has some weakness on examination of some muscles. This class recognizes that some patients who otherwise meet the definition of CSR or PR do have weakness that is only detectable by careful examination.
MM-0	The patient has received no MG treatment for at least 1 year.
MM-1	The patient continues to receive some form of immunosuppression, but no cholinesterase inhibitors or other symptomatic therapy.
MM-2	The patient has received only low-dose cholinesterase inhibitors (<120 mg pyridostigmine/day) for at least 1 year.
MM-3	The patient has received cholinesterase inhibitors or other symptomatic therapy and some form of immunosuppression during the past year.
Change in Status	
Improved (I)	A substantial decrease in pretreatment clinical manifestations or a sustained substantial reduction in MG medications as defined in the protocol. In prospective studies, this should be defined as a specific decrease in QMG score.
Unchanged (U)	No substantial change in pretreatment clinical manifestations or reduction in MG medications as defined in the protocol. In prospective studies, this should be defined in terms of a maximum change in QMG score.
Worse (W)	A substantial increase in pretreatment clinical manifestations or a substantial increase in MG medications as defined in the protocol. In prospective studies, this should be defined as a specific increase in QMG score.
Exacerbation (E)	Patients who have fulfilled criteria of CSR, PR, or MM, but subsequently developed clinical findings greater than permitted by these criteria.
Died of MG (D of MG)	Patients who died of MG, of complications of MG therapy, or within 30 days after thymectomy. List the cause (see Morbidity and Mortality data).

NOTE: From ref. 3 with permission.

MG Manual Muscle Test (MG-MMT)

Investigators at Duke University Medical Center have developed an MG-specific manual muscle test that is performed at the bedside by a physician. Thirty muscle groups (8 cranial nerve/22 limb-axial) are measured on a scale of 0 to 4 (0: normal; 1: 25% weak/mild impairment; 2: 50% weak/moderate impairment; 3: 75% weak/severe impairment; 4: paralyzed/unable to do). The MG-MMT was used in an open-label pilot study of mycophenolate mofetil in MG with the QMG Score and MG-ADL.[20] The MG-MMT has been shown to have acceptable interrater reliability and correlates strongly with the QMG Score.[21] Advantages of the MG-MMT over the QMG Score are that it does not require additional personnel to administer other than the physician and that it can be performed in less time. The MG-MMT awaits further use in prospective clinical trials.

Fatigue Testing

Quantification of static fatigue during isometric strength testing has been studied in diseases such as multiple sclerosis and amyotrophic lateral sclerosis, but surprisingly has received little attention in MG. We recently performed static fatigue testing in 77 MG patients by comparing the maximum force generated in the initial 2- to 7-s time epoch with the 25- to 30-s epoch.[22] Our initial results suggest static fatigue testing correlates better with a decremental response on repetitive stimulation than the QMG Score or the MG-ADL; however, further study of this tool in MG is needed.

REFERENCES

1. Jaretzki, A., III, A.S. Penn, D.S. Younger *et al.* 1988. "Maximal" thymectomy for myasthenia gravis: results. J. Thorac. Cardiovasc. Surg. **95:** 747–757.
2. Jaretzki, A., III. 1997. Thymectomy for myasthenia gravis: analysis of the controversies regarding technique and result. Neurology **48**(suppl. 5)**:** S52–S63.
3. Task Force of the Medical Scientific Advisory Board of the Myasthenia Gravis Foundation of America. 2000. Myasthenia gravis: recommendations for clinical research standards. Neurology **55:** 16–23.
4. Osserman, K.E. 1958. Clinical aspects. *In* Myasthenia Gravis, pp. 79–80. Grune & Stratton. New York.
5. Osserman, K.E., P. Kornfeld, E. Cohen *et al.* 1958. Studies in myasthenia gravis: review of two hundred eighty-two cases at the Mount Sinai Hospital, New York City. Arch. Int. Med. **102:** 72–81.
6. Osserman, K.E. & G. Genkins. 1971. Studies in myasthenia gravis: review of a twenty-year experience in over 1200 patients. Mt. Sinai J. Med. **38:** 497–537.
7. Drachman, D.B., R.N. Adams, L.F. Josifek & S.G. Self. 1982. Functional activities of autoantibodies to acetylcholine receptors and the clinical severity of myasthenia gravis. N. Engl. J. Med. **307:** 769–775.
8. Oosterhuis, H.J. 1981. Observations of the natural history of myasthenia gravis and the effect of thymectomy. Ann. N.Y. Acad. Sci. **377:** 678–690.
9. Barohn, R.J. & C.E. Jackson. 1994. New classification system for myasthenia gravis [abstract]. J. Child Neurol. **9:** 205.
10. Wolfe, G.I. & R.J. Barohn. 1999. Neuromuscular junction disorders of childhood. *In* Swaiman's Pediatric Neurology: Principles and Practice. Third edition, pp. 1216–1234. Mosby. Philadelphia.
11. Olanow, C.W., A.S. Wechsler, M. Sirotkin-Roses *et al.* 1987. Thymectomy as primary therapy in myasthenia gravis. Ann. N.Y. Acad. Sci. **505:** 595–606.

12. BESINGER, U.A., K.V. TOYKA, K. HEININGER *et al.* 1981. Long-term correlation of clinical course and acetylcholine receptor antibody in patients with myasthenia gravis. Ann. N.Y. Acad. Sci. **377:** 812–815.
13. BESINGER, U.A., K.V. TOYKA, M. HOMBERG *et al.* 1983. Myasthenia gravis: long-term correlation of binding and bungarotoxin blocking antibodies against acetylcholine receptors with changes in disease severity. Neurology **33:** 1316–1321.
14. TINDALL, R.S.A., J.A. ROLLINS, J.T. PHILLIPS *et al.* 1987. Preliminary results of a double-blind, randomized, placebo-controlled trial of cyclosporine in myasthenia gravis. N. Engl. J. Med. **316:** 719–724.
15. TINDALL, R.S.A., T. PHILLIPS, J.A. ROLLINS *et al.* 1993. A clinical therapeutic trial of cyclosporine in myasthenia gravis. Ann. N.Y. Acad. Sci. **681:** 539–551.
16. BAROHN, R.J., D. MCINTIRE, L. HERBELIN *et al.* 1998. Reliability testing of the quantitative myasthenia gravis score. Ann. N.Y. Acad. Sci. **841:** 769–772.
17. WOLFE, G.I., R.J. BAROHN, B.M. FOSTER *et al.* 2003. Randomized controlled trial of intravenous immunoglobulin in myasthenia gravis. Muscle Nerve. In press.
18. BAROHN, R.J. & L. HERBELIN. 1996. How to Administer the Quantitative Myasthenia Test [Video]. Myasthenia Gravis Foundation of America. Chicago.
19. WOLFE, G.I., L. HERBELIN, S.P. NATIONS *et al.* 1999. Myasthenia gravis activities of daily living profile. Neurology **52:** 1487–1489.
20. CIAFALONI, E., J.M. MASSEY, B. TUCKER-LIPSCOMB & D.B. SANDERS. 2001. Mycophenolate mofetil for myasthenia gravis: an open-label pilot study. Neurology **56:** 97–99.
21. SANDERS, D.B., B. TUCKER-LIPSCOMB & J.M. MASSEY. 2003. A simple manual muscle test for myasthenia gravis: validation and comparison with the QMG score. This volume.
22. HERBELIN, L.L., S.P. NATIONS, G.I. WOLFE *et al.* 2001. The correlation between static fatigue testing and the quantitative myasthenia gravis score and activities of daily living profile. Neurology **56:** A63.

A Simple Manual Muscle Test for Myasthenia Gravis

Validation and Comparison with the QMG Score

DONALD B. SANDERS, BERNADETTE TUCKER-LIPSCOMB, AND JANICE M. MASSEY

Duke University Medical Center, Durham, North Carolina 27710, USA

KEYWORDS: myasthenia gravis (MG); QMG; activities of daily living; manual muscle testing; scoring systems

A Task Force of the Myasthenia Gravis Foundation of America recommended that the quantitative myasthenia gravis (QMG) score or a similar scoring system be used in treatment trials for MG.[1] We describe a manual muscle test (MMT) specific for MG and compare it with the QMG score, as modified and validated by Barohn *et al.*[2] We compare both scores with the clinical severity.

METHODS

The MMT score is the sum of strength or function values assigned by the examining physician to 30 muscle groups usually affected by MG (TABLE 1). To assess interobserver variability of the MMT score, independent assessments were made by a senior physician and a neuromuscular fellow at the same clinic visit in 274 patients. The linear correlation between the independent MMT assessments was calculated (FIG. 1). The QMG score is administered by the clinic nurse coordinator, who is blinded to the MMT results. The correlation between MMT and QMG scores was calculated for all clinic visits at which both scores were determined (FIG. 2). At each clinic visit, the senior physician assigns each patient to a class of disease severity (TABLE 2). The severity of disease was compared with QMG and MMT scores in 234 and 227 patient visits, respectively.

Address for correspondence: Donald B. Sanders, M.D., Duke University Medical Center, Durham, NC 27710. Voice: 919-684-6078; fax: 919-660-3853.
donald.sanders@duke.edu

Ann. N.Y. Acad. Sci. 998: 440–444 (2003). © 2003 New York Academy of Sciences.
doi: 10.1196/annals.1254.057

TABLE 1. Manual muscle testing work sheet

	Right	Left	Sum
Lid ptosis	___	___	___
Diplopia	___	___	___
Eye closure	–	–	___
Cheek puff	–	–	___
Tongue protrusion	–	–	___
Jaw closure	–	–	___
Neck flexion	–	–	___
Neck extension	–	–	___
Shoulder abduction (deltoid)	___	___	___
Elbow flexion (biceps)	___	___	___
Elbow extension (triceps)	___	___	___
Wrist extension	___	___	___
Grip	___	___	___
Hip flexion (iliopsoas)	___	___	___
Knee extension (quadriceps)	___	___	___
Knee flexion (hamstrings)	___	___	___
Ankle dorsiflexion (tib ant +)	___	___	___
Ankle plantar flexion (triceps surae)	___	___	___
TOTAL			___

NOTE: Score each function as follows: 0, normal; 1, 25% weak/mild impairment; 2, 50% weak/moderate impairment; 3, 75% weak/severe impairment; 4, paralyzed/unable to do. In addition, record any conditions other than MG causing weakness in any of these muscles.

TABLE 2. Definitions of disease severity

Remission—The patient has no symptoms of MG, and the examination demonstrates no weakness from MG. Weakness of eyelid closure may be present.

Ocular—There is weakness from MG limited to muscles of ocular motility or eyelid opening.

Mild generalized—There is weakness from MG in any muscle other than those defined as ocular (above) or bulbar (below), which is not judged to be disabling or life-threatening. There may also be weakness in ocular muscles.

Bulbar—There is weakness or there are symptoms of dysfunction involving muscles of speech, swallowing, or respiration. Ocular or generalized weakness may also be present.

Severe generalized—There is disabling or life-threatening weakness from MG. There may also be weakness in ocular muscles.

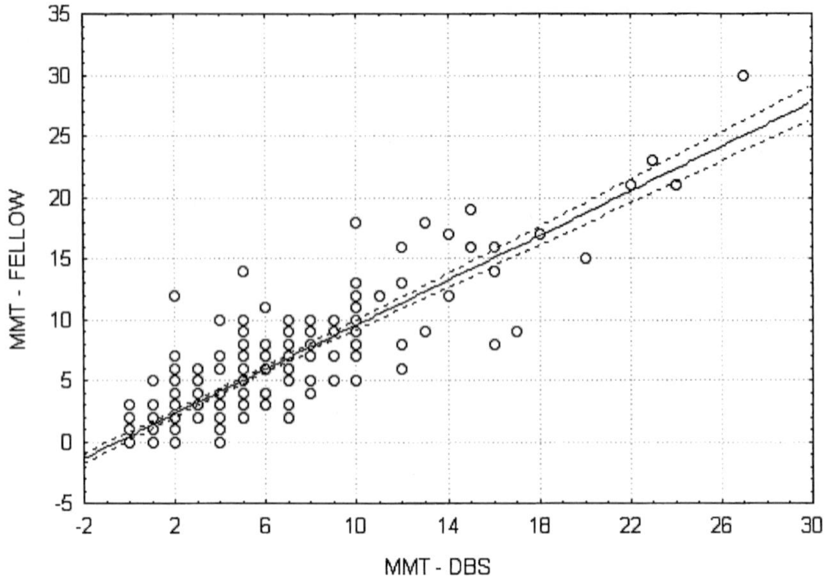

FIGURE 1. The linear correlation between the MMT scores obtained independently by a senior physician (D.B.S.) and a neuromuscular fellow at the same clinic visit in 274 patients. The correlation is highly significant (r = 0.898). The regression lines and 95% confidence limits are shown.

RESULTS

There was a strong correlation between the 274 independent MMT scores (correlation coefficient $r = 0.898$; $p < 0.05$), demonstrating acceptable interrater reliability (see FIG. 1). The mean difference between scores was 1.3 ± 1.8 (SD) points, and the neuromuscular fellow's score was, on average, 0.07 points greater than that determined by the senior physician. There was also a strong correlation between the QMG and MMT scores obtained at 1655 clinic visits (r = 0.69) (see FIG. 2). The mean values of both scores increased with disease severity, but there was wide scatter of values within the same class of clinical severity, and great overlap of values between groups (FIGS. 3 and 4).

CONCLUSIONS

The MMT score has acceptable interrater reliability and correlates strongly with the QMG score. The mean values of both scores increase with overall disease severity, but the scatter of values among patients with similar disease severity and the overlap of values among patients with different severity indicate that neither score can be used to determine severity at one point in time. These findings suggest that the MMT score could be used as an alternative to QMG to assess the change in

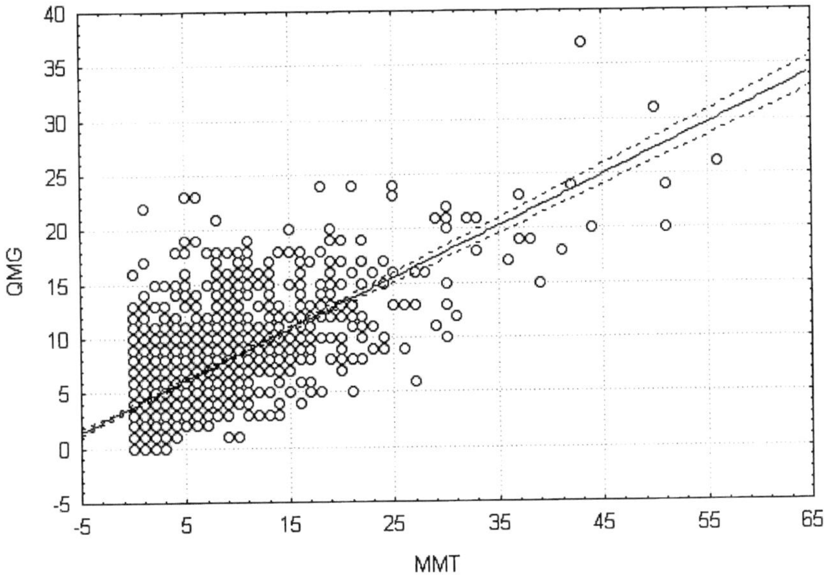

FIGURE 2. The linear correlation between the QMG and MG-MMT scores performed in 303 patients at 1655 clinic visits. The regression lines and 95% confidence limits are shown.

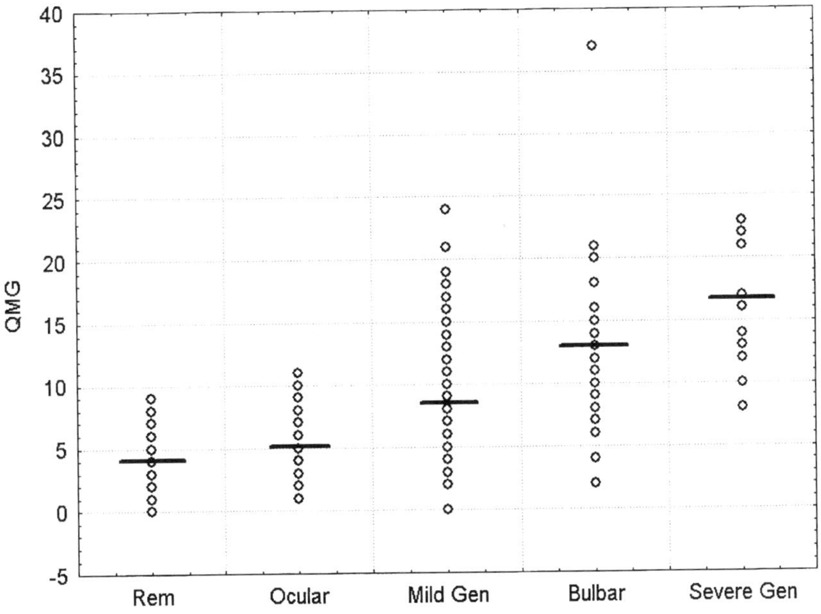

FIGURE 3. Severity of disease versus QMG score in 234 patients. Horizontal lines indicate mean values for each group. Rem: remission; Gen: generalized.

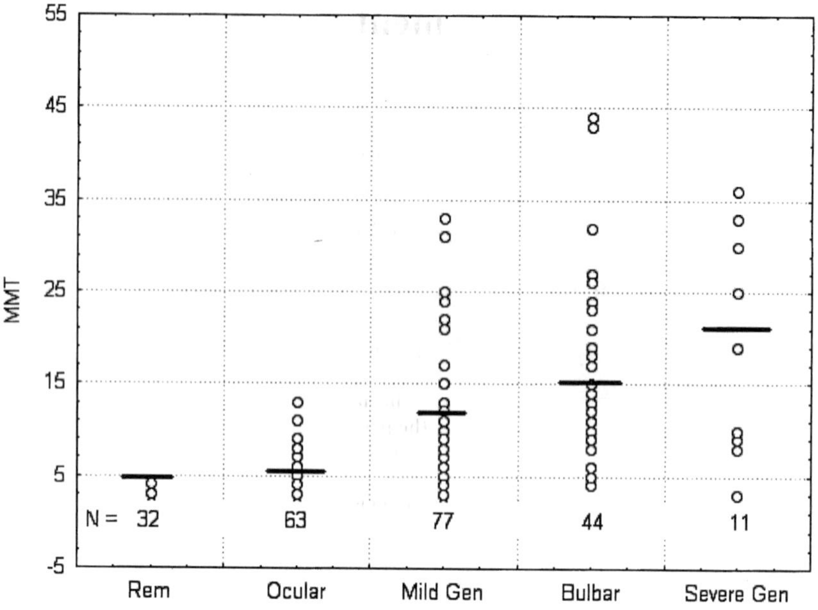

FIGURE 4. Severity of disease versus MMT score in 227 patients. Horizontal lines indicate mean values for each group. Rem: remission; Gen: generalized.

severity in clinical trials. The MMT score is performed by the physician and requires no extra time or personnel. The QMG score takes approximately 20 min and is performed by trained paramedical personnel.

REFERENCES

1. JARETZKI, A. *et al.* 2000. Myasthenia gravis: recommendations for clinical research standards. Neurology **55:** 16–23.
2. BAROHN, R.J. *et al.* 1998. Reliability testing of the quantitative myasthenia gravis score. Ann. N.Y. Acad. Sci. **841:** 769–772.

Standards of Measurements in Myasthenia Gravis

P. GAJDOS,[a] T. SHARSHAR,[a] AND S. CHEVRET[b]

[a]*Service de Réanimation Médicale, Hôpital Raymond Poincaré, Garches, France*

[b]*Département de Biostatistique et Informatique Médicale, Hôpital Saint Louis, Paris, France*

ABSTRACT: Valid and reliable measurements of muscle impairment are needed to assess therapeutic efficacy in patients with generalized myasthenia gravis. Several muscle scoring systems have been proposed for assessing muscle strength in such patients. The aim of the present study is to assess the validity and interobserver agreement of these muscle scores.

KEYWORDS: measurement; muscle; myasthenia gravis; reliability; validity

INTRODUCTION

Valid and reliable measurements of muscle impairment are needed to assess therapeutic efficacy in patients with generalized myasthenia gravis (MG). Several muscle scoring systems have been proposed for assessing muscle strength in such patients. We have assessed the validity and reliability of two muscle scores commonly used. The quantified myasthenia gravis score (QMGS) commonly used in the United States (TABLE 1) was developed by Tindall *et al.*[1] in 1987 as a modification of the quantified MG score previously proposed by Besinger *et al.*[2] in 1983. It is derived from 13 independent observations of the strength of limbs, neck, cranial muscles, and respiratory muscles (vital capacity) that, when summed, yield an overall numerical rating between 0 (normal) and 39.

The myasthenic muscle score (MMS) commonly used in France (TABLE 2) was developed by Gajdos *et al.*[3] in 1983. It is a sum of 9 independent observations of trunk, limbs, neck, and cranial muscles that, when summed, yield an overall numerical rating between 0 and 100 (normal).

The aim of the present study was to assess the validity and interobserver agreement of these muscle scores.

Address for correspondence: Philippe Gajdos, Service de Réanimation Médicale, Hôpital Raymond Poincaré, Assistance Publique-Hôpitaux de Paris, 104 Boulevard Raymond Poincaré, F-92380 Garches, France. Voice: +33-(0)-147-10-77-80; fax: +33-(0)-147-10-77-83.
philippe.gajdos@rpc.ap-hop-paris.fr

Ann. N.Y. Acad. Sci. 998: 445–452 (2003). © 2003 New York Academy of Sciences.
doi: 10.1196/annals.1254.058

TABLE 1. Quantified myasthenia gravis score

	Grade of weakness			
Test items	None (0)	Mild (1)	Moderate (2)	Severe (3)
Double vision (lateral gaze) (s)	>60	>10–60	>1–10	Spontaneous heterotropia
Ptosis (upward gaze) (s)	>60	>10–60	>1–10	Spontaneous
Facial muscles	Normal	Mild weakness on lid closure, snarl	Incomplete lid closure	No mimic expressions
Chewing	Normal	Fatigue after solid foods	Only soft foods	Gastric tube
Swallowing	Normal	Fatigue after normal foods	Incomplete palatal closure, nasal speech	Gastric tube
Head lifting (45°, supine) (s)	>120	>30–120	>0–30	0
Outstretching of right arm (90°, standing) (s)	>240	>90–240	>10–90	≤10
Outstretching of left arm (90°, standing) (s)	>240	>90–240	>10–90	≤10
Vital capacity				
Male	>3.5	>2.5–3.5	>1.5–2.5	<1.5
Female	>2.5	>1.8–2.5	>1.2–1.8	<1.2
Outstretching of right leg (45°, standing) (s)	>100	>30–100	>0–30	0
Outstretching of left leg (45°, standing) (s)	>100	>30–100	>0–30	0
Right grip (kgW) (5.0, male; 4.5, female)				
Male	>45	>15–45	5–15	<5
Female	>31	>10–30	5–10	<5
Left grip (kgW)				
Male	>35	>15–35	5–15	<5
Female	>25	>10–25	5–10	<5

PATIENTS AND METHODS

All consecutive patients with generalized MG referred to the Service de Réanimation Médicale de l'Hôpital Raymond Poincaré (Garches, France) were eligible to participate in our study, provided they gave oral consent. Diagnosis of MG was confirmed by elevation titer of AChR antibodies. Patients with any other neurological disease or requiring sedation were excluded.

TABLE 2. Myasthenic muscle score

Task	Score
Maintain upper limbs horizontally outstretched: 1 point per 10 s	0–15
Maintain lower limbs above bed plane, while lying on back: 1 point per 5 s	0–15
Raise head above bed plane, while lying on back	
Against resistance	10
Without resistance	5
Impossible	0
Sit up from lying position	
Without help of hands	10
Impossible	0
Extrinsic ocular musculature	
Normal	10
Ptosis	5
Double vision	0
Eyelid occlusion	
Complete	10
Mild weakness	7
Incomplete with corneal covering	5
Incomplete without corneal covering	0
Chewing	
Normal	10
Weak	5
Impossible	0
Swallowing	
Normal	10
Impaired without aspiration	5
Impaired with aspiration	0
Speech	
Normal	10
Nasal	5
Slurred	0

Concurrent validity was assessed by calculating the correlation of the scores with a five-grade functional scale: 1, complete remission; 2, minor symptoms allowing normal, nonexertional activity; 3, moderate symptoms allowing occupational or partial daily activity; 4, major disability requiring discontinuation of occupational activity; 5, major disability requiring continuous help or mechanical ventilation.

Interobserver variability was assessed by comparison of repeated measurements of the muscle scores. Two neurologists and two residents were combined to form six different, randomly chosen pairs of observers. All observers were trained to use the two scores by an independent coordinator before the onset of the study.

Assessing the strength of limbs requires an effort that can increase a patient's general weakness and induces a bias in the measurement of a second score. Thus, to assess QMGS and MMS, two standardized forms differing in the order of items of the QMGS and MMS evaluations were randomly used. (In form 1, the items of the QMGS and those of the MMS assessing the strength of limbs and trunk were at the beginning and at the end, respectively. In form 2, the order was reversed.) The same form was used by the selected pair of observers.

The examinations were performed in the morning and scheduled 90 and 150 min after the last injection of anticholinesterasic drug. At each examination, the observer checked whether the patient cleaned or dressed himself alone; ate solid food, mixed food, or was fed by a gastric tube; walked farther than 10 m, less than 10 m, or was bedfast or chair-bound; and breathed freely or required mechanical ventilation.

Swallowing was assessed by asking the patient to drink a glass of water; chewing was assessed by asking the patient to bite a tongue depressor. Vital capacity was measured spirographically by an independent physiotherapist. A vigorimeter (Martin Medizin Technik, Tuttlingen, Germany) assessed the decrease after 10 maximal closures of right- and left-grip strength.

The functional scale was established by each observer. At the end of the examination, each observer asked the patient to indicate his or her own clinical state on a numerical scale ranging from 0 (very bad) to 100 (very good).

STATISTICAL ANALYSIS

To assess the validity of the two muscle scores, the correlation between them and the functional and self-evaluation scales was calculated by the nonparametric Spearman's coefficient, using average measurements on each score obtained by the two observers for each patient. The reliability of ordinal data used the weighted K.[4] To analyze reliability of semiquantitative data (QMGS, MMS, and the self-evaluation), we used statistical methods previously described.[5] Intraclass correlation coefficients and their 95% confidence intervals were computed using a two-way, random-effect analysis of variance. To examine the pattern of agreement visually and to investigate any relationship between the measurement error (estimated by the difference) and the true value (estimated by the mean), we also used the graphic analysis proposed by Bland and Altman,[6] which consists of plotting the differences between repeated measurements against their mean. Median differences were also calculated.

Finally, to further assess the relative importance of each item in the overall reliability of the scores, we deleted one item at a time from the original data set and recalculated the intraclass correlation coefficient based on the rest of the data. Analysis was performed on the SAS software package (SAS, Cary, NC).

RESULTS

From February to October 1997, 22 patients were enrolled in the study. The median time between the ingestion of anticholinesterasic drug and the first examina-

TABLE 3. Main characteristics at baseline of the 22 patients with MG according to observers

	Observer 1	Observer 2
Cleaning alone	17	17
Dressing alone	18	18
Walking		
>10 m	17	15
<10 m	0	2
Chair-bound	5	5
Ate		
Solid food	12	12
Mixed food	5	5
Gastric tube	5	5
Mechanical ventilation	4	4
Functional scale		
Class 1	1	2
Class 2	3	6
Class 3	7	6
Class 4	7	3
Class 5	4	5
Self-evaluation, median (range)	62.5 (5–100)	60 (2–100)
QMGS, median (range)	10 (0–31)	10.5 (3–30)
MMS, median (range)	69.5 (18–100)	64.5 (18–100)

tion was 90 min (range: 90–150); the median time between the ingestion of anticholinesterasic drug and the second examination was 150 min (range: 150–260). The median length of rest before the first examination was 30 min (range: 25–120); the median length of rest before the second examination was 30 min (range: 15–150).

TABLE 3 shows the main findings at each examination. The correlation between mean QMGS and mean MMS was 0.869. Each muscle score was correlated with the functional scale, but was less closely associated with the patient self-evaluation (TABLE 4).

QMGS

Agreement between observers in measuring the QMGS was high, with an intraclass correlation coefficient of 0.905 (TABLE 4). Differences between measurements of the two observers ranged from −5.0 to +6.0, with a median difference of −0.50. There was no apparent relationship between the difference and the mean of the measurements from the two observers.

The intraclass correlation of QMGS ranged from 0.86 to 0.93 when items of the QMGS were deleted in turn. As shown in TABLE 5, items of the QMGS assessing

TABLE 4. Correlation between average measures of muscle scores and functional scales

	Correlation	*p*
QMGS and:		
MMS	–0.869	0.0001
Functional scale	0.713	0.0002
Self-evaluation	0.611	0.0025
MMS and:		
QMGS	–0.869	0.0001
Functional scale	–0.582	0.0045
Self-evaluation	0.529	0.011

strength of the upper and lower limbs, chewing, swallowing, and vital capacity were more reliable because, when they were removed, the intraclass correlation coefficient decreased. In contrast, the intraclass correlation coefficient increased when items assessing the strength of the neck and facial muscles, double vision in lateral gaze, and ptosis in vertical gaze were excluded, suggesting that these items are less reliable. Removing the items assessing grip strength modified the intraclass correlation only slightly.

MMS

Agreement between observers was slightly higher on the MMS ($r = 0.906$) than on the QMGS (TABLE 4). The differences between the two measures of the observers ranged from –28 to +20, with a median difference of –3.0.

The intraclass correlation of MMS (TABLE 5) ranged from 0.86 to 0.93 when items were deleted in turn. Items of the MMS assessing the strength of upper and lower limbs and those of the neck and trunk were more reliable because, when they were removed, the intraclass correlation coefficient decreased. In contrast, the intraclass correlation coefficient increased when items assessing eyelid occlusion, extrinsic ocular musculature, chewing, and swallowing were excluded, suggesting that these items are less reliable. Removing the item assessing speech modified the intraclass correlation only slightly.

Functional and Self-Evaluation Scales

Intrapatient agreement on self-evaluation was –0.068; that is, there was no agreement at all. The weighted K for the functional scale was 0.582 (TABLE 6), indicating moderate agreement. It is noteworthy that agreement was reached only for 11 patients out of 22 and that the distinction between minor and moderate symptoms or moderate symptoms and severe disability appeared difficult to observe.

TABLE 5. Intraclass correlation of QMGS and MMS in MG

Variable	Intraclass correlation
QMGS	
Whole score	0.905
Incomplete, minus:	
Outstretching of legs	0.87
Outstretching of arms	0.86
Head lifting	0.91
Facial muscles	0.91
Chewing	0.89
Swallowing	0.89
Double vision	0.92
Ptosis	0.93
Vital capacity	0.89
Grip strength	0.90
MMS	
Whole score	0.906
Incomplete, minus:	
Outstretching of legs	0.89
Outstretching of arms	0.87
Head lifting	0.87
Sit up from lying position	0.86
Eyelid occlusion	0.91
Chewing	0.91
Swallowing	0.93
Speech	0.90
Extrinsic ocular musculature	0.93
Further complete, with addition of:	
Vital capacity	0.92
Vital capacity and grip strength	0.91

TABLE 6. Agreement on functional scale (FS)

	Observer 1					
Observer 2	FS	1	2	3	4	5
	1	1				
	2		2	1		
	3	1	3	2	1	
	4		1	3	2	1
	5					4

NOTE: Weighted *K*: 0.582.

DISCUSSION

The first assessment of reliability of the QMGS was reported by Besinger *et al.*[2] on 12 MG patients, with 3 neurologist observers and with student observers without experience in neuromuscular diseases. The measure of agreement used was the coefficient of variation, at below 10%, which in fact actually refers to dispersion rather than agreement of measurements.

Reliability of QMGS was tested by Barohn *et al.*[7] on 5 MG patients and 4 normal subjects examined by 7 clinical evaluators. The overall measure of reliability was based on a weighted average of the standard deviations of interobserver measures. This value was 1.342. Thus, it was estimated that, at the 95% confidence level, QMGS did not differ from the observed values by more than ± 2.63. However, these results are based on a small and very heterogeneous sample (normal and myasthenic subjects).

We compared the validity and reliability of QMGS and MMS using a randomized design. Intraobserver agreement would have required at least one more measurement, increasing the weakness of these patients and thus inducing an important bias. Results exhibited high agreement between observers regardless of the score that was used. The fact that high interobserver agreement did not rely markedly on any of the constituent items suggests a high reliability of each item. This indicates that both scores provide reliable information on the main muscle function in generalized MG.

In contrast with QMGS, MMS does not account for measurement of vital capacity. In spite of this, interobserver agreement did not differ. Addition of this measurement in MMS did not improve its reliability. However, measurement of vital capacity provides irreplaceable information upon respiratory status of MG patients. Thus, measurement of vital capacity, whether included in a score or not, is essential.

Therefore, our findings support the use of either QMGS or MMS for assessing the muscular strength of patients with MG as the end point in clinical trial and in routine practice. Functional scales are to be used cautiously.

REFERENCES

1. TINDALL, R.S.A., J.A. ROLLINS, J.T. PHILLIPS *et al.* 1987. Preliminary results of a double-blind, randomized, placebo-controlled trial of cyclosporine in myasthenia gravis. N. Engl. J. Med. **316:** 719–724.
2. BESINGER, U.A., V.T. KLAUS, M. HOMBERG *et al.* 1983. Myasthenia gravis: long-term correlation of binding and bungarotoxin blocking antibodies against acetylcholine receptors with changes in disease severity. Neurology **33:** 1316–1321.
3. GAJDOS, P., N. SIMON, P. DE ROHAN CHABOT & M. GOULON. 1983. Effets à long terme des échanges plasmatiques au cours de la myasthénie. Résultats d'une étude randomisée. Presse Med. **12:** 939–942.
4. FLESS, J. & J. COHEN. 1973. The equivalence of weighted kappa statistic and the intraclass correlation coefficient as a measure of reliability. Educ. Psychol. Meas. **33:** 613–619.
5. DONNER, A. 1986. A review of inference procedures for the intraclass correlation coefficient in the one-way random effects model. Int. Stat. Rev. **54:** 67–82.
6. BLAND, J.M. & D.G. ALTMAN. 1986. Statistical methods for assessing agreement between two methods of clinical measurements. Lancet **i:** 307–310.
7. BAROHN, R.J., D. MCINTIRE, L. HERBELIN *et al.* 1998. Reliability testing of the quantitative myasthenia gravis score. Ann. N.Y. Acad. Sci. **841:** 769–772.

Three Forms of Immune Myasthenia

MARK A. AGIUS,[a] DAVID P. RICHMAN,[a] ROBERT H. FAIRCLOUGH,[a]
JOHAN AARLI,[b] NILS ERIK GILHUS,[b] AND FREDRIK ROMI[b]

[a]*Department of Neurology, University of California at Davis, Davis, California 95616, USA*

[b]*Department of Neurology, University of Bergen, Bergen, Norway*

ABSTRACT: We propose a new classification for immune myasthenia based on antibody pattern. The types of immune myasthenia presently characterized by known antibody targets segregate into three groups: type 1, in which the muscle target is the acetylcholine receptor only; type 2, in which titin antibodies are present in addition to acetylcholine receptor antibodies; and type 3, in which muscle-specific kinase antibodies are present in the absence of acetylcholine receptor antibodies. The immune target is unknown in the patients with immune myasthenia not associated with these antibodies. This classification has advantages over the present classifications as regards homogeneity of groups, etiology, mechanism of disease, and prognosis.

KEYWORDS: immune myasthenia (IM); antibody (Ab); acetylcholine receptor (AChR); pathogenicity

INTRODUCTION

The neuromuscular junction provides multiple targets for biochemical defects that result in clinical disease. Apart from genetic and toxic disorders, these biochemical defects also include distinct forms of immune myasthenia (IM). Whereas the acetylcholine receptor (AChR) represents the main target in most individuals with IM, complement-fixing striated muscle antibodies (Abs), which were first described in 1960 by Strauss *et al.*,[1] also appear to be important pathogenically. Furthermore, approximately 15% of IM patients do not have detectable AChR Abs. In 1980, Compston *et al.*[2] discussed the heterogeneity of IM and proposed a classification based on age of onset and thymic pathology that subdivided patients into three groups: those with early onset, those with late onset, and those with thymoma. A current working classification of IM contains two additional subgroups: those patients with purely ocular myasthenia and those with seronegative myasthenia.

We propose a revised, simplified classification of IM based on the detected Abs. This classification implies distinct mechanisms of disease.

Address for correspondence: Mark A. Agius, Department of Neurology, University of California at Davis, 1515 Newton Court, Room 510, Davis, CA 95616-8603. Voice: 530-754-5020; fax: 530-754-5036.

maagius@ucdavis.edu

Ann. N.Y. Acad. Sci. 998: 453–456 (2003). © 2003 New York Academy of Sciences.
doi: 10.1196/annals.1254.059

TABLE 1. Ab patterns in immune myasthenia (IM)

IM type	Ab specificities
1	AChR (high)
2	AChR (low), titin
3	Muscle-specific kinase
4	Undefined

REVISED CLASSIFICATION OF IMMUNE MYASTHENIA

Patients with type 1 IM (TABLE 1) have an Ab pattern characterized by relatively high serum concentrations of AChR Abs (up to 100 nM or more) without associated striated muscle Abs. These patients may have other autoimmune diseases and other auto-Abs, including those to thyroid antigens. Germinal centers are generally present in the thymic medulla.

Patients with type 2 IM have an Ab pattern also characterized by the presence of serum AChR Abs. However, the concentration of the AChR Abs tends to be low compared to those of patients with type 1 disease, often less than 20 nM. In addition, type 2 disease is characterized by the presence of titin Ab (TABLE 1). These patients often have a cortical or mixed cortical/medullary thymoma or carcinoma. Aarli and his colleagues[3] documented that the main target for the striated muscle Abs is the N-terminal domain of the intracytoplasmic protein titin. Furthermore, they described an association between thymoma and the Abs to the voltage-gated ryanodine receptor. All patients with IM and a thymic tumor have AChR Abs; almost all also have titin Abs and half have ryanodine receptor Abs. Patients with type 2 disease (with AChR and titin Abs) in the absence of a detectable thymoma may also possess ryanodine receptor Abs. The myasthenia in patients with type 2 disease without a thymoma often demonstrates a late onset, that is, an onset after the age of 50 years.

Patients with type 3 disease possess muscle-specific kinase Abs in the absence of AChR or striated muscle Abs. We have previously demonstrated that Abs directed at cytoskeletal elements of the AChR clustering mechanism, including rapsyn, constituted additional targets for the immune system in patients with IM.[4] Vincent and her colleagues[5] have since demonstrated that muscle-specific kinase is an Ab target in up to a third of patients with seronegative IM. These patients with type 3 IM do not possess AChR or titin Abs; conversely, patients with type 1 and type 2 IM do not possess muscle-specific kinase Abs. Patients with type 4 disease include patients with Abs to targets other than AChR and muscle-specific kinase, but which are as yet undefined.

Types 2 and 3 IM may be associated with a more severe course (TABLE 2). Type 3 is associated with muscle atrophy, whereas type 2 is associated with cardiomyopathy and myositis. The myasthenia associated with type 2 IM does not appear to respond well to thymectomy.[6] In addition, as with type 3, it does not appear to respond as well to immunosuppressive therapy.

TABLE 2. Ab-specific disease manifestations

Ab specificity	Severe course	Myocarditis	Myositis	Muscle atrophy	Poor response to thymectomy
AChR	+	–	–	–	–
Titin, RyR	++	+	+	–	+
MuSK	++	–	–	+	?

ANTIBODY PATHOGENICITY

The pathogenicity of AChR Abs is established by means of passive and active immunization. Most serum AChR Abs are directed at the extrasynaptic portion. In addition, however, Abs to AChR cytoplasmic components occur and appear to be important in pathogenicity. The pathogenicity of titin and muscle-specific kinase Abs is suggested by their association with IM in the absence of AChR Abs. The pathogenicity of titin and ryanodine receptor Abs is suggested by their association with myositis and cardiomyopathy. This pathogenicity, though, needs confirmation in animal models.

ADDITIONAL CANDIDATE ANTIGENS IN IMMUNE MYASTHENIA

Additional candidate antigens at the neuromuscular junction include rapsyn and other peripheral membrane proteins. Thus, rapsyn Abs were detected in 2 of 15 myasthenic patients tested.[4] One of the patients also possessed reactivity with proteins of 58-kDa and 87-kDa molecular weight as well as with proteins of lower molecular weight. In a blinded, coded manner, we detected rapsyn Abs in 1 of 10 patients with high positive AChR Ab titers, 1 of 10 patients with borderline elevated AChR titers, 3 of 17 patients with AChR Ab-negative IM, and 2 of 17 patients with IM and thymoma with AChR Abs.[4] Rapsyn Abs were not present in healthy controls. They were not specific to IM and were present in 1 of 10 patients with other autoimmune neurological disease and in 7 of 9 patients with systemic lupus erythematosus.

Animals immunized with alkali extract of electric organ from *Torpedo californica* develop clinical weakness within 3 weeks of immunization. They also developed AChR Abs within 5 weeks of immunization. When tested at 4 months, they were found to have a significant decrease in AChR content.[4]

EPITOPE SPREAD IN IMMUNE MYASTHENIA

Epitope spread refers to the exposure and presentation to the immune system of novel antigenic targets subsequent to an initial immune attack directed at a localized epitope. The presentation of cytoplasmic AChR peptides to T cells resulting in their activation would constitute a form of intramolecular epitope spread. Similarly, damage of associated peripheral membrane proteins such as rapsyn would result in intermolecular epitope spread. The lack of AChR Abs in patients with type 3 IM would suggest that, in most individuals, muscle-specific kinase Abs do not arise as a consequence of spread from an AChR immune response.

We have previously documented that intermolecular epitope spreading at a humoral (and consequently likely also at a T cell) level occurs in experimental IM.[7] When we immunized female Lewis rats with peptides corresponding to *Torpedo* α chain 192–212 and α chain 127–145, we generated monoclonal Abs that were directed against the β and γ subunits, respectively, that did not cross-react with the original peptide or with the α subunit.

CONCLUSIONS

The proposed classification of IM on the basis of the Ab target identifies three defined and nonoverlapping types of IM. In contrast, most of the subgroups identified in the currently employed classifications are heterogeneous and demonstrate overlap with each other. It is suggested that the Abs that characterize the proposed classification are pathogenic; however, formal proof in appropriate animal models still needs to be obtained for targets other than the AChR and rapsyn. The origins of the Abs and consequently the etiologies of the immune process are likely to be different in the three IM types. Cross-reactivity, including molecular mimicry, is suggested to underlie their development. Epitope spread may complicate the immune response and represents an argument towards early treatment with immunosuppression even in those with mild disease.

The fourth type of IM in the present classification probably represents multiple additional types. The term seronegative IM should be replaced by AChR Ab-negative IM.

REFERENCES

1. STRAUSS, A.J.L., B. SEEGAL, J.C. HSU *et al.* 1960. Immunofluorescence demonstration of a muscle binding, complement fixing serum globulin fraction in myasthenia gravis. Proc. Soc. Exp. Biol. **1195:** 184–191.
2. COMPSTON, D.A., A. VINCENT, J. NEWSOM-DAVIS & J.R. BATCHELOR. 1980. Clinical, pathological, HLA antigen, and immunological evidence for disease heterogeneity in myasthenia gravis. Brain **103:** 579–601.
3. AARLI, J.A. *et al.* 1990. Patients with myasthenia gravis and thymoma have in their sera IgG autoantibodies against titin. Clin. Exp. Immunol. **82:** 284–288.
4. AGIUS, M.A., S. ZHU, C.A. KIRVAN *et al.* 1998. Rapsyn antibodies in myasthenia gravis. Ann. N.Y. Acad. Sci. **841:** 516–521.
5. HOCH, W., J. MCCONVILLE, S. HELMS *et al.* 2001. Auto-antibodies to the receptor tyrosine kinase MuSK in patients with myasthenia gravis without acetylcholine receptor antibodies. Nat. Med. **7:** 365–368.
6. ROMI, F., N.E. GILHUS, J.E. VARHAUG *et al.* 2002. Thymectomy and anti-muscle autoantibodies in late-onset myasthenia gravis. Eur. J. Neurol. **9:** 55–61.
7. AGIUS, M.A., G.M. TWADDLE & R.H. FAIRCLOUGH. 1998. Epitope spreading in experimental autoimmune myasthenia gravis. Ann. N.Y. Acad. Sci. **841:** 365–367.

Treatment Principles in the Management of Autoimmune Myasthenia Gravis

DAVID P. RICHMAN AND MARK A. AGIUS

Department of Neurology, University of California, Davis, Davis, California 95616, USA

ABSTRACT: The pathogenesis of myasthenia gravis (MG) involves a T cell–directed antibody-mediated autoimmune attack on the nicotinic acetylcholine receptor (AChR) or, occasionally, on other postsynaptic antigens. The antibodies induce their effects through complement-mediated destruction of the postsynaptic endplate membrane with resultant reduction in endplate AChR, and to a lesser degree by increased turnover of endplate AChR or blockade of AChR function. Considerable progress in the treatment of MG has accrued from so-called symptomatic treatments, including improved critical care of seriously ill patients and medications (e.g., cholinesterase inhibitors) increasing the concentration of acetylcholine at the remaining endplate AChRs. Information from other autoimmune diseases and from the response of the normal immune system to invading pathogens supports the view that the course of MG is characterized by exacerbations and remissions. Therefore, the goal in MG treatment is to induce and maintain a remission. This usually involves combinations of short-term and long-term immunosuppressive agents. Selection of the particular combinations of agents in a given patient is guided by the goal of minimizing the cost/benefit ratio of the regimen in an individual patient. In general, the plan involves an initial forceful attack followed by a slow and measured withdrawal.

KEYWORDS: myasthenia gravis; treatment; autoimmune; acetylcholine receptor; acetylcholinesterase; neuromuscular junction; immunosuppression; plasma exchange; intravenous immunoglobulin

INTRODUCTION

Autoimmune myasthenia gravis (MG) is a serious disease that has become amenable to treatment. This success has resulted primarily from the remarkable advances in our understanding of the biology of neuromuscular transmission and of the pathogenic processes underlying this disorder. The various treatments available to clinicians caring for MG patients can be readily listed and discussed. In most patients, use of these agents and modalities can result in improvement in their symptoms and increased functionality. However, most of these treatments have considerable side effects so that, in many patients, the treatment of their MG may

Address for correspondence: David P. Richman, Department of Neurology, University of California, Davis, 1515 Newton Court, Room 510, Davis, CA 95616. Fax: 530-754-5036. dprichman@ucdavis.edu

Ann. N.Y. Acad. Sci. 998: 457–472 (2003). © 2003 New York Academy of Sciences.
doi: 10.1196/annals.1254.060

involve trading one disease for another—the second disease consisting of the set of side effects of the treatment. The future will involve the development of agents with greater specificity so that the side effects are reduced, thereby reducing the cost/benefit ratio of the treatment. For the present, efforts must be made to tailor the treatment of the disease, in many cases in an individualized manner, to improve this ratio.

MG can be considered the model human antibody-mediated autoimmune disease, primarily because its pathogenesis is so well understood. Much of this information has been applicable to similar autoimmune diseases. Advances made in those disorders, many of which affect larger numbers of patients, in turn, have been useful in the development of treatments for MG. For these diseases as well as for MG, clinicians have made use of both scientific and empiric information to improve the care of affected patients. One theme of the analysis that follows is the interplay between these two forms of information in the practical treatment of MG.

PATHOGENESIS OF MG—ROLE OF THE ACETYLCHOLINE RECEPTOR

MG is an acquired autoimmune disease of the neuromuscular junction. The major target of the autoimmune attack is the nicotinic acetylcholine receptor (AChR) located in the postsynaptic muscle endplate membrane (FIG. 1). AChR is an intrinsic (transmembrane) protein that functions as a ligand-gated ion channel. It is made up of four subunits in the following stoichiometry, $\alpha_2\beta\gamma\delta$. All four subunits are homologous, with an extracellular portion, a membrane-spanning region that contributes to the lining of the ion channel, and an intracellular portion. Both T helper cells and B cells are involved in the autoimmune response, but the effector arm of the immune response solely comprises anti-AChR antibodies.[1–3] That is, whereas T cells play a crucial role in this disease, the attack upon the neuromuscular junction is carried out exclusively by antibodies. The target of these antibodies is primarily, but not exclusively, the extracellular portion of the AChR. It is the α subunit, two copies of which are present in each AChR molecule, that is the major target. It appears that most of these anti-α subunit antibodies are directed against the so-called main immunogenic region (MIR), α67–76.[4] Three mechanisms have been identified by which the anti-AChR antibodies, once they bind to their target, produce disordered neuromuscular transmission. The first is the blockade of AChR function. Although this represents a potent mechanism,[5] antibodies with this property are present in very small amounts and probably play a minor role in most cases.[6,7] The other two mechanisms result in reduction in the number of AChRs in the postsynaptic membrane. The first of these is so-called antigenic modulation (increased turnover) induced by cross-linking of adjacent AChR molecules by a single bivalent antibody molecule. This mechanism also appears to play a relatively minor role as well.[1,8] It is the third effector mechanism of these autoantibodies that appears to be the most effective in reducing neuromuscular transmission. The AChR antibodies induce destructive and inflammatory changes in the postsynaptic membrane, both reducing the concentration of AChRs and producing morphologic changes in the entire postsynaptic (endplate) membrane. These destructive changes are mediated primarily through activation of the complement cascade. The complement activation in MG produces both the membrane

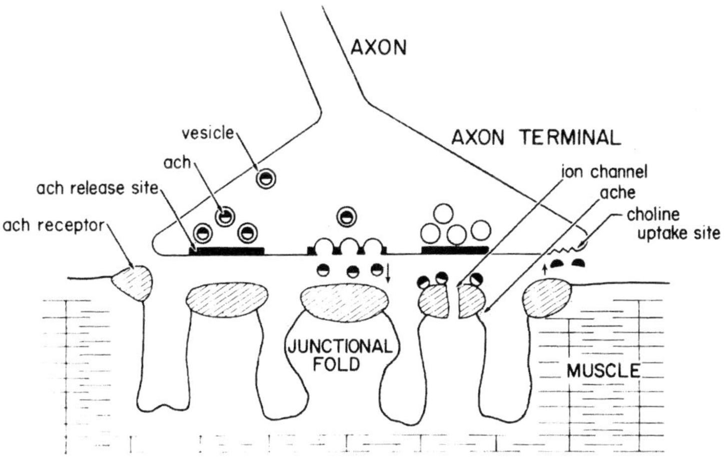

FIGURE 1. Diagram of the presynaptic and postsynaptic components of the neuromuscular junction.

attack complex, which lyses the membrane to which the antibody is bound, and chemotactic products, which attract inflammatory macrophages.[1,9–11]

There are several associations between the autoimmune attack on the neuromuscular junction in this disease and other abnormalities in the immune system. The most studied have been the abnormalities in the thymus in patients with MG.[3,12] About 15% of MG patients have a thymoma. Another 60% have the non-neoplastic histological changes involving germinal centers in the gland medulla, referred to as thymic hyperplasia. In addition, patients with MG appear to have a propensity to autoimmunity. There is a marked increase in the presence of other autoantibodies and other autoimmune diseases.[13–16] Moreover, there is an increased incidence of autoimmune diseases in relatives of MG patients.[13,14]

OTHER ANTIGENS IN MG

Other neuromuscular junction antigens, distinct from AChR, also play a role in autoimmune attack in MG. In about 10% of patients with acquired MG, anti-AChR antibodies are not detected in serum, whereas the characteristics of the disorder appear to be very similar to those in which anti-AChR antibodies are detected.[3,4,12] Vincent and colleagues have recently demonstrated the presence, in about half of these so-called seronegative patients, of serum antibodies directed against a distinct endplate membrane intrinsic protein, muscle-specific receptor tyrosine kinase.[17,18] In addition, it has been known since 1960 that patients with thymoma have antibodies that react with both thymoma cells and muscle striations.[19] These antibodies appear to be directed against the striational cytoskeleton protein titin.[20,21] Many patients with striational antibodies also have antibodies to the intracellular ryanodine receptor.[22] Patients with this group of antibodies, including many older patients without thymoma, tend to have a more severe form of the disease.[23] In particular, their response to thymectomy is less. An additional autoantigen in the muscle endplate has also been identified in acquired MG. In 15% of MG patients, antibodies directed against a small intracellular AChR-associated protein, rapsyn, have been detected.[24] Rapsyn has been shown to play a role in the dense "clustering" of AChR molecules in the endplate membrane.

LESSONS FROM OTHER AUTOIMMUNE DISEASES

In the course of an immune attack on an antigen or autoantigen, the immune response begins to be directed against other antigenic regions (epitopes) on the original antigen or even against neighboring antigens on the target.[25] These phenomena are referred to as epitope spreading. This phenomenon results in a widening of the autoimmune attack and increased damage to the target. Intramolecular epitope spreading has been demonstrated in experimental autoimmune MG.[26] Animals immunized with a peptide from a portion of the α subunit of the AChR that is not present on the other subunits were used for the development of α subunit–specific monoclonal antibodies (mAbs). In addition to several α subunit–specific mAbs that were obtained from these animals, some mAbs were isolated that bound specifically to either the β or γ AChR subunits, but not to the α subunit. There is also information from human MG suggesting the presence of intermolecular epitope spreading.[24]

Many autoimmune diseases follow a relapsing and remitting course.[27,28] Periods of exacerbation are followed by periods of relative quiescence. This appears to relate to the mechanisms involved in the major activity of the normal immune system, response to infection (FIG. 2). The response builds very rapidly beginning with the activation of the innate immune system and is quickly followed by the recruitment of the components of the adaptive immune system, antigen-specific T cells and antibody-producing B cells. The effector agents, cytotoxic T cells, and antibodies lead to efficient destruction of most invading organisms. Once the invading organism is eliminated, the reduction in the immune response is also rapid, limiting the damage to host tissue.[29] Eventually, only memory cells remain to provide the basis for a secondary antigen-specific response in the future if such a response were to become necessary.[30] In autoimmune disorders, the tissue damage may not completely subside, but periods of reduced damage are common. In a general sense, the goal of treatment of these diseases is to induce and support the quiescent stage and to prevent the exacerbation stage.

While it is difficult to obtain information on the natural history of MG,[31–34] the data suggest that the natural history of MG is also characterized by exacerbations and remissions.[35] It is quite clear in the present era of symptomatic and immune-directed treatments (see below) that patients do experience exacerbations. The most striking initiating factors in the relatively recent past have been infection and surgery.[15,16,34–39] Currently, the most common initiator is reduction in the dose of immunosuppressant.

The roles of epitope spreading and the exacerbating/remitting nature of autoimmune diseases have been addressed in patients with a more common disease, rheumatoid arthritis. Large clinical trials have demonstrated the effectiveness in this disease of early vigorous treatment with combinations of agents.[40,41] The data suggest that the earlier in the course of rheumatoid arthritis a complete remission of

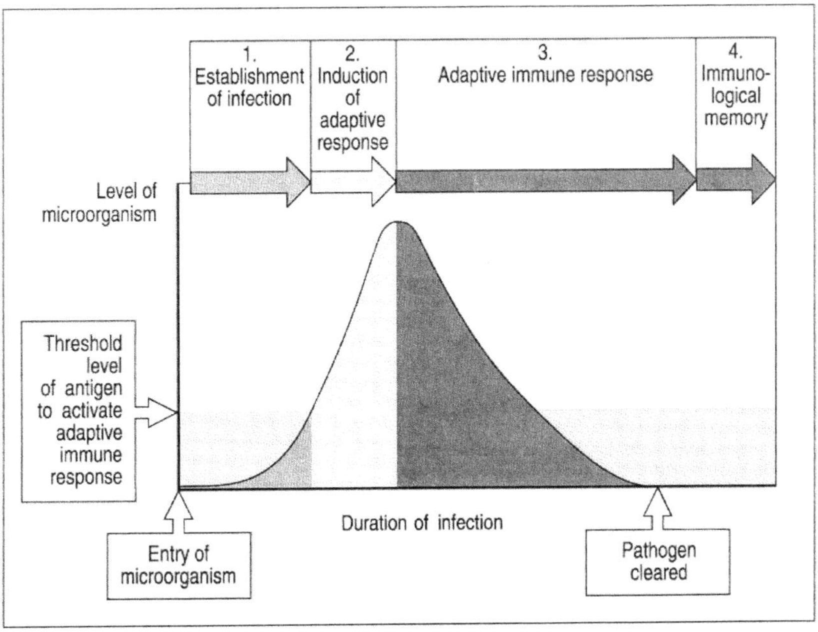

FIGURE 2. Time course of the "normal" immune response to an invading pathogen (©2001 from *Immunobiology* by C. A. Janeway. Reproduced by permission of Routledge, Inc., part of Taylor & Francis Group).

symptoms can be induced, the less joint damage will occur in the long run.[42–44] Stated in another way, the earlier a remission can be induced and maintained, the better the long-term prognosis.

TREATMENT OF AUTOIMMUNE MG

Considerable progress has been made in reducing morbidity and mortality in MG through the use of several symptomatic treatments (TABLE 1) aimed at treating the aftermath of the antibody attack without directly affecting the attack itself.[37] A significant reduction in the mortality of autoimmune MG has been the result of improved methods in critical care.[15] However, the bedrock of symptomatic treatment of autoimmune MG is the cholinesterase inhibitors,[45] especially pyridostigmine. These agents block the acetylcholinesterase in the extracellular matrix of the folded endplate membrane (FIG. 1), increasing the concentration of ACh at the remaining AChRs. Such treatment is usually effective early in the disease or in mild cases, presumably because there are still adequate numbers of AChRs present. The side effects are relatively mild and related to the high concentrations of ACh at both nicotinic and muscarinic synapses. Common muscarinic effects of pyridostigmine are gut hypermotility (stomach cramps, diarrhea), excessive perspiration, excessive respiratory and gastrointestinal secretions, and bradycardia. The nicotinic effects

TABLE 1. Symptomatic treatments of MG

(1) General critical care
Ventilatory support
Infection management
(2) Cholinesterase inhibitors
Maximize receptor activation
Muscarinic effects
(3) Presynaptic agents
Ephedrine
3,4-Diaminopyridine (no approved indication)

TABLE 2. Immune-directed treatments

(1) Long-term treatments
Thymectomy
Corticosteroids
Azathioprine
Cyclophosphamide
Cyclosporine
Newer agents
(2) Short-term treatments
Plasmapheresis
Intravenous immunoglobulin

can be muscle fasciculations and increased blockade of neuromuscular transmission (so-called cholinergic crisis).

There are two additional symptomatic medical treatments available. Both appear to increase the amount of acetylcholine released from the presynaptic nerve terminal. From the perspective of the endplate membrane, this is an identical effect to that of cholinesterase inhibitors. On the basis of limited data, it appears that neither is as effective or safe as pyridostigmine. One of these, ephedrine,[46] is available, but difficult to obtain. The second, 3,4-diaminopyridine,[47] is experimental and has not been approved for any medical indication.

The more effective treatments of MG are those that directly target the autoimmune response (TABLE 2). They may either modify anti-AChR antibody production or modify the damage to the neuromuscular junction induced by the binding of these antibodies. In general, there are two sets of treatments: those that have a rapid, but relatively short-lived, effect on the disease and those that have a long-term effect. The use of these two groups of treatments should be considered in the context of the overall treatment strategy in MG. As discussed above, the natural history of MG, like that of other autoimmune diseases, tends to be characterized by exacerbations and remissions. The strategy of treatment is to first induce a remission and then to maintain the remission, the latter with the least possible cost/benefit ratio (TABLE 3).

TABLE 3. Immune-directed treatments: general principles

- Natural history of exacerbations and remissions, like other autoimmune diseases
- Strategy: First induce remission; then maintain the remission with lowest possible cost/benefit ratio
- Begin with high doses and perhaps multiple agents
- Taper doses slowly to prevent re-exacerbation
- Remember the goal is to maintain remission

TABLE 4. Thymectomy

- No prospective controlled studies
- Meta-analysis of other studies suggests it is effective
- Full effect after 5 years
- More effective if done in first 2 years
- Less effective in older patients with skeletal muscle antibodies
- Possibility of reducing exposure to immunosuppressive medications
- Since all risk is at time of surgery, cost/benefit ratio diminishes with time

LONG-TERM IMMUNE-DIRECTED TREATMENTS

Thymectomy is the classical long-term treatment (TABLE 4). Its effect is usually not apparent until 1 year, and the full effect is not felt for 5 years.[15,36,39,48,49] There are two histologic abnormalities of the thymus that occur in MG. With frankly neoplastic thymoma, removal of the tumor is usually indicated because of the risk of extension of the tumor into adjacent structures in the mediastinum. In these cases, the concurrent removal of other thymic tissue may be less effective in treating the MG than is the case in patients without thymoma. In the second group of patients, there is frequently the presence of germinal centers within the medulla of the gland, so-called thymic hyperplasia. Thymectomy is the single treatment of MG in which the cost/benefit ratio appears to diminish with time. The effectiveness of thymectomy in MG is based on data from nonrandomized studies. Most of these were not controlled. A review of these studies showed that the majority demonstrated efficacy, but that the inability to control for confounding variables in these studies prevented definitive conclusions.[50] Aarli and coworkers have noted that the reduced effectiveness appears to occur in those patients in this group who have thymoma or have anti-skeletal muscle antibodies, but no thymoma.[51] A number of studies have suggested that, in all patients, the earlier in the course of the disease thymectomy is performed, the more effective it is—with 2 years suggested as a goal.[52]

Corticosteroids are currently the mainstay of the immune-directed treatment of MG (TABLE 5). Their major effect is anti-inflammatory by reducing expression of inflammatory cytokines and adhesion molecules and reducing trafficking of inflammatory cells. Very high doses may also induce apoptosis in immune cells.[53,54] These medications, when applied appropriately, appear to be effective in inducing remission in at least 50% of patients, but perhaps as many as 80%. Remarkably, the effi-

TABLE 5. Corticosteroids

- Inhibit expression of cytokines and adhesion molecules
- Mainstay of treatment of MG
- No large adequately controlled trial
- Cost/benefit ratio important issue: use limited by side effects
- Start with high doses; use short-term treatments if patient develops worsening at 7–14 days to tide them over
- Usually remission occurs at 4–8 weeks
- Begin tapering as soon as patient clearly improving
- Taper slowly especially at lower doses (5–10% per month)
- If re-exacerbation occurs during tapering, dose will need to be significantly increased
- Steroid-sparing medications (and perhaps thymectomy) result in improved tapering
- Biphosphonates very effective in preventing osteoporosis

TABLE 6. Azathioprine

- Blocks cell proliferation by inhibiting purine synthesis
- Affects the most rapidly dividing cell populations (e.g., lymphocytes)
- No large controlled studies on use as a single agent
- Large placebo-controlled, double-blind study has shown its effectiveness as steroid-sparing agent
- Low risk/benefit ratio

cacy of these medications in MG has never been studied in an adequate double-blind, placebo-controlled trial.[55] They have significant side effects, making the cost/benefit ratio an important issue in individual patients. Common side effects include weight gain, hypertension, diabetes, anxiety/depression/insomnia ("steroid psychosis"), glaucoma, osteoporosis, cataracts, ulcer/gastrointestinal perforations, myopathy, opportunistic infections, and avascular necrosis of large joints. In many ways, this treatment is the equivalent of "trading one disease for another". Some of these complications can now be prevented or treated. Osteoporosis, with associated compression fractures, can now be readily prevented with the addition of bisphosphonates to the regimen.[56] Peptic ulcers can be prevented using any of the array of acid-reducing medications now available.

Azathioprine has been used extensively in MG (TABLE 6). It acts by inhibiting purine synthesis and, hence, cell proliferation.[57] A few studies have suggested that it is useful alone in inducing a remission, but most studies have described its use in conjunction with corticosteroids.[58–64] A large double-blind, randomized study has demonstrated its effectiveness as a steroid-sparing agent.[61] Its use along with high-dose steroids may increase the risk of opportunistic infections. Azathioprine has considerably fewer side effects than corticosteroids. It can induce leukopenia or thrombocytopenia, intractable vomiting, or hepatic dysfunction.[62] Occasionally, individuals with inborn errors of metabolism, such as thiopurine methyltransferase deficiency, may develop bone marrow suppression at lower doses.[63,64]

TABLE 7. Cyclophosphamide

- Alkylating agent that blocks cell proliferation, predilection for lymphocytes—especially B cells
- No large controlled studies
- Small studies suggest it may be almost as effective as corticosteroids
- Probably has a higher cost/benefit ratio than corticosteroids
- Useful in patients intolerant to corticosteroids or patients not responding to high doses

TABLE 8. Cyclosporine

- Calcineurin inhibitor that blocks cytokine activation of T helper cells
- Large double-blind, placebo-controlled trial demonstrated mild effectiveness as steroid-sparing agent
- Smaller studies suggest mild effectiveness as single agent
- Relatively high cost/benefit ratio

TABLE 9. Newer immune-directed treatments

- No large controlled trials in MG
- Useful in transplantation and other autoimmune diseases
- Mycophenolate
    - High specificity for lymphocytes
    - Inhibits B and T cell proliferation by blocking inosine monophosphate dehydrogenase (purine synthesis)
    - Few small uncontrolled MG trials promising low cost/benefit ratio
- Mitoxantrone and Rituxan—useful in other autoimmune diseases

Cyclophosphamide is also useful in the treatment of MG. It is a strong alkylating agent that acts on DNA (TABLE 7),[57] inhibiting cell proliferation. The effect is greater on B cells than on T cells, making it an excellent agent for antibody-mediated diseases.[65] It appears to be nearly as effective as corticosteroids in inducing remissions, although there are no controlled studies of this drug in induction of remission in MG.[66,67] The risks of the side effects of this medication are even greater than those of steroids, including severe bone marrow suppression with risk of opportunistic infections, bladder toxicity, and a dose-related risk of neoplasms.

Cyclosporin A (TABLE 8) has been marginally effective in MG, primarily as a steroid-sparing medication in steroid-dependent patients.[68] It is an inhibitor of T cell function through inhibition of calcineurin signaling.[69] It has not been shown to be better than azathioprine in this situation, but has a much higher cost/benefit ratio than azathioprine, with side effects including hypertension and renal damage. It is reasonable to consider cyclosporine in patients who are intolerant to azathioprine.

Newer agents (TABLE 9): A number of newer immunosuppressant agents are presently being studied in MG. The best studied is mycophenolate mofetil. It is an

TABLE 10. Short-term immune-directed treatments

- Rapid response, but short-lived
- Plasmapheresis
  - One plasma volume every other day × 5
  - Usual replacement: albumin and saline
- Intravenous immunoglobulin
  - Total dose: 2 g/kg
  - Usually given in divided doses over 5 days
  - Can be given over 3 or 4 days

TABLE 11. Plasmapheresis

- No large controlled studies
- Many smaller studies showing efficacy
- Considerable medical cost/benefit ratio
- Considerable financial cost
- Appears more effective and long-lasting when used with immunosuppressants

inhibitor of the pathway for *de novo* purine synthesis by directly blocking the enzyme inosine monophosphate dehydrogenase. It is highly specific for proliferating lymphocytes, which do not make use of the purine salvage pathway.[70] In two relatively small, uncontrolled studies involving a variety of types of MG patients, it has appeared to be effective.[68,71,72] In patients with poorly controlled disease on the combinations described above, addition of the mycophenolate has resulted in remission of the disease. It also appears to be useful as a steroid-sparing medication. It is unclear whether it is useful as a sole agent in inducing a remission. Mitoxantrone and Rituximab are B cell–directed agents that have been effective in other autoimmune diseases, making them reasonable candidates for study in MG.

SHORT-TERM IMMUNE-DIRECTED TREATMENTS

Plasmapheresis and infusion of intravenous immunoglobulin (IVIG) are two immune-directed treatments that have a rapid onset of effect, but a relatively short duration of action (TABLE 10). The rationale for plasmapheresis was that, because MG was mediated by circulating anti-AChR antibody, the bulk removal of antibody (by removing plasma) would reduce the autoimmune attack at the neuromuscular junction. Uncontrolled studies have demonstrated efficacy with the onset of improvement within the first week (TABLE 11).[73–75] In general, the effect lasts for 1 to 2 months.

IVIG has a very similar effect to plasmapheresis (TABLE 12). Considerable speculation has been made concerning the mechanism of action of this agent with little data to support any of the possibilities.[76] The process involves daily infusions of polyclonal human immunoglobulin, usually 0.4 g/kg per day for 5 consecutive days.[77] Improvement usually begins within a few days of the onset of the treatment.

TABLE 12. Intravenous immunoglobulin

- Large controlled study demonstrated efficacy equal to plasmapheresis
- Same study demonstrated lower medical cost/benefit ratio
- Very considerable financial cost
- May be more effective and long-lasting when used with immunosuppressants

TABLE 13. Role of short-term modalities

- Prevent or treat myasthenic crisis
- Impending surgery (e.g., thymectomy) or medical illness
- Worsening occurring with initiation of corticosteroid treatment
- Boost the effect of immunosuppressant medication during induction of remission
- Treat acute exacerbation (usually during tapering of immunosuppressant medication)
- Rarely, chronic treatment in patients intolerant to immunosuppressants

A multicenter randomized, controlled study comparing plasmapheresis to IVIG has demonstrated equal efficacy, but significantly fewer, and less severe, side effects for the IVIG treatment.[78,79] Hence, the latter is the modality of choice. As with plasmapheresis, the effect of IVIG treatment is usually short-lived, from 1 to 2 months, and seems to be enhanced if the patient is taking immunosuppressive medications.

Therefore, these treatments tend to be used for acute worsening of the MG—such as actual or impending myasthenic crisis (TABLE 13). In severe crisis, more than one course of plasmapheresis or IVIG may be necessary. Occasionally, when plasmapheresis or IVIG is performed in a patient taking an immunosuppressive medication, the effect is one of remission that may last indefinitely. Presumably, in this instance, the plasmapheresis or IVIG is able to push the overall immunosuppression over the threshold needed to induce a remission. This effect seems to occur also in patients whose disease is beginning to flare up as a result of reduction in the dose of immunosuppressive medication. Hence, the first response to a flare-up that occurs during the tapering phase of steroids, or of other immunosuppressive agents, is to hold the dose of the immunosuppressant steady and begin a course of plasmapheresis or IVIG. If these short-term treatments are not effective, then the dose of the immunosuppressant will need to be increased significantly, with or without a second course of plasmapheresis or IVIG.

A PROTOCOL FOR THE TREATMENT OF MG

Most of the principles of the treatment of MG are those of medical treatment of most diseases and in some sense seem self-evident. However, it is useful to state them explicitly so that the basis of the treatment scheme may be readily understood (TABLE 14).

As noted above, the goal of the protocol discussed here is to optimize the use of the various treatments described above by taking into account our knowledge of the

TABLE 14. General principles of treatment in MG

(1) The best data to guide treatment decisions are those from applicable randomized double-blind, placebo-controlled clinical studies. In situations in which such information is not available, decisions should be made and actions taken based on less definitive clinical studies and on our knowledge of the pathogenesis of MG.
(2) Decision making on any particular aspect of the treatment plan is a partnership between the informed patient and the treating physician.
(3) In general, the safest regimen that will *adequately* treat the disease should be employed.
(4) The duration of treatment is as important as the intensity of treatment in considering both efficacy and side effects.

TABLE 15. Specific treatment principles in MG

(1) Make use of immune-directed treatments as early as possible to reduce the likelihood of epitope spreading.
(2) Aim for complete remission (absence of symptoms).
(3) It is likely that the autoantigen cannot be completely removed, but aim for minimizing tissue destruction.
(4) Maintenance of remission usually requires slow tapering of immunosuppressive treatment.

pathogenesis of MG and the nature of the autoimmune attack. In many individual patients, the agents and their combinations will have to be appropriately tailored. Several specific treatment goals can be derived from the information discussed above concerning the roles of epitope spreading and of exacerbations and remissions in MG and other autoimmune diseases (TABLE 15).

The following is a treatment protocol, designed on the basis of these principles, for generalized acquired MG. The patient is treated with anticholinesterase medication until it is clear that this treatment alone does not produce remission. Each step requires that the cost/benefit ratio for the individual patient be lower than other alternatives. The patient is started on high-dose daily prednisone, in divided doses (commonly 20 mg three times per day), with the goal of inducing a remission. Any worsening in symptoms in the first 2 weeks is treated with a course of either IVIG or plasmapheresis. These two short-term treatments appear to be effective in overcoming the worsening that can occur in this period after initiation of high-dose corticosteroids. They may also assist in the induction of the remission. Therefore, it is also reasonable to start the short-term treatment concomitantly with the initiation of the steroids. Once remission is established, the tapering of the prednisone is begun, aimed at an alternate-day dosing schedule. In this phase, the goal is to reach the minimum dose of prednisone that will maintain the remission. Once some reduction in prednisone dose has been accomplished, a steroid-sparing agent, such as azathioprine or mycophenolate mofetil, is added. (A major role for thymectomy is as a steroid-sparing treatment. Its timing is discussed above.) It is important also to begin a bisphosphonate to prevent steroid-induced osteoporosis. Any other side effects of the prednisone or of the other immunosuppressants are treated as they appear, and the anticholinesterase medications are tapered as tolerated. The slow tapering of the prednisone is continued. If MG symptoms return during the tapering phase, the dose of prednisone at that time is held steady for a few weeks to allow spontaneous reestablishment of the remission to occur. If there is no improvement after several weeks or if the worsening accelerates, a full course of IVIG or plasma exchange is begun. If this does not help, it will require significant increases in the steroid dose to reestablish the remission. A minor increase in dose, for example, to a level that was the last that successfully maintained the remission, is usually not effective. Once the remission is established again, the slow tapering of the prednisone is begun. If the prednisone can eventually be tapered to zero, the other immunosuppressant medication is then very slowly tapered.

REFERENCES

1. Richman, D.P., M.A. Agius, C.A. Kirvan *et al.* 1998. Antibody effector mechanisms in myasthenia gravis: the complement hypothesis. Ann. N.Y. Acad. Sci. **841:** 450–465.
2. Lisak, R.P. 1999. Myasthenia gravis. Curr. Treat. Options Neurol. **1:** 239–250.
3. Vincent, A., J. Palace & D. Hilton-Jones. 2001. Myasthenia gravis. Lancet **357:** 2122–2128.
4. Lindstrom, J.M. 2000. Acetylcholine receptors and myasthenia. Muscle Nerve **23:** 453–477.
5. Gomez, C.M. & D.P. Richman. 1983. Anti-acetylcholine receptor antibodies directed against the alpha-bungarotoxin binding site induce a unique form of experimental myasthenia. Proc. Natl. Acad. Sci. USA **80:** 4089–4093.
6. Lefvert, A.K., S. Cuenoud & B.W. Fulpius. 1981. Binding properties and subclass distribution of anti-acetylcholine receptor antibodies in myasthenia gravis. J. Neuroimmunol. **1:** 125–135.
7. Fulpius, B.W., A.K. Lefvert, S. Cuenoud & A. Mourey. 1981. Properties and serum levels of specific populations of anti-acetylcholine receptor antibodies in myasthenia gravis. Ann. N.Y. Acad. Sci. **377:** 307–315.
8. Richman, D.P. & M.A. Agius. 1994. Myasthenia gravis: pathogenesis and treatment. Semin. Neurol. **14:** 106–110.
9. Engel, A.G. & K. Arahata. 1987. The membrane attack complex of complement at the endplate in myasthenia gravis. Ann. N.Y. Acad. Sci. **505:** 326–332.
10. Maselli, R.A., D.P. Richman & R.L. Wollmann. 1991. Inflammation at the neuromuscular junction in myasthenia gravis. Neurology **41:** 1497–1504.
11. Nakano, S. & A.G. Engel. 1993. Myasthenia gravis: quantitative immunocytochemical analysis of inflammatory cells and detection of complement membrane attack complex at the end-plate in 30 patients. Neurology **43:** 1167–1172.
12. Drachman, D.B. 1994. Myasthenia gravis. N. Engl. J. Med. **330:** 1797–1810.
13. Simpson, J.A. 1966. Myasthenia gravis as an autoimmune disease: clinical aspects. Ann. N.Y. Acad. Sci. **135:** 506–516.
14. Wolf, S.M., L.P. Rowland, D.L. Schotland *et al.* 1966. Myasthenia as an autoimmune disease: clinical aspects. Ann. N.Y. Acad. Sci. **135:** 517–535.
15. Oosterhuis, H.J.G.H. 1997. Myasthenia Gravis. Groningen Neurologic Press. Groningen.
16. Grob, D. 1999. Natural history of myasthenia gravis. *In* Myasthenia Gravis and Myasthenic Disorders, pp. 131–145. Oxford University Press. Oxford.
17. Hoch, W., J. McConville, S. Helms *et al.* 2001. Auto-antibodies to the receptor tyrosine kinase MuSK in patients with myasthenia gravis without acetylcholine receptor antibodies. Nat. Med. **7:** 365–368.

18. LIYANAGE, Y., W. HOCH, D. BEESON & A. VINCENT. 2002. The agrin/muscle-specific kinase pathway: new targets for autoimmune and genetic disorders at the neuromuscular junction. Muscle Nerve **25:** 4–16.
19. STRAUSS, A.J., B.C. SEEGAL, K.C. HSU *et al.* 1960. Immunofluorescence demonstration of a muscle-binding complement-fixing serum globulin fraction in myasthenia gravis. Proc. Soc. Exp. Biol. Med. **105:** 184–191.
20. AARLI, J.A., K. STEFANSSON, L.S. MARTON & R.L. WOLLMANN. 1990. Patients with myasthenia gravis and thymoma have in their sera IgG autoantibodies against titin. Clin. Exp. Immunol. **82:** 284–288.
21. VOLTZ, R.D., W.C. ALBRICH, A. NAGELE *et al.* 1997. Paraneoplastic myasthenia gravis: detection of anti-MGT30 (titin) antibodies predicts thymic epithelial tumor. Neurology **49:** 1454–1457.
22. MYGLAND, A., J.A. AARLI, R. MATRE & N.E. GILHUS. 1994. Ryanodine receptor antibodies related to severity of thymoma associated myasthenia gravis. J. Neurol. Neurosurg. Psychiatry **57:** 843–846.
23. ROMI, F., G.O. SKEIE, J.A. AARLI & N.E. GILHUS. 2000. The severity of myasthenia gravis correlates with the serum concentration of titin and ryanodine receptor antibodies. Arch. Neurol. **57:** 1596–1600.
24. AGIUS, M.A., S. ZHU, C.A. KIRVAN *et al.* 1998. Rapsyn antibodies in myasthenia gravis. Ann. N.Y. Acad. Sci. **841:** 516–521.
25. VANDERLUGT, C.L. & S.D. MILLER. 2002. Epitope spreading in immune-mediated diseases: implications for immunotherapy. Nat. Rev. Immunol. **2:** 85–95.
26. AGIUS, M.A., G.M. TWADDLE & R.H. FAIRCLOUGH. 1998. Epitope spreading in experimental autoimmune myasthenia gravis. Ann. N.Y. Acad. Sci. **841:** 365–367.
27. HAHN, B.H. 2001. Systemic lupus erythematosis. *In* Harrison's Principles of Internal Medicine, pp. 1922–1928. McGraw–Hill. New York.
28. LIPSKY, O.E. 2001. Rheumatoid arthritis. *In* Harrison's Principles of Internal Medicine, pp. 1928–1935. McGraw–Hill. New York.
29. VERHASSELT, V. & M. GOLDMAN. 2001. From autoimmune responses to autoimmune disease: what is needed? J. Autoimmun. **16:** 327–330.
30. VAN PARIJS, L. & A.K. ABBAS. 1998. Homeostasis and self-tolerance in the immune system: turning lymphocytes off. Science **280:** 243–248.
31. CAMPBELL, H. & E. BRAMWELL. 1900. Myasthenia gravis. Brain **23:** 277–337.
32. KENNEDY, F.S. & F.P. MOERSCH. 1937. Myasthenia gravis: a clinical review of eighty-seven cases observed between 1915 and the early part of 1932. Can. Med. Assoc. J. **37:** 216–223.
33. VIETS, H.R. 1953. A historical review of myasthenia gravis from 1672 to 1900. J. Am. Med. Assoc. **153**(14): 1273–1280.
34. ROWLAND, L.P., P.F.A. HOEFER, H. ARANOW & H.H. MERRITT. 1956. Fatalities in myasthenia gravis: a review of 39 cases with 26 autopsies. Neurology **6:** 307–326.
35. VERMA, P. & J. OGER. 1992. Treatment of acquired autoimmune myasthenia gravis: a topic review. Can. J. Neurol. Sci. **19:** 360–375.
36. PERLO, V.P., D.C. POSKANZER, R.S. SCHWAB *et al.* 1966. Myasthenia gravis: evaluation of treatment in 1,355 patients. Neurology **16:** 431–439.
37. GROB, D., N.G. BRUNNER & T. NAMBA. 1981. The natural course of myasthenia gravis and effect of therapeutic measures. Ann. N.Y. Acad. Sci. **377:** 652–669.
38. OOSTERHUIS, H.J. 1981. Observations of the natural history of myasthenia gravis and the effect of thymectomy. Ann. N.Y. Acad. Sci. **377:** 678–690.
39. GROB, D., E.L. ARSURA, N.G. BRUNNER & T. NAMBA. 1987. The course of myasthenia gravis and therapies affecting outcome. Ann. N.Y. Acad. Sci. **505:** 472–499.
40. BOERS, M., A.C. VERHOEVEN, H.M. MARKUSSE *et al.* 1997. Randomised comparison of combined step-down prednisolone, methotrexate and sulphasalazine with sulphasalazine alone in early rheumatoid arthritis. Lancet **350:** 309–318.
41. KREMER, J.M. 2001. Rational use of new and existing disease-modifying agents in rheumatoid arthritis. Ann. Intern. Med. **134:** 695–706.
42. BATHON, J.M., R.W. MARTIN, R.M. FLEISCHMANN *et al.* 2000. A comparison of etanercept and methotrexate in patients with early rheumatoid arthritis. N. Engl. J. Med. **343:** 1586–1593.

43. LANDEWE, R.B., M. BOERS, A.C. VERHOEVEN *et al.* 2002. COBRA combination therapy in patients with early rheumatoid arthritis: long-term structural benefits of a brief intervention. Arthritis Rheum. **46:** 347–356.
44. O'DELL, J.R. 2002. Treating rheumatoid arthritis early: a window of opportunity? Arthritis Rheum. **46:** 283–285.
45. WALKER, M.B. 1934. Treatment of myasthenia gravis with physostigmine. Lancet **1:** 1200–1201.
46. SIEB, J.P. & A.G. ENGEL. 1993. Ephedrine: effects on neuromuscular transmission. Brain Res. **623:** 167–171.
47. LUNDH, H., O. NILSSON & I. ROSEN. 1985. Improvement in neuromuscular transmission in myasthenia gravis by 3,4-diaminopyridine. Eur. Arch. Psychiatry Neurol. Sci. **234:** 374–377.
48. PERLO, V.P., B. ARNASON, D. POSKANZER *et al.* 1971. The role of thymectomy in the treatment of myasthenia gravis. Ann. N.Y. Acad. Sci. **183:** 308–315.
49. BUCKINGHAM, J.M., F.M. HOWARD, JR., P.E. BERNATZ *et al.* 1976. The value of thymectomy in myasthenia gravis: a computer-assisted matched study. Ann. Surg. **184:** 453–458.
50. GRONSETH, G.S. & R.J. BAROHN. 2000. Practice parameter: thymectomy for autoimmune myasthenia gravis (an evidence-based review): report of the Quality Standards Subcommittee of the American Academy of Neurology. Neurology **55:** 7–15.
51. ROMI, F., N.E. GILHUS, J.E. VARHAUG *et al.* 2002. Thymectomy and anti-muscle autoantibodies in late-onset myasthenia gravis. Eur. J. Neurol. **9:** 55–61.
52. DEFILIPPI, V.J., D.P. RICHMAN & M.K. FERGUSON. 1994. Transcervical thymectomy for myasthenia gravis. Ann. Thorac. Surg. **57:** 194–197.
53. CASE, J.P. 2001. Old and new drugs used in rheumatoid arthritis: a historical perspective. Part 1: The older drugs. Am. J. Ther. **8:** 123–143.
54. BARNES, P.J. 2001. Molecular mechanisms of corticosteroids in allergic diseases. Allergy **56:** 928–936.
55. BRUNNER, N.G., C.L. BERGER, T. NAMBA & D. GROB. 1976. Corticotropin and corticosteroids in generalized myasthenia gravis: comparative studies and role in management. Ann. N.Y. Acad. Sci. **274:** 577–595.
56. SAAG, K.G., R. EMKEY, T.J. SCHNITZER *et al.* 1998. Alendronate for the prevention and treatment of glucocorticoid-induced osteoporosis: Glucocorticoid-Induced Osteoporosis Intervention Study Group. N. Engl. J. Med. **339:** 292–299.
57. POHANKA, E. 2001. New immunosuppressive drugs: an update. Curr. Opin. Urol. **11:** 143–151.
58. BROMBERG, M.B., J.J. WALD, D.A. FORSHEW *et al.* 1997. Randomized trial of azathioprine or prednisone for initial immunosuppressive treatment of myasthenia gravis. J. Neurol. Sci. **150:** 59–62.
59. KUKS, J.B., S. DJOJOATMODJO & H.J. OOSTERHUIS. 1991. Azathioprine in myasthenia gravis: observations in 41 patients and a review of literature. Neuromuscul. Disord. **1:** 423–431.
60. WITTE, A.S., D.R. CORNBLATH, G.J. PARRY *et al.* 1984. Azathioprine in the treatment of myasthenia gravis. Ann. Neurol. **15:** 602–605.
61. PALACE, J., J. NEWSOM-DAVIS & B. LECKY. 1998. A randomized double-blind trial of prednisolone alone or with azathioprine in myasthenia gravis: Myasthenia Gravis Study Group. Neurology **50:** 1778–1783.
62. KISSEL, J.T., R.J. LEVY, J.R. MENDELL & R.C. GRIGGS. 1986. Azathioprine toxicity in neuromuscular disease. Neurology **36:** 35–39.
63. EVANS, W.E., Y.Y. HON, L. BOMGAARS *et al.* 2001. Preponderance of thiopurine *S*-methyltransferase deficiency and heterozygosity among patients intolerant to mercaptopurine or azathioprine. J. Clin. Oncol. **19:** 2293–2301.
64. MCLEOD, H.L. & C. SIVA. 2002. The thiopurine *S*-methyltransferase gene locus: implications for clinical pharmacogenomics. Pharmacogenomics **3:** 89–98.
65. ZHU, L.P., T.R. CUPPS, G. WHALEN & A.S. FAUCI. 1987. Selective effects of cyclophosphamide therapy on activation, proliferation, and differentiation of human B cells. J. Clin. Invest. **79:** 1082–1090.
66. PEREZ, M.C., W.L. BUOT, C. MERCADO-DANGUILAN *et al.* 1981. Stable remissions in myasthenia gravis. Neurology **31:** 32–37.

67. NIAKAN, E., Y. HARATI & L.A. ROLAK. 1986. Immunosuppressive drug therapy in myasthenia gravis. Arch. Neurol. **43:** 155–156
68. TINDALL, R.S., J.T. PHILLIPS, J.A. ROLLINS *et al.* 1993. A clinical therapeutic trial of cyclosporine in myasthenia gravis. Ann. N.Y. Acad. Sci. **681:** 539–551.
69. MATSUDA, S. & S. KOYASU. 2000. Mechanisms of action of cyclosporine. Immunopharmacology **47:** 119–125.
70. ALLISON, A.C. & E.M. EUGUI. 2000. Mycophenolate mofetil and its mechanisms of action. Immunopharmacology **47:** 85–118.
71. CHAUDHRY, V., D.R. CORNBLATH, J.W. GRIFFIN *et al.* 2001. Mycophenolate mofetil: a safe and promising immunosuppressant in neuromuscular diseases. Neurology **56:** 94–96.
72. CIAFALONI, E., J.M. MASSEY, B. TUCKER-LIPSCOMB & D.B. SANDERS. 2001. Mycophenolate mofetil for myasthenia gravis: an open-label pilot study. Neurology **56:** 97–99.
73. PINCHING, A.J. & D.K. PETERS. 1976. Remission of myasthenia gravis following plasma-exchange. Lancet **2:** 1373–1376.
74. DAU, P.C., J.M. LINDSTROM, C.K. CASSEL *et al.* 1977. Plasmapheresis and immunosuppressive drug therapy in myasthenia gravis. N. Engl. J. Med. **297:** 1134–1140.
75. PINCHING, A.J., D.K. PETERS & J.N. DAVIS. 1977. Plasma exchange in myasthenia gravis. Lancet **1:** 428–429.
76. FERRERO, B. & L. DURELLI. 2002. High-dose intravenous immunoglobulin G treatment of myasthenia gravis. Neurol. Sci. **23**(suppl. 1)**:** S9–S24.
77. ARSURA, E.L., A. BICK, N.G. BRUNNER *et al.* 1986. High-dose intravenous immunoglobulin in the management of myasthenia gravis. Arch. Intern. Med. **146:** 1365–1368.
78. GAJDOS, P., S. CHEVRET, B. CLAIR *et al.* 1997. Clinical trial of plasma exchange and high-dose intravenous immunoglobulin in myasthenia gravis: Myasthenia Gravis Clinical Study Group. Ann. Neurol. **41:** 789–796.
79. RONAGER, J., M. RAVNBORG, I. HERMANSEN & S. VORSTRUP. 2001. Immunoglobulin treatment versus plasma exchange in patients with chronic moderate to severe myasthenia gravis. Artif. Organs **25:** 967–973.

Development of a Thymectomy Trial in Nonthymomatous Myasthenia Gravis Patients Receiving Immunosuppressive Therapy

GIL I. WOLFE,[a] HENRY J. KAMINSKI,[b] ALFRED JARETZKI III,[c] ANTHONY SWAN,[d] AND JOHN NEWSOM-DAVIS[e]

[a]*Department of Neurology, University of Texas Southwestern Medical School, Dallas, Texas, USA*

[b]*Case Western Reserve University, University Hospitals of Cleveland, Louis Stokes Cleveland Veteran Affairs Medical Center, Cleveland, Ohio, USA*

[c]*Department of Surgery, Columbia Presbyterian Medical Center, New York, New York, USA*

[d]*Guy's, Kings, and St. Thomas's Medical School, London, United Kingdom*

[e]*University of Oxford, John Radcliffe Hospital, Oxford, United Kingdom*

ABSTRACT: Thymectomy has been regularly used in the management of nonthymomatous autoimmune myasthenia gravis (MG), but its benefits have not been established in a randomized, controlled trial. The widespread use of thymectomy in MG patients without thymoma is largely based on retrospective, nonrandomized case series that have produced a consensus that the procedure is sometimes beneficial. Still, the benefits and utilization of thymectomy are actively debated among MG experts. In this paper, we describe the development of a multicenter, international trial to determine whether extended transsternal thymectomy reduces corticosteroid requirements for patients with generalized AChR antibody-positive nonthymomatous MG.

KEYWORDS: myasthenia gravis (MG); thymectomy; nonthymomatous; trial

INTRODUCTION

For more than 60 years, thymectomy has been regularly used in the management of nonthymomatous autoimmune myasthenia gravis (MG), but its benefits have not been established in a randomized, controlled trial.[1] The widespread use of thymectomy in MG patients without thymoma is largely based on retrospective, nonrandomized case series that have produced a consensus that the procedure is sometimes beneficial. Still, the benefits and utilization of thymectomy are actively debated among MG experts. In a 1990 survey, only 3 of 56 experts expressed no reservation

Address for correspondence: Gil I. Wolfe, Department of Neurology, University of Texas Southwestern Medical School, 5323 Harry Hines Boulevard, Dallas, TX 75390-8897. Voice: 214-648-9082; fax: 214-648-9311.
gil.wolfe@utsouthwestern.edu

**Ann. N.Y. Acad. Sci. 998: 473–480 (2003). © 2003 New York Academy of Sciences.
doi: 10.1196/annals.1254.061**

in using thymectomy in patients with generalized MG.[2] Over 20% of the experts surveyed had significant reservations about recommending the procedure.

Thymectomy, although now performed with low morbidity and almost no mortality, is not risk-free and can result in significant complications. MG outcomes in many retrospective studies have varied widely.[1] Some of the reasons for this variation, which include differences in the surgical technique used, have been critically analyzed.[3] A recent evidence-based review determined that the benefit of thymectomy in nonthymomatous MG has not been established conclusively.[1] Recommendations from this practice parameter were that, for the current time, thymectomy be considered a treatment *option* and that a prospective, controlled, randomized study be performed with standardized medical therapy for all patients. Similar calls for a randomized, controlled study have been made in the past.[4,5]

Corticosteroids and other immunosuppressive agents are effective therapies for MG and are routinely prescribed in its management, although their use may be associated with complications. The role of thymectomy in the common clinical context of coexistent therapy is particularly unclear. Whether thymectomy reduces the need for immunosuppression has never been rigorously studied. In this paper, we describe the development of a multicenter, international trial to determine whether extended transsternal (XTS) thymectomy reduces corticosteroid requirements for patients with generalized acetylcholine receptor (AChR) antibody-positive nonthymomatous MG.

METHODS

Formal planning for the study began in October 2000 under the direction of John Newsom-Davis, who had assembled a group of interested investigators. The initial discussion took place in Boston during that year's annual meeting of the American Neurological Association. Three more investigator meetings were held in 2001, in Philadelphia, London, and Chicago. Based on feedback from these meetings, the protocol underwent several modifications. Further revisions to the study plan were made in response to peer reviews of grant applications to the Medical Research Council of the United Kingdom and the National Institutes of Health in 2001, and following a March 2002 meeting with the clinical trials section of the National Institute of Neurological Disorders and Stroke.

There is some evidence to support the view that the more aggressive the thymic resection, the better the results.[3] The XTS approach was selected for this study because it provides the greatest resection with low morbidity and limited risk of nerve injury. This approach is already in use at all centers participating in this study, and the surgeons enlisted are experienced in the method.

Sample size calculations were based on the primary outcome measure for the trial, the mean area under the dose-time curve (AUDTC) for prednisone at 2 years. The investigators formed a consensus that a reduction by thymectomy of prednisone dose requirements by 30% or more would provide justification for recommending the procedure. That higher doses of corticosteroids are more likely to produce adverse effects is generally understood.[6] A similar outcome measure was used in a recent placebo-controlled trial comparing prednisolone plus azathioprine versus prednisolone alone.[7] The sample size calculation assumes a two-group comparison of the treatment means, with the distribution of the areas assumed to be adequately

TABLE 1. Study eligibility criteria

Inclusion criteria	Exclusion criteria
(1) Onset of generalized MG within the last 3 years.	(1) Ocular MG without generalized weakness or mild generalized weakness that would not require corticosteroids (MGFA class I and some class II patients).[10]
(2) Age 18–60 years. (Thymectomy is not regularly performed in nonthymomatous MG patients over 60 years of age, and the thymus is often atrophic in these patients.)	(2) Myasthenic weakness requiring intubation (MGFA class V)[10] in the prior month.
(3) Positive serum anti-AChR binding antibodies (specifically, AChR antibody ≥ 1.0 nmol/L) within the previous 3 months.	(3) Immunosuppressive therapy other than corticosteroids in the preceding year.
(4) Clinical grade of class II–IV using the MGFA classification[10] who in routine practice would require corticosteroids and/or thymectomy to manage their disease.	(4) Medically unfit for thymectomy.
	(5) Chest CT or MRI evidence of thymoma.
	(6) Pregnancy or lactation.
	(7) Unwillingness to use contraception.

normal. Also assumed is a dropout rate of no more than 20% at year 2. On this basis, for 80% power to obtain a significant result at the 5% level, if the true difference between the treatment effects on the AUDTC at 2 years is 30% of the baseline mean, the trial requires 55 subjects in the surgical and nonsurgical arms, or 110 total. For 90% power, 148 patients would be needed.

Preliminary data regarding patient recruitment were compiled from chart and database reviews at the individual centers. Analyses (*t* test) of the Quantitative MG score (QMG)[8] and MG Activities-of-Daily-Living Profile (MG-ADL)[9] as they relate to clinical MG status were performed on a population of 85 patients from UT Southwestern (Dallas, TX).

RESULTS

Plan of Study

The proposed study is a single-blinded, randomized, controlled trial to determine whether XTS thymectomy confers added benefits to treatment with corticosteroid therapy alone in nonthymomatous generalized MG. The study includes over 40 MG centers in North America, South America, Europe, and South Africa. Inclusion and exclusion criteria are presented in TABLE 1. The study design is outlined in FIGURE 1.

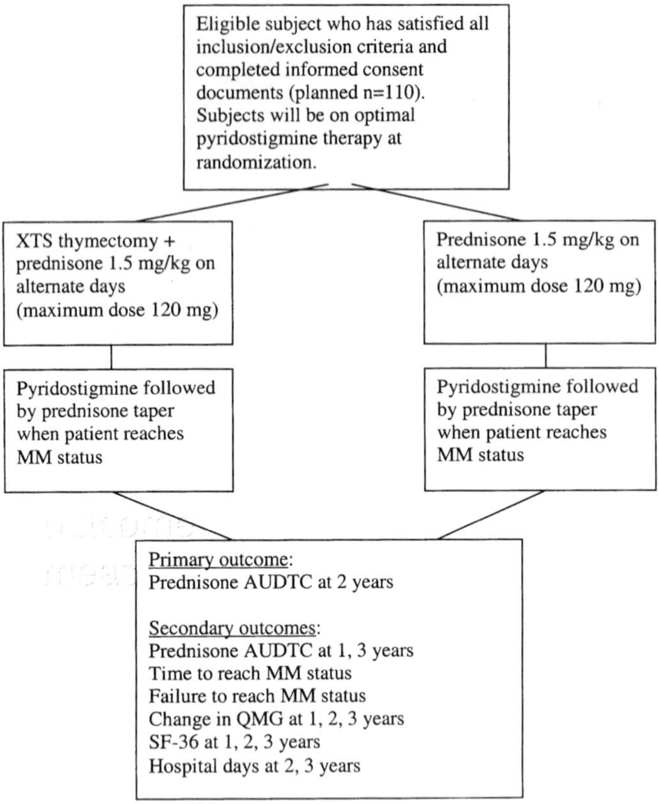

Eligible subject who has satisfied all inclusion/exclusion criteria and completed informed consent documents (planned n=110). Subjects will be on optimal pyridostigmine therapy at randomization.
XTS thymectomy + prednisone 1.5 mg/kg on alternate days (maximum dose 120 mg)
Prednisone 1.5 mg/kg on alternate days (maximum dose 120 mg)
Pyridostigmine followed by prednisone taper when patient reaches MM status
Pyridostigmine followed by prednisone taper when patient reaches MM status
Primary outcome:
Prednisone AUDTC at 2 years
Secondary outcomes:
Prednisone AUDTC at 1, 3 years
Time to reach MM status
Failure to reach MM status
Change in QMG at 1, 2, 3 years
SF-36 at 1, 2, 3 years
Hospital days at 2, 3 years

FIGURE 1. Flow diagram of the study plan.

A brief summary of the study plan follows. Patients will be on optimal oral anticholinesterase treatment at randomization. The trial treatment will begin on day 0, which will be within 30 days of randomization. Thymectomy will be performed on day 1. XTS thymectomy will be the surgical procedure used at all centers. Both groups will receive alternate-day prednisone (or prednisolone) beginning on day 0 according to a set protocol. The initial target dose is 1.5 mg/kg or 120 mg on alternate days, whichever is lower. Patients will be evaluated by an unblinded clinical manager (CM) at months 1 and 2 because blinding in the immediate postoperative period is not feasible. From month 3 onwards, the patient will be evaluated by a blinded CM who is masked as to whether the patient underwent thymectomy or not. The blinded CM will be responsible for all medication adjustments according to the protocol. Unblinded research personnel will ensure that patients are appropriately clothed with full-length shirts/tops so as not to unmask the blinded CM regarding their surgical status. Patients will be instructed prior to each blinded encounter not to reveal whether they underwent thymectomy to the blinded CM. Patients will be followed for 3 years.

TABLE 2. Schedule of patient evaluations

	Year 1									Years 2 and 3							
	R	D0	M1[a]	M2[a]	M3	M4	M6	M9	M12	M15	M18	M21	M24	M27	M30	M33	M36
Clinical assess-ment	+	+	+	+	+	+	+	+	+	+	+	+	+	+	+	+	+
QMG/ MG-ADL		+	+	+	+	+	+	+	+	+	+	+	+	+	+	+	+
Adverse events			+	+	+	+	+	+	+	+	+	+	+	+	+	+	+
Blood sample[b]		+			+		+		+		+		+		+		+
SF 36		+			+		+	+	+				+				+

NOTE—R: randomization day; D0: day 0 (initiation of the trial treatment protocol); M: month. Thymectomy is on day 1.

[a]Assessments by unblinded CM. All others to be performed by blinded CM.

[b]Blood and serum sample for AChR antibody assay and other immunological studies.

Clinic evaluations (TABLE 2) will be aimed at determining whether the patient has reached minimal manifestation (MM) status, defined as no symptoms or functional limitations from MG.[10] The QMG[8] will be employed to provide objective support for MM status. A QMG ≤ 13 will be required for a patient to satisfy MM status.

Once a patient is judged to have reached MM status, the daily dose of anticholinesterase medication will be withdrawn at a rate of 60 mg per week. This will be followed by a scheduled reduction of prednisone at a rate of 10 mg per month to a dose of 30 mg on alternate days, and then by 5 mg per month. A defined schedule for dose increments is in place should MM status not be maintained. Patients failing to enter MM status by the end of year 1 or who are experiencing intolerable side effects from prednisone will receive azathioprine at a dose of 2.5 mg/kg. Standards for laboratory monitoring are included in the protocol, and adverse events will be assessed at every clinic evaluation (TABLE 1).

The trial includes several management options for patients who are treatment failures: (1) patients intolerant of azathioprine will be offered cyclosporine; (2) plasma exchange or intravenous gamma globulin can be administered when clinically indicated in the period between randomization and day 0, but may not be used to maintain MM status—after initial MM status is achieved, plasma exchange or intravenous gamma globulin are permitted to control serious, life-threatening MG exacerbations; and (3) a late thymectomy after 2 years is an option for nonsurgical patients who continue to have substantial weakness or are unable to tolerate full implementation of the protocol because of adverse events.

Major Revisions to the Protocol

The current protocol addresses several concerns raised in peer reviews of grant applications to federal funding agencies in North America and Europe. Major changes to the study plan include (1) the introduction of a blinded CM to reduce bias in medication dose adjustments, on which the primary outcome is based; (2) moving the primary outcome measure from year 1 to year 2 to address concerns on the time it takes for benefits from thymectomy to become evident; (3) elimination of azathioprine in the first 12 months to reduce potential risks from multiple concomitant immunosuppressive agents; (4) specification that enrollment is open only to those Myasthenia Gravis Foundation of America (MGFA) class II–IV patients who in routine practice would be managed with corticosteroids and/or thymectomy, to ensure that subjects with milder disease will not be subjected to these treatments' risks; (5) the introduction of a maximum QMG score to provide some degree of objectivity to the MM status, a declaration that is largely based on clinical impression; and (6) the requirement that all patients receive prednisone on an alternate-day schedule. In prior versions of the protocol, either daily or alternate-day regimens were permitted, per investigator preference, as long as the total dose over 2 days was equivalent.

Relating QMG to MM Status

Initial QMG and MG-ADL encounters in 85 MG patients were analyzed. The mean QMG score for patients not in MM status was 12.07 (SD: 4.38) and for those in MM status was 6.12 (SD: 3.85). The mean MG-ADL score for patients not in MM status was 7.25 (SD: 4.28) and for those in MM status was 3.92 (SD: 2.40). Although these differences were statistically significant for both the QMG ($p < 0.0001$) and MG-ADL ($p < 0.0005$), considerable overlap existed in the MM status and non-MM status categories. In another strategy, if all 13 items on the QMG were scored 0 (normal) or 1 (mild impairment), patients were almost always in MM status. Specificity using this methodology was high—no worse than 83.8% and as high as 98.15%. However, the sensitivity was low, with confidence limits between 38.7% and 78.9%. Thus, many patients in MM status would be missed with this strategy. Of 25 encounters satisfying MM status, the highest QMG score was 13. As a result, to provide some objectivity to the MM status classification, a QMG score ≤ 13 will be required.

Patient Recruitment

Preliminary data indicate that it is essential to enlist many centers to enroll an adequate study sample in a reasonable amount of time. The mean number of eligible patients encountered at each center on an annual basis is approximately 5 (36 centers responding). For a study with 40 active centers, it is estimated that 110 MGFA class II, 92 MGFA class III, and 8 MGFA class IV subjects will be encountered annually.

A small sample of eligible patients was surveyed at UT Southwestern to determine whether patients would be willing to enroll in a randomized study of thymectomy. Consent documents approved by the local institutional review board were included in the survey. Three of 4 eligible subjects who had been surveyed to this point would hypothetically agree to enter the study.

Informal surveys of 86 patients at other centers indicate that one-half to two-thirds of subjects would potentially enroll. These results suggest that recruitment of subjects into a randomized thymectomy study is feasible, but that an 18- to 24-month period will likely be necessary to recruit an adequate population.

CONCLUSIONS

We have summarized the development of a randomized, single-blinded, controlled study of XTS thymectomy in nonthymomatous MG patients receiving immunosuppressive therapy. Revisions to the protocol reflect majority opinions generated by a large group of investigators with expertise in MG management and address concerns raised by study section reviews of grant proposals. There is considerable enthusiasm to perform a randomized, controlled study of thymectomy in this clinical setting, on the basis of the many investigators who are participating and on the feedback received from federal granting agencies. Planning and organizational support has already been received from the Muscular Dystrophy Association and Myasthenia Gravis Foundation of America. Recruitment of MG patients into a randomized trial of thymectomy appears feasible, although many centers are required to recruit an adequate population. The trial leadership is finalizing a grant resubmission to the National Institutes of Health for full funding of the trial.

It is of historical interest that Blalock *et al.*[11] expressed caution in the first report of thymectomy as intended therapy in MG. They wrote, "We wish to emphasize again the absence of conclusive proof that the improvement noted in our patient is due to the removal of the tumor from the thymic region." While thymectomy for essentially all patients with thymoma is not debated, questions persist on many fronts regarding the therapeutic role of thymectomy in MG. The objective of the proposed trial is to begin addressing some of these lingering questions in a scenario that commonly confronts clinicians who care for patients with MG.

ACKNOWLEDGMENTS

This work was supported by a Neuromuscular Disease Research Grant from the Muscular Dystrophy Association and funding from the Myasthenia Gravis Foundation of America.

REFERENCES

1. GRONSETH, G.S. & R.J. BAROHN. 2000. Thymectomy for non-thymomatous autoimmune myasthenia gravis (an evidence-based review). Neurology **55:** 7–15.
2. LANSKA, D.J. 1990. Indications for thymectomy in myasthenia gravis. Neurology **40:** 1828–1829.
3. JARETZKI, A., III. 1997. Thymectomy for myasthenia gravis: analysis of the controversies regarding technique and results. Neurology **48**(suppl. 5)**:** S52–S63.
4. MCQUILLEN, M.P. & M.G. LEONE. 1977. A treatment carol: thymectomy revisited. Neurology **27:** 1103–1106.
5. MASAOKA, A. & M. MONDEN. 1981. Comparison of the results of transsternal simple, transcervical simple, and extended thymectomy. Ann. N.Y. Acad. Sci. **377:** 755–765.
6. BOWYER, S., M. LAMOTHE & J. HOLLISTER. 1985. Steroid myopathy: incidence and detection in a population with asthma. J. Allergy Clin. Immunol. **76:** 234–242.

7. PALACE, J., J. NEWSOM-DAVIS & B. LECKY. 1998. A randomized double-blind trial of prednisolone alone or with azathioprine in myasthenia gravis. Neurology **50:** 1778–1783.
8. BAROHN, R.J., D. MCINTIRE, L. HERBELIN *et al.* 1998. Reliability testing of the Quantitative Myasthenia Gravis Score. Ann. N.Y. Acad. Sci. **841:** 769–772.
9. WOLFE, G.I., L. HERBELIN, S.P. NATIONS *et al.* 1999. Myasthenia gravis activities of daily living profile. Neurology **52:** 1487–1489.
10. JARETZKI, A., III, R.J. BAROHN, R.M. ERNSTOFF *et al.* FOR THE MEDICAL SCIENTIFIC ADVISORY BOARD OF THE MYASTHENIA GRAVIS FOUNDATION OF AMERICA. 2000. Myasthenia gravis: recommendations for clinical research standards. Neurology **55:** 16–23.
11. BLALOCK, A., M.F. MASON, H.J. MORGAN & S.S. RIVEN. 1939. Myasthenia gravis and tumors of the thymic region: report of a case in which the tumor was removed. Ann. Surg. **110:** 544–561.

Thymectomy and Antimuscle Antibodies in Nonthymomatous Myasthenia Gravis

FREDRIK ROMI,[a] NILS E. GILHUS,[a] JAN E. VARHAUG,[b] ANDREAS MYKING,[c] GEIR O. SKEIE,[a] AND JOHAN A. AARLI[a]

Departments of [a]Neurology, [b]Surgery, and [c]Pathology, Haukeland University Hospital, N-5021 Bergen, Norway

ABSTRACT: The clinical effect of thymectomy in early- and late-onset myasthenia gravis (MG) and the correlation to MG severity, pharmacological treatment, and antimuscle antibodies were examined in two series of consecutive acetylcholine receptor (AChR) antibody-positive nonthymoma MG patients. The results indicate a benefit of thymectomy in early-onset MG, but no obvious clinical benefit in late-onset MG. The presence of muscle autoantibodies did not influence the outcome of thymectomy in early-onset MG. In late-onset MG, improvement is least likely in patients with titin and/or RyR antibodies. Thymectomy should always be considered shortly after MG onset in early-onset MG patients and might only be considered in late-onset patients who have early-onset-like immunological characteristics.

KEYWORDS: thymectomy; myasthenia gravis; muscle autoantibodies

INTRODUCTION

Thymectomy was introduced as a treatment for myasthenia gravis (MG) in the 1950s. Although no randomized controlled studies exist, it is widely carried out for MG patients.

There is clinical support for postthymectomy improvement in younger MG patients, but the role of thymectomy in early-onset MG as a well-defined subgroup is not completely elucidated. The evidence for a positive effect of thymectomy in late-onset MG is even more equivocal.[1,2] Age alone should not be the most critical factor for the outcome after thymectomy. Pathogenic differences in the various MG subgroups are probably much more important. Nonacetylcholine receptor (AChR) muscle autoantibodies, against titin[3] and ryanodine receptor (RyR),[4] are mainly found in sera from patients with thymoma or late-onset MG and very infrequently in early-onset MG.[5–7] They are more common in severe MG.[8–10] It is unknown whether a possible therapeutic effect of thymectomy is linked to the presence of AChR or non-AChR muscle antibodies. Our objective in these two studies was therefore to study the clinical effect of thymectomy in well-defined early- and late-onset MG subgroups and to correlate the presence and concentration of circulating muscle

Address for correspondence: Fredrik Romi, Department of Neurology, Haukeland University Hospital, N-5021 Bergen, Norway. Voice: +47-55-97-50-69; fax: +47-55-97-51-65. fredrik.romi@haukeland.no

Ann. N.Y. Acad. Sci. 998: 481–490 (2003). **© 2003 New York Academy of Sciences.**
doi: 10.1196/annals.1254.062

autoantibodies against AChR, titin, and RyR to MG severity and pharmacological treatment in a long-term follow-up.

MATERIALS AND METHODS

Patients

Fifty-two early-onset (13 males, 39 females) and 43 late-onset (23 males, 20 females) consecutive MG patients treated at Haukeland University Hospital, Bergen, from 1951 to 2000, with available clinical data and blood samples, were included in the studies (TABLE 1). Patients with purely ocular MG, AChR antibody-negative patients, and MG patients with thymoma were not included.

Thirty-four out of the 52 early-onset and 21 out of the 43 late-onset MG patients were thymectomized, all with an open transsternal approach. Thymectomies were carried out soon after MG onset and diagnosis, when there was a poor clinical response to standard pharmacological treatment with acetylcholinesterase inhibitors, and no contraindications to surgery. No patients were treated with corticosteroids or azathioprine until 3 months after thymectomy. Thymectomized and nonthymectomized patients were treated along the same principles concerning pharmacological immunosuppression. Corticosteroids were always used initially and were given on alternate days, usually by slowly increasing the dose to 60–80 mg initially and then with a gradual and slow reduction to 20 mg or lower. Azathioprine was introduced when long-term treatment was necessary.

Severity Assessment and Study Design

The clinical disease severity in all patients was scored annually starting from the onset year of MG. Severity assessment was done blindly for the muscle autoantibody results. Forty-five early-onset patients were assessed for 5 consecutive years, 40 for 10 consecutive years, 27 for 15 consecutive years, and 18 for 20 consecutive years after the year of MG onset. Forty-two late-onset MG patients were assessed for 2 consecutive years, 29 for 3 consecutive years, and 19 for 5 consecutive years after the year of MG onset.

For comparing patient groups, the severity of MG was graded using a modified Osserman's scale:[11,12] 0 = no MG symptoms; 1 = MG with purely ocular muscle weakness; 2 = MG with mild generalized weakness, without bulbar involvement; 3 = MG with mild generalized weakness, including bulbar involvement with dysarthria, dysphagia, and poor mastication; 4 = MG with moderate generalized weakness; 5 = MG with severe generalized, bulbar, and respiratory muscle weakness, or death caused by an MG-related complication.

Complete MG remission was defined as the disappearance of all myasthenic symptoms and without any ongoing treatment, and with persistence for at least 1 year (according to MGFA postintervention status classification).[13] MG pharmacological remission is defined as the disappearance of all myasthenic symptoms with ongoing immunosuppressive treatment and pyridostigmine.[13]

The severity of MG in thymectomized and nonthymectomized patients was compared by three different methods:

TABLE 1. Clinical and immunological data of early- and late-onset thymectomized (T) and nonthymectomized (NT) MG patients

	Early onset			Late onset		
	T	NT	Total	T	NT	Total
Number of patients	34	18	52	21	22	43
Male/female	9/25	4/14	13/39	10/11	10/12	20/23
Age at MG onset	25 (± 11)	27 (± 9)	26 (± 10)	63 (± 8)	69 (± 7)	66 (± 8)
Age at MG diagnosis	27 (± 11)	31 (± 7)	28 (± 10)	64 (± 7)	69 (± 8)	67 (± 8)
Age at thymectomy	32 (± 11)			64 (± 8)		
MG severity:						
At onset	2.7	2.2	2.2	2.9	2.6	2.7
At blood sampling	2	2.4	2.2	2.9	2.6	2.7
AChR antibody concentration	88.2 (± 190)	104 (± 187)	93.7 (± 187)	24.8 (± 64.1)	36.6 (± 59.3)	30.2 (± 61.2)
Titin antibodies:						
Number of positive	4	2	6	10	12	22
Mean titer	1200 (± 1347)	1000 (± 849)	1133 (± 1115)	8080 (± 7335)	6333 (± 9237)	7127 (± 7344)
RyR antibodies:						
Number of positive	0	0	0	5	1	6
Mean titer				2240 (± 2360)	3200	2400 (± 2147)

(1) The first method used a study design of the follow-up groups with the thymectomized and nonthymectomized patients in an open cohort frame.[14] Each patient was moved from the nonthymectomized to the thymectomized group when thymectomized. As thymectomies were carried out successively, the number of thymectomized patients increased gradually, while the number of nonthymectomized patients fell. This design minimized any expected bias due to the clinical differences between thymectomized and nonthymectomized patients since each patient served as a nonthymectomized control before thymectomy. It also allowed a clear illustration of the effect of thymectomy on MG severity in the cohort of MG patients as they were thymectomized.

(2) The second method used a study design of the follow-up groups with the thymectomized and nonthymectomized patients in a closed cohort frame.[14] All patients who underwent thymectomy during the study were compared to those who did not undergo thymectomy. With this design, the number of patients in the two groups remained constant during each of the three follow-up periods, while the number of thymectomies increased yearly. This design gave very similar results to the first study design, and the results obtained by this study design are thus not illustrated by figures.

(3) The severity of MG in the thymectomized patients was also assessed and compared at MG onset, immediately before thymectomy, and yearly after thymectomy. To evaluate the clinical outcome of thymectomy in the individual patient, MG severity was also assessed using the MGFA clinical classification.[13]

To study the impact of AChR antibody concentration on the outcome of thymectomy, the thymectomized patients were divided into two groups: those with AChR antibody concentrations below and above the median AChR antibody concentration in thymectomized patients. The severity of MG was assessed and compared at MG onset, immediately before thymectomy, and after thymectomy in the high and low AChR antibody groups.

Muscle Autoantibody Assays

Sera

Sera were obtained from all patients. Control sera were collected from 24 healthy subjects comparable for age and sex.

AChR Antibodies

AChR antibodies were measured by a standard radioimmunoassay (RIA) method with human [^{125}I]AChR as the antigen and using AChR RRA kits (IBL, Hamburg, Germany).[7,15]

Titin Antibodies

Titin antibodies were detected by ELISA using purified titin fragment MGT-30 as the antigen.[9,10]

RyR Antibodies

RyR antibodies were detected by Western blot using pc2 Ry1 fusion protein as the antigen.[16,17] RyR antibodies were also assayed in ELISA using the same antigen, and antibody titers were obtained.[10,16]

Statistical Analysis

Mean AChR concentrations and mean titin and RyR antibody titers were compared using the *t* test for difference between population means. The proportions of titin and RyR antibody-positive patients were compared using the χ^2 test of independence with Yates' correction. MG severity was compared using the χ^2 test of independence, comparing the real numbers of patients in the various severity groups, and not mean severity; *p* values less than 0.05 were considered significant.

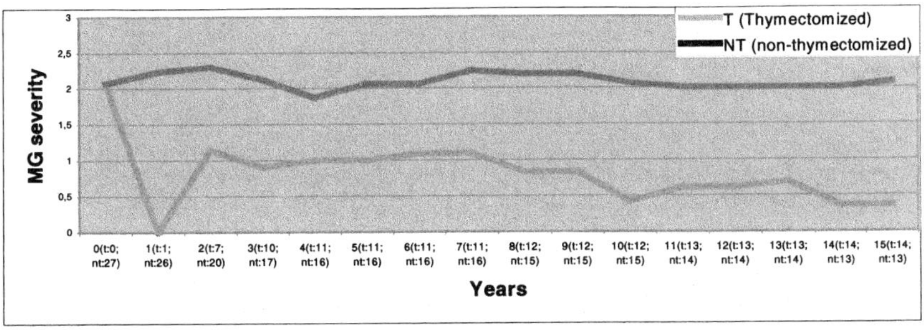

A

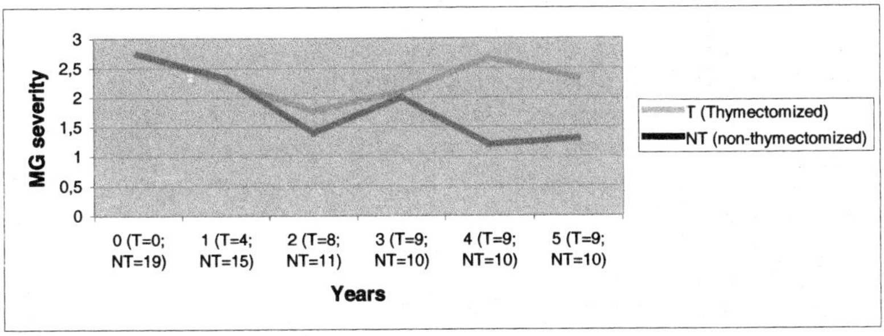

B

FIGURE 1. MG severity assessed yearly in thymectomized and nonthymectomized early-onset **(A)** and late-onset **(B)** MG patients in an open cohort design.

RESULTS

Clinical Data

MG Severity

Remission was seen in 21 thymectomized (17 complete and 4 pharmacological remissions) and 4 nonthymectomized (2 complete and 2 pharmacological remissions) early-onset MG patients. Remission was also seen in 6/11 titin and RyR antibody-negative thymectomized and in 2/10 nonthymectomized late-onset MG patients. No titin antibody-positive thymectomized late-onset MG patients had remission, but 5/12 nonthymectomized had remission.

Thymectomized early-onset MG patients had significantly less severe MG than nonthymectomized, showing from 2 years after MG onset ($p = 0.005$) (FIG. 1A). In late-onset MG, there was no difference in MG severity between thymectomized and nonthymectomized patients during the first years, but MG was more severe in the thymectomized group at 4 years after MG onset ($p = 0.001$) (FIG. 1B).

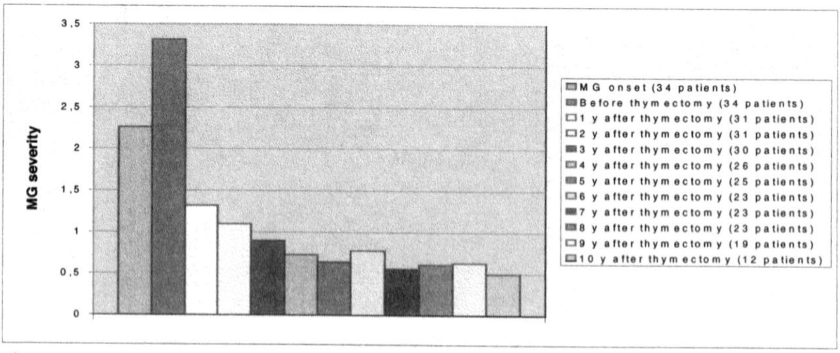

A

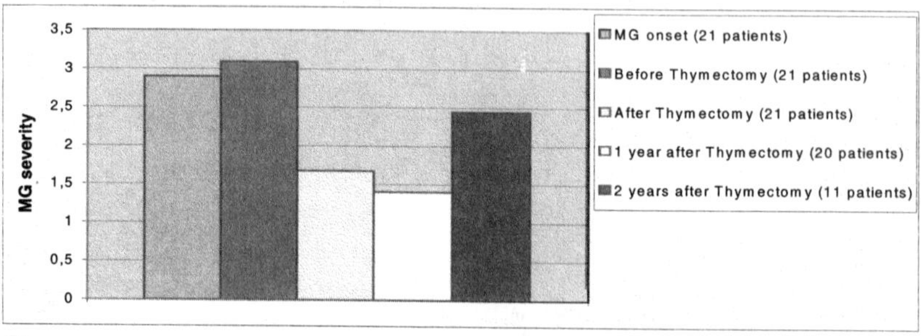

B

FIGURE 2. MG severity assessed at MG onset, before thymectomy, and yearly after thymectomy in thymectomized early-onset **(A)** and late-onset **(B)** MG patients. (The number of patients is diminishing each year because patients are entering the study at different time points, and the baseline is adjusted to the time point of thymectomy.)

Thymectomized early-onset MG patients had significant and long-lasting improvement already 1 year after thymectomy compared to before thymectomy and at MG onset ($p = 0.001$) (FIG. 2A). Thymectomized late-onset MG patients had only short-lasting improvement after thymectomy, which was probably mainly the effect of prethymectomy plasmapheresis treatment (FIG. 2B).

In early-onset MG, there was no MG-related mortality and only 1 patient died from non-MG-related disease during the observation period. Three thymectomized late-onset MG patients died from MG-related respiratory insufficiency; all had titin antibodies.

Pharmacological Treatment

All the MG patients were treated with pyridostigmine. Thymectomized patients received immunosuppressive pharmacological treatment when insufficient improvement was achieved by pyridostigmine alone after thymectomy. The number of patients treated with immunosuppressive drugs increased in early-onset MG from 2/12 thymectomized and 0/33 nonthymectomized at 2 years after MG onset to 5/14 thymectomized and 2/13 nonthymectomized at 15 years after MG onset. The number of patients treated with immunosuppressive drugs increased in late-onset MG from 5/12 thymectomized and 8/30 nonthymectomized at 1 year after MG onset to 8/9 thymectomized and 5/10 nonthymectomized at 5 years after MG onset.

From 3 years after MG onset, when most of the thymectomies were carried out, plasmapheresis treatment was given to 5 thymectomized and 2 nonthymectomized early-onset MG patients, and 3 thymectomized and 3 nonthymectomized late-onset MG patients, due to MG exacerbation.

Immunological Data

MG severity did not differ in patients with low or high AChR antibody concentration. No early-onset MG patients had RyR antibodies and only 6 had titin antibodies, while both antibodies were common in late-onset MG (TABLE 1). The occurrence of titin/RyR antibodies could not predict the outcome of thymectomy with statistical significance.

Thymus Histology

Histological examination of thymus tissue showed hyperplasia with germinal centers in all thymectomized early-onset MG patients, and atrophy in all thymectomized late-onset MG patients. Germinal centers were seen in 6 atrophic thymuses. Titin and RyR antibodies tended to occur more frequently in patients with atrophic thymus lacking germinal centers (8/16) than in those with germinal centers (2/6).

DISCUSSION

In early-onset MG, thymectomy gave a rapid, highly significant, and long-lasting amelioration of MG severity. The rate of remissions increased significantly after thymectomy, both in younger and in older early-onset MG patients. Late-onset MG patients improved initially after thymectomy, either as a result of the thymectomy itself or more probably due to the prior plasmapheresis; this improvement was transitory and no longer detectable at 2 years after thymectomy.

The outcome of thymectomy in late-onset MG was not statistically predictable from presence or concentration of non-AChR muscle antibodies. However, all 3 late-onset MG-related deaths were thymectomized patients with titin antibodies, and the 6 thymectomized late-onset MG patients with remission (4 complete and 2 pharmacological) were all titin antibody-negative. In early-onset MG, the low occurrence of titin and RyR antibodies makes their influence on thymectomy outcome insignificant. The concentration of AChR antibody early after MG onset had no impact on the outcome of thymectomy.

As early as 1949, Keynes suspected that the effect of thymectomy was less pronounced in older MG patients.[18] Simpson suggested that the earlier the onset of the disease, the better was the response to thymectomy.[19] Perlo *et al.* explicitly stated that it was unlikely that attempts to remove the thymus of elderly patients could be rewarding,[20] whereas Slater *et al.* concluded that even patients thymectomized after 40 years of age did benefit, but this without considering the age at MG onset.[21] In a more recent study, the outcome was less favorable in patients older than 45 years.[22] In a recent review paper, it is clearly stated that any benefit of thymectomy for late-onset MG patients remains to be established.[2] Our present results are comparable to those found in these earlier studies. However, in our opinion, the age at MG onset is a more important factor than the age at thymectomy.[7,10] It is the age at MG onset that reflects the pathogenesis of the disease.

There are a number of differences between early-onset and late-onset MG, apart from a different age of MG onset. While the concentration of AChR antibodies is highest in early-onset MG,[7] the occurrence of titin and RyR antibodies is highest in late-onset MG[5,6,10] and is accompanied by a more severe disease in late-onset MG.[8–10,23] Histologically, thymic hyperplasia is seen in thymuses from early-onset MG patients, while thymuses from late-onset MG patients are atrophic;[20,24–26] this clear distinction is confirmed by us in these studies. There is a correlation between thymic hyperplasia and the HLA genotype DR3, while the presence of titin antibodies in nonthymoma MG patients has been reported to correlate with DR7.[27,28] While thymectomy is an effective treatment in early-onset MG, it has no clinically evident effect in late-onset MG. On the contrary, while standard immunosuppressive therapy was needed in only 25% of early-onset patients in this study, the majority of both thymectomized and nonthymectomized late-onset MG patients responded equally well to this treatment. In a previous study, 70% of the late-onset MG patients received pharmacological immunosuppression.[29] The age at MG onset therefore seems to be one of the most important factors to take into consideration when treating a patient with nonthymoma MG.

These studies are retrospective, and the patients were not randomized to thymectomy versus nonthymectomy treatment. However, there was no significant difference in MG severity at the onset or year of diagnosis between thymectomized and nonthymectomized patients, and both groups were treated similarly with standard therapy except for prethymectomy plasmapheresis. One main reason for a large group of nonthymectomized MG patients is that we included patients with MG debut beginning from the 1950s, and our policy regarding thymectomy has changed during the last 50 years. The multiple design of the studies and the open cohort design also reduce possible bias. Our results strongly indicate a benefit of thymectomy in early-onset MG patients. The concentration of muscle autoantibodies does not influence the outcome of thymectomy in early-onset MG. While our results do not give any firm answers regarding the effect of thymectomy in late-onset MG in general, any potential benefits seem definitely to be less likely in cases with titin and/or RyR antibodies.

REFERENCES

1. Venuta, F., E.A. Rendina, T. De Giacomo *et al.* 1999. Thymectomy for myasthenia gravis: a 27-year experience. Eur. J. Cardiothorac. Surg. **15:** 621–625.
2. Gronseth, G.S. & R.J. Barohn. 2000. Practice parameter: thymectomy for autoimmune myasthenia gravis (an evidence-based review). Neurology **55:** 7–15.
3. Aarli, J.A., K. Stefansson, L.S.G. Marton & R.L. Wollmann. 1990. Patients with myasthenia gravis and thymoma have in their sera IgG autoantibodies against titin. Clin. Exp. Immunol. **82:** 284–288.
4. Mygland, Å., O-B. Tysnes, J.A. Aarli *et al.* 1992. Myasthenia gravis patients with a thymoma have antibodies against a high molecular weight protein in sarcoplasmatic reticulum. J. Neuroimmunol. **37:** 1–7.
5. Aarli, J.A., N.E. Gilhus & H. Hofstad. 1987. CA-antibody: an immunological marker of thymic neoplasia in myasthenia gravis? Acta Neurol. Scand. **63:** 55–57.
6. Voltz, R.D., W.C. Albrich, A. Nägele *et al.* 1997. Paraneoplastic myasthenia gravis: detection of anti-MGT30 (titin) antibodies predicts thymic epithelial tumor. Neurology **49:** 1454–1457.
7. Romi, F., G.O. Skeie, J.A. Aarli & N.E. Gilhus. 2000. Muscle autoantibodies in subgroups of myasthenia gravis patients. J. Neurol. **247:** 369–375.
8. Mygland, Å., J.A. Aarli, R. Matre & N.E. Gilhus. 1994. Ryanodine receptor antibodies related to severity of thymoma associated myasthenia gravis. J. Neurol. Neurosurg. Psychiatry **57:** 843–846.
9. Skeie, G.O., Å. Mygland, J.A. Aarli & N.E. Gilhus. 1995. Titin antibodies in patients with late onset myasthenia gravis: clinical correlations. Autoimmunity **20:** 99–104.
10. Romi, F., G.O. Skeie, J.A. Aarli & N.E. Gilhus. 2000. The severity of myasthenia gravis correlates with the serum concentration of titin and ryanodine receptor antibodies. Arch. Neurol. **57:** 1596–1600.
11. Osserman, K. & G. Genkins. 1981. Studies in myasthenia gravis: review of a twenty-year experience in over 1200 patients. Mt. Sinai J. Med. **38:** 497–537.
12. Detterbeck, F.C., W.W. Scott, J.F. Howard *et al.* 1996. One hundred consecutive thymectomies for myasthenia gravis. Ann. Thorac. Surg. **62:** 242–245.
13. Jaretzki, A., III, R.J. Barohn, R.M. Ernstoff *et al.* 2000. Myasthenia gravis: recommendations for clinical research standards. Task Force of the Medical Scientific Advisory Board of the Myasthenia Gravis Foundation of America. Neurology **55:** 16–23.
14. MacMahon, B. 1996. Cohort studies. *In* Epidemiology Principles and Methods, pp. 168–223. Little, Brown. Boston.
15. Lefvert, A.K., K. Bergstrøm, G. Matell *et al.* 1978. Determination of acetylcholine receptor antibody in myasthenia gravis—clinical usefulness and pathogenic implications. J. Neurol. Neurosurg. Psychiatry **41:** 394–403.
16. Skeie, G.O., Å. Mygland, S. Treves *et al.* 2003. Ryanodine receptor antibodies in myasthenia gravis: epitope mapping and effect on calcium release *in vitro*. Muscle Nerve **27:** 81–89.
17. Mygland, Å., O-B. Tysnes, R. Matre *et al.* 1992. Ryanodine receptor autoantibodies in myasthenia gravis patients with thymoma. Ann. Neurol. **32:** 589–591.
18. Keynes, G. 1949. The results of thymectomy in myasthenia gravis. Br. Med. J. **2:** 611–616.
19. Simpson, J.A. 1958. An evaluation of thymectomy in myasthenia gravis. Brain **81:** 112–144.

20. PERLO, V.P., B. ARNASON & B. CASTLEMAN. 1975. The thymus gland in elderly patients with myasthenia gravis. Neurology **25:** 294–295.
21. SLATER, G., A.E. PAPATESTAS, G. GENKINS *et al.* 1978. Thymectomy in patients more than forty years of age with myasthenia gravis. Surg. Gynecol. Obstet. **146:** 54–56.
22. FRIST, W.H., S. THIRUMALAI, C.B. DOEHRING *et al.* 1994. Thymectomy for the myasthenia gravis patient: factors influencing outcome. Ann. Thorac. Surg. **57:** 334–338.
23. SKEIE, G.O., E. BARTOCCIONI, A. EVOLI *et al.* 1996. Ryanodine receptor antibodies are associated with severe myasthenia gravis. Eur. J. Neurol. **3:** 136–140.
24. MÜLLER-HERMELINK, H.K., A. MARX & T. KIRCHNER. 1993. The pathological basis of thymoma associated myasthenia gravis. Ann. N.Y. Acad. Sci. **681:** 56–65.
25. WILLCOX, N. & A. VINCENT. 1988. Myasthenia gravis as an example of organ specific autoimmune disease. *In* B Lymphocytes in Human Disease, pp. 469–506. Oxford University Press. Oxford.
26. MYKING, A.O., G.O. SKEIE, J.E. VARHAUG *et al.* 1998. The histomorphology of the thymus in late onset, non-thymoma myasthenia gravis. Eur. J. Neurol. **5:** 401–405.
27. GIRAUD, M., G. BEAURAIN, A.M. YAMAMOTO *et al.* 2001. Linkage of HLA to myasthenia gravis and genetic heterogeneity depending on anti-titin antibodies. Neurology **57:** 1555–1560.
28. YAMAMOTO, A.M., P. GAJDOS, B. EYMARD *et al.* 2001. Anti-titin antibodies in myasthenia gravis: tight association with thymoma and heterogeneity of nonthymoma patients. Arch. Neurol. **58:** 885–890.
29. SLESAK, G., A. MELMS, F. GERNETH *et al.* 1998. Late-onset myasthenia gravis: follow-up of 113 patients diagnosed after age 60. Ann. N.Y. Acad. Sci. **841:** 777–780.

Prognostic Factors of Thymectomy in Patients with Myasthenia Gravis

A Cohort of 132 Patients

JOSÉ FRANCISCO TÉLLEZ-ZENTENO,[a] JOSE MARÍA REMES-TROCHE,[a] GUILLERMO GARCÍA-RAMOS,[a] BRUNO ESTAÑOL,[a] AND JUAN GARDUÑO-ESPINOZA[b]

[a]*Department of Neurology, Instituto Nacional de Ciencias Médicas y Nutrición, "Salvador Zubirán", Delegación Tlalpan, Mexico*

[b]*Medical Investigation Unit in Clinical Epidemiology, National Institute of Social Security, "Centro Médico Nacional Siglo XXI", Mexico City, Mexico*

KEYWORDS: myasthenia gravis; prognosis; age; response; thymectomy; steroids; pyridostigmine; thymic atrophy; nested case-control study

Our objective was to identify the response to thymectomy and the factors associated with a poor response. We used a nested case-control study, and the study units were 132 patients with the established diagnosis of myasthenia gravis who had a thymectomy between 1987 and 1997, and who had at least three years of follow-up. In order to assess the response to thymectomy, the following two points were taken into account before and after the thymectomy: (i) the dose of pyridostigmine and other drugs (steroids, azathioprine) and (ii) the Osserman classification. The patients were divided into four groups: (1) patients in remission, (2) patients experiencing improvement, (3) patients with no change, and (4) patients who worsened before thymectomy. The results showed that 91 patients had a good response (69%) and that 41 patients had a poor response (31%). The response by groups was as follows: 50 patients were found in remission, 41 had improvement, 34 had no change, and 7 got worse. The most important variables associated with poor prognosis were being more than 60 years old (OR 4.6; CI 1.11–20.32; $p < 0.01$), having Osserman I (OR 4.97; CI 1.02–26.83; $p < 0.01$), having thymoma (OR 3.51; CI 0.43–31.5; $p < 0.15$), having thymic atrophy (OR 2.19; CI 0.93–5.16; $p < 0.04$), and the use of steroids before the

Address for correspondence: José Francisco Téllez-Zenteno, Department of Neurology, Instituto Nacional de Ciencias Médicas y Nutrición, "Salvador Zubirán", Vasco de Quiroga No. 15, Colonia Sección XVI, Delegación Tlalpan, Mexico, D.F. Fax: +52-5-6430741.
jftellez@quetzal.innsz.mx

**Ann. N.Y. Acad. Sci. 998: 491–493 (2003). © 2003 New York Academy of Sciences.
doi: 10.1196/annals.1254.063**

thymectomy (OR 2.26; CI 0.99–5.18; $p < 0.03$). We conclude the following: The response to thymectomy was high (69%). The variables that had the most prognostic importance were age and the Osserman stage. Other variables were high doses of pyridostigmine and the use of steroids before the surgery, the duration of the disease between diagnosis and the surgical procedure, and the presence of thymic atrophy and thymoma. (See TABLES 1 and 2.)[1–9]

TABLE 1. Factors associated with poor response of the thymectomy

	OR	CI	*p*
Gender			
Female	1.15	0.44–2.95	0.75
Age			
>60 years old	4.60	1.11–20.32	0.01
Evolution (from the beginning of symptoms until thymectomy)			
>3 years of evolution	2.07	0.79–5.39	0.09
>4 years of evolution	2.53	0.89–7.55	0.02
Evolution (since the diagnosis until thymectomy)			
>3 years of evolution	2.02	0.69–5.90	0.15
>4 years of evolution	2.53	0.83–7.70	0.06
Osserman			
I	4.97	1.02–26.83	0.01
IIA	0.61	0.26–1.41	0.20
IIB	0.83	0.37–1.85	0.61
Dose of Mestinon			
>240	2.79	1.12–7.13	0.01
>360	3.33	1.23–9.15	0.007
Previous thymectomy			
Yes	4.62	0.31–132.7	0.17
Use of steroids before the surgery			
Yes	2.26	0.99–5.18	0.03
Type of thymectomy			
Transcervical	1.13	0.45–2.84	0.77
Use of plasmapheresis after surgery			
Yes	3.46	2.64–4.54	0.002
Pathology findings			
Hyperplasia	0.30	0.13–0.71	0.002
Thymoma	3.51	0.45–31.5	0.15
Thymic atrophy	2.19	0.93–5.16	0.04

TABLE 2. Response to thymectomy

	n	%
General response to thymectomy (*n* = 132)		
Good response	91	69%
Poor response	41	31%
Response by groups (*n* = 132)		
Remission	50	38%
Improvement	41	31%
No change	34	26%
Worsening	7	5%

REFERENCES

1. TÉLLEZ-ZENTENO, J.F., L.E. MORALES BUENROSTRO & A. TORRE DELGADILLO. 2000. Patogénesis de la miastenia gravis. Rev. Invest. Clin. **52:** 78–83.
2. DRACHMAN, D. 1994. Myasthenia gravis. N. Engl. J. Med. **330:** 1797–1810.
3. HATTON, P., J. DIEHL, B. DALY *et al.* 1988. Transsternal radical thymectomy for myasthenia gravis; a 15-year review. Ann. Thorac. Surg. **47:** 438–440.
4. BUSCH, C., A. MACHENS, U. PICHLMEIER *et al.* 1996. Long-term outcome and quality of life after thymectomy for myasthenia gravis. Ann. Surg. **224:** 225–232.
5. FRIST, W., S. THIRUMALAI, C. DOEHRING *et al.* 1991. Thymectomy for the myasthenia gravis patient: factors influencing outcome. J. Neurol. Neurosurg. Psychiatry **54:** 406–411.
6. DEFILIPPI, V., D. RICHMAN & M. FERGUSON. 1994. Transcervical thymectomy for myasthenia gravis. Ann. Thorac. Surg. **57:** 194–197.
7. JARETZKI, A., A. PENN, D. YOUNGER *et al.* 1988. Maximal thymectomy for myasthenia gravis. J. Thorac. Cardiovasc. Surg. **95:** 747–757.
8. DURRELI, L., G. MAGGI, C. CASADIO *et al.* 1991. Actuarial analysis of the occurrence of remissions following thymectomy for myasthenia gravis in 400 patients. J. Neurol. Neurosurg. Psychiatry **54:** 406–411.
9. OOSTERHUIS, H. 1989. The natural course of myasthenia gravis: a long term follow up study. J. Neurol. Neurosurg. Psychiatry **52:** 1121–1127.

Mycophenolate Mofetil for Myasthenia Gravis

A Double-Blind, Placebo-Controlled Pilot Study

MATTHEW N. MERIGGIOLI, JULIE ROWIN, JUDITH G. RICHMAN, AND SUE LEURGANS

Department of Neurological Sciences, Rush University and Rush–Presbyterian–St. Luke's Medical Center, Chicago, Illinois 60612, USA

ABSTRACT: Mycophenolate mofetil (MM) is an immunosuppressive agent developed and originally used to prevent acute rejection of solid-organ transplantation. There have been preliminary reports of its successful use in the treatment of autoimmune myasthenia gravis (MG). We conducted a double-blind, placebo-controlled pilot trial of MM in the treatment of suboptimally controlled, stable MG. Results of this pilot study are promising and suggestive of greater improvement in the patients who received MM compared to placebo.

KEYWORDS: myasthenia gravis; mycophenolate mofetil; quantitative myasthenia gravis score

INTRODUCTION

Mycophenolate mofetil (MM) is an immunosuppressive agent developed and originally used to prevent acute rejection of solid-organ transplantation. There have been preliminary reports of its successful use in the treatment of autoimmune myasthenia gravis (MG).[1–3] We conducted a double-blind, placebo-controlled pilot trial of MM in the treatment of suboptimally controlled, stable MG.

METHODS

Patients

Patients with autoimmune MG between the ages of 18 and 80, with or without prior thymectomy, were eligible for the study. The diagnosis of MG was made on the basis of the clinical presentation and confirmed either by positive acetylcholine-receptor-binding antibodies (AChRAbs) or by electrodiagnostic testing demonstrating a primary defect in neuromuscular transmission [abnormal single-fiber electromyography (SFEMG) in the setting of normal nerve conduction studies and conventional electromyography]. If patients had undergone thymectomy, the procedure

Address for correspondence: Matthew N. Meriggioli, M.D., Department of Neurological Sciences, Rush University, 1725 West Harrison Street, Suite 1106, Chicago, IL 60612. Voice: 312-942-4500; fax: 312-942-2380.
matthew_n_meriggioli@rush.edu

Ann. N.Y. Acad. Sci. 998: 494–499 (2003). © 2003 New York Academy of Sciences.
doi: 10.1196/annals.1254.064

must have been performed at least 12 months prior to entry into the study. Patients could be on concomitant immunotherapy with prednisone or cyclosporine. If on prednisone, the dose was required to be stable for a period of 4 weeks. If on cyclosporine, a stable dose for 3 months prior to entry was required. Patients on azathioprine were excluded. Plasmapheresis or intravenous immune globulin was prohibited during the study and for 1 month prior to entry into the study.

Patients who met the above criteria and had suboptimally controlled disease as defined by persistent daily symptoms of fatigable weakness involving ocular, bulbar, or extremity muscles were recruited for the study. We excluded patients with purely ocular disease (MGFA class I),[4] with severe respiratory or bulbar weakness (MGFA classes IVb and V),[4] and with a history of thymoma. Patients with severe concurrent medical or psychiatric illness and women who were pregnant or not practicing reliable birth control methods were also excluded.

Study Design

Stability of disease was assessed during a 1-month, pretreatment observation period. Quantitative myasthenia gravis (QMG) scores[5] were obtained at the beginning and end of this 1-month period. Patients whose QMG scores varied by more than 2 points were disqualified. The clinical evaluator was blinded to the patient's previous QMG scores. The baseline QMG score was defined as the average of the two scores obtained during the observation period. A QMG score greater than or equal to 5 was also required to be eligible to be randomized. The purpose of this requirement was to eliminate patients with very mild disease in whom measurement of a change in disease state would be difficult.

Other baseline assessments included vital signs, physical examination, manual muscle testing (MMT),[6] SFEMG, AChRAbs, serum chemistries, urinalysis (UA), and complete blood count (CBC). Female patients of childbearing age underwent pregnancy testing. Patients who qualified for the study were assigned to the treatment group (1 g MM twice daily) or placebo group by a random allocation system. Patients were seen and assessed monthly during a 5-month treatment period. QMG scores, MMT scores, CBC, chemistries, and UA were performed at all visits. All study procedures were performed in the morning, and patients were instructed to withhold their morning dose of pyridostigmine (if applicable) until after the testing was completed. AChRAb and SFEMG tests were performed only at baseline and at month 4 of the treatment period.

The study protocol was approved by the Rush University Institutional Review Board, and approved informed consent procedures were followed.

Measures of Efficacy

The primary measure of efficacy was the change in the QMG score compared to the baseline value. Secondary measures included the change in the MMT score, the change in the AChRAb titer, and the change in the magnitude of the SFEMG abnormalities. For all efficacy measures, the *change* was defined as baseline measurements minus measurements at the time of exit from the study. An intention-to-treat analysis was used.

Statistical Analysis

Data were summarized as percentages, means, or medians (AChRAbs) as appropriate. Wilcoxon rank-sum tests comparing the MM and placebo groups were conducted for quantitative measures. Qualitative characteristics were compared using Fisher's exact test. All tests were two-sided, and the significance level was set at $\alpha = 0.05$.

RESULTS

The results of the randomization process are illustrated in FIGURE 1. Eighteen patients were screened for entry into the study. Of these, 1 was disqualified because of a variation of greater than 2 QMG points during the observation period. Three were disqualified because of mild disease (QMGS $\leq$ 5). Fourteen patients were randomly assigned to receive either MM or placebo. One patient in the MM group developed worsening of her disease after 27 days on study drug. She was removed from the study, received appropriate therapy (plasmapheresis), and was classified as a treatment failure. One patient in the placebo group developed gross hematuria, subsequently found to be due to nephrolithiasis, and was withdrawn after 3 months of treatment. A single patient in the placebo group was disqualified after 3 months because of protocol violation. Baseline characteristics in the treatment and placebo groups are shown in TABLES 1 and 2.

Patients who received MM improved by an average of 2.86 QMG points, compared to 0.29 points for the placebo group ($p = 0.30$). The results of secondary measures of efficacy also revealed greater improvement in the MM group. The data

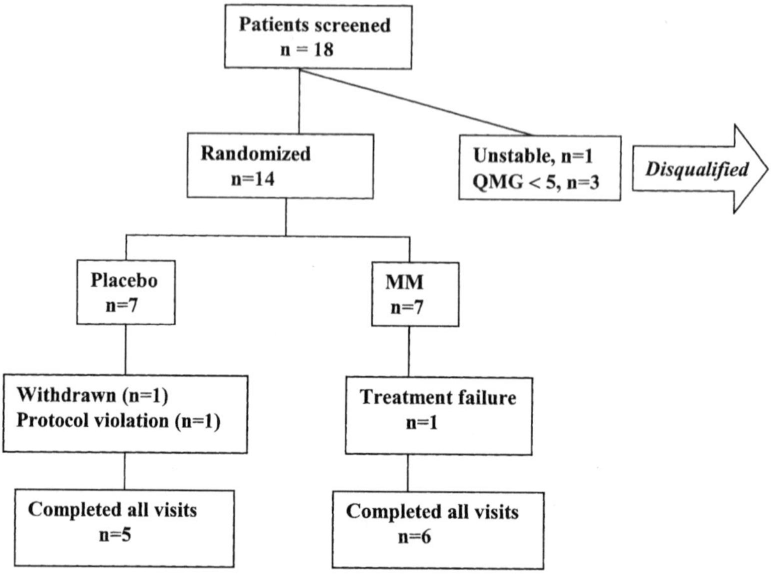

FIGURE 1. Trial randomization.

TABLE 1. Baseline characteristics

Characteristic	MM	Placebo	*p* value
Age (years)			
Mean	57.7	51.3	0.48
Range	39–74	23–74	
Sex	2M/5F	2M/5F	1.00
Duration of disease (months, group means)	107.9	118.9	0.95
Baseline QMG score (group means)	15.86	16.71	0.75
AChRAbs (group medians)	1.3	1.4	0.70
Thymectomy	3	5	0.59

TABLE 2. Baseline characteristics—disease severity and treatment

Characteristic	MM	Placebo
MGFA class		
2A	4	3
2B	0	0
3A	2	3
3B	1	1
Medications		
Prednisone	5	5
Cyclosporine	1	1
No immunosuppressants	2	2

for all 14 patients are shown in TABLE 3 and are summarized in TABLE 4. The difference in the SFEMG measure was statistically significant ($p = 0.030$) despite the small number of patients.

DISCUSSION

MM treatment resulted in greater improvement than that due to placebo on all four efficacy criteria in our pilot study in suboptimally controlled MG patients. The difference reached statistical significance only for the SFEMG measure of efficacy. The small sample size is the main limitation of our study and may explain the failure to reach statistically significant differences on the other efficacy measures.

Our data prompted several notable observations: (1) AChRAbs in 3 patients in the MM group converted from positive to negative (TABLE 3), compared to 0 in the placebo group ($p = 0.19$); (2) all 6 MM patients who had baseline and posttreatment SFEMG studies showed improvement in mean jitter values, compared to 1 of 5 in the placebo group ($p = 0.015$); and (3) while 3 patients in the MM group improved by 3 or more QMG points, 2 patients in the placebo group also demonstrated this level of improvement.

TABLE 3. Data table

Patient	Base QMG	Exit QMG	Base MMT	Exit MMT	Base AChRAbs	Exit AChRAbs	Base SFEMG	Exit SFEMG
MM								
1	12	9	5	3	1.3	0.0	50.2	39.4
2	26	24[a]	38	36[a]	0.0	–	45.5	–
3	7	7	5	5	4.1	4.9	56.8	51.1
4	14	12	18	15	1.1	0.0	107.9	99.6
5	15	9	16	4	2.6	0.0	76.4	46.0
6	18	11	12	7	56.0	14.5	97.6	78.8
7	19	19	40	38	0.0	0.0	66.4	48.2
Mean	*15.86*	*13.0*	*19.14*	*15.43*	*9.30*	*3.23*	*71.54*	*60.52*
Placebo								
8	14	23	27	41	12.9	12.4	87.7	88.8
9	17	18	28	26	1.2	1.5	44.9	–
10	15	15	15	14	1.4	1.3	59.9	43.9
11	19	17	24	21	0.0	0.0	43.7	41.4
12	22	22	41	41	0.9	1.1	118.9	–
13	13	10	16	12	9.9	6.7	82.5	118.8
14	17	10	10	8	4.4	3.7	52.4	53.4
Mean	*16.71*	*16.43*	*23.00*	*23.29*	*4.39*	*3.81*	*70.00*	*69.26*

[a]Treatment failure (see text).

TABLE 4. Summary of results for all efficacy criteria

	ΔQMG	ΔMMT	ΔAChRAbs, (nmol/L)	ΔSFEMG, mean MCD (μs)
MM	2.86	3.71	1.1	15.37
Placebo	0.29	–1.14	0.1	–4.02
p value	0.30	0.10	0.52	0.03

NOTE: Δ = mean change (baseline minus exit) for all except AChRAbs, which are medians. Wilcoxon rank-sum tests were used to determine *p* values.

There were no serious adverse events consistent with previous uncontrolled case series.[1–3] Diarrhea (2 patients), insomnia (1 patient), and urinary tract infections (2 patients) were side effects that occurred in the MM group and not in the placebo group. One patient with a history of diverticulosis in the MM group (patient 1) developed diverticulitis that was not believed to be treatment-related.

Considerations for future trials examining MM as a treatment for MG include the following: (1) existing information on MM in MG[1–3] would indicate that the onset of clinical benefit may occur anywhere from as soon as 3 weeks to as long as 9 months or more after starting treatment, suggesting that a longer treatment period may be necessary; (2) the optimal dose of MM for treatment of MG is not known, and options for dose adjustment should be considered in future trials; (3) monitoring of mycophenolic acid levels[7] may be helpful in determining appropriate dosing in individual patients; (4) the precise role of MM in the therapy of MG (i.e., steroid-sparing, initial immunotherapy) requires specific investigation.

CONCLUSIONS

The results of this pilot study are promising and suggestive of greater improvement in the patients who received MM compared to placebo. Larger scale, multicenter, randomized controlled clinical trials are necessary to confirm the efficacy of MM in the treatment of MG and to define its specific therapeutic role. Finally, in any therapeutic trial involving patients with MG, it is important to recognize the potential for spontaneous improvement as illustrated by 2 of our placebo patients. This emphasizes the need for randomized controlled clinical trials in assessing therapeutic interventions in this fluctuating disease.

ACKNOWLEDGMENTS

This work was supported in part by Roche Pharmaceuticals (Grant No. CEL 132) and by a grant from the Myasthenia Gravis Foundation of Illinois.

REFERENCES

1. Chaudhry, V., D.R. Cornblath, J.W. Griffin *et al.* 2001. Mycophenolate mofetil: a safe and promising immunosuppressant in neuromuscular diseases. Neurology **56:** 94–96.
2. Ciafaloni, E., J.M. Massey, B. Tucker-Lipscomb & D.B. Sanders. 2001. Mycophenolate mofetil for myasthenia gravis: an open-label pilot study. Neurology **56:** 97–99.
3. Cos, L., A.K. Mankodi, R. Tawil & C.A. Thornton. 2000. Neurology **54**(suppl. 3)**:** A137.
4. Jaretzki, A., R.J. Barohn, R.M. Ernstoff *et al.* 2000. Myasthenia gravis: recommendations for clinical research standards. Neurology **55:** 16–23.
5. Barohn, R.J., D. McIntire, L. Herbelin *et al.* 1998. Reliability testing of the quantitative myasthenia gravis score. Ann. N.Y. Acad. Sci. **841:** 769–772.
6. Sanders, D.B., B. Tucker-Lipscomb & J.M. Massey. 2003. A simple manual muscle test for myasthenia gravis: validation and comparison with the QMG score. This volume.
7. Mourad, M., P. Wallemacq, J. Konig *et al.* 2002. Therapeutic monitoring of mycophenolate mofetil in organ transplant recipients: is it necessary? Clin. Pharmacokinet. **41:** 319–327.

Lambert-Eaton Myasthenic Syndrome

Diagnosis and Treatment

DONALD B. SANDERS

Duke University Medical Center, Durham, North Carolina 27710, USA

ABSTRACT: A high index of suspicion is essential in arriving at the correct diagnosis of Lambert-Eaton myasthenic syndrome (LEMS). LEMS should be considered in the differential in any patient who has proximal weakness, reduced or absent muscle stretch reflexes, and dry mouth. Weakness predominates in hip and shoulder muscles, but may also affect ocular and oropharyngeal muscles to a lesser extent. The diagnosis is confirmed by demonstrating characteristic electromyographic findings—low-amplitude muscle responses that increase dramatically after activation. Most patients also have circulating antibodies to the voltage-gated calcium channel. Half the patients with LEMS have a malignancy, usually small-cell lung cancer. The diagnosis should trigger an intensive search for malignancy, especially in older patients with a history of smoking. Younger, nonsmoking patients are likely to have LEMS as part of a more general autoimmune state. Successful treatment of the underlying cancer leads to improvement in many patients. More than 85% of patients have clinically significant benefit from 3,4-diaminopyridine (DAP). In over half of these, the improvement is marked. If severe weakness persists despite DAP, immunotherapy should be considered. Plasma exchange and high-dose immunoglobulin induce transient improvement in many patients, but function rarely becomes normal. Combinations of prednisone, azathioprine, or cyclosporine have been used with variable success. Improvement, if any, occurs only after many months and requires chronic administration of immunosuppressive medications at significant doses. The long-term prognosis in LEMS is determined by the presence of cancer or other autoimmune disease.

KEYWORDS: Lambert-Eaton myasthenic syndrome; voltage-gated calcium channel antibodies; electromyography; aminopyridines; 3,4-diaminopyridine; guanidine

CLINICAL FEATURES

LEMS usually begins in mid to late life, although it has been reported rarely in children. In recent series, 53% of the patients are male.[1] Symptoms usually begin insidiously, and many patients go for months or years before the diagnosis is made. The major symptoms are weakness in the legs and generalized fatigue. The weak muscles frequently ache and may be tender. Oropharyngeal and ocular muscles are usually spared or only mildly affected. Although respiratory symptoms are probably

Address for correspondence: Donald B. Sanders, M.D., Duke University Medical Center, Box 3403, Durham, NC 27710. Voice: 919-684-6078; fax: 919-660-3853.
donald.sanders@duke.edu

**Ann. N.Y. Acad. Sci. 998: 500–508 (2003). © 2003 New York Academy of Sciences.
doi: 10.1196/annals.1254.065**

not more common than expected from underlying lung disease, breathing function is usually reduced, and occasional patients present with respiratory failure.[2]

Most patients have dry mouth, which frequently precedes other symptoms of LEMS, but many do not mention this unless specifically questioned. Many patients are also aware of an unpleasant metallic taste. Impotence is common in males, and other symptoms of autonomic dysfunction, such as postural hypotension, may also be seen. Pupils may be dilated and respond poorly to light.[3] Autonomic function tests are abnormal in most LEMS patients, even when there are no clinical signs of autonomic dysfunction.[4] These tests usually show evidence of sympathetic as well as parasympathetic dysfunction.[5–7] Because dry mouth and other autonomic symptoms are also common in cancer patients in general, they are not specific for LEMS.[8]

The weakness demonstrated on examination is usually relatively mild compared to the patient's complaints. Strength may improve after exercise and then weaken as activity is sustained, but this is not seen in all patients and is easily demonstrable in only about half. Edrophonium or pyridostigmine may improve strength, but this improvement is rarely as dramatic as the one seen in myasthenia gravis. Tendon reflexes are reduced or absent, but can frequently be brought out by having the patient briefly contract the appropriate muscle.[9] Potentiation of hypoactive tendon reflexes in this manner is virtually diagnostic of LEMS.

LEMS patients with underlying small-cell lung cancer (SCLC) may have other paraneoplastic syndromes: inappropriate ADH secretion, sensorimotor neuropathy, or cerebellar degeneration.[10]

Muscle biopsy in LEMS frequently shows type-II muscle fiber atrophy, as in disuse, which is not diagnostic.

Cancer is present when the disease begins or is found later in 40% of patients. SCLC is by far the most common underlying cancer, and smoking and age at onset are the major risk factors for this neoplasm. Lymphoproliferative malignancies, especially non-Hodgkin's lymphoma, are found in occasional LEMS patients. The association with other cancers has not been established. What is the likelihood that a patient with LEMS has an underlying cancer? If a tumor is not found within the first 2 years after LEMS symptom onset, then it is unlikely. In practical terms, this means that a patient less than age 50 at onset of LEMS symptoms with no known tumor after 2 years is unlikely to have an underlying cancer. However, a chronic smoker with LEMS beginning after age 50 almost certainly has an underlying lung cancer.

EPIDEMIOLOGY

Several factors impede accurate determination of the true incidence of LEMS: in patients with cancer, the symptoms of LEMS may erroneously be attributed to cachexia, peripheral neuropathy, or the effects of treatment. In patients without evident cancer, LEMS symptoms may be dismissed without explanation if little weakness is found on examination, or they may be attributed to myopathy, neuropathy, or myasthenia gravis. Considering all these factors, it is probable that most patients with LEMS are undiagnosed.

It has been estimated that up to 3% of patients with SCLC have LEMS,[8] which gives a LEMS prevalence of 5 per 1,000,000 in the United States. Since only half the patients with LEMS have a tumor, the total prevalence would be double this figure, or 1 per 100,000.

ELECTRODIAGNOSIS

The diagnosis of LEMS is confirmed by demonstrating characteristic abnormalities on electromyographic studies: the compound muscle action potentials (CMAPs) recorded with surface electrodes are small, often less than 10% of normal, and fall further with repetitive nerve stimulation at frequencies between 1 and 5 Hz. During stimulation at frequencies from 20 to 50 Hz, the CMAP increases in size and characteristically becomes at least twice the size of the initial response. A similar increase in CMAP size is seen immediately after the patient contracts the muscle maximally for 5 to 10 s. The electrodiagnostic abnormalities may be partially masked by low muscle temperature;[11] thus, the muscle should be warmed and rested for several minutes before testing.

The following statements regarding the electrodiagnosis of LEMS are based on our experience with 61 patients:[12]

(1) Almost all patients have a decrementing response to low-frequency nerve stimulation in at least one hand muscle. This finding is not specific for LEMS because it occurs typically in myasthenia gravis and rarely in some nerve and muscle diseases.
(2) The CMAP amplitude is low in most muscles tested. This is also a nonspecific finding, commonly seen in nerve or muscle disease.
(3) A reproducible postexercise increase in CMAP amplitude of at least 100% is considered to be typical of LEMS.[13] We found this degree of facilitation in at least one hand or foot muscle in about 90% of our LEMS patients. The amount of facilitation varies considerably among muscles, but is always greater in distal muscles. If facilitation is greater than 100% in most muscles tested or is greater than 400% in any muscle, the patient almost certainly has LEMS. If facilitation is less than 50% in all muscles tested, the patient still may have LEMS, especially if symptoms have been present for only a short time.

When LEMS is mild, the electrodiagnostic findings may resemble those of myasthenia gravis, with normal CMAP amplitudes, a decrementing response to repetitive nerve stimulation at low rates, and little facilitation. A helpful observation is that, in myasthenia gravis, the electromyographic findings are frequently less severe than the clinical findings would suggest, whereas the opposite is usually the case in LEMS.[14]

Conventional needle electromyography in LEMS demonstrates markedly unstable motor unit action potentials, which vary in shape during voluntary activation. This variability is a manifestation of abnormal neuromuscular transmission and can be quantified by single-fiber electromyography measurements of jitter. The jitter is markedly increased in LEMS, frequently out of proportion to the severity of weakness, and there is frequent impulse blocking. In many endplates, the jitter and blocking decrease as the firing rate increases.[15,16] However, this pattern is not seen in all endplates or in all patients with LEMS.[15,17]

CALCIUM CHANNEL ANTIBODIES

Human neuronal cell lines and SCLC cell lines both express voltage-gated calcium channels (VGCCs) that bind the Ω-conotoxin from the snail *Conus geographus*. (This toxin binds with high affinity to the P/Q form of VGCC, which is associated with neurotransmitter release.) Assays for antibodies to VGCCs have been developed using human neuroblastoma or SCLC cell lines as the source of VGCCs, which are labeled by binding to $[^{125}I]\Omega$-conotoxin. Immunoprecipitation of conotoxin-bound VGCC complexes has demonstrated antibodies in close to 100% of patients with LEMS who have primary lung cancer, and in over 90% of those without evident cancer.[18] Low titers of these antibodies are also found in non-LEMS patients with systemic lupus erythematosus or rheumatoid arthritis, conditions in which there are high levels of circulating immunoglobulins,[19] and in less than 5% of patients with myasthenia gravis.[18]

Because VGCC antibodies may disappear in patients receiving immunosuppressive therapy, the assay is most informative when performed before such treatment. Levels of VGCC antibodies do not correlate with disease severity among patients with LEMS, but the levels do fall in individual patients as the disease improves.[20]

Organ-specific autoantibodies (to thyroid, gastric parietal cells, or skeletal muscle) are found more frequently in LEMS patients without cancer than in a control population. Nonorgan-specific autoantibodies (antinuclear, antismooth muscle, antimitochondrial antibodies) are found more frequently in LEMS patients who have cancer than in those without cancer.[21]

PATHOPHYSIOLOGY

The physiology of neuromuscular transmission is studied by measuring the subsynaptic events at the neuromuscular junction with microelectrodes inserted into muscle fibers *in vitro*. Normally, single quanta of acetylcholine released from the motor nerve terminal produce localized depolarizations of the peri-endplate muscle membrane. The amplitude of these miniature endplate potentials reflects the size of each acetylcholine quantum, as well as the responsiveness of the postsynaptic muscle membrane to acetylcholine. Such studies demonstrate that miniature endplate potential amplitude is normal in LEMS muscle, but that the number of quanta released by each nerve depolarization is reduced from normal.[22]

IMMUNOPATHOLOGY

Active zone particles, which represent the VGCCs, are normally arranged in regular parallel arrays on the presynaptic muscle membrane. In LEMS patients and in mice injected with LEMS IgG, the active zone particles lose this regular pattern and become clustered and reduced in number.[23,24] Divalent IgG antibodies against the VGCCs cross-link the calcium channels, bringing them together and disrupting the parallel arrays. Ultimately, the active zone particles become clustered and reduced in number.

SCLC cells are of neuroectodermal origin, share several antigens with peripheral nervous system tissue, and contain high concentrations of VGCCs. Calcium influx into these cells is inhibited by LEMS IgG,[25] and the degree of suppression of calcium influx correlates with the severity of LEMS.[26] Antibodies to VGCC are found in the serum of most patients with LEMS. These observations suggest that, in patients with LEMS, VGCC antibodies downregulate VGCCs. In those LEMS patients who have SCLC, the cancer cells induce the production of VGCC antibodies. In LEMS patients without cancer, these antibodies are produced as part of a more general autoimmune state.

TREATMENT OF LEMS

Therapy must be tailored for each patient, on the basis of severity of weakness, underlying disease(s), life expectancy, and response to previous treatment. The treatment plan that follows may serve as a general guide, but will require modification for many patients.

When the diagnosis of LEMS has been confirmed, an extensive search for malignancy should be carried out, including radiographs and computed tomography scans of the chest. I recommend bronchoscopy during the initial evaluation of patients with LEMS who have a significant risk of lung cancer, especially in smokers and when symptoms have been present for less than 2 years. We have found cancer on bronchoscopy in several LEMS patients after results of chest computed tomography and magnetic resonance imaging were normal.

The initial treatment should be aimed at any tumor present because the weakness frequently improves with effective cancer therapy,[27,28] in which case no further treatment may be necessary for LEMS. If no tumor is found, the search for an occult malignancy should be repeated periodically; the frequency of these evaluations is determined by the patient's risk of cancer. Patients less than 50 without a history of chronic smoking have a low risk of associated malignancy, especially if there is evidence for a coexisting autoimmune disease. In these patients, extensive surveillance for cancer may not be necessary. Patients over 50 with a history of chronic smoking almost certainly have an underlying lung cancer, which must be assiduously sought.

In patients with cancer, LEMS is usually not the major therapeutic concern, nor does it represent the major threat to life. Experience has shown that immunotherapy of LEMS without effective treatment of an underlying cancer usually produces little or no improvement in strength. There is also a theoretical concern that immunosuppression may reduce the immunologic suppression of tumor growth. In patients with LEMS who do not have cancer, aggressive immunotherapy is more readily justified.

Cholinesterase inhibitors do not usually produce significant improvement in LEMS, although they may improve dry mouth. Pyridostigmine (Mestinon®) (30 or 60 mg every 4 to 6 hours) is the preferred agent and should be given for several days before assessing the response.

Guanidine hydrochloride inhibits mitochondrial calcium uptake, which increases the intracellular calcium concentration. This increases the release of acetylcholine from the motor nerve terminal, which produces improvement in strength in many patients with LEMS. Guanidine is taken orally, beginning with a dose of 5 to 10 mg per kg per day, divided throughout the waking hours. The dose may be increased to a maximum of 30 mg per kg per day, depending upon the clinical response, but side effects may be severe at doses greater than 1 g per day. The dose of guanidine should not be increased more often than every 3 days because the maximum response to a given dose may not be seen for 2 to 3 days. Pyridostigmine enhances the therapeutic response to guanidine and permits use of a lower dose. Side effects of guanidine include bone marrow suppression, renal tubular acidosis, chronic interstitial nephritis, cardiac arrhythmia, hepatic toxicity, pancreatic dysfunction, peripheral paresthesias, ataxia, confusion, alterations of mood, and behavioral changes. Deaths have been attributed to the drug. Blood tests of hematologic, hepatic, and renal function must be performed frequently as long as patients are taking guanidine.

Aminopyridines increase neurotransmitter release at central and peripheral synapses by blocking the delayed potassium conductance.[29] 4-Aminopyridine and 3,4-diaminopyridine (DAP) improve strength and autonomic function in most patients with LEMS,[30–33] but the clinical utility of 4-aminopyridine is limited by seizures, which occur at therapeutic doses.[34] DAP has less penetrance through the blood-brain barrier and does not share this limitation.

In our experience, more than 85% of LEMS patients have significant clinical benefit from DAP; in over half of these, the improvement is marked.[12] The effect of DAP begins about 20 min after an oral dose, the effect of each dose lasts about 4 h, and the maximum response to a given dosage may not be seen for 2 to 3 days. DAP is given orally in dosages of 5 to 25 mg, three or four times a day. The optimal dose and dosing schedule vary considerably and can be determined for each patient as follows: Begin DAP at 10 mg TID or QID and observe the response for 2 weeks. The dose is then increased in 5-mg increments at 2-week intervals until the maximum benefit is obtained, not to exceed 100 mg/day. Pyridostigmine at 30 or 60 mg is then added TID, and the effect on maximum response and duration of action of each dose of DAP is noted. The dose of DAP is then reduced in 5-mg decrements until the lowest effective dose is determined. In most patients, pyridostigmine enhances and prolongs the duration of action of DAP and permits use of lower doses. The optimal dose of DAP, taken with pyridostigmine, is usually between 15 and 60 mg per day. This may change and should be reassessed periodically by reducing the dose slowly to again determine the minimum dose that produces the maximum response.

Patients with or without underlying cancer benefit from DAP. Side effects are minimal and usually are limited to brief perioral and digital paresthesias if the dose is 10 to 15 mg or more. Gastrointestinal cramps and diarrhea may occur when DAP is taken with pyridostigmine and can be minimized by reducing the dose of pyridostigmine. Seizures may occur with doses greater than 100 mg/day, and asthma attacks have been induced in patients with preexisting asthma. A patient who inadvertently took six times the therapeutic dose (60 mg $\times$ 6) had seizures and cardiac arrhythmia, which cleared within 24 h.[35]

DAP should not be given to patients with known seizures. There is also a theoretical possibility that it could cause cardiac arrhythmia, although no such effects have been reported, and we found no effect on the electrocardiogram.[36] We recommend that DAP not be given to patients with known cardiac rhythm irregularities and that all patients undergo a screening electrocardiogram before starting. Organ toxicity has not been reported, even in patients who have taken aminopyridines for more than 10 years. However, because the clinical experience with these agents is still limited, periodic blood tests of liver, kidney, and hematologic function should be performed to assure that no such side effects develop. We recommend that liver function tests, measurements of BUN and creatinine, and complete blood counts be performed every 3 months for the first year after beginning DAP, and every 6 to 12 months thereafter.

When DAP is given in this way, experience indicates that it is a safe, effective, and valuable treatment for LEMS.[32,36] It has not been approved for clinical use in the United States, but is available on a compassionate-use basis for individual patients with LEMS. Information about the application process can be obtained from Jacobus Pharmaceutical (Princeton, NJ).

If the previously discussed treatments are not effective and the weakness is relatively mild, the physician must determine if aggressive immunotherapy is justified, bearing in mind that, even with optimum immunosuppression, most LEMS patients continue to be weak. When weakness is severe, plasma exchange or high-dose intravenous immunoglobulin (IVIg) may be used to induce relatively rapid, albeit transitory, improvement (see below). Immunosuppressants can be added in an attempt to produce more sustained improvement. Prednisone and azathioprine are the most frequently used immunosuppressants, and they are given alone or together.[37]

Plasma exchange produces improvement in many patients with LEMS, but this improvement is only temporary unless the patient is also receiving immunosuppression.[38] Repeated courses are usually necessary to maintain the improvement. IVIg also induces clinically significant temporary improvement in many patients with LEMS.[39] The frequency with which improvement occurs and the response to repeated courses of treatment have yet to be determined. In patients treated with plasma exchange or IVIg, we frequently note that improvement lasts for longer and longer periods after each treatment.

MEDICATIONS/SITUATIONS THAT EXACERBATE LEMS

Drugs that compromise neuromuscular transmission frequently exacerbate weakness in LEMS. Competitive neuromuscular blocking agents, such as *d*-tubocurarine and pancuronium, have an exaggerated and prolonged effect in patients with LEMS. In fact, the disease may initially be recognized when prolonged weakness or apnea follows administration of neuromuscular blocking agents given during anesthesia.[40] Some antibiotics, particularly the aminoglycosides, have significant neuromuscular blocking effects.[41] Some antiarrhythmics (quinine, quinidine, and procainamide) also worsen myasthenic weakness, as do β-adrenergic and calcium channel blocking drugs.[42] There are isolated reports of LEMS becoming worse after administration of a number of other agents, including magnesium and intravenous iodinated radiographic contrast agents.[43–45] In general, patients with LEMS should be observed for clinical worsening after any new medication is begun.

The weakness of LEMS may be worse when the ambient temperature is elevated or when the patient is febrile. Patients may need to avoid hot showers or baths. Systemic illness of any sort may cause transient worsening of weakness in patients with LEMS.

REFERENCES

1. Sanders, D.B. 1995. Lambert-Eaton myasthenic syndrome: clinical diagnosis, immune-mediated mechanisms, and update on therapy. Ann. Neurol. **37**(suppl. 1)**:** S63–S73.
2. Smith, A.G. & J. Wald. 1996. Acute ventilatory failure in Lambert-Eaton myasthenic syndrome and its response to 3,4-diaminopyridine. Neurology **46:** 1143–1145.

3. Wirtz, P.W. *et al.* 2001. Tonic pupils in Lambert-Eaton myasthenic syndrome. Muscle Nerve **24:** 444–445.
4. Khurana, R.K. 1993. Paraneoplastic autonomic dysfunction. *In* Clinical Autonomic Disorders, pp. 506–511. Little, Brown. Boston.
5. Baker, M.K. *et al.* 1994. Quantification of autonomic dysfunction in Lambert-Eaton syndrome by composite autonomic scoring scale. Neurology **44**(suppl. 2)**:** A220.
6. Khurana, R.K. *et al.* 1988. Autonomic dysfunction in Lambert-Eaton myasthenic syndrome. J. Neurol. Sci. **85:** 77–86.
7. O'Suilleabhain, P. *et al.* 1998. Autonomic dysfunction in the Lambert-Eaton myasthenic syndrome: serologic and clinical correlates. Neurology **50:** 88–93.
8. Elrington, G.M. *et al.* 1991. Neurological paraneoplastic syndromes in patients with small cell lung cancer: a prospective survey of 150 patients. J. Neurol. Neurosurg. Psychiatry **54:** 764–767.
9. Nilsson, O. & I. Rosén. 1978. The stretch reflex in the Eaton-Lambert syndrome, myasthenia gravis, and myotonic dystrophy. Acta Neurol. Scand. **57:** 350–357.
10. Kobayashi, H. *et al.* 1988. Bronchogenic carcinoma with subacute cerebellar degeneration and Eaton-Lambert syndrome: an autopsy case. Jpn. J. Med. **27:** 203–206.
11. Ward, C.D. & N.M.F. Murray. 1979. Effect of temperature on neuromuscular transmission in the Eaton-Lambert syndrome. J. Neurol. Neurosurg. Psychiatry **42:** 247–249.
12. Tim, R.W. *et al.* 2000. Lambert-Eaton myasthenic syndrome: electrodiagnostic findings and response to treatment. Neurology **54:** 2176–2178.
13. AAEM Quality Assurance Committee and American Association of Electrodiagnostic Medicine. 2001. Practice parameter for repetitive nerve stimulation and single fiber EMG evaluation of adults with suspected myasthenia gravis or Lambert-Eaton myasthenic syndrome: summary statement. Muscle Nerve **24:** 1236–1238.
14. Lambert, E.H. 1987. General discussion. Ann. N.Y. Acad. Sci. **505:** 380–381.
15. Sanders, D.B. 1992. The effect of firing rate on neuromuscular jitter in Lambert-Eaton myasthenic syndrome. Muscle Nerve **15:** 256–258.
16. Trontelj, J.V. & E. Stålberg. 1991. Single motor end-plates in myasthenia gravis and LEMS at different firing rates. Muscle Nerve **14:** 226–232.
17. Trontelj, J.V. & E. Stålberg. 1992. The effect of firing rate on neuromuscular jitter in Lambert-Eaton myasthenic syndrome: a reply. Muscle Nerve **15:** 258.
18. Lennon, V.A. 1997. Serological profile of myasthenia gravis and distinction from the Lambert-Eaton myasthenic syndrome. Neurology **48:** S23–S27.
19. Lang, B. *et al.* 1993. Autoantibody specificities in Lambert-Eaton myasthenic syndrome. Ann. N.Y. Acad. Sci. **681:** 382–393.
20. Leys, K. *et al.* 1991. Calcium channel autoantibodies in the Lambert-Eaton myasthenic syndrome. Ann. Neurol. **29:** 307–314.
21. Lennon, V.A. 1994. Serological diagnosis of myasthenia gravis and the Lambert-Eaton myasthenic syndrome. *In* Handbook of Myasthenia Gravis and Myasthenic Syndromes, pp. 149–164. Dekker. New York.
22. Elmqvist, D. & E.H. Lambert. 1968. Detailed analysis of neuromuscular transmission in a patient with the myasthenic syndrome sometimes associated with bronchogenic carcinoma. Mayo Clin. Proc. **43:** 689–713.
23. Fukunaga, H. *et al.* 1983. Passive transfer of Lambert-Eaton myasthenic syndrome with IgG from man to mouse depletes the presynaptic membrane active zones. Proc. Natl. Acad. Sci. USA **80:** 7636–7640.
24. Fukunaga, H. *et al.* 1982. Paucity and disorganization of presynaptic membrane active zones in the Lambert-Eaton myasthenic syndrome. Muscle Nerve **5:** 686–697.
25. Roberts, A. *et al.* 1985. Paraneoplastic myasthenic syndrome IgG inhibits $^{45}Ca^{2+}$ flux in a human small cell carcinoma line. Nature **317:** 737–739.
26. Lang, B. *et al.* 1989. Lambert-Eaton myasthenic syndrome: immunoglobulin G inhibition of Ca^{++} flux in tumor cells correlates with disease severity. Ann. Neurol. **25:** 265–271.
27. Chalk, C.H. *et al.* 1990. Response of the Lambert-Eaton myasthenic syndrome to treatment of associated small-cell lung carcinoma. Neurology **40:** 1552–1556.
28. Jenkyn, L.R. *et al.* 1980. Remission of the Lambert-Eaton syndrome and small cell anaplastic carcinoma of the lung induced by chemotherapy and radiotherapy. Cancer **46:** 1123–1127.

29. YEH, J.Z. *et al.* 1976. Interactions of aminopyridines with potassium channels of squid axon membranes. Biophys. J. **16:** 77–81.
30. AGOSTON, S. *et al.* 1978. Effects of 4-aminopyridine in Eaton-Lambert syndrome. Br. J. Anaesth. **50:** 383–385.
31. LUNDH, H. *et al.* 1983. Novel drug of choice in Eaton-Lambert syndrome. J. Neurol. Neurosurg. Psychiatry **46:** 684–687.
32. MCEVOY, K.M. *et al.* 1989. 3,4-Diaminopyridine in the treatment of Lambert-Eaton myasthenic syndrome. N. Engl. J. Med. **321:** 1567–1571.
33. SANDERS, D.B. *et al.* 1993. 3,4-Diaminopyridine in Lambert-Eaton myasthenic syndrome and myasthenia gravis. Ann. N.Y. Acad. Sci. **681:** 588–590.
34. SANDERS, D.B. *et al.* 1980. Eaton-Lambert syndrome: a clinical and electrophysiological study of a patient treated with 4-aminopyridine. J. Neurol. Neurosurg. Psychiatry **43:** 978–985.
35. BOERMA, C.E. *et al.* 1995. Cardiac arrest following an iatrogenic 3,4-diaminopyridine intoxication in a patient with Lambert-Eaton myasthenic syndrome. J. Toxicol. Clin. Toxicol. **33:** 249–251.
36. SANDERS, D.B. *et al.* 2000. A randomized trial of 3,4-diaminopyridine in Lambert-Eaton myasthenic syndrome. Neurology **54:** 603–607.
37. MADDISON, P. *et al.* 2001. Long-term outcome in Lambert-Eaton myasthenic syndrome without lung cancer. J. Neurol. Neurosurg. Psychiatry **70:** 212–217.
38. NIH CONSENSUS CONFERENCE STATEMENT. 1986. The utility of therapeutic plasmapheresis for neurological disorders. J. Am. Med. Assoc. **256:** 1333–1337.
39. RICH, M.M. *et al.* 1997. Treatment of Lambert-Eaton syndrome with intravenous immunoglobulin. Muscle Nerve **20:** 614–615.
40. ANDERSON, H.J. *et al.* 1953. Bronchial neoplasm with myasthenia: prolonged apnea after administration of succinylcholine. Lancet **ii:** 1291–1293.
41. SCHOTTLAND, J.R. 1999. Ofloxacin in the Lambert-Eaton myasthenic syndrome. Neurology **52:** 435.
42. UENO, S. & Y. HARA. 1992. Lambert-Eaton myasthenic syndrome without anti-calcium channel antibody: adverse effect of calcium antagonist diltiazem. J. Neurol. Neurosurg. Psychiatry **55:** 409–410.
43. GUTMANN, L. & M. TAKAMORI. 1973. Effect of Mg^{++} on neuromuscular transmission in the Eaton-Lambert syndrome. Neurology **23:** 977–980.
44. STREIB, E.W. 1977. Adverse effects of magnesium salt cathartics in a patient with the myasthenic syndrome (Lambert-Eaton syndrome). Ann. Neurol. **2:** 175–176.
45. VAN DEN BERGH, P. *et al.* 1986. Intravascular contrast media and neuromuscular junction disorders. Ann. Neurol. **19:** 206–207.

Abnormal Single-Fiber Electromyography in Patients Not Having Myasthenia

Risk for Diagnostic Confusion?

RUDY MERCELIS

University Hospital, Antwerp, Belgium

KEYWORDS: **single-fiber electromyography; myasthenia gravis; sensitivity; specificity**

Single-fiber electromyography (SFEMG) is the most sensitive diagnostic tool in the evaluation of patients suspected for myasthenia gravis (MG), showing abnormalities of neuromuscular transmission in up to 99%.[1] However, abnormal neuromuscular transmission as shown by SFEMG is not specific for MG. It occurs in other primary disorders of neuromuscular transmission such as the Lambert-Eaton myasthenic syndrome (LEMS), congenital myasthenia, and botulism, and also in more common conditions such as peripheral neuropathies, radiculopathies, motor neuron disorders, and myopathies. The risk for diagnostic confusion is difficult to measure and depends heavily on the composition of the patient group.

PATIENTS AND METHODS

Between September 1989 and October 1997, 391 patients had stimulated SFEMG for confirmation or exclusion of suspected MG. This was the only indication for SFEMG in our laboratory. Before 1989, the technique with voluntary activation was used. The group included 157 males and 234 females, with a mean age of 49.9 and a range of 3 to 93 years. One hundred seventy-two patients had only ptosis or double vision. With all available information (symptoms, clinical findings, EMG, anti-acetylcholine-receptor antibodies, response to therapy, and clinical follow-up), the diagnosis of MG was retained in 78 patients, including 39 males and 39 females with a different age distribution and a predominance of older patients in both sexes. For women only, there was a second peak between age 20 and 40. Exclusively ocular symptoms were found in 31 patients. Most of the other patients had ocular complaints too. Seven patients had only bulbar complaints, and only 3 patients had neither ocular nor bulbar symptoms.

Address for correspondence: Rudy Mercelis, University Hospital, Antwerp, Belgium. Voice: +32/38.21.34.18; fax: +32/38.21.43.12.
rudy.mercelis@ua.ac.be

Ann. N.Y. Acad. Sci. 998: 509–511 (2003). © 2003 New York Academy of Sciences.
doi: 10.1196/annals.1254.066

Stimulated SFEMG was performed in the extensor digitorum communis (EDC) muscle in 227 patients and in the orbicularis oculi (OO) in 233 patients, while both muscles were examined in 69 patients. In patients with only ocular symptoms, examination was always done in the OO.

Stimulation was at 10 Hz with a Teflon-coated needle electrode, and registration with a Medelec single-fiber electrode. Jitter was measured as the mean of consecutive differences (MCD), mostly of 100 discharges; in most patients, at least 20 potentials were recorded. Jitter measurement was semiautomatic with a Medelec Mystro specialist application module. Conventional criteria for abnormality were used:[2] a study was considered as abnormal when the mean jitter was >20 μs in OO or >25 μs in EDC, or when at least 2 of the individual potentials had a jitter of >30 μs in OO or >40 μs in EDC.

RESULTS

First, patients with MG: SFEMG was abnormal in 71/78 patients or 91%. Two studies were normal in the EDC: 1 patient had a thymoma and only respiratory complaints; the other was in clinical remission from his MG, but developed chronic fatigue. The 5 patients with normal studies in the OO had only intermittent ocular symptoms with no abnormality on clinical examination. In 2 of them, the diagnosis was based on past clinical findings; 3 of them developed more severe symptoms in the weeks following the initial examination and showed abnormalities on a second SFEMG. In most patients, the abnormalities were very pronounced. In 2 patients with ocular MG, minimal abnormalities were found in the OO with only 1 or 2 abnormal individual potentials and borderline values for the mean jitter.

Second, other patients (no MG): this group contained 1 patient with LEMS, 1 amyotrophic lateral sclerosis (ALS), 8 chronic progressive external ophthalmoplegias (CPEO), 2 oculopharyngeal muscular dystrophies, 2 inflammatory myopathies, and 11 blepharospasms, of whom 2 proved to have had botulinum toxin injections previously. The majority of patients in this group had no definite diagnosis. Fifty-three of them complained only of chronic fatigue.

SFEMG was normal in 293/313 patients (specificity 94%). As expected, the jitter was severely increased in the patient with LEMS. The jitter was slightly increased in the patient with ALS and moderately in 3/8 CPEO. A slight to moderate increase was found in 5/11 blepharospasms, including the 2 with previous botulinum toxin injections. A slight increase was found in the 2 inflammatory myopathies. In the group without definite diagnosis, the jitter was abnormal in 8/290 patients and abnormalities were always very mild. With a minor adaptation of the criteria of abnormality, requiring at least 3 abnormal individual potentials instead of 2, these 8 patients became normal and the specificity of the test increased to 96%, while the sensitivity for MG decreased to 68/78 or 87%.

DISCUSSION AND CONCLUSIONS

First, the sensitivity of SFEMG for MG is high. The sensitivity of 87% to 91% in our series is somewhat lower than previously reported rates.[1] This is probably due to the high proportion of patients with only intermittent ocular symptoms, referred by ophthalmologists.

Second, in this selected group of patients referred with clinical suspicion of MG, the specificity of SFEMG is very high (94%; 96% after a minor modification of the criteria of abnormality), with only "false-positive" results in patients with other neuromuscular disorders such as LEMS, ALS, and CPEO and in a few patients with blepharospasm. These patients can be distinguished from MG mostly on clinical grounds, sometimes after conventional EMG or muscle biopsy. The lack of specificity of SFEMG is not a major problem in its use in the diagnosis of MG.

Third, the age distribution of this group shows a majority of older patients. Stimulated SFEMG proves especially efficient in confirming MG in older patients with limited ocular disease.

REFERENCES

1. Sanders, D.B. & E.V. Stalberg. 1996. AAEM minimonograph no. 25: single-fiber electromyography. Muscle Nerve **19:** 1069–1083.
2. Stalberg, E. & J.V. Trontelj. 1994. Single Fiber Electromyography: Studies in Healthy and Diseased Muscle. Second edition. Raven Press. New York.

Treatment of Autoimmune Disease by Adoptive Cellular Gene Therapy

INGO H. TARNER,[a] ANTHONY J. SLAVIN,[a] JACQUELINE McBRIDE,[a] ALENKA LEVICNIK,[a] RICHARD SMITH,[b] GARRY P. NOLAN,[b] CHRISTOPHER H. CONTAG,[c] AND C. GARRISON FATHMAN[a]

[a]*Department of Medicine, Division of Immunology and Rheumatology,*
[b]*Baxter Laboratory for Genetic Pharmacology, Department of Microbiology and Immunology, and* [c]*Department of Pediatrics,*
Stanford University School of Medicine, Stanford, California 94305, USA

ABSTRACT: Autoimmune disorders represent inappropriate immune responses directed at self-tissue. Antigen-specific CD4+ T cells and antigen-presenting dendritic cells (DCs) are important mediators in the pathogenesis of autoimmune disease and thus are ideal candidates for adoptive cellular gene therapy, an *ex vivo* approach to therapeutic gene transfer. Using retrovirally transduced cells and luciferase bioluminescence, we have demonstrated that primary T cells, T cell hybridomas, and DCs rapidly and preferentially home to the sites of inflammation in animal models of multiple sclerosis, arthritis, and diabetes. These cells, transduced with retroviral vectors to drive expression of various "regulatory proteins" such as IL-4, IL-10, IL-12p40, and anti-TNF scFv, deliver these immunoregulatory proteins to the inflamed lesions, providing therapy for experimental autoimmune encephalitis (EAE), collagen-induced arthritis (CIA), and nonobese diabetic mice (NOD).

KEYWORDS: gene therapy; retrovirus; adoptive cell transfer; autoimmunity; arthritis; diabetes; multiple sclerosis; CIA; NOD; EAE; cytokines; IL-12p40; IL-4; anti-TNF scFv; T cells; dendritic cells; bioluminescence imaging

INTRODUCTION

Autoimmune diseases affect about 3–5% of the U.S. population.[1] Their chronic nature and their complex and insufficiently understood etiopathogenesis make them a special challenge for clinical therapy. In the battle against autoimmune disease, different therapies have been tried with varying success. Among these, gene therapy has developed over the last decade as a particularly interesting and promising approach. Gene therapy offers the unique chance of providing long-term expression of immune-modulating molecules *in vivo* that can antagonize the chronic inflammatory processes in autoimmune diseases. Besides long-term efficacy, a successful treatment

Address for correspondence: C. Garrison Fathman, M.D., Department of Medicine, Division of Immunology and Rheumatology, Stanford University School of Medicine, CCSR Building, Room 2225, 269 Campus Drive, Stanford, CA 94305-5166. Voice: 650-723-7887; fax: 650-725-1958. cfathman@stanford.edu

Ann. N.Y. Acad. Sci. 998: 512–519 (2003). © 2003 New York Academy of Sciences.
doi: 10.1196/annals.1254.067

for autoimmune diseases should also be safe with a low side effect profile and should specifically target known pathogenic mechanisms.

In an effort to fulfill these criteria, our laboratory has developed adoptive cellular gene therapy. This *ex vivo* approach utilizes antigen-specific T cells and dendritic cells (DCs) for the targeted and safe delivery of immune-regulatory molecules to sites of autoimmune inflammation after retroviral transduction of the vehicle cells *in vitro* and adoptive transfer by intravenous (i.v.) injection. It has become evident that T cells and their cytokines play a central role in the initiation as well as the perpetuation of organ-specific autoimmune disease.[2–4] Because of their importance as mediators in the pathogenesis of autoimmune disease, CD4+ T cells were considered to be ideal candidates for cell-based gene therapy. Several models of autoimmunity involve a Th1-based progression of immune responses against self-antigens that is probably responsible for much of the tissue destruction that occurs in autoimmune diseases. Numerous studies have demonstrated successful prevention or amelioration of autoimmune diseases by blocking Th1 cytokines with specific antagonists or by counteracting the inflammatory response with immune-regulatory cytokines.[2,5] Systemic administrations of transforming growth factor (TGF)–β, interleukin-1 receptor antagonist (IL-1ra), IL-4, IL-10, IL-12p40, or anti-TNF serve as effective therapies in models of autoimmune disease such as collagen-induced arthritis (CIA),[6–9] EAE,[10–13] and NOD.[14–16] These protocols appear to work by shifting the cytokine balance away from Th1 dominance. Indeed, cytokine-induced immune deviation has been investigated as potential therapy for autoimmune diseases because cytokines present at the time of activation may alter the pathogenicity of effector T cells.[17] However, systemic cytokine therapy can lead to deleterious side effects as exemplified by IL-4.[18,19] Therefore, recent approaches have explored targeting cytokine delivery to the site of inflammation as an alternative to systemic therapeutic regimens.[5]

Various approaches are used to introduce DNA into host cells, including nonviral systems such as naked DNA and DNA complexed with liposomes or peptides, as well as various viral vectors.[5,20] The nonviral systems are not very target tissue–specific, and gene expression does not last long.[20] Of the viral vectors, adenoviruses have commonly been used for gene delivery.[21] However, they afford only transient expression in infected cells and have been associated with severe immune reactions and fatality in a recent clinical trial.[22,23] Safe and site-specific gene delivery requires an appropriate vehicle, and we and others have shown that the cells involved in the inflammation themselves, T cells and DCs, may serve as such vehicles.[9,13,24,25] Retroviral-mediated gene transfer into T cells and DCs allows stable integration of transgenes with resultant long-term expression.[26,27] Furthermore, retroviral gene delivery has been used safely to treat human disease[28] and has avoided the viral protein immunogenicity that occurs with the use of adenoviral gene delivery.

ADOPTIVE CELLULAR GENE THERAPY

Retroviral Gene Transfer

Gene transfer into target cells via retroviruses utilizes the ability of murine retroviruses to bind cell surface molecules in the initial stages of the infection process. After binding, a fusion event occurs that allows the retroviral core and genome access into the infected cell. Within the cytoplasm of infected cells, retroviral reverse transcription occurs with subsequent integration into the genome after cell division. Thus, the genetic modifications and the expression of the transferred genes are maintained through target cell division. Pioneered by Richard Mulligan and David Baltimore,[29] defective packaging lines are capable of producing all the necessary proteins required for packaging, processing, reverse transcription, and integration of recombinant genomes. Virions are produced through transfection of packaging cell lines with the retroviral vectors expressing recombinant gene products cloned downstream of the psi packaging sequence. The producer cells will encapsulate or "package" only the transcripts containing the psi signal and release the viral particles into the culture supernatant, which is then harvested and used for transduction of target cells.

In the past, effective use of antigen-specific T cells and DCs was impeded by a low retroviral transduction efficiency. Our group has developed a novel retroviral construct, termed pGCy,[26] that contains an internal ribosomal entry site (IRES) between the gene of interest and a gene encoding a fluorescent marker (yellow fluorescent protein, YFP). This bicistronic expression vector allows coexpression of the two genes on one mRNA. Using our novel construct, we have been able to stably and durably transduce primary T cells and T cell hybridomas with up to 80% efficiency[9,26] and DCs with up to 40% efficiency (Tarner, McBride, and Levicnik, unpublished data). Moreover, by using bioluminescence imaging, which allows repeated *in vivo* real-time imaging of the homing behavior of retrovirally transduced, luciferase-expressing T cells and DCs, we have been able to demonstrate site-specific homing of our gene therapy vehicles to inflamed joints in murine CIA,[9] to the central nervous system (CNS) in EAE,[13] and to the pancreas in NOD mice (Urbanek-Ruiz, manuscript submitted).

Treatment of Autoimmune Disease Using T Cells

As mentioned above, regulatory cytokines and cytokine antagonists such as IL-4, IL-10, and anti-TNF antibodies or soluble TNF receptors as well as chemokine antagonists and complement antagonists, which antagonize proinflammatory autoimmune reactions, have been used successfully in treatment studies of autoimmune disease.[5] We and others have used antigen-specific CD4+ T cells and T cell hybridomas to deliver regulatory cytokines and cytokine inhibitors to autoimmune lesions,[9,11,30,31] showing that T cells are suitable vehicles for targeted immunotherapy. We originally described amelioration of EAE with IL-4.[11] Recently, our laboratory has demonstrated effective prevention of EAE and of CIA by adoptive cellular gene therapy using autoantigen-specific T cells and T cell hybridomas retrovirally transduced to express the IL-12 receptor blocker IL-12p40,[9,13] the regulatory cytokine IL-4 (Tarner *et al.*, 2002. *Clin. Immunol.* **105:** 304–314), and TNF-antagonizing anti-TNF scFv (Smith, Tarner & Levicnik, submitted). We demonstrated that amelioration of CIA was due to local delivery of IL-12p40, IL-4, or anti-TNF scFv to the inflamed joint based on the following findings. First, analysis of the cytokine profile and the proliferative response to antigen of draining lymph node cells and spleen cells was unaffected in the treatment groups compared with untreated and vector-only treated animals. This finding is also consistent with a good safety profile of our adoptive cellular gene therapy approach in terms of low systemic side effects. Second, antigen specificity was required for effective treatment. To this effect, when retrovirally transduced collagen type II (CII)–reactive and myelin basic protein (MBP)–reactive T cell hybridomas that expressed equivalent amounts of IL-12p40 were injected into both CIA mice and EAE mice, only CII-reactive T cell hybridomas were therapeutic in CIA and only MBP-reactive cells were therapeutic in EAE. Interestingly, both cell types were found to migrate to inflamed paws as confirmed by *in vivo* real-time bioluminescence imaging (described below) and PCR detection of YFP marker mRNA in joint tissue homogenates. However, bioluminescence imaging showed that only the CII-specific cells persisted in the inflammatory lesions, while the homing of the MBP-specific cells was transient. Of note, the CII-specific cells persisted in the joints long-term because YFP mRNA could be detected by PCR up to 55 days after adoptive cell transfer. Based on the chemokine receptor expression profile of our antigen-specific T cell hybridomas and their ability to migrate *in vitro* in response to chemokines that were found to be expressed in inflamed joints in CIA, we hypothesize that these vehicle cells home to sites of inflammation by means of chemotaxis independent of their antigen specificity. Retention in inflammatory lesions, however, occurs only upon recognition of antigen by the specific T cell receptor (TCR). Third, PCR analysis of joint tissue homogenates showed that in animals that received anti-TNF scFv expressing T cell hybridomas, IL-6 transcription was suppressed. Taken together, these results strongly suggest that T cell–mediated adoptive cellular gene therapy works based on site-specific homing and retention of the vehicle cells and local effects of the delivered immune-modulating molecules.

Using Dendritic Cells as Vehicles

DCs not only provide a common set of signals to initiate clonal expansion of T cells, but also provide T cells with selective signals that lead to either Th1 or Th2 immunity. Menges and colleagues recently demonstrated that transfer of TNF-treated, incompletely matured DCs (semimature DCs) induces peptide-specific IL-10-producing T cells *in vivo* and prevents EAE.[32] Similarly, injection of immature DCs, infected with IL-4-encoding adenovirus into mice with established CIA resulted in almost complete suppression of disease with no disease recurrence for up to 4 weeks posttreatment.[25] We have found that DCs transduced to express either IL-12p40 or IL-10 are effective in suppressing CIA (Seroogy, Nakajima, and Tarner, unpublished data). These data are in excellent agreement with Morita *et al.*,[24] who demonstrated reduced CIA disease incidence and severity by injecting bone marrow–derived DCs retrovirally transduced to express IL-4 before disease onset. These experiments raise the exciting possibility of using DCs for adoptive cellular gene therapy of autoimmune disease. Regarding the mechanism of DC action, both Kim *et al.*[25] and Morita *et al.*[24] found that the adoptive transfer of IL-4-expressing DCs leads to suppression of Th1-type immune responses in the lymph nodes and spleen and diminished the associated humoral immune responses. The authors concluded that the therapeutic DCs migrated to the lymphoid tissues and modulated T cell immune responses by expression of the regulatory cytokine IL-4 and through specific DC–T cell interactions. Our own studies of bone marrow–derived DC migration in CIA using bioluminescence imaging suggested that i.v. injected DCs not only home to lymphoid organs, but also accumulate in inflamed joints (McBride and Tarner, unpublished observations) and therefore could be used to deliver anti-inflammatory molecules directly to the site of inflammation. A possible local action of transduced

DCs, in addition to their effects in lymphoid organs, is suggested by studies from Robbins and colleagues on the role of DCs in the so-called contralateral effect after local intra-articular gene expression in various models of arthritis. This phenomenon is characterized by the clinical improvement of both the injected and the noninjected joints.[33–35] Further investigation of the contralateral effect in arthritis models and a delayed-type hypersensitivity (DTH) model suggested that locally injected adenovirus encoding IL-4 or vIL-10 leads to transduction of local DCs that then leave the injected joint, migrate to the local lymph nodes and to distant joints, and affect immune responses in those sites.[25,33,36] Results from the DTH study also indicate that a potential mechanism of the therapeutic DC–T cell interaction is through silencing or anergizing T cells to antigen. Taken together, these results indicate that the use of genetically engineered DCs is a very promising approach for adoptive cellular gene therapy of autoimmune disease.

Bioluminescence Imaging

Specific homing to sites of autoimmune inflammation is the central principle of adoptive cellular gene therapy. In order to ascertain that our vehicle cells would exhibit the assumed homing behavior *in vivo*, we made use of whole-body bioluminescence imaging. This novel and powerful technique allows tracking of cells *in vivo* in real time. It has been used to monitor tumor cell growth and bacterial colonization *in vivo*, demonstrating very good sensitivity.[37,38] For our purposes, T cell hybridomas and DCs are transduced with a retrovirus encoding luciferase and transferred to recipients. The mice are anesthetized and receive the substrate luciferin by intraperitoneal injection. The enzymatic reaction between luciferase and luciferin causes emission of photons from within the animal. Photons that are transmitted through the tissue can be detected by a cooled charge-coupled device camera. A pseudocolor image representing light intensity of the emission is superimposed on a gray-scale body-surface reference image collected under weak illumination, and the data are acquired and analyzed using appropriate software. Transfer of luciferase expressing T cell hybridomas and DCs into arthritic CIA mice, EAE-affected mice, and NOD mice confirmed the assumed homing behavior. Three days after the cell transfer, photons emitted from the cells were detected in arthritic joints from all mice tested in the CIA model,[9] while five of six mice with EAE demonstrated luciferase-positive cells in the brain within three days of adoptive transfer.[13] Similarly, cellular homing to the pancreas was found in the NOD mouse (Urbanek-Ruiz, manuscript submitted; and McBride, unpublished data). No luciferase-positive cells were detected in the paws, CNS, or pancreas, respectively, in naïve control mice at any time.

CONCLUSIONS

Although a complete mechanistic understanding of autoimmune diseases has not been achieved, gene therapy offers a platform by which to study the effects of various immune-modulating proteins on disease pathogenesis. Retroviral-mediated adoptive cellular gene therapy has been developed as an efficient novel strategy for the therapy of autoimmune diseaes. The use of a replication-defective retrovirus for gene transfer obviates a critical safety issue because the presence of replication-competent virus could become a potential health risk, most notably by an increased risk of proviral insertional mutagenesis. Hence, prior to reinfusion of transduced cells, rigorous safety issues must be undertaken to ensure the absence of replication-competent retroviruses. To date, approximately 3500 patients have been entered into gene therapy trials. The majority of human gene therapy protocols utilize replication-incompetent retroviruses due to the fact that the retroviral-mediated gene transfer process is relatively well understood, particularly for the murine retroviruses, and safety has been rigorously studied.[39,40] A phase-I clinical trial of gene therapy for rheumatoid arthritis was recently completed and showed safe and successful gene expression after *ex vivo* retroviral transduction and intra-articular injection of autologous synovial cells.[41,42]

Antigen-specific T cells and DCs hold promise as effective gene delivery vehicles for adoptive cellular gene therapy as shown by our studies described above. As a further step to enhance homing capabilities, novel engineered chemokine receptor-bearing cells that can more specifically follow chemokine gradients to inflammatory lesions may be studied in the future. Finally, as some very encouraging results have been obtained in studies combining various gene products and/or gene delivery strategies, future research should look further into combination therapy in order to achieve potentiated therapeutic effectiveness and reduced side effects. Improved adoptive cellular gene therapy delivering optimized combinations of immune-regulatory molecules will undoubtedly be informative in characterizing the underlying immune mechanisms in organ-specific autoimmune diseases and will potentially lead to new therapeutic options for treating human autoimmune diseases.

ACKNOWLEDGMENTS

I. H. Tarner was funded by the German Academic Exchange Service (Deutscher Akademischer Austauschdienst, DAAD-Stipendium im Rahmen des Gemeinsamen Hochschulprogramms III von Bund und Ländern). C. G. Fathman was funded in part by a contract from the National Institute of Arthritis and Musculoskeletal and Skin Diseases to explore the use of gene therapy in murine arthritis, the Juvenile Diabetes Research Foundation, and the National Institute of Diabetes and Digestive and Kidney Diseases for studies on type 1 diabetes.

REFERENCES

1. JACOBSON, D.L. *et al.* 1997. Epidemiology and estimated population burden of selected autoimmune diseases in the United States. Clin. Immunol. Immunopathol. **84:** 223–243.
2. HARRISON, L.C. & D.A. HAFLER. 2000. Antigen-specific therapy for autoimmune disease. Curr. Opin. Immunol. **12:** 704–711.
3. LIBLAU, R.S., S.M. SINGER & H.O. MCDEVITT. 1995. Th1 and Th2 CD4+ T cells in the pathogenesis of organ-specific autoimmune diseases. Immunol. Today **16:** 34–38.
4. MAURI, C. *et al.* 1996. Relationship between Th1/Th2 cytokine patterns and the arthritogenic response in collagen-induced arthritis. Eur. J. Immunol. **26:** 1511–1518.
5. TARNER, I.H. & C.G. FATHMAN. 2001. Gene therapy in autoimmune disease. Curr. Opin. Immunol. **13:** 676–682.
6. HORSFALL, A.C. *et al.* 1997. Suppression of collagen-induced arthritis by continuous administration of IL-4. J. Immunol. **159:** 5687–5696.

7. WOODS, J.M. *et al.* 2001. IL-4 adenoviral gene therapy reduces inflammation, proinflammatory cytokines, vascularization, and bony destruction in rat adjuvant-induced arthritis. J. Immunol. **166:** 1214–1222.
8. KIM, S.H. *et al.* 2000. Gene therapy for established murine collagen-induced arthritis by local and systemic adenovirus-mediated delivery of interleukin-4. Arthritis Res. **2:** 293–302.
9. NAKAJIMA, A. *et al.* 2001. Antigen-specific T cell–mediated gene therapy in collagen-induced arthritis. J. Clin. Invest. **107:** 1293–1301.
10. INOBE, J. *et al.* 1998. IL-4 is a differentiation factor for transforming growth factor-beta secreting Th3 cells and oral administration of IL-4 enhances oral tolerance in experimental allergic encephalomyelitis. Eur. J. Immunol. **28:** 2780–2790.
11. SHAW, M.K. *et al.* 1997. Local delivery of interleukin 4 by retrovirus-transduced T lymphocytes ameliorates experimental autoimmune encephalomyelitis. J. Exp. Med. **185:** 1711–1714.
12. CROXFORD, J.L. *et al.* 2000. Gene therapy for chronic relapsing experimental allergic encephalomyelitis using cells expressing a novel soluble p75 dimeric TNF receptor. J. Immunol. **164:** 2776–2781.
13. COSTA, G.L. *et al.* 2001. Adoptive immunotherapy of experimental autoimmune encephalomyelitis via T cell delivery of the IL-12 p40 subunit. J. Immunol. **167:** 2379–2387.
14. TOMINAGA, Y. *et al.* 1998. Administration of IL-4 prevents autoimmune diabetes, but enhances pancreatic insulitis in NOD mice. Clin. Immunol. Immunopathol. **86:** 209–218.
15. PENNLINE, K.J., E. ROQUE-GAFFNEY & M. MONAHAN. 1994. Recombinant human IL-10 prevents the onset of diabetes in the nonobese diabetic mouse. Clin. Immunol. Immunopathol. **71:** 169–175.
16. KOH, J.J. *et al.* 2000. Degradable polymeric carrier for the delivery of IL-10 plasmid DNA to prevent autoimmune insulitis of NOD mice. Gene Ther. **7:** 2099–2104.
17. RACKE, M.K. *et al.* 1994. Cytokine-induced immune deviation as a therapy for inflammatory autoimmune disease. J. Exp. Med. **180:** 1961–1966.
18. LEACH, M.W. *et al.* 1997. Safety evaluation of recombinant human interleukin-4. I. Preclinical studies. Clin. Immunol. Immunopathol. **83:** 8–11.
19. LEACH, M.W., M.E. RYBAK & I.Y. ROSENBLUM. 1997. Safety evaluation of recombinant human interleukin-4. II. Clinical studies. Clin. Immunol. Immunopathol. **83:** 12–14.
20. BALICKI, D. & E. BEUTLER. 2002. Gene therapy of human disease. Medicine (Baltimore) **81:** 69–86.
21. EVANS, C.H. *et al.* 2001. Future of adenoviruses in the gene therapy of arthritis. Arthritis Res. **3:** 142–146.
22. SMAGLIK, P. 2000. Gene Therapy Institute denies that errors led to trial death. Nature **403:** 820.
23. MARSHALL, E. 2000. Gene therapy on trial. Science **288:** 951–957.
24. MORITA, Y. *et al.* 2001. Dendritic cells genetically engineered to express IL-4 inhibit murine collagen-induced arthritis. J. Clin. Invest. **107:** 1275–1284.
25. KIM, S.H. *et al.* 2001. Effective treatment of established murine collagen-induced arthritis by systemic administration of dendritic cells genetically modified to express IL-4. J. Immunol. **166:** 3499–3505.
26. COSTA, G.L. *et al.* 2000. Targeting rare populations of murine antigen-specific T lymphocytes by retroviral transduction for potential application in gene therapy for autoimmune disease. J. Immunol. **164:** 3581–3590.
27. TARNER, I.H. *et al.* 2001. Retroviral gene therapy of collagen-induced arthritis by local delivery of immunoregulatory molecules using antigen-specific T-cells and dendritic cells. Arthritis Rheum. **44:** S149.
28. CAVAZZANA-CALVO, M. *et al.* 2000. Gene therapy of human severe combined immunodeficiency (SCID)-X1 disease. Science **288:** 669–672.
29. MANN, R., R.C. MULLIGAN & D. BALTIMORE. 1983. Construction of a retrovirus packaging mutant and its use to produce helper-free defective retrovirus. Cell **33:** 153–159.
30. MATHISEN, P.M. *et al.* 1997. Treatment of experimental autoimmune encephalomyelitis with genetically modified memory T cells. J. Exp. Med. **186:** 159–164.

31. ANNENKOV, A. & Y. CHERNAJOVSKY. 2000. Engineering mouse T lymphocytes specific to type II collagen by transduction with a chimeric receptor consisting of a single chain Fv and TCR zeta. Gene Ther. **7:** 714–722.
32. MENGES, M. *et al.* 2002. Repetitive injections of dendritic cells matured with tumor necrosis factor alpha induce antigen-specific protection of mice from autoimmunity. J. Exp. Med. **195:** 15–21.
33. GHIVIZZANI, S.C. *et al.* 1998. Direct adenovirus-mediated gene transfer of interleukin 1 and tumor necrosis factor alpha soluble receptors to rabbit knees with experimental arthritis has local and distal anti-arthritic effects. Proc. Natl. Acad. Sci. USA **95:** 4613–4618.
34. LECHMAN, E.R. *et al.* 1999. Direct adenoviral gene transfer of viral IL-10 to rabbit knees with experimental arthritis ameliorates disease in both injected and contralateral control knees. J. Immunol. **163:** 2202–2208.
35. WHALEN, J.D. *et al.* 1999. Adenoviral transfer of the viral IL-10 gene periarticularly to mouse paws suppresses development of collagen-induced arthritis in both injected and uninjected paws. J. Immunol. **162:** 3625–3632.
36. WHALEN, J.D. *et al.* 2001. Viral IL-10 gene transfer inhibits DTH responses to soluble antigens: evidence for involvement of genetically modified dendritic cells and macrophages. Mol. Ther. **4:** 543–550.
37. EDINGER, M. *et al.* 1999. Noninvasive assessment of tumor cell proliferation in animal models. Neoplasia **1:** 303–310.
38. CONTAG, C.H. *et al.* 1995. Photonic detection of bacterial pathogens in living hosts. Mol. Microbiol. **18:** 593–603.
39. ANDERSON, W.F., G.J. MCGARRITY & R.C. MOEN. 1993. Report to the NIH Recombinant DNA Advisory Committee on murine replication-competent retrovirus (RCR) assays (February 17, 1993). Hum. Gene Ther. **4:** 311–321.
40. MILLER, A.D. 1992. Human gene therapy comes of age. Nature **357:** 455–460.
41. EVANS, C.H. *et al.* 2000. Clinical trials in the gene therapy of arthritis. Clin. Orthop. Relat. Res. **379S:** 300–307.
42. ROBBINS, P.D., C.H. EVANS & Y. CHERNAJOVSKY. 1998. Gene therapy for rheumatoid arthritis. Springer Semin. Immunopathol. **20:** 197–209.

Specific Immunotherapy of Experimental Myasthenia by Genetically Engineered APCs

The "Guided Missile" Strategy

D. B. DRACHMAN, J-M. WU, A. MIAGKOV, M. A. WILLIAMS, R. N. ADAMS, AND B. WU

Neuromuscular Laboratory, Department of Neurology, Johns Hopkins School of Medicine, Baltimore, Maryland 21287-7519, USA

ABSTRACT: Although treatment of MG with general immunosuppressive agents is often effective, it has important drawbacks, including suppression of the immune system as a whole, with the risks of infection and neoplasia, and numerous other adverse side effects. Ideally, treatment of MG should eliminate the specific pathogenic autoimmune response to AChR, without otherwise suppressing the immune system or producing other adverse side effects. Although antibodies to AChR are directly responsible for the loss of AChRs at neuromuscular junctions in MG, the AChR antibody response is T cell–dependent, and immunotherapy directed at T cells can abrogate the autoantibody response, with resulting benefit. As in other autoimmune diseases, the T cell response in MG is highly heterogeneous. The design of specific immunotherapy must take this heterogeneity into account and target the entire repertoire of AChR-specific T cells. We describe our investigation of a novel strategy for specific immunotherapy of MG, involving gene transfer to convert antigen-presenting cells (APCs) to "guided missiles" that target AChR-specific T cells, and that induce apoptosis and elimination of those T cells. This strategy uses the ability of APCs from a given individual to present the entire spectrum of AChR epitopes unique for that individual, and thereby to target the entire repertoire of antigen-specific T cells of the same individual. Using viral vectors, we have genetically engineered the APCs to process and present the most important domain of the AChR molecule, and to express a "warhead" of Fas ligand (FasL) to eliminate the activated AChR-specific T cells with which they interact. Our results show that the APCs express the appropriate gene products, and effectively and specifically eliminate AChR-specific T cells by the Fas/FasL pathway, while sparing T cells of other specificities.

KEYWORDS: experimental myasthenia gravis; genetically engineered APCs; "guided missiles"; Fas ligand; specific immunotherapy

At present, the majority of patients with myasthenia gravis (MG) can be treated effectively and safely with conventional immunosuppressive agents, if used judiciously and skillfully. Agents that are in current clinical use include adrenal

Address for correspondence: D. B. Drachman, Neuromuscular Laboratory, Department of Neurology, Johns Hopkins School of Medicine, 600 N. Wolfe Street, Baltimore, MD 21287-7519. Voice: 410-955-5406; fax: 410-955-1961.
dandrac@aol.com

Ann. N.Y. Acad. Sci. 998: 520–532 (2003). © 2003 New York Academy of Sciences.
doi: 10.1196/annals.1254.068

corticosteroids, azathioprine, cyclosporin A, mycophenolate mofetil, and cyclophosphamide.[1–3] Newer agents, such as tacrolimus (FK506), rapamycin, and leflunomide, are being tested experimentally as well and may soon contribute to the practical treatment of MG. However, these agents have certain important drawbacks. The list of their potential adverse side effects is long, and treatment in most patients must be continued indefinitely.[2,4] Since they produce generalized suppression of the immune system, there is an increased risk of infection, or rarely of malignancy.

Ideally, treatment of MG should specifically delete the immune response to the autoantigen, acetylcholine receptor (AChR), while leaving the immune system otherwise intact. Treatment should avoid toxic side effects, and the results should be long-lasting or permanent. Although autoantibodies are directly responsible for the loss of AChRs at neuromuscular junctions in MG,[5–8] therapeutic strategies directed at AChR-specific B cells, such as those that have previously been described,[9–11] are not practicable in ongoing disease.[12] However, the AChR antibody response is T cell–dependent,[13–20] and immunotherapy directed at T cells can abrogate the autoantibody response, with resulting benefit.[1,21–23] An important challenge in designing specific immunotherapy for MG—and undoubtedly for other autoimmune diseases as well—is the marked heterogeneity that the T cell response presents. Each individual's T cells respond to multiple AChR epitopes, and there are significant differences in the patterns of epitopes to which different individuals' T cells respond, both in MG in humans[16,18,24–29] and in experimental MG (EAMG) in animals.[30–32] The design of specific immunotherapy must take this into account and allow targeting of the entire spectrum of AChR-specific T cells. Efforts to identify key pathogenic epitopes or T cell receptors in MG have generally been unrewarding because the inherent resourcefulness of the immune system results in a broad and unpredictable immune response. Even in animals inbred to have only a single MHC class II, there is significant heterogeneity of T cell responses to AChR.[32] The situation is much more complicated in humans since APCs of humans express 10 to 20 different MHC class II molecules, and the polymorphism of class II from individual to individual varies enormously.[33] A wide variety of different epitopes derived from the AChR subunits are recognized by T cells, and the repertoire of AChR-related T cells is therefore potentially very large. Thus, the prospect of actually identifying and targeting the T cells that are pathologically relevant in individual patients with MG is daunting. In designing a specific immunotherapeutic strategy for MG, the necessity to outguess the immune system can be avoided by using the individual's own immune system to target the AChR-specific T cells and turn off the autoimmune response. In that sense, it represents a kind of "immunological jiujitsu." We have devised a strategy using genetically engineered APCs as "missiles" to eliminate the AChR-specific T cells. The APC constitutes the missile body itself; a special AChR gene construct serves as the guidance system; and Fas ligand (FasL) is the payload or "warhead."

(1) *The individual's own APCs are used to target the AChR-specific T cells.* Since the natural function of APCs is to process and present a given antigen to the entire spectrum of that individual's antigen-specific T cells, the APCs can be co-opted to carry out the same function for the purpose of targeting the relevant T cells, and inhibiting rather than stimulating them.

(2) *The guidance system.* To guide the APCs to the AChR-specific T cells, we provide them with a gene construct consisting of the immunologically most impor-

tant part of the AChR molecule, plus signals that direct it to the APC's mechanism for processing and presentation.

(3) *The warhead.* In order to eliminate the targeted T cells, the APCs are armed with FasL, which is capable of inducing apoptosis of activated T cells. When activated, T cells express Fas on their surface membranes. Interaction of Fas with FasL induces activation of apoptosis-promoting caspase enzymes and results in elimination of the T cells.[34–36]

(4) *Viral vectors for gene transfer.* Transfer of the genes of interest into the APCs can be efficiently accomplished by the use of viral vectors. We initially used vaccinia virus (VV) for this purpose and are now developing more clinically suitable adeno-viral and adeno-associated viral vectors. VV has been used for more than 15 years as a vector for expression of genes in mammalian cells,[37] including APCs.[38] Vaccinia has several valuable characteristics, including (i) the ability to transfer multiple genes simultaneously; (ii) high level production of the proteins encoded by the transferred genes; (iii) the ability to be attenuated (by treatment with psoralen and UV light [PUVA]),[39,40] so that the VV does not replicate and therefore does not escape to infect other cells, but does direct expression of the gene products by the infected cells. We have learned that the need for attenuation and the cytopathic potential of vaccinia are somewhat limiting, leading to our current use of other viral vectors. However, VV has been been extremely useful in establishing proof of principle of the guided missile strategy.

ANTIGEN PRESENTATION: TARGETING OF T CELLS BY GENETICALLY ENGINEERED APCs

Under normal circumstances, APCs acquire antigen from the external environment, which is internalized and shunted to a trafficking pathway where it is processed. The antigen-derived peptides are combined with MHC class II, and the MHC class II/peptide complexes are presented on the APC's surface membrane. For our purpose of targeting the antigen-specific T cells, it is desirable for the APCs to present the antigen continuously. This can be accomplished by providing the APCs with a special gene construct that produces AChR internally and induces it to be processed and presented. For efficient processing and presentation, endogenously produced antigen must be flanked by peptides derived from the lysosomal-associated membrane protein (LAMP-1), consisting of a signal sequence (*sig*) and a transmembrane/cytoplasmic tail (*Tm*/*Cyt*). The *sig* sequence directs entry of the protein into the endoplasmic reticulum; the *Tm*/*Cyt* tail directs it into the endosomal/lysosomal processing compartment, where it enters the MHC class II trafficking pathway.[41–43] Although the exact nature of this pathway is unresolved, studies have demonstrated that routing antigen through the LAMP trafficking pathway of APCs results in highly efficient MHC class II presentation to $CD4^+$ T cells.[38,44,45] We prepared a chimeric gene construct consisting of the extracellular domain of the α subunit of *Torpedo* AChR flanked by *sig* at the 5′ end, and by LAMP-1 *Tm*/*Cyt* at the 3′ end. We then tested the ability of this construct to induce APCs to target and stimulate AChR-specific T cells. We transfected APCs derived from BALB/c mice (A20 cells) with the gene construct and coincubated them with an AChR-specific T cell line prepared, as previously described,[46] from BALB/c mice. Our results confirmed that APCs transfected with the AChR presentation gene construct powerfully stimulated the AChR-specific T cells. As few as 200 to 1000 transfected APCs were capable of maximally stimulating 2.5×10^4 AChR-specific T cells. Addition of exogenous AChR did not increase the [^{3}H]TdR incorporation in the cocultures. By contrast, T cells specific for an unrelated antigen (influenza hemagglutinin [HA]) were not stimulated by the transfected APCs. These results demonstrated that APCs engineered with the *sig*–AChR–LAMP-1 *Tm/Cyt* construct are capable of powerfully and uniquely targeting AChR-specific T cells.

FasL INDUCES LETHAL DAMAGE TO Fas-EXPRESSING CELLS

We next tested the ability of FasL to kill the activated T cells via Fas-FasL interaction. We added two different Fas-binding agents—soluble recombinant human FasL or antibody to mouse Fas—to cocultures of AChR-specific T cells that were stimulated as above with transfected APCs. The results showed that FasL or anti-Fas antibody inhibited T cell proliferation by 70% to 100%, indicating that the stimulated T cells are powerfully inhibited by Fas-FasL interaction.[47]

To evaluate the killing ability of cells genetically engineered to express FasL, we prepared a vaccinia virus vector with the gene for FasL by homologous recombination technology.[37,48] We used the FasL vaccinia vector to transduce mouse fibroblast cells (MC57G) and thereby induced highly efficient expression of FasL in over 80% of the cells. To test the functional activity of the FasL gene product expressed in this way, we used Fas-positive A20 lymphoblastoid cells as targets and cocultured them with the FasL-expressing MC57G cells. After overnight incubation, 40% to 80% of the target cells' DNA was fragmented, indicating that the recombinant VV effectively induced expression of functional FasL, leading to apoptosis of Fas-positive target cells.[48] In our current experiments, we have modified the FasL cDNA, as described by Tanaka,[49] to increase the potency of the expressed FasL, which is membrane bound, rather than being secreted.

THE GUIDANCE SYSTEM AND THE WARHEAD MUST BE IN THE SAME APC

It is essential that the key components of the guided missile be delivered at the same time, rather than separately. Thus, if AChR were presented by APCs that did not also express FasL, it would result in stimulation of AChR-specific T cells, thereby increasing—rather than inhibiting—the autoimmune response. On the other hand, if FasL were expressed by APCs in the absence of AChR presentation, the APCs might target and kill unrelated T cells, or nonimmunologic Fas-expressing cells, such as hepatocytes.[50] The viral vectors that we are using in these experiments—VV, adenovirus, and adeno-associated virus—can all induce expression of at least two gene constructs.

PROTECTION OF APCs FROM FasL-INDUCED "SUICIDE"

We initially used splenocytes depleted of T cells as APCs. This cell population is enriched in B cells, which are vulnerable to FasL-mediated cell death (Wu *et al.*, unpublished results). To use these cells as guided missiles, they must be protected from self-destruction by the FasL warhead they carry. To develop a robust strategy for preventing Fas-mediated death of APCs, we relied on studies of the role of FADD (Fas-associated death domain).[51,52] The FADD protein is directly associated with the cytoplasmic portion of Fas and normally participates as an intermediary in the Fas-mediated cell death pathway. However, a truncated form of FADD lacking amino acids 1–79 can powerfully inhibit Fas-mediated cell death.[51,52] To avoid Fas-mediated self-destruction of the APCs, we obtained cDNA for this truncated FADD (TrFADD) mutant (gift of V. Dixit, Genentech) and recombined it as a third gene in our vaccinia vector, which already contained the gene construct for presentation of antigen, and the gene for FasL. We have used APCs transduced with this 3-gene VV as our guided missiles.

GUIDED MISSILE APCs KILL ONLY THE TARGETED T CELLS

We carried out critical experiments to evaluate the specificity of T cell killing by guided missile APCs.[53] We first prepared a dually specific rat T cell line by immunizing rats with both AChR and an unrelated antigen, keyhole limpet hemocyanin (KLH), in complete Freund's adjuvant. Six weeks later, the lymph nodes were removed and lymphocytes were stimulated in culture with optimal concentrations of both AChR and KLH, and then expanded in medium containing IL2. This dually specific T cell line responded with closely similar proliferation when stimulated with either antigen alone (AChR or KLH) in the presence of added APCs. We prepared AChR-specific guided missile APCs as follows. Vaccinia vectors with three genes, (1) *sig*–AChRα1–210–LAMP-1 *Tm*/*Cyt*, (2) FasL, and (3) TrFADD, were attenuated with PUVA and used to transduce rat splenic APCs. Two types of control APCs were also prepared: one was transduced with VV that contained only the targeting gene construct *sig*–AChRα1–210–LAMP-1 *Tm*/*Cyt*; the other was infected with wild-type vaccinia. The dually specific AChR + KLH T cell line was coincubated for 48 hours with APCs infected with each of these three VV preparations. At the end of the coculture period, the live T cells were harvested and tested for their ability to proliferate in response to stimulation with either AChR or KLH, with fresh rat splenocytes added as APCs. The results (FIG. 1) showed that T cells that had been coincubated with the AChR 3-gene VV did not proliferate in response to exogenous AChR, with only a background level of $[^3H]$TdR incorporation. In contrast, stimulation with KLH resulted in a strong proliferative response, with only a 14% reduction in Δcpm. This demonstrates the functional ability of APCs transduced with the AChR 3-gene VV (i.e., guided missiles) to eliminate the T cell AChR response, presumably by inducing apoptosis of AChR-specific T cells. Most important, it shows the specificity of the effect since the KLH-specific T cells were virtually unaffected even *in vitro*, where the effector and T cells were in close proximity. T cells from control cultures that had been coincubated with APCs transduced with the stimulating gene construct, *sig*–AChRα1–210–LAMP-1 *Tm*/*Cyt*, or

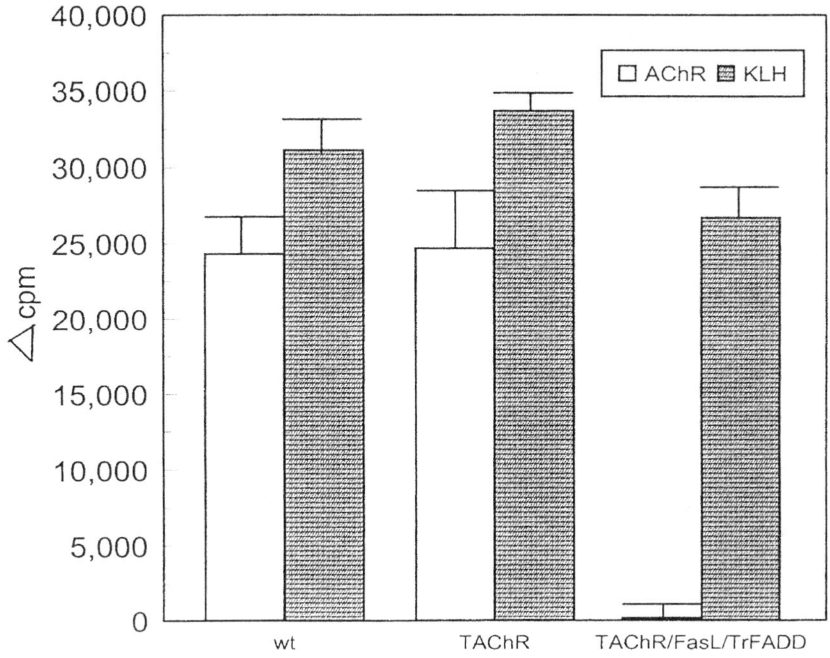

FIGURE 1. Specificity of 3-gene VV "guided missiles". A Lewis rat T cell line that was dually specific for AChR and for KLH was coincubated for two days with APCs transduced with (1) wild-type [wt] VV, (2) VV with *sig*–AChRα1–210–LAMP-1 *Tm*/*Cyt* [TAChR], or (3) the 3-gene "guided missile" VV (*sig*–AChRα1–210–LAMP-1 *Tm*/*Cyt*; FasL; and TrFADD). The T cells from each coculture were restimulated with either AChR or KLH, in the presence of fresh rat splenic APCs, and pulsed with [^{3}H]TdR. Note that coincubation with the guided missile APCs eliminated the AChR-specific T cell response, but only minimally affected the KLH-specific T cell response. This figure is reproduced with permission of ref. 53.

infected with control wild-type VV, proliferated normally in response to AChR stimulation. These controls confirmed that elimination of AChR-specific T cells by the guided missile 3-gene APCs could not be attributed either to the VV itself or to prior stimulation by AChR-presenting APCs. The latter control is especially important because it excludes the possibility that the effect was due to AICD (activation induced cell death).

CELL DEATH INDUCED BY GUIDED MISSILES IS MEDIATED BY THE FAS/FASL PATHWAY

We used mutant mice lacking Fas (*lpr*/*lpr* mice) to evaluate the role of FasL in killing AChR-specific T cells. Since *lpr*/*lpr* mice do not express Fas, their T cells should not be killed by FasL. We prepared AChR-specific T cell lines in parallel, derived from *lpr*/*lpr* mice (on a C57Bl/6 background) and from congenic wild-type

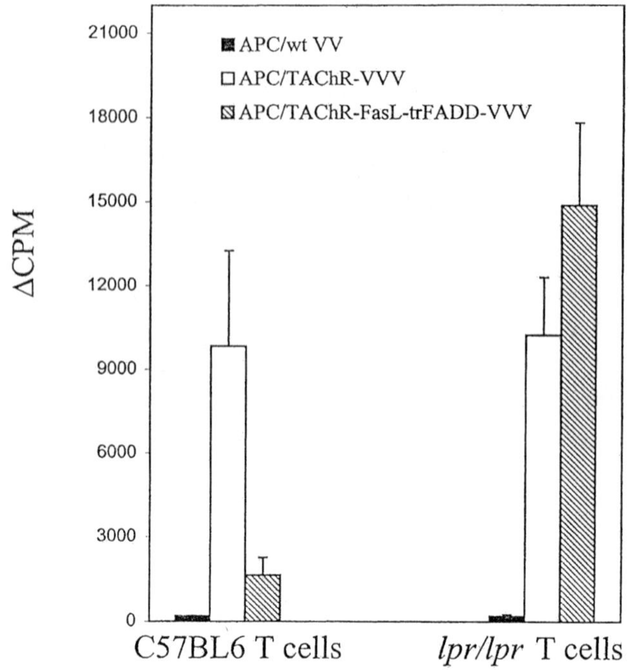

FIGURE 2. Essential role of FasL in elimination of AChR-specific T cells by 3-gene "guided missile". AChR-specific T cell lines were prepared from C57Bl/6 mice or *lpr*/*lpr* mice (lacking Fas expression). APCs from C57Bl/6 mice were transduced with (1) wild-type [wt] VV, (2) VV with *sig*–AChRα1–210–LAMP-1 *Tm*/*Cyt* [TAChR], or (3) the 3-gene "guided missile" VV (*sig*–AChRα1–210–LAMP-1 *Tm*/*Cyt*; FasL; and TrFADD). These APCs were coincubated with the AChR-specific T cells from C57Bl/6 mice or *lpr*/*lpr* mice for 5 days, followed by pulsing with [^{3}H]TdR. Note that the T cells from C57Bl/6 mice were markedly inhibited by the guided missiles, while T cells from *lpr*/*lpr* mice were not inhibited and were actually stimulated by the guided missiles. Lacking Fas, the *lpr*/*lpr* T cells are not subject to apoptosis induced by FasL. This demonstrates the essential role of FasL in the effect of the guided missiles. This figure is reproduced with permission of ref. 53.

C57Bl/6 mice, as previously described.[46] We transduced spleen cells from naïve C57Bl/6 mice with the same attenuated VVs as above and coincubated them with AChR-specific T cells from the C57Bl/6 T cell line or the *lpr*/*lpr* T cell line. The results (FIG. 2) showed that APCs with the control wild-type VV had no intrinsic stimulatory or inhibitory effect on either C57Bl/6 T cells or *lpr* T cells. APCs transduced with the stimulatory AChR VV (*sig*–AChR–LAMP-1 *Tm*/*Cyt*) stimulated both the C57Bl/6 T cell line and the *lpr* T cell line. APCs transduced with the 3-gene VV inhibited the C57Bl/6 line dramatically. By contrast, they did not inhibit the *lpr* line cells, but instead stimulated them. These findings indicate that the inhibitory effect of APCs transduced with the 3-gene VV is due to its expressed FasL, which interacts with Fas-expressing T cells to cause apoptosis.

THE GUIDED MISSILE CAN BE USED TO ELIMINATE T CELLS OF OTHER SPECIFICITIES

We tested the effectiveness of the guided missile strategy in eliminating T cells specific for HA, an antigen that is unrelated to AChR. For this purpose, VV were prepared with the targeting construct consisting of cDNA for HA, rather than for AChR. HA-specific T cells were obtained from BALB/c mice that were transgenic for the α and β chains of the T cell receptor for HA.[54] Approximately 40% to 60% of $CD4^+$ T cells from these mice express HA-specific T cell receptors. Guided missile APCs that were transduced with 3-gene VV specific for HA induced apoptosis of HA-specific T cells, characterized by fragmentation of DNA, and marked inhibition of proliferation of HA-specific T cells.[48] In contrast, T cells specific for an unrelated antigen (ovalbumin) were not affected by coincubation with the HA-specific APCs, demonstrating antigen specificity of the effect in the HA system. A time course experiment demonstrated that the HA-specific T cells were first stimulated and then killed by the guided missiles.[48] This is consistent with the concept that the T cells must be activated to be killed by the Fas-FasL pathway.

IN VIVO EFFECT OF GUIDED MISSILES

In a preliminary experiment, we injected a limited number of HA transgenic mice with either 5×10^7 3-gene APCs or with an equal number of APCs transduced with FasL and TrFADD (but not the HA-LAMP targeting construct). Two days after injection with the 3-gene guided missile APCs, the percentage of HA-specific $CD4^+$ T cells fell to 9.4% and gradually increased to 24.5% by 8 days (FIG. 3, top). A mouse that was injected with the FasL/TrFADD APCs showed only a modest decrease of HA-specific $CD4^+$ cells to ~40% at 5 and 8 days. Twelve days after injection of the APCs, the mice were killed, and proliferation of lymph node cells and splenocytes was tested after stimulation with HA *in vitro* (FIG. 3, bottom). Proliferation of lymph node cells was reduced by more than twofold, and proliferation of splenocytes was reduced by more than threefold, as compared with responses of lymphocytes from control mice. Although these are only preliminary results in a very limited experiment, they suggest that the guided missile strategy should be useful *in vivo*. Further, they suggest that a single treatment may have an incomplete effect and may need to be repeated in order to be most effective.

WORK IN PROGRESS

As noted above, there are certain limitations imposed by the use of splenocytes as APCs and by our choice of VV as the vehicle for gene transfer. Splenic APCs consist of a mixed population of B cells, macrophages, dendritic cells (DCs), and T cells. For use as APCs, they must first be depleted of T cells. B cells are vulnerable to killing by FasL, requiring protection by the use of TrFADD. Finally, there is no comparable population of APCs for use in human immunotherapy. Fortunately, it is now possible to obtain large numbers of DCs, both from experimental animals and from humans.

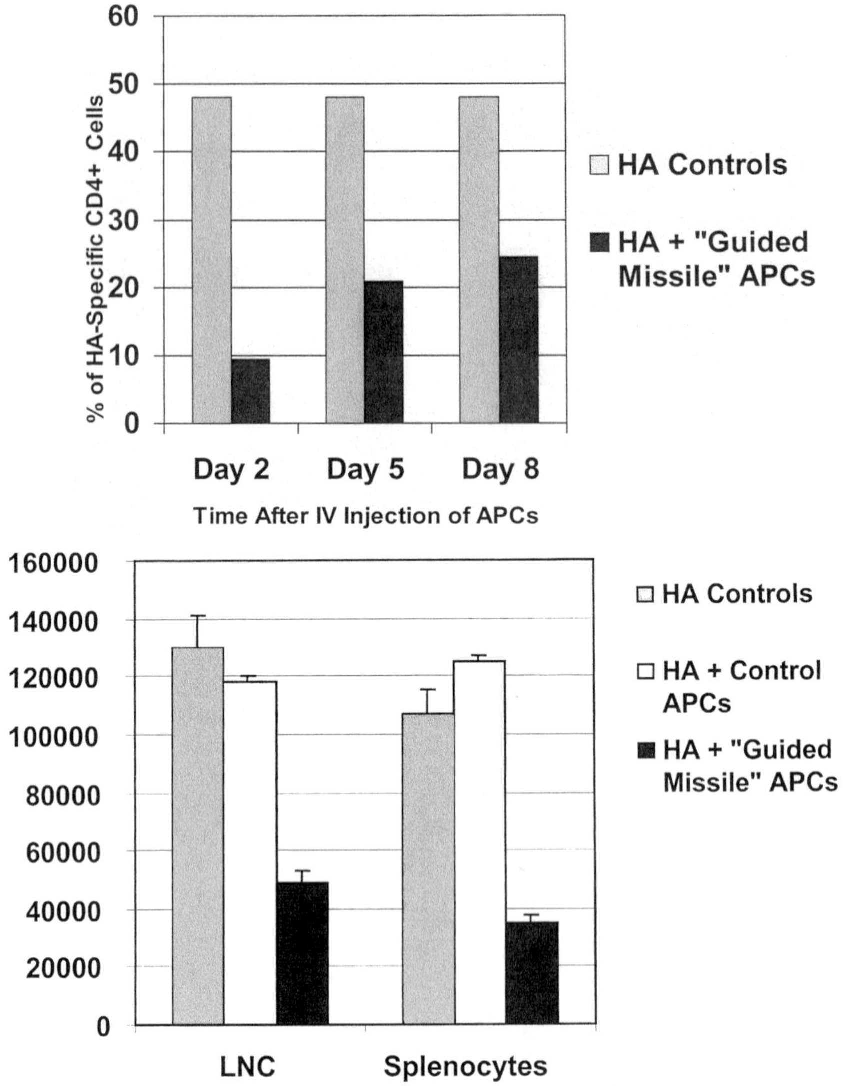

FIGURE 3. *In vivo* effects of "guided missiles". HA-specific "guided missiles" were prepared by transducing splenic APCs from BALB/c mice with 3-gene VV (see text). Control APCs were transduced with FasL + TrFADD. HA-transgenic mice were injected with 5×10^7 of these cells. **(Top)** The percentage of HA-specific $CD4^+$ T cells in peripheral blood was evaluated by flow cytometry, using the clonotypic mAb 6.5 and anti-CD4 antibody, at three time points. Note the marked decrease in HA-specific T cells as compared with control untreated HA transgenic mice. **(Bottom)** Twelve days after injection of the transduced APCs, the mice were killed, and proliferation of lymph node cells (LNC) or splenocytes in response to AChR was measured. Note the marked reduction of T cell proliferation after injection of 3-gene "guided missile" APCs.

Dendritic Cells Have Several Advantages

DCs are the most efficient professional APCs.[55] A relatively uniform population of cells can be obtained by culture of bone marrow cells or peripheral monocytic cells.[56,57] DCs are not as vulnerable to apoptosis by FasL. On the other hand, DCs have the disadvantage of being damaged or killed by infection with VV. For the above reasons, we have decided to switch to the use of DCs as APCs in our animal experiments. Vaccinia has two major disadvantages: It must be attenuated with PUVA to prevent unwanted replication. This treatment reduces its transduction efficiency and is difficult to reproduce in a uniform manner. Second, VV damages DCs and thus cannot be used to transduce them. In contrast to VV, adenovirus does not damage DCs and has been used previously to transduce DCs.[58] Furthermore, "defective" adenoviral vectors that are capable of infecting cells, but do not proliferate except in special packaging cell lines, are in general use for gene transfer. At present, we have invested considerable time and effort in developing the methods for culturing and expanding mouse DCs, and for producing adenoviral vectors that can transfer the AChR targeting gene construct plus the gene for FasL. Preliminary studies show that the adenoviral vector with the targeting gene construct is effective in transducing DCs, which then stimulate AChR-specific T cells. Our current goals are to test the adenoviral vectors and DCs first *in vitro* and then to use them *in vivo*. For the *in vivo* studies, we have also developed a transgenic mouse with a high proportion of T cells that express receptors specific for the immunodominant epitope of *Torpedo* AChR[59] (also see Miagkov *et al.*, this volume). In the future, we plan to use the adeno-associated virus (AAV), which is safer, in human subjects.[60]

CONCLUSIONS

Thus far, we have clearly demonstrated proof of principle for the guided missile strategy. *Targeting*: The *sig*–AChR–LAMP *Tm*/*Cyt* construct uniquely stimulates AChR-specific T cells. *FasL warhead*: The FasL gene is expressed after gene transfer and is functionally effective in killing Fas-expressing cells. *Specificity*: Only antigen-specific T cells are killed by the guided missile APCs. *Viral vector*: Vaccinia transfers genes effectively. Likewise, adenovirally transferred genes are expressed and effective. *In vivo effect*: In preliminary experiments, guided missile APCs reduce the percent of antigen-specific $CD4^+$ cells.

SCHEME FOR USE IN HUMAN MG

Although the *ex vivo* gene transfer treatment scheme must be custom-tailored to the individual patient, it is no more labor-intensive or risky than many other medical and surgical procedures that are now considered virtually routine.[61] We envision the plan as follows: The patient's lymphocytes are collected by leukopheresis. DCs are expanded from this population by culture. They are transduced *ex vivo* using the viral vector (adenovirus or AAV). The transduced DCs are then reinfused. This procedure can be repeated as necessary to achieve clinically beneficial results.

ACKNOWLEDGMENTS

This work was supported by the NIH (Grant Nos. R01NS40778 and NS07368) and the Muscular Dystrophy Association. Generous support was provided by the C. W. Parke Family Foundation, the Ann and Donald Brown Family Foundation, and the Eleanor Denmead Ingram Foundation.

REFERENCES

1. DRACHMAN, D.B. 1996. Immunotherapy in neuromuscular disorders: current and future strategies. Muscle Nerve **19:** 1239–1251.
2. DRACHMAN, D.B. 1999. The ten most frequently asked questions about myasthenia gravis. Neurologist **5:** 350–355.
3. CHAUDHRY, V.V., D.R. CORNBLATH, J.W. GRIFFIN *et al.* 2001. Mycophenolate mofetil: a safe and promising immunosuppressant in neuromuscular diseases. Neurology **56:** 94–96.
4. HOHLFELD, R. & K.V. TOYKA. 1993. Therapies. *In* Myasthenia Gravis, pp. 235–261. CRC Press. Boca Raton, FL.
5. KAO, I. & D.B. DRACHMAN. 1977. Myasthenic immunoglobulin accelerates acetylcholine receptor degradation. Science **196:** 527–529.
6. TOYKA, K.V., D.B. DRACHMAN, D.E. GRIFFIN *et al.* 1977. Myasthenia gravis: study of humoral immune mechanisms by passive transfer to mice. N. Engl. J. Med. **296:** 125–131.
7. DRACHMAN, D.B., C.W. ANGUS, R.N. ADAMS *et al.* 1978. Myasthenic antibodies cross-link acetylcholine receptors to accelerate degradation. N. Engl. J. Med. **298:** 1116–1122.
8. PINCHING, A., D. PETERS & J. NEWSOM-DAVIS. 1976. Remission of myasthenia gravis following plasma exchange. Lancet **2:** 1373–1376.
9. STERZ, R.K., G. BIRO, K. RAJKI *et al.* 1985. Experimental autoimmune myasthenia gravis: can pretreatment with ^{125}I-labeled receptor prevent functional damage at the neuromuscular junction? J. Immunol. **134:** 841–846.
10. OLSBERG, C.A., T.M. MIKITEN & K.A. KROLICK. 1985. Selective *in vitro* inhibition of an antibody response to purified acetylcholine receptor by using antigen-ricin A chain immunotoxin. J. Immunol. **135:** 3062–3067.
11. KILLEN, J.A. & J.M. LINDSTROM. 1984. Specific killing of lymphocytes that cause experimental autoimmune myasthenia gravis by ricin toxin–acetylcholine receptor conjugates. J. Immunol. **133:** 2549–2553.
12. DRACHMAN, D.B. 1998. Myasthenia gravis. *In* The Autoimmune Diseases, pp. 637–662. Academic Press. San Diego.
13. CONTI-FINE, B.M., M.P. PROTTI, M. BELLONE & J.F. HOWARD. 1997. Myasthenia Gravis: The Immunobiology of an Autoimmune Disease. Neuroscience Intelligence Unit. R. G. Landes Co. Austin.
14. LENNON, V.A., J.M. LINDSTROM & M.E. SEYBOLD. 1976. Experimental autoimmune myasthenia gravis: cellular and humoral immune responses. Ann. N.Y. Acad. Sci. **274:** 283–289.
15. RICHMAN, D.P., J.P. ANTEL, J.W. PATRICK & B.G. ARNASON. 1979. Cellular immunity to acetylcholine receptor in myasthenia gravis: relationship to histocompatibility type and antigenic site. Neurology **29:** 291–296.
16. BROCKE, S., C. BRAUTBAR *et al.* 1988. *In vitro* proliferative responses and antibody titers specific to human acetylcholine receptor synthetic peptides in patients with myasthenia gravis and relation to HLA class II genes. J. Clin. Invest. **82:** 1894–1900.
17. HOHLFELD, R., K.V. TOYKA, M. MICHELS *et al.* 1987. Acetylcholine receptor–specific human T-lymphocyte lines. Ann. N.Y. Acad. Sci. **505:** 27–37.
18. NEWSOM-DAVIS, J., G. HARCOURT, N. SOMMER *et al.* 1989. T-cell reactivity in myasthenia gravis. J. Autoimmun. **2**(suppl.)**:** 101–108.
19. WANG, Z.Y., D.K. OKITA, J. HOWARD, JR. & B.M. CONTI-FINE. 1997. Th1 epitope repertoire on the alpha subunit of human muscle acetylcholine receptor in myasthenia gravis. Neurology **48:** 1643–1653.

20. KAUL, R., M. SHENOY, E. GOLUSZKO & P. CHRISTADOSS. 1994. Major histocompatibility complex class II gene disruption prevents experimental autoimmune myasthenia gravis. J. Immunol. **152:** 3152–3157.
21. WRAITH, D.C., H.O. MCDEVITT, L. STEINMAN & H. ACHA-ORBEA. 1989. T cell recognition as the target for immune intervention in autoimmune disease. Cell **57:** 709–715.
22. MCINTOSH, K.R., P.S. LINSLEY, P.A. BACHA & D.B. DRACHMAN. 1998. Immunotherapy of experimental autoimmune myasthenia gravis: selective effects of CTLA4Ig and synergistic combination with an IL2-diphtheria toxin fusion protein. J. Neuroimmunol. **87:** 136–146.
23. CHRISTADOSS, P. & M.J. DAUPHINEE. 1986. Immunotherapy for myasthenia gravis: a murine model. J. Immunol. **136:** 2437–2440.
24. HOHLFELD, R., K.V. TOYKA, L.L. MINER *et al.* 1988. Amphipathic segment of the nicotinic receptor alpha subunit contains epitopes recognized by T lymphocytes in myasthenia gravis. J. Clin. Invest. **81:** 657–660.
25. OSHIMA, M., T. ASHIZAWA, M.S. POLLACK & M.Z. ATASSI. 1990. Autoimmune T cell recognition of human acetylcholine receptor: the sites of T cell recognition in myasthenia gravis on the extracellular part of the alpha subunit. Eur. J. Immunol. **20:** 2563–2569.
26. MELMS, A., G. MALCHEREK, U. GERN *et al.* 1992. T cells from normal and myasthenic individuals recognize the human acetylcholine receptor: heterogeneity of antigenic sites on the alpha-subunit. Ann. Neurol. **31:** 311–318.
27. MOIOLA, L., M.P. PROTTI, A.A. MANFREDI *et al.* 1993. T-helper epitopes on human nicotinic acetylcholine receptor in myasthenia gravis. Ann. N.Y. Acad. Sci. **681:** 198–218.
28. PROTTI, M.P., A.A. MANFREDI, R.M. HORTON *et al.* 1993. Myasthenia gravis: recognition of a human autoantigen at the molecular level [see comments]. Immunol. Today **14:** 363–368.
29. NAVANEETHAM, D., A.S. PENN, J. HOWARD & B.M. CONTI-FINE. 1998. TCR-Vbeta usage in the thymus and blood of myasthenia gravis patients. J. Autoimmun. **11:** 621–633.
30. YEH, T.M. & K.A. KROLICK. 1987. Influence of T cell specificity on the heterogeneity and disease-causing capability of antibody against the acetylcholine receptor. J. Neuroimmunol. **17:** 17–34.
31. INFANTE, A.J., P.A. THOMPSON, K.A. KROLICK & K.A. WALL. 1991. Determinant selection in murine experimental autoimmune myasthenia gravis: effect of the bm12 mutation on T cell recognition of acetylcholine receptor epitopes. J. Immunol. **146:** 2977–2982.
32. YANG, B., K.R. MCINTOSH & D.B. DRACHMAN. 1998. How subtle differences in MHC class II affect the severity of experimental myasthenia gravis. Clin. Immunol. Immunopathol. **86:** 45–58.
33. ABBAS, A.K., A.H. LICHTMAN & J.S. POBER. 2000. Cellular and Molecular Immunology. Saunders. Philadelphia.
34. ALDERSON, M.R., R.J. ARMITAGE, E. MARASKOVSKY *et al.* 1993. Fas transduces activation signals in normal human T lymphocytes. J. Exp. Med. **178:** 2231–2235.
35. DRAPPA, J., N. BROT & K.B. ELKON. 1993. The Fas protein is expressed at high levels on CD4+CD8+ thymocytes and activated mature lymphocytes in normal mice, but not in the lupus-prone strain, MRL lpr/lpr. Proc. Natl. Acad. Sci. USA **90:** 10340–10344.
36. BOISE, L.H. & C.B. THOMPSON. 1996. Hierarchical control of lymphocyte survival. Science **274:** 67–68.
37. MACKETT, M., G. SMITH & B. MOSS. 1982. Vaccinia virus: a selectable eukaryotic cloning and expression vector. Proc. Natl. Acad. Sci. USA **79:** 7415–7419.
38. WU, T.C., F.G. GUARNIERI, K.F. STAVELEY-O'CARROLL *et al.* 1995. Engineering an intracellular pathway for major histocompatibility complex class II presentation of antigens. Proc. Natl. Acad. Sci. USA **92:** 11671–11675.
39. TSUNG, K., J.H. YIM, W. MARTI *et al.* 1996. Gene expression and cytopathic effect of vaccinia virus inactivated by psoralen and long-wave UV light. J. Virol. **70:** 165–171.
40. OERTLI, D., W.R. MARTI, J.A. NORTON & K. TSUNG. 1996. Non-replicating recombinant vaccinia virus encoding murine B-7 molecules elicits effective costimulation of naive $CD4^+$ splenocytes *in vitro*. J. Gen. Virol. **77:** 3121–3125.

41. CHEN, J.W., Y. CHA, K.U. YUKSEL *et al.* 1988. Isolation and sequencing of a cDNA clone encoding lysosomal membrane glycoprotein mouse LAMP-1: sequence similarity to proteins bearing onco-differentiation antigens. J. Biol. Chem. **263:** 8754–8758.
42. GUARNIERI, F.G., L.M. ARTERBURN, M.B. PENNO *et al.* 1993. The motif Tyr-X-X-hydrophobic residue mediates lysosomal membrane targeting of lysosome-associated membrane protein 1. J. Biol. Chem. **268:** 1941–1946.
43. MELLMAN, I., P. PIERRE & S. AMIGORENA. 1995. Lonely MHC molecules seeking immunogenic peptides for meaningful relationships. Curr. Opin. Cell Biol. **7:** 564–572.
44. ROWELL, J.F., A.L. RUFF, F.G. GUARNIERI *et al.* 1995. Lysosome-associated membrane protein-1-mediated targeting of the HIV-1 envelope protein to an endosomal/lysosomal compartment enhances its presentation to MHC class II–restricted T cells. J. Immunol. **155:** 1818–1828.
45. NAIR, S.K., D. BOCZKOWSKI, M. MORSE *et al.* 1998. Induction of primary carcinoembryonic antigen (CEA)–specific cytotoxic T lymphocytes *in vitro* using human dendritic cells transfected with RNA. Nat. Biotechnol. **16:** 364–369.
46. MCINTOSH, K.R., P.S. LINSLEY & D.B. DRACHMAN. 1995. Immunosuppression and induction of anergy by CTLA4Ig *in vitro*: effects on cellular and antibody responses of lymphocytes from rats with experimental autoimmune myasthenia gravis. Cell. Immunol. **166:** 103–112.
47. WU, J.M., B. WU, F. GUARNIERI *et al.* 2000. Targeting antigen-specific T cells by genetically engineered antigen presenting cells: a strategy for specific immunotherapy of autoimmune disease. J. Neuroimmunol. **106:** 145–153.
48. WU, B., J.M. WU, A. MIAGKOV *et al.* 2001. Specific immunotherapy by genetically engineered APCs: the "guided missile" strategy. J. Immunol. **166:** 4773–4779.
49. TANAKA, M., T. ITAI, M. ADACHI & S. NAGATA. 1998. Downregulation of Fas ligand by shedding [see comments]. Nat. Med. **4:** 31–36.
50. GREEN, D.R. & C.F. WARE. 1997. Fas-ligand: privilege and peril. Proc. Natl. Acad. Sci. USA **94:** 5986–5990.
51. CHINNAIYAN, A.M., K. O'ROURKE, M. TEWARI & V.M. DIXIT. 1995. FADD, a novel death domain–containing protein, interacts with the death domain of Fas and initiates apoptosis. Cell **81:** 505–512.
52. HSU, H., H.B. SHU, M.G. PAN & D.V. GOEDDEL. 1996. TRADD-TRAF2 and TRADD-FADD interactions define two distinct TNF receptor 1 signal transduction pathways. Cell **84:** 299–308.
53. WU, J.M., B. WU, A. MIAGKOV *et al.* 2001. Specific immunotherapy of experimental myasthenia gravis *in vitro*: the "guided missile" strategy. Cell. Immunol. **208:** 137–147.
54. STAVELEY-O'CARROLL, K., E. SOTOMAYOR, J. MONTGOMERY *et al.* 1998. Induction of antigen-specific T cell anergy: an early event in the course of tumor progression. Proc. Natl. Acad. Sci. USA **95:** 1178–1183.
55. STEINMAN, R.M. 1991. The dendritic cell system and its role in immunogenicity. Annu. Rev. Immunol. **9:** 271–296.
56. HILL, M.E., D.J. FERGUSON J.M. AUSTYN *et al.* 1999. Potent immunostimulatory dendritic cells can be cultured in bulk from progenitors in normal infant and adult myasthenic human thymus. Immunology **97:** 325–332.
57. MIN, Y.H., S.T. LEE, K.M. CHOI *et al.* 1998. *Ex vivo* generation of functional dendritic cells from mobilized CD34+ hematopoietic stem cells. Yonsei Med. J. **39:** 328–338.
58. ZHANG, H.G., D. LIU, Y. HEIKE *et al.* 1998. Induction of specific T-cell tolerance by adenovirus-transfected, Fas ligand–producing antigen presenting cells [see comments]. Nat. Biotechnol. **16:** 1045–1049.
59. LOBITO, A.A., B. YANG, M.F. LOPES *et al.* 2002. T cell receptor transgenic mice recognizing the immunodominant epitope of the *Torpedo californica* acetylcholine receptor. Eur. J. Immunol. **32:** 2055–2067.
60. KAPTURCZAK, M.H., T. FLOTTE & M.A. ATKINSON. 2001. Adeno-associated virus (AAV) as a vehicle for therapeutic gene delivery: improvements in vector design and viral production enhance potential to prolong graft survival in pancreatic islet cell transplantation for the reversal of type 1 diabetes. Curr. Mol. Med. **1:** 245–258.
61. PAP, T., R.E. GAY, U. MULLER-LADNER & S. GAY. 2002. *Ex vivo* gene transfer in the years to come. Arthritis Res. **4:** 10–12.

Suppression of Myasthenia Gravis by Antigen-Specific Mucosal Tolerance and Modulation of Cytokines and Costimulatory Factors

MIRIAM C. SOUROUJON,[a,b] PRASANTA K. MAITI,[a] TALI FEFERMAN,[a] SIN-HYEOG IM,[a,c] LILY RAVEH,[d] AND SARA FUCHS[a]

[a]*Department of Immunology, Weizmann Institute of Science, Rehovot 76100, Israel*

[b]*Open University of Israel, Tel Aviv 61392, Israel*

ABSTRACT: We have shown that mucosal administration of recombinant fragments corresponding to the human acetylcholine receptor (AChR) α subunit suppresses chronic ongoing experimental autoimmune myasthenia gravis (EAMG) in rats. Treated animals exhibit a Th1 to Th2/Th3 shift in their cytokine profile and downregulation of costimulatory factors. However, application of a xenogeneic recombinant fragment may have limitations when considered as a possible approach for the treatment of MG in humans. We therefore tested the potential of a syngeneic fragment and of long synthetic peptides to suppress EAMG. We found that a syngeneic fragment corresponding to the extracellular region of the rat AChR α subunit was as effective as the formerly described human xenogeneic fragment in suppressing ongoing EAMG. This is encouraging in view of the potential use of mucosally administered recombinant AChR fragments for the treatment of MG in humans. However, in severely affected individuals, this antigen-specific approach may need to be supported by direct modulation of cytokines and costimulatory factors known to be involved in the pathogenesis of EAMG. To test the potential of this approach, myasthenic rats were injected by antibodies either to the proinflammatory cytokine IL-18 or to the costimulatory factor CD40L. These treatments act via different mechanisms, but both lead to the alleviation of clinical symptoms even when given at the chronic phase of EAMG. We suggest that antagonists to key cytokines and/or costimulatory factors be used to augment antigen-specific treatments of myasthenia such as mucosal administration of AChR recombinant fragments.

KEYWORDS: mucosal tolerance; cytokines; costimulatory factors; syngeneic recombinant fragments; synthetic peptides; suppression of ongoing EAMG

Address for correspondence: Prof. Miriam C. Souroujon, Open University of Israel, 16 Klausner Street, Tel Aviv 61392, Israel. Voice: +972-3-6460233; fax: +972-3-6465465.
miriso@oumail.openu.ac.il

[c]Permanent address: S-H. Im, Department of Life Science, Kwangju Institute of Science and Technology, Kwangju 500-712, Korea.

[d]Permanent address: L. Raveh, Israel Institute for Biological Research, Ness-Ziona 74100, Israel.

Ann. N.Y. Acad. Sci. 998: 533–536 (2003). © 2003 New York Academy of Sciences.
doi: 10.1196/annals.1254.069

SUPPRESSION OF ONGOING EAMG BY A SYNGENEIC AChR RECOMBINANT FRAGMENT

We have recently shown that experimental autoimmune myasthenia gravis (EAMG) in rats could be suppressed by mucosal administration of a recombinant fragment (Hα1–205) corresponding to the extracellular domain of the human acetylcholine receptor (AChR) α subunit.[1–3] This treatment is effective when initiated at the acute or even at the chronic phase of disease and is accompanied by a shift of the anti-AChR immune response from Th1 to Th2/Th3 regulation. The application of a xenogeneic AChR fragment may have limitations for the future treatment of MG in humans. We have thus investigated the possibility of suppressing EAMG in rats by oral administration of a syngeneic recombinant AChR fragment, rat α1–205 (Rα1–205). Rats were fed with 1 mg/rat of Rα1–205 on alternate days starting either at the acute phase or at the chronic phase of EAMG (1 and 4 weeks after EAMG induction, respectively) and were followed for clinical signs and weight loss.

Oral administration of Rα1–205 led to significant suppression of EAMG. T cell proliferative responses to AChR were decreased in Rα1–205-treated rats as compared to ovalbumin-treated controls, but overall anti-AChR IgG levels were not reduced (in contrast to what we observed in rats fed by the xenogeneic fragment Hα1–205). The underlying mechanism of immunomodulation by Rα1–205 was similar, but not identical, to that of the xenogeneic human fragment. It induced a shift from a Th1 response to Th2 regulation as evidenced by a decreased AChR-specific delayed-type hypersensitivity response, upregulated mRNA expression level of IL-10, and down-regulated IL-2, IFN-γ, and TNFα levels. There was no elevation of the Th3-type cytokine TGF-β, which was increased in Hα1–205-treated rats. Moreover, IgG1, which is regulated by Th2-type cells in rats, was found to be significantly increased, and IgG2a, regulated by Th1-type cells, was decreased in rats treated with Rα1–205 starting at the acute phase. In addition, reduced expression levels of CD28 at both treatment protocols (acute and chronic) and CTLA4 and B7.1 levels at the acute phase treatment protocol suggest that the CD28/CTLA4:B7.1 signaling pathway, which is thought to deliver a Th1 response,[4,5] is less effective in rats treated with Rα1–205. The ability of a syngeneic fragment of AChR to suppress EAMG as effectively as the formerly described xenogeneic human fragment is encouraging in view of its potential application for the treatment of MG in humans.

PREVENTION OF EAMG BY LONG PEPTIDES CORRESPONDING TO THE EXTRACELLULAR DOMAIN OF THE AChR α SUBUNIT

If we consider the preparation of a future antigen-specific drug for therapy of human patients with MG, peptides would have a clear advantage over recombinant fragments. We therefore addressed the question whether mucosal administration of a mixture of long, partially overlapping, peptides (50–60 amino acids long) covering the entire extracellular portion of the α subunit would have a suppressive effect on EAMG. We first tested the ability of such a mixture to protect rats against subsequently induced EAMG. The peptide mixture was administered to rats either nasally (1 or 25 μg/rat on 12 consecutive days) or orally (0.5 or 1.5 mg/rat on 6 alternating days) prior to *Torpedo* AChR injection for EAMG induction. Nasal administration of the peptide mixture before EAMG induction had a certain protective effect (25 μg was more effective than 1 μg). Nasal administration of peptides after disease induction (at the acute phase) had no significant effect on the course of EAMG. Oral administration of 0.5 mg peptide mixture had no significant protective effect, and 1.5 mg peptide mixture led to exacerbation of clinical symptoms in treated rats.

These observations seem to indicate that peptides cannot replace recombinant fragments for the suppression of ongoing EAMG via mucosal tolerance. Since we have previously demonstrated the importance of tolerogen conformation for mucosal tolerance induction,[6] the failure of peptides to suppress ongoing EAMG could stem from their inability to meet conformation requirements, even when they are relatively long.

DIRECT MODULATION OF CYTOKINES AND COSTIMULATORY FACTORS

Mucosal tolerance induction by recombinant fragments corresponding to the extracellular domain of the AChR α subunit is an effective antigen-specific immunotherapy for ongoing EAMG. However, treatment of severely affected animals needs to be improved, for instance, by modulation of cytokines and costimulatory factors that were shown by us to be involved in the antigen-specific mucosal tolerance.[1–3,6] We first checked whether blockade of a representative cytokine (IL-18) and a representative costimulatory factor (CD40-ligand; CD40L), both of which are known to be involved in the pathogenesis of myasthenia,[7,8] can affect the course of disease. For that, we injected myasthenic rats with antibodies either to IL-18 or to CD40L, starting at the acute or chronic phase of disease, and found that both treatments resulted in a suppression of disease that was marked during the first period after initiation of treatment and diminished later.[9,10]

TABLE 1 summarizes our results with blockade of IL-18 and CD40L and compares them to our observations following mucosal tolerance induction by fragments corresponding to the extracellular domain of the human AChR (Hα1–205). As can be seen, the effects of anti-IL-18 and anti-CD40L on humoral and cellular AChR-specific responses complement each other: anti-CD40L affects the humoral response as expected, whereas it has no effect on the T cell proliferation; and anti-IL-18 affects

TABLE 1. Effects of antigen-specific mucosal tolerance and blockade of cytokines and costimulatory factors

Treatment	EAMG suppression	T cell response	Ab titer	Cytokines Th1	Th2	Th3	CTLA4
Ag-specific mucosal tolerance	+++	↓	↓↓	↓	↑	↑	↓
Anti-CD40L	++	–	↓↓	↓	–	–	↑
Anti-IL-18	++	↓	±	↓	–	↑	↑

NOTE: When mucosal tolerance was induced by the syngeneic rat fragment Rα1–205, anti-AChR antibody titers were not affected and Th3-type cytokine levels were not increased.

the T cell proliferative response. The antigen-specific treatment leads to a shift from a Th1- to a Th2/Th3-type response to AChR, whereas blockade of IL-18 and CD40L decreases Th1, but has no effect on Th2. Anti-IL-18 treatment increased the expression of the Th3-type suppressive anti-inflammatory cytokine TGF-β and led to the elicitation of regulatory cells as suggested also by the ability of splenocytes of treated rats to adoptively transfer protection against EAMG. A possible added value of direct modulation of cytokine networks and costimulatory signaling could be the upregulation of the negative immunomodulator, CTLA4, which was not induced by recombinant AChR fragments.

Therefore, targeting of CD40/CD40L-mediated signaling as well as blockade of IL-18 activity can be potentially suitable for immunotherapy of myasthenia, but should be used in conjunction with an antigen-specific therapy such as mucosal tolerance by AChR recombinant fragments.

ACKNOWLEDGMENTS

This work was supported by grants from the Muscular Dystrophy Association of America (MDA), the Association Française Contre les Myopathies (AFM), and the European Commission (EC) (Nos. QLG1-CT-2001-10918 and QLRT-2001-00225).

REFERENCES

1. Barchan, D., M.C. Souroujon, S-H. Im *et al.* 1999. Antigen-specific modulation of experimental myasthenia gravis: nasal tolerization with recombinant fragments of the human acetylcholine receptor α-subunit. Proc. Natl. Acad. Sci. USA **96:** 8086–8091.
2. Im, S-H., D. Barchan, S. Fuchs & M.C. Souroujon. 1999. Suppression of ongoing experimental myasthenia by oral treatment with an acetylcholine receptor recombinant fragment. J. Clin. Invest. **104:** 1723–1728.
3. Im, S-H., D. Barchan, S. Fuchs & M.C. Souroujon. 2000. Mechanism of nasal tolerance induced by a recombinant fragment of acetylcholine receptor for treatment of experimental myasthenia gravis. J. Neuroimmunol. **111:** 161–168.
4. Kuchroo, V.K., M.P. Das, J.A. Brown *et al.* 1995. B7-1 and B7-2 costimulatory molecules activate differentially the Th1/Th2 developmental pathways: application to autoimmune disease therapy. Cell **80:** 707–718.
5. Thompson, C.B. 1995. Distinct roles for the costimulatory ligands B7-1 and B7-2 in T helper cell differentiation. Cell **81:** 979–982.
6. Im, S-H., D. Barchan, M.C. Souroujon & S. Fuchs. 2000. Role of tolerogen conformation in induction of oral tolerance in experimental autoimmune myasthenia gravis. J. Immunol. **165:** 3599–3605.
7. Shi, F.D., H.B. Wang, H. Li *et al.* 2000. Natural killer cells determine the outcome of B cell–mediated autoimmunity. Nat. Immunol. **1:** 245–251.
8. Shi, F.D., B. He, H. Li *et al.* 1998. Differential requirements for CD28 and CD40 ligand in the induction of experimental autoimmune myasthenia gravis. Eur. J. Immunol. **28:** 3587–3593.
9. Im, S-H., D. Barchan, P.K. Maiti *et al.* 2001. Blockade of CD40 ligand suppresses chronic experimental myasthenia by downregulation of Th1 differentiation and upregulation of CTLA-4. J. Immunol. **166:** 6893–6898.
10. Im, S-H., D. Barchan, P.K. Maiti *et al.* 2001. Suppression of experimental myasthenia gravis, a B cell–mediated autoimmune disease, by blockade of IL-18. FASEB J. **15:** 2140–2148.

Suppression of EAMG in Lewis Rats by IL-10-Exposed Dendritic Cells

H. LINK, Y. M. HUANG, AND B. XIAO

Division of Neurology, Karolinska Institute, Huddinge University Hospital, SE-141 86 Stockholm, Sweden

KEYWORDS: EAMG; dendritic cells (DC); tolerance; IL-10; treatment

INTRODUCTION

Dendritic cells (DC) are specialized to take up and process antigen (Ag), to present Ag peptide–MHC conjugates, and to activate T and B cells, thereby initiating immunity. In this way, DC protect us, for example, from infections. It has been proposed that DC also play a major role in silencing self-reactive T cells.[1] DC functions are partly dependent on the maturation state of DC: immature DC may be tolerogenic, while DC maturation enhances immunogenicity reflected by augmented cell membrane expression of CD80 and CD86, and by synthesis of cytokines that influence T and even B cell proliferation and differentiation.

EAMG is a suitable animal model to examine whether DC can be rendered tolerogenic *in vitro* for subsequent use to prevent or treat EAMG. We observed that DC prepared from healthy Lewis rats, upon *in vitro* exposure to TGF-β, effectively prevented clinical EAMG and body weight loss when administered to rats during the incipient phase of EAMG.[2] Although important, this observation is not easily transferable to the human situation where DC are not available before MG onset. IL-10 is known to prevent DC maturation. In the present study, we prepared DC from Lewis rats with severe EAMG, exposed the EAMG DC *in vitro* to IL-10, and transferred the IL-10-exposed EAMG DC to rats with incipient EAMG.

MATERIALS AND METHODS

Previously described procedures of active EAMG induction, DC preparation, flow cytometry, proliferation assays, ELISA to determine IL-10 and IFN-γ levels in cell culture supernatants, and enumeration of anti-AChR antibody (Ab) secreting cells by ELISPOT assays were used.[2] Splenic DC were prepared with >85% purity from EAMG rats on day 39 postimmunization (p.i.), exposed to recombinant human IL-10 (82% homology with rat IL-10) at 200 ng/mL for 72 h, washed, and trans-

Address for correspondence: H. Link, Division of Neurology, Karolinska Institute, Huddinge University Hospital, SE-141 86 Stockholm, Sweden.
hans.link@neurotec.ki.se

Ann. N.Y. Acad. Sci. 998: 537–538 (2003). © 2003 New York Academy of Sciences.
doi: 10.1196/annals.1254.070

ferred intraperitoneally (i.p.) to rats at a dose of 1×10^6 cells/rat on day 5 p.i. Control EAMG rats received 1×10^6 untreated DC or the same volume (1 mL) of serum-free medium only. Rats were sacrificed on day 37 p.i. Each of the three groups consisted of five rats.

RESULTS AND DISCUSSION

Administration of IL-10-exposed EAMG DC to Lewis rats on day 5 p.i. with AChR + FCA effectively ameliorated clinical signs of EAMG and prevented body weight loss. Untreated EAMG DC or medium had no effect.

Lymph node mononuclear cells (MNC) were prepared from rats on day 37 p.i. and incubated with or without AChR for 48 h. CD80 and CD86 were downregulated in rats receiving IL-10-exposed DC compared to untreated DC or medium. Spontaneous and AChR-specific T cell proliferation were also decreased in rats receiving IL-10-exposed DC compared to both control groups. Both Th1 cytokine IFN-γ and Th2 cytokine IL-10 production were markedly reduced in rats receiving IL-10-exposed DC. IL-10 is usually considered an anti-inflammatory cytokine, but has B cell stimulatory effects. Administration of IL-10 aggravates EAMG.[3] The reduced IL-10 production induced by IL-10-exposed DC is in line with the alleviation of clinical EAMG achieved with IL-10-exposed DC.

Also in line with the observed amelioration of clinical EAMG induced by IL-10-exposed DC is the low ($p < 0.001$) number of anti-AChR IgG Ab secreting cells in thus-treated rats compared to the two control groups. Specificity of data was confirmed by lack of responses to the control Ag myelin basic protein (MBP). The relative affinity of serum anti-AChR IgG Ab, measured by KSCN-ELISA, was lower ($p < 0.001$) in rats that had received IL-10-exposed DC compared to rats injected with medium.

Trials with autologous DC that have been exposed *in vitro* to anti-inflammatory cytokines to induce tolerogenicity are a new option for treatment of severe MG.

REFERENCES

1. Steinman, R.M. & M.C. Nussenzweig. 2002. Avoiding horror autotoxicus: the importance of dendritic cells in peripheral T cell tolerance. Proc. Natl. Acad. Sci. USA **99:** 351–358.
2. Yarilin, D. *et al.* 2002. Dendritic cells exposed *in vitro* to TGF-β1 ameliorate experimental autoimmune myasthenia gravis. Clin. Exp. Immunol. **127:** 214–219.
3. Zhang, G.X. *et al.* 2001. IL-10 aggravates experimental autoimmune myasthenia gravis through inducing Th2 and B cell responses. J. Neuroimmunol. **113:** 10–18.

Future Therapeutic Strategies in Autoimmune Myasthenia Gravis

LOUKIA PSARIDI-LINARDAKI,[a] AVGI MAMALAKI,[a]
AND SOCRATES J. TZARTOS[a,b]

[a]*Department of Biochemistry, Hellenic Pasteur Institute, 11521 Athens, Greece*

[b]*Department of Pharmacy, University of Patras, 26504 Patras, Greece*

ABSTRACT: Antibodies against muscle acetylcholine receptor (AChR) undoubtedly play a critical role in the pathology of most myasthenia gravis (MG) cases. Selective elimination of the majority of these antibodies should result in a considerable improvement of the MG symptoms. Such a specific elimination could be achieved by AChR-based immunoadsorbents. However, sufficient quantities of native human AChR are not available while bacterially expressed recombinant domains of the AChR are unable to bind satisfactorily MG antibodies. We have undertaken the production of the extracellular domains of human AChR subunits in eukaryotic systems, in native-like conformation, for their use as potent immunoadsorbents. The N-terminal extracellular domain (amino acids 1–210; α_{1-210}) of the α_1 subunit of the human muscle AChR was expressed in the yeast *Pichia pastoris*. The polypeptide was water-soluble, glycosylated, and in monomer form. The α_{1-210} bound ^{125}I-α-bungarotoxin (^{125}I-α-BTX) with a high affinity (K_d = 5.1 ± 2.4 nM), and this binding was blocked by unlabeled *d*-tubocurarine and gallamine. Several conformation-dependent anti-AChR antibodies were able to bind α_{1-210} as did antibodies from a large proportion of MG patients. The purified protein was subsequently immobilized on Sepharose-CNBr and was used to immunoadsorb anti-AChR antibodies from 64 MG sera. It eliminated more than 50% (50–94%) of the anti-AChR antibodies in 20% of the sera, whereas from another 30% of the sera it eliminated 20–60% of their anti-AChR antibodies. Work is in progress for the expression of the extracellular domain of all other muscle AChR subunits. It is expected that their combined use may eliminate the great majority of the anti-AChR antibodies from most MG patients.

KEYWORDS: myasthenia gravis; acetylcholine receptor; immunoadsorption; anti-AChR autoantibodies; α subunit

INTRODUCTION

Myasthenia gravis (MG) is a well-characterized neurological autoimmune disease. It affects at least 1 out of 8000–10,000 people. In MG, the characteristic weakness and fatigability of the voluntary muscles result mainly from antibody-mediated loss

Address for correspondence: Socrates J. Tzartos, Department of Biochemistry, Hellenic Pasteur Institute, 127 Vas Sofias Avenue, 11521 Athens, Greece. Voice: +30-1-6478844; fax: +30-1-6478842.
tzartos@mail.pasteur.gr

**Ann. N.Y. Acad. Sci. 998: 539–548 (2003). © 2003 New York Academy of Sciences.
doi: 10.1196/annals.1254.071**

of the acetylcholine receptors (AChRs) at the neuromuscular junction.[1] If swallowing and breathing muscles are involved, it can be life-threatening. The pathogenic role of serum antibodies is clearly demonstrated by the dramatic clinical improvement that follows plasma exchange and immunosuppressive treatments. The AChR is a transmembrane glycoprotein consisting of five homologous subunits with the stoichiometry of $\alpha_2\beta,\gamma,\delta$ or $\alpha_2\beta,\varepsilon,\delta$.[2,3] Effector mechanisms responsible for antibody-dependent AChR loss are (a) cross-linking of AChRs by bivalent antibodies; (b) activation of complement; and, less importantly, (c) direct interference with the ion channel.[4,5] The mechanism that triggers the autoimmune response to the AChR is not known. Current treatments of MG include anticholinesterase and immunosuppressive agents, thymectomy, plasmapheresis, and intravenous human Ig.[6] Although these therapies are often successful, they are nonspecific and can be associated with severe side effects. Ideally, therapy should be antigen-specific and aimed at preventing the induction of specific antibodies or eliminating them.

Plasmapheresis is an efficient short-term treatment for MG, and clinical improvement correlates well with the reduction in circulating anti-AChR antibodies.[7,8] However, plasmapheresis is very expensive because of the need to replace serum proteins, and removes nonpathogenic (protective) antibodies and other important molecules. An affinity column made of AChR or appropriate AChR fragments that bind selectively the anti-AChR antibodies would overcome many of these problems. Since native AChR is available only in very small quantities, specific immunoadsorption can only be achieved by the use of columns with recombinant AChR fragments.

Recombinant subunits, or their fragments, of nonhuman muscle AChRs have been produced in mammalian cells, but in small amounts. The α subunit has been extensively studied in several laboratories since its N-terminal extracellular domain (α_{1-210}) contains both the binding sites for cholinergic ligands[9] and the main immunogenic region (MIR), the major target for autoantibodies in both MG and experimental models of MG.[10,11] Large amounts of water-soluble human recombinant α subunit fragments with conformations close to that of the native protein could be used as a potent autoantigen in the study of MG. Two different approaches have been used to try to achieve this goal, namely, expression in mammalian cell lines and in bacteria. The extracellular domain of the mouse AChR α subunit has been expressed in CHO cells,[12] but at low expression level. The human α_{1-210} polypeptide has been expressed in *E. coli* and reconstituted using the "artificial chaperone" approach,[13] while another human α subunit fragment (1–210 aa), also expressed in *E. coli*, was shown to have protective activity against experimentally acquired myasthenia gravis (EAMG).[14] The recombinant α subunit fragments that have been reported bind some conformation-dependent AChR monoclonal antibodies, but their ability to bind MG sera was not satisfactory or not tested. Nonhuman AChR subunits have been also produced in Sf9 cells by the baculovirus expression system and in the yeast *Saccharomyces* expression system;[15,16] no binding of MG antibodies was determined. The yeast expression systems combine the advantages of both expression systems (mammalian cell lines and bacteria) because they allow post-translational modifications, including glycosylation, thus resulting in correct protein folding, while the ease of manipulation, short doubling time, and high yield of protein expression are approaching those using bacteria. Moreover, the methylotropic yeast strain, *Pichia pastoris*, has a strong inducible promoter and it is less prone to hyperglycosylation than *Saccharomyces cerevisiae*.[17,18]

Our approach aims at the production of a recombinant human AChR α subunit fragment capable of binding a major fraction of the MG autoantibodies. We have expressed the extracellular domain of the human AChR α subunit (α_{1-210}) in yeast *Pichia pastoris*. The recombinant protein is water-soluble and has a native-like conformation, as shown by the high binding affinity for several cholinergic ligands and for conformation-dependent anti-AChR mAbs. We also studied the binding of α_{1-210} to MG autoantibodies and the ability of the immobilized polypeptide to immunoadsorb these antibodies. The binding of the expressed molecule to human autoantibodies suggests that it could be used as highly specific immunoadsorbent for the *ex vivo* selective elimination of the patients' anti-AChR antibodies.

EXPRESSION OF THE EXTRACELLULAR DOMAIN OF HUMAN MUSCLE AChR α SUBUNIT IN YEAST *PICHIA PASTORIS* AS A SOLUBLE, GLYCOSYLATED MOLECULE

The N-terminal extracellular domain of the human muscle nicotinic AChR α subunit (α_{1-210}) was expressed in yeast *Pichia pastoris*.[19] α_{1-210} was enzymatically amplified by PCR using a full-length α cDNA clone. The purified cDNA fragment was subcloned into the expression vector pPICZαA (Invitrogen, San Diego, CA) and the resulting construct was transformed into the *Pichia pastoris* host strain GS115. Several colonies were tested for expression of α_{1-210} after induction for 3 days with daily addition of methanol (0.5% v/v). The clone with the highest protein yield was used for large-scale protein expression.

The recombinant protein was purified from the culture supernatant by affinity chromatography on an Ni^{2+}-NTA column, elution being performed with increasing concentrations of imidazole at 40, 70, and 100 mM. As shown in FIGURE 1, most of the produced protein was eluted at 40 mM imidazole, while about 30% was eluted at 70 mM. Almost no protein was detected at 100 mM imidazole. The yield of purified α_{1-210} was 0.2–0.3 mg/L. The molecular weight of the product is estimated as higher than that predicted from the amino acid sequence, this difference being due to glycosylation of the molecule at residue 141, because enzymatic deglycosylation using peptide N-glycosidase F results in a reduction in the apparent molecular weight (FIG. 2). These results show that, like the native receptor α subunit, α_{1-210} is glycosylated.[20]

The solubility and the size of the recombinant protein were further studied by gel chromatography (FPLC) analysis, which showed that α_{1-210} migrated as a monomer with a molecular weight consistent with that estimated by SDS-PAGE.

HIGH-AFFINITY BINDING OF α-BTX AND OTHER SMALL CHOLINERGIC LIGANDS TO α_{1-210}

Binding studies of α-BTX to the AChR α subunit are used to indicate correct folding of the recombinant molecule because the formation of a high-affinity binding site requires the coordination of several posttranslational events that draw together different regions of the α subunit. We tested α-BTX binding on α_{1-210} in filter assay experiments using several concentrations of ^{125}I-α-BTX (FIG. 3). By Scatchard plot

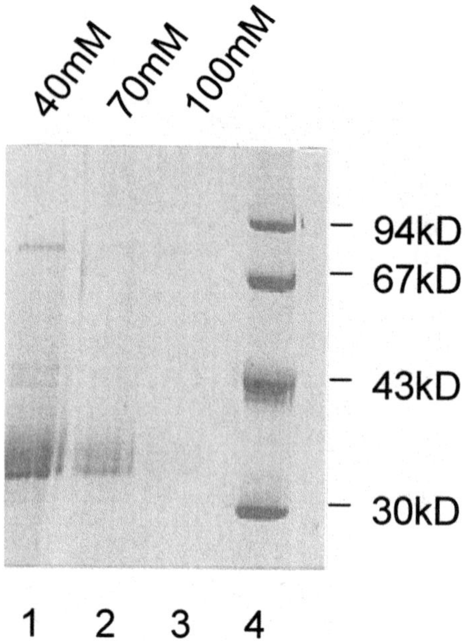

FIGURE 1. Purification of α_{1-210} using Ni-NTA metal-affinity chromatography performed with increasing imidazole concentrations of 40, 70, and 100 mM. The eluates were analyzed by 12% SDS-PAGE (lanes 1, 2, and 3, respectively) and the proteins stained with Coomassie Brilliant Blue; the positions of molecular weight markers are indicated (lane 4).

TABLE 1. ^{125}I-α-BTX binding (% of control) in competition with unlabeled ligands

	Concentration of unlabeled ligand (mM)				
	0.1	1	5	10	20
d-Tubocurarine	97	77	54	36	20
Carbamylcholine	106	104	95	95	93
Nicotine	90	98	92	88	86
Gallamine	103	81	52	40	26
NaCl	111	101	105	107	103

analysis, we estimated that the K_d is 5.1 ± 2.4 nM. This affinity is one order of magnitude lower than that of the native human AChR.[21,22]

The specificity of α-BTX binding to α_{1-210} was confirmed by competition experiments with unlabeled α-BTX. In these experiments, we also studied the binding of small cholinergic ligands such as carbamylcholine, nicotine, gallamine, or *d*-tubocurarine. Different amounts of these unlabeled ligands were added together with ^{125}I-α-BTX, and the percentage of the inhibition in ^{125}I-α-BTX binding to α_{1-210} is

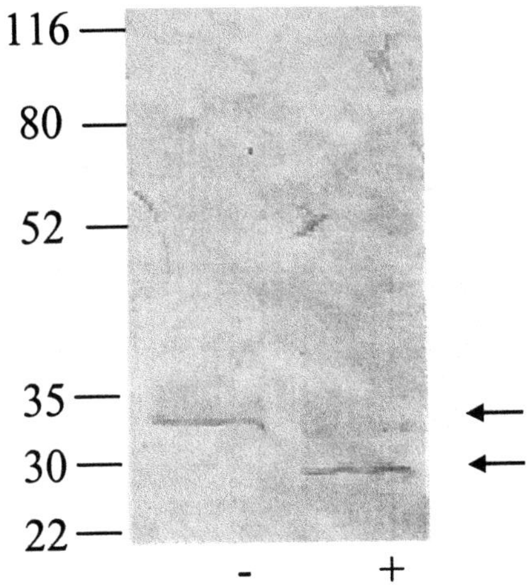

FIGURE 2. Deglycosylation of α_{1-210} by peptide N-glycosidase F. Purified α_{1-210} treated with N-glycosidase F (+) or without it (−) was analyzed by 12% SDS-PAGE followed by Western blotting using anti-myc 9E.10 mAb. The *arrows* indicate the bands corresponding to the glycosylated (*upper*) and deglycosylated (*lower*) forms of α_{1-210}.

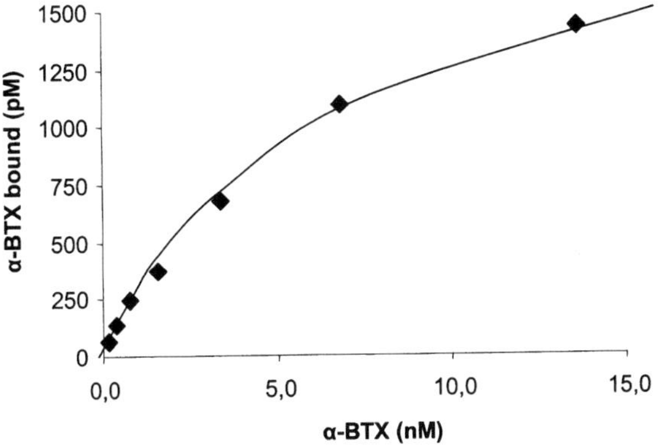

FIGURE 3. High-affinity binding of α-BTX to α_{1-210}. Culture supernatant containing α_{1-210} was incubated with various concentrations of ^{125}I-α-BTX. The K_d in the experiment shown, estimated by Scatchard plot, is 3.3 nM, while the average K_d of a series of experiments was 5.1 ± 2.4 nM.

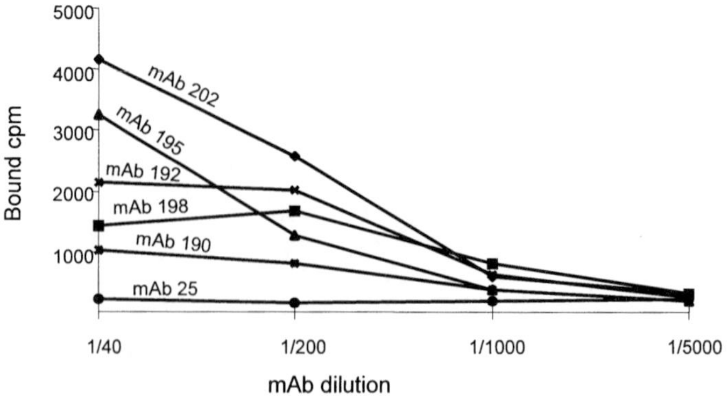

FIGURE 4. Conformation-dependent and partially conformation-dependent mAbs bind to α_{1-210} fragment. Two groups of mAbs were used in RIA assays: (i) anti-MIR mAbs, the binding of which is partially conformation-dependent (mAbs 198, 202, 195); (ii) anti-MIR mAbs that bind only to native receptor (mAbs 192, 190). mAb 25 was used as a negative control.

shown in TABLE 1. In these experiments, the small competitive antagonists, *d*-tubocurarine and gallamine, but not the agonists, nicotine and carbamylcholine, inhibited α-BTX binding to α_{1-210} at mM concentrations.

BINDING OF MONOCLONAL ANTIBODIES TO α_{1-210}

The binding to α_{1-210} of several anti-MIR mAbs would provide useful information about the protein conformation because some of the mAbs are known to bind exclusively to the native nondenatured AChR, while the binding of others is only partially conformation-dependent. We used five different anti-MIR mAbs derived from rats immunized with intact AChR from human muscle, namely, mAbs 190, 192, 195, 198, and 202. The binding of mAbs 190 and 192 is characterized as conformation-dependent, while that of mAbs 195, 198, and 202 as only partially conformation-dependent.[23] In addition, we used mAb 25, which does not bind to mammalian AChR, as a negative control.

We performed radioimmunoassay experiments with ^{125}I-α-BTX-labeled α_{1-210} using serial mAb dilutions (FIG. 4). All the tested mAbs (with the exception of the negative control) were able to bind to recombinant α_{1-210}, at least in dilutions 1:40 and 1:200, suggesting a nearly correct protein conformation.

BINDING OF MG ANTI-AChR ANTIBODIES TO ^{125}I-α-BTX-LABELED α_{1-210}

The binding of anti-AChR autoantibodies from MG sera is, in general, highly conformation-dependent. We tested 70 human sera from 50 MG patients and 20 healthy controls. The MG sera were distinguished in two groups: patients containing

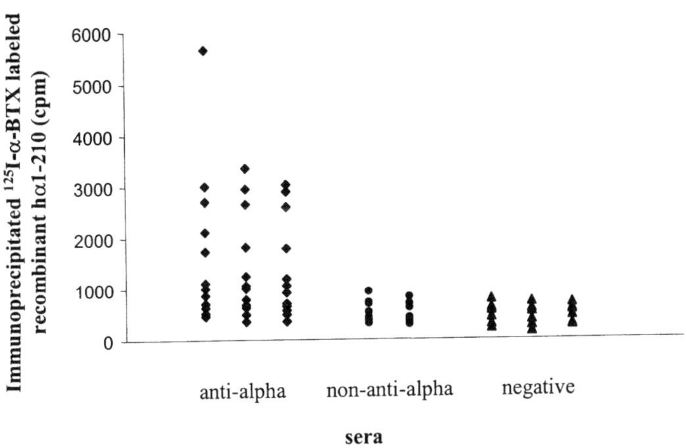

FIGURE 5. Anti-α autoantibodies from a high proportion of MG sera can bind to recombinant α_{1-210}. Seventy human sera were assayed for binding to α_{1-210} labeled with ^{125}I-α-BTX: 50 from MG patients and 20 from healthy controls. The MG sera were distinguished in two groups: patients with anti-α autoantibodies and patients with antibodies against the other (non-α) subunits.

autoantibodies directed against the α subunit and patients with antibodies mainly against the non-α subunits. As shown in FIGURE 5, a high percentage of the anti-α MG patients (24 out of 36) recognized the recombinant α_{1-210} (i.e., they immunoprecipitated an amount of radiolabeled recombinant molecule greater than the mean of the controls + 3 standard deviations of that immunoprecipitated by healthy control sera), while no binding was shown in the non–anti-α sera, suggesting the specific binding of anti-α antibodies from MG sera to recombinant α_{1-210}.

IMMUNOADSORPTION OF ANTI-AChR ANTIBODIES FROM MG SERA USING IMMOBILIZED α_{1-210}

To immunoadsorb autoantibodies from MG patient sera, purified α_{1-210} mixed with BSA was covalently bound to CNBr-Sepharose. In parallel, BSA alone was bound on CNBr-Sepharose under the same conditions as a control. MG patient sera were incubated with immobilized α_{1-210} mixed with BSA or the same amount of immobilized BSA. A portion of these treated MG sera was subsequently used in a typical MG diagnostic test. The percentage of immunoadsorption was estimated as the ratio between the reduction in immunoprecipitated radiolabeled human AChR after incubation with α_{1-210} Sepharose and the immunoprecipitated radiolabeled human AChR without incubation with α_{1-210} (incubation with just BSA-Sepharose). Sixty-four MG positive sera were assayed for binding to human AChR after incubation with immobilized α_{1-210} or BSA. As shown in FIGURE 6, in 13 of the 64 MG sera (20%), more than 60% (60–94%) of the anti-AChR antibodies were found to be eliminated, while in another 19 sera (30%) the immunoadsorption was 20–60%.

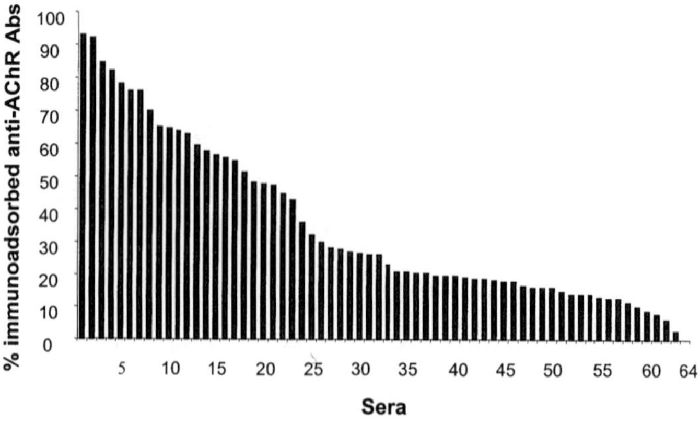

FIGURE 6. Immunoadsorption of anti-AChR antibodies from MG sera using immobilized α_{1-210}. Sixty-four MG positive sera were assayed for binding to human AChR after incubation with α_{1-210} immobilized to CNBr-Sepharose or with BSA immobilized to the same insoluble matrix. The percentage of immunoadsorption was estimated as the ratio between the reduction in immunoprecipitated radiolabeled human AChR after incubation with Sepharose-α_{1-210} and the immunoprecipitated radiolabeled human AChR without incubation with α_{1-210} (incubation with just Sepharose-BSA).

CONCLUSIONS

Recombinant α_{1-210} expressed in *Pichia pastoris* appears to be correctly folded because it is water-soluble, glycosylated, and in monomer form. In addition, α-BTX, *d*-tubocurarine, and gallamine, as well as several anti-MIR mAbs (strictly or partially conformation-dependent), bind to the recombinant molecule. Interestingly, this folded molecule binds autoantibodies from a high proportion of MG sera. This reaction is specific because α_{1-210} can react only with MG sera from patients who have autoantibodies against α subunit. Most importantly, the immobilized α_{1-210} is able to immunoadsorb more than 60% of the anti-AChR antibodies in several MG sera. Since plasmapheresis has beneficial effects with even partial withdrawal of the anti-AChR antibodies and partial reduction of the patient's titer, and since it is known that for a single patient anti-AChR antibody titers correlate well with MG symptoms, it is expected that elimination of even 60% of the anti-AChR antibodies will be highly beneficial to the patients. Moreover, we have already started the expression of the other (non-α) human AChR subunits in *Pichia pastoris*. The combined use of α_{1-210} with the extracellular parts of the non-α subunits should increase the efficiency of the immunoadsorbents and thus lead to a very efficient therapeutic approach by the extracorporeal removal of the anti-AChR autoantibodies from the circulation of MG patients.

ACKNOWLEDGMENTS

This work was supported by the Biotechnology Program of the EU (Grant No. BIO4-CT98-0110); the Quality of Life Program of the EU (Grant Nos. QLG3-CT-2001-00902 and QLG3-CT-2001-00225); programs of the Greek General Secretariat for Research and Technology, PENED 99ED 417 (Research Potential Strengthening Program) and EPET 104 (Operational Program for Research and Technology); and the Association Française contre les Myopathies.

REFERENCES

1. KARLIN, A. & M.H. AKABAS. 1995. Toward a structural basis for the function of nicotinic acetylcholine receptors and their cousins. Neuron **15:** 1231–1244.
2. DEVILLERS-THIERY, A. *et al.* 1993. Functional architecture of the nicotinic acetylcholine receptor: a prototype of ligand-gated ion channels. J. Membr. Biol. **136:** 97–112.
3. KARLIN, A. 1993. Structure of nicotinic acetylcholine receptors. Curr. Opin. Neurobiol. **3:** 299–309.
4. WILLCOX, N. 1993. Myasthenia gravis. Curr. Opin. Immunol. **5:** 910–917.
5. TZARTOS, S.J. *et al.* 1998. Anatomy of the antigenic structure of a large membrane autoantigen, the muscle-type nicotinic acetylcholine receptor. Immunol. Rev. **163:** 89–120.
6. MASSEY, J.M. 1997. Acquired myasthenia gravis. Neurol. Clin. **15:** 577–595.
7. BATOCCHI, A.P. *et al.* 2000. Therapeutic apheresis in myasthenia gravis. Ther. Apher. **4:** 275–279.
8. TAKAMORI, M. & Y. IDE. 1996. Specific removal of anti-acetylcholine receptor antibodies in patients with myasthenia gravis. Transfus. Sci. **17:** 445–453.
9. ARIAS, H.R. 1997. Topology of ligand binding sites on the nicotinic acetylcholine receptor. Brain Res. Brain Res. Rev. **25:** 133–191.
10. TZARTOS, S.J. & J.M. LINDSTROM. 1980. Monoclonal antibodies used to probe acetylcholine receptor structure: localization of the main immunogenic region and detection of similarities between subunits. Proc. Natl. Acad. Sci. USA **77:** 755–759.
11. TZARTOS, S.J., M.E. SEYBOLD & J.M. LINDSTROM. 1982. Specificities of antibodies to acetylcholine receptors in sera from myasthenia gravis patients measured by monoclonal antibodies. Proc. Natl. Acad. Sci. USA **79:** 188–192.
12. WEST, A.P., JR. *et al.* 1997. Expression and circular dichroism studies of the extracellular domain of the alpha subunit of the nicotinic acetylcholine receptor. J. Biol. Chem. **272:** 25468–25473.
13. TSOULOUFIS, T. *et al.* 2000. Reconstitution of conformationally dependent epitopes on the N-terminal extracellular domain of the human muscle acetylcholine receptor alpha subunit expressed in *Escherichia coli*: implications for myasthenia gravis therapeutic approaches. Int. Immunol. **12:** 1255–1265.
14. BARCHAN, D. *et al.* 1998. Modulation of the anti-acetylcholine receptor response and experimental autoimmune myasthenia gravis by recombinant fragments of the acetylcholine receptor. Eur. J. Immunol. **28:** 616–624.
15. JANSEN, K.U. *et al.* 1989. Expression of the four subunits of the *Torpedo californica* nicotinic acetylcholine receptor in *Saccharomyces cerevisiae*. J. Biol. Chem. **264:** 15022–15027.
16. FUJITA, N. *et al.* 1986. Biosynthesis of the *Torpedo californica* acetylcholine receptor alpha subunit in yeasts. Science **231:** 1284–1287.
17. CREGG, J.M. *et al.* 2000. Recombinant protein expression in *Pichia pastoris*. Mol. Biotechnol. **16:** 23–52.
18. GELLISSEN, G. 2000. Heterologous protein production in methylotrophic yeasts. Appl. Microbiol. Biotechnol. **54:** 741–750.
19. PSARIDI-LINARDAKI, L., A. MAMALAKI, M. REMOUNDOS & S.J. TZARTOS. 2002. Expression of soluble ligand- and antibody-binding extracellular domain of human muscle

acetylcholine receptor alpha subunit in yeast *Pichia pastoris*: role of glycosylation in alpha-bungarotoxin binding. J. Biol. Chem. **277:** 26980–26986.
20. CLAUDIO, T. 1987. Stable expression of transfected *Torpedo* acetylcholine receptor alpha subunits in mouse fibroblast L cells. Proc. Natl. Acad. Sci. USA **84:** 5967–5971.
21. CONROY, W.G., M.S. SAEDI & J. LINDSTROM. 1990. TE671 cells express an abundance of a partially mature acetylcholine receptor alpha subunit which has characteristics of an assembly intermediate. J. Biol. Chem. **265:** 21642–21651.
22. LUKAS, R.J. *et al.* 1981. Radiolabeled alpha-bungarotoxin derivatives: kinetic interaction with nicotinic acetylcholine receptors. Biochemistry **20:** 7373–7378.
23. TZARTOS, S. *et al.* 1983. Demonstration of a main immunogenic region on acetylcholine receptors from human muscle using monoclonal antibodies to human receptor. FEBS Lett. **158:** 116–118.

Index of Contributors